DEMENTIA

CONTEMPORARY NEUROLOGY SERIES AVAILABLE:

DEMENTIA

Editor

PETER J. WHITEHOUSE, M.D., Ph.D.
Associate Professor of Neurology
Case Western Reserve University School of Medicine
Director, Alzheimer Center and Division of
    Behavioral and Geriatric Neurology
University Hospitals of Cleveland
Cleveland, Ohio

Editor-in-Chief

FRED PLUM, M.D.

Series Editors

**SID GILMAN, M.D., JOSEPH B.
MARTIN, M.D., Ph.D., F.R.C.P.(C),
ROBERT B. DAROFF, M.D., STEPHEN
G. WAXMAN, M.D., Ph.D. and
M-MARSEL MESULAM, M.D.**

 F.A. Davis Company • Philadelphia

Last digit indicates print number: 10 9 8 7 6 5 4 3 2 1

acquisitions editor: Robert H. Craven
developmental editor: Bernice M. Wissler
production editor: Crystal S. McNichol

As new scientific information becomes available through basic and clinical research, recommended treatments and drug therapies undergo changes. The author(s) and publisher have done everything possible to make this book accurate, up to date, and in accord with accepted standards at the time of publication. The authors, editors, and publisher are not responsible for errors or omissions or for consequences from application of the book, and make no warranty, expressed or implied, in regard to the contents of the book. Any practice described in this book should be applied by the reader in accordance with professional standards of care used in regard to the unique circumstances that may apply in each situation. The reader is advised always to check product information (package inserts) for changes and new information regarding dose and contraindications before administering any drug. Caution is especially urged when using new or infrequently ordered drugs.

Library of Congress Cataloging-in-Publication Data

Dementia / editor, Peter J. Whitehouse.
    p.   cm.
    Includes bibliographical references and index.
    ISBN 0-8036-9271-4 (hardbound : alk. paper)
    1. Dementia. I. Whitehouse, Peter J.
    [DNLM: 1. Dementia. WT 150 D3751]
  RC521.D45 1992
  616.8′3 — dc20
  DNLM/DLC
  for Library of Congress   92-49876
                                                    CIP

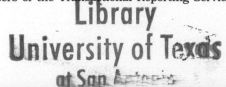

INTRODUCTION TO THE FOREWORDS

The challenge to our society of Alzheimer's disease and related disorders requires the response of the private, professional, and political sectors. I am grateful, therefore, that representatives from these three parts of our society, who themselves have made substantial contributions to research and to the clinical care of patients with Alzheimer's disease and related disorders, have agreed to introduce the reader to our book.

Mr. Edward F. Truschke, President of the National Alzheimer's Association, together with its Board, local chapters, and individual members, has made substantial contributions to bringing the needs of patients and their families to the attention of clinicians and policy makers. All clinicians reading this book are urged to imagine themselves in the position of the family suffering from this disease in order to be most helpful to them in dealing with their day-to-day challenges.

Dr. Joseph M. Foley has been a personal role model for the editor and many of the authors in his unswerving commitment to his patients and the quality of their care. In the tumultuous world of health care reform and the bewildering complexities of new, molecular medicine, Dr. Foley's emphasis on his patient is an important reminder to physicians of their primary responsibility to care in a compassionate and humanitarian fashion.

Dr. Zaven S. Khachaturian, of the National Institute on Aging, has been an exceedingly effective scientific administrator, channeling the public's concern about these devastating disorders into the development of effective programs of research.

Building links among academia, industry, and government will continue to be key to our society's (and the world's) response to dementia. Future success will continue to depend on partnerships among citizens, patients, professionals of all kinds, and policy makers.

PETER J. WHITEHOUSE, M.D., PH.D.

FOREWORD

Each year, thousands of American families receive the devastating news that a loved one is suffering with some form of dementia. Most have no understanding of the long, hard journey they face — caring for a family member who has lost, or will lose, the ability to control his or her life, make decisions, form new memories, do a day's work, be self-supporting, drive a car, or care for himself or herself.

The challenges of dementia, as Dr. Peter J. Whitehouse so aptly describes in this book, go beyond the research laboratory. They fall most heavily on families, who must make tremendous emotional and financial sacrifices to directly provide and pay for the care a dementia patient receives throughout his or her illness.

The Alzheimer's Association, dedicated to serving those affected by the most common form of dementia, Alzheimer's disease, recognized early that the most devastating impact of dementia is on families. In fact, family need was the underlying factor that led to the formation of the Alzheimer's Association in 1980.

Most persons with dementia live at home, where they receive care and support from family and friends. The patient's need for continuous care places a great burden on the primary caregiver, usually a spouse or adult child. As a result, caregiver stress is a key issue impacting care of dementia patients.

The cost of dementia care, which is the sole responsibility of the family, can be catastrophic. For example, the cost of caring for an Alzheimer patient at home averages $18,000 a year. The average annual cost of professional care in a nursing home — where half of all residents have dementia — is $30,000. These are not one-time costs. From the time of diagnosis, a patient can live from 3 to 20 years — or more.

As a service organization, we have tried to help professional caregivers truly understand the problems of dementia families. Although families appreciate the optimistic reports of the scientific community about dementia research, they especially need to know that medical professionals understand the burden of families and are sensitive to the frustrations they face.

The Association stands ready to help physicians and other health care professionals care for patients with Alzheimer's disease. Educational brochures and videotapes are available to assist the physician and help plan families' responses to this devastating disease. A partnership among professionals to improve the quality of care, as well as other important aspects of our mission, including public policy, advocacy, and the promotion of research, are major themes of our activities.

Physicians play a key role in the process of helping families and patients deal with Alzheimer's disease and related disorders. Taking the extra time to explain the diagnostic process and the importance of early planning for medical, legal, and social care is crucial. Maintaining a balance of planning for the worst-case scenario of progressive cognitive deterioration, as well as maintaining an optimistic view about what appropriate planning and research efforts can contribute, is important. Emphasizing that research is progressing and that new medications and other health care interventions are being developed that will help the family in the future offers hope to the families. Often families find that participation in research can give them a sense of fighting back against the disorder, which otherwise can be frustrating in terms of what patients and families think they can do to combat the relentless progression. More information about our programs and about research opportunities can be obtained by calling 1-800-272-3900 or writing to the Association at 919 North Michigan Avenue, Suite 1000, Chicago, Illinois 60611-1676.

Dr. Whitehouse, a 6-year member of the Alzheimer's Association's Medical and Scientific Advisory Board (MSAB), has been in the forefront of this effort. He played a strong leadership role in educating professionals about the special care needs of dementia patients and their families. Through his service on the Association's Patient and Family Services Committee, Dr. Whitehouse has helped to build professional partnerships with such organizations as the Robert Wood Johnson Foundation, the Administration on Aging Dementia Care and Respite Service Program, and the Brookdale Foundation to create dementia-specific day care programs at the community level.

Most importantly, he has helped forge a bridge between scientists and families. As chair of the MSAB's Treatment Committee, he is involved in efforts to find both pharmacologic and nonpharmacologic treatments that will facilitate the care of Alzheimer patients.

This book, which contributes greatly to the understanding of dementia, will be of tremendous benefit to those who care for the afflicted patients. As Dr. Whitehouse notes, we have achieved a much greater scientific understanding of dementia during the past decade but still must provide for those who are afflicted through a health care system poorly organized to deliver that care.

Dementia provides a humanistic view of how family members and health care professionals can work together to create a dementia-specific health care program that works. For this book, and many other contributions, the Alzheimer's Association is most grateful to Dr. Whitehouse.

EDWARD F. TRUSCHKE
PRESIDENT
ALZHEIMER'S ASSOCIATION
CHICAGO, ILLINOIS

FOREWORD

Dementia is a clinical state that, although described in many different ways, is in essence a sustained decline from a previously attained intellectual level. It is producible by a whole multitude of disease states, from Tay-Sachs to Alzheimer's, from trauma to AIDS, from cardiac arrest to intoxication. Some dementia is reversible, some arrestable. Its prevention is one of the reasons for the existence of intensive care units. Numerically the most significant cause, and the most pressing public health problem, is the category of progressive degenerative dementia, the most important of which is Alzheimer's disease.

Research on disease must involve study of cause and cure and study of effect. The cause of dementia is well understood. Enough involvement, directly or indirectly, of the association areas of the cerebral cortex will produce it. The "cause and cure" research, then, must concern itself with the dementing diseases, and in this sense, research is almost exclusively biologic, from epidemiology to molecular biology. Cause and cure is the Holy Grail of research in the progressive degenerative diseases capable of producing dementia.

"Effect" research must look at the phenomena of dementia — the many different presentations, manifestations, and modes of evolution. It must look at the effect the dementing disease and the dementia have on the afflicted individual — not only on cognitive state but also on emotional life — and find ways of making life gratifying despite the presence of the disease of the brain. Effect research must also explore the social effect, most importantly on the family, but also on the broader society. These social effects include important and urgent ethical issues.

Dr. Whitehouse is a happy choice to edit this volume. He is one of the few who has made contributions in the biologic, phenomenologic, psychological, and social aspects of dementia. Among the social concerns, he has credibility even in the areas of health care delivery and the formulation of institutional and public policy. He has the inestimable advantages of a clinician: seeing patients regularly, being stimulated constantly by their needs, and developing and conveying that passion for the possible, known as hope.

ix

The future depends on the talent working in the field, and this volume gives a good sample of that elite group, as it describes accomplishments to date and the multipronged drive to bring this destructive epidemic of dementia under control.

JOSEPH M. FOLEY, M.D.
PROFESSOR EMERITUS
DEPARTMENT OF NEUROLOGY
CASE WESTERN RESERVE UNIVERSITY
CLEVELAND, OHIO

FOREWORD

As we stand on the threshold of the 21st century, a Demographic Revolution faces the world — a period unparalleled in history since the Industrial Revolution. Our society will be greatly challenged by the dynamic changes of this revolution, which will result in a greater number and proportion of older individuals in the population. In fact, our abilities to adapt to different life-styles, dictated by our older population, will require a complete change in perceptions, attitudes, thinking, and priorities.

In the past, we have enjoyed immense technical accomplishments in the areas of science, engineering, art, music, and other intellectual achievements. Today, the scientific and technical knowledge gained through the ages has allowed us to enter into many previously inaccessible areas and learn about our world. We have examined the universe and explored outer space, observed the hidden depths of the oceans, exposed tightly held secrets of particle physics, peered into the mysteries of genetics, and in some cases practically eliminated killer diseases. With this awe-inspiring display of accomplishments, would it be unreasonable to deduce that we either have the necessary technical information at hand or the potential to produce needed scientific knowledge to solve most problems associated with an aging world population?

Indeed, the critical issue is: *Will we have the conviction, courage, and wisdom to allocate the necessary resources to address these problems?* These challenges must be confronted to create a new order, a more humane society. I hope we will have the determination to resolve these problems that affect the quality of life of older people. Without a doubt, the spectrum of issues associated with an aging society are vast and varied, including health, income, nourishment, housing, transportation, work-retirement, and pension. Among these concerns, factors that influence one's health, well-being, and the quality of life are, perhaps, the most critical problems the world must face. The biologic, behavioral, and psychosocial processes associated with normal aging and the diseases of older people must be explored further with great intensity if humankind plans to improve the quality of life.

During the last 10 to 12 years, remarkable progress has been made in understanding the biologic basis of normal aging and some of the age-associated disorders. In particular, research on dementing disorders has capitalized on the rapid advances under way in neuroscience and molecular biology. This volume provides a comprehensive review of the progress made in a relatively short period with respect to the dementias of old age.

The fields of neuroscience, neurology, psychiatry, neuropathology, and psychology have every reason to feel proud of their contributions for dramatically improving our knowledge of Alzheimer's disease, but these fields cannot afford to be complacent. The resources devoted to the study of Alzheimer's disease must be increased substantially. The pool of investigators should be enlarged to include a broader spectrum of scientific disciplines that may contribute to a better understanding of Alzheimer's disease.

During the next decade, it is my expectation that we will be able to solve some of the most difficult scientific problems associated with the dementias of old age, provided that we are able to maintain the current momentum and enthusiasm within the scientific community. It is no longer a question of *whether* we can solve the puzzle of Alzheimer's disease, it is a question of *when* we will solve it. The answers to these questions can only be determined by society's resolve to commit the necessary resources to fight this battle.

ZAVEN S. KHACHATURIAN, PH.D.
ASSOCIATE DIRECTOR
NEUROSCIENCE AND NEUROPSYCHOLOGY OF AGING
NATIONAL INSTITUTE ON AGING
BETHESDA, MARYLAND

PREFACE

Our current concept of dementia as a clinical syndrome of acquired, global cognitive impairment emerged from the fog of confusing psychiatric terminology approximately 150 years ago.[2,5] Until recently, however, most individuals did not live long enough to reach the age at which dementia is most likely to occur (over 65). Nevertheless, the roots of our current understanding of dementia and our current care system go back to before the turn of the century, when average life expectancy was less than 50 years. Although cognitive impairment in the elderly was acknowledged in antiquity, it was not until the middle of the 19th century that clinical descriptions were offered that match our current use of the term "dementia." For example, in his book, *Treatise on Insanity* (1837), J.C. Prichard[8] described dementia as a loss of global intellectual abilities occurring in stages. He differentiated dementia from mental retardation, in that dementia represented a *decline* in intellectual abilities from a previous baseline, whereas mental retardation was present at birth. Prichard was also well aware of the poor prognosis associated with most cases. Two French psychiatrists, Pinel and Esquirol, also clarified the differences among dementia, delirium, and other psychiatric illnesses.[5]

Approximately 50 years after the original clinical descriptions of dementia, sectioning and staining techniques were developed to study brain tissue. The belief that psychiatry should become a branch of neuropathology motivated the studies of "brain psychiatrists" such as Theodor Meynert.[13] For example, most of the content of Meynert's textbook on psychiatry, published in 1874, was neuroanatomy.[6] Weigert, Nissl, and Bielschowski, among others, developed stains that allowed microscopic evaluation of neural tissues. Alois Alzheimer was one of the more productive investigators of the time; he not only characterized the disease that came to bear his name, but also made fundamental contributions to understanding vascular disease, Huntington's disease, and Pick's disease. Emil Kraepelin, Professor of Psychiatry in Munich, where Alzheimer practiced, was a progenitor of modern psychiatric nosology. He suggested that the term "Alzheimer's disease" be applied to the presenile form of dementia that his faculty member described. Kraepelin had begun his career as a neuroanatomist, but ended working with Wilhelm Wundt, who had established the first experimental psychology laboratory in Leipzig during this pivotal time in the development of clinical neuroscience.[1]

As new methods for neuropathologic analysis of brain tissue were being developed, so too the field of brain chemistry began. Johann Thudichum, a German who later moved to England, was one of the pioneers. Thudichum's book, written in 1884, is sometimes cited as the first textbook of neurochemistry.[9,11] At the turn of the century, neurotransmitters, such as acetylcholine and noradrenaline, were first described, and the basis for our current understanding of how transmitters interact with receptors was developed.

At the same time that the clinical phenomenology and biology of dementia were being described by the neurologists and psychiatrists, changes were occurring in the philosophy of care for the mentally ill.[1] More humane attitudes led to better quality of care in mental institutions. Pinel developed separate wards for patients with dementia. Patients were usually cared for in the home, however, with the exception of the poor, who were more frequently admitted to chronic care institutions.

Shortly after the turn of the century, the number of hospitals began to grow rapidly, as they changed from providing care to the chronically ill poor to caring for the acutely ill from a wider range of social classes. Antisepsis and improved surgical procedures revolutionized the treatment of acute illness. As a result, chronically ill patients were moved from the hospital to other institutions. The development of nursing homes followed this rapid growth and change in the focus of hospitals. Yet, for a number of reasons, including the power of the medical model for treating acute illnesses, nursing homes were modeled after hospitals.

As we face this "Decade of the Brain" and the next millenium with anticipation, we are fortunate to be able to build on a century of progress. A short 100 years of microscopic and neurochemical investigation of the brain has led to much knowledge and also to a greater appreciation of our ignorance. We have also inherited a health care system unprepared for its new primary consumer, the chronically ill elder, often suffering from cognitive impairment. With these tools and this history, we face the challenges ahead.

THE CHALLENGES OF DEMENTIA

From the biologic point of view, the demented state can be caused by a set of diseases that challenge our basic understanding of how individual neurons work and how they are connected to form coordinated neural systems that produce behavior. For family members and health care professionals caring for individual patients, dementia creates a challenge in dealing with conditions that rob the patient of individuality and autonomy yet leave the body intact. When "self" identity is radically compromised, what is the goal of medical care? For the medical sociologist and health care planner, the challenge, in a time of cost constraint, is to modify health care delivery systems that are almost universally perceived as grossly unsatisfactory. What are the major aspects of these biologic, psychological, and societal challenges that lie ahead?

Biologic Challenges

Although many diseases can cause cognitive impairment, dementing diseases share common biologic features. The first is that most dementing conditions, notably the degenerative type, show changes in specific neuronal populations. The cause of cell dysfunction varies in different conditions from genetically programmed death to exogenous or environmental toxins. The challenge, at the individual cellular level, is to understand the mechanisms by which cells become sick and die. In the several dementing illnesses where genetic factors play a strong role, the molecular biologic puzzle is to relate abnormalities in specific genes to the neural dysfunction. The different disease processes are selective; characterizing which populations of neurons are affected in which diseases is essential. Understanding the nature of the neural failure at a systems level tests our ability to map the anatomic interconnections among different subsystems in the nervous system. Thus, dementia challenges us to understand how the functions of these normal neural circuits break down gradually as a particular disease progresses. Determining how the neural system abnormalities cause the clinically apparent behavioral and cognitive abnormalities will depend on fundamental breakthroughs in our understanding of how mind and brain relate.

Psychological Challenges

Dementia represents a challenge to the clinical researcher attempting to organize the clinical symptoms around a model of normal cognition and behavior. Dementia is characterized by dysfunction in more than one cognitive system, yet our understanding of how normal cognitive systems operate and interrelate is only rudimentary.

Diagnostic problems exist in dementia. Diseases of blood vessels (Chapter 7), viral and nonviral infectious diseases (Chapters 8 and 9), systemic metabolic dysfunction (Chapter 10), and certain psychiatric disorders (Chapter 12) have been identified as causing generalized cognitive impairment. Specific diagnostic tests exist for some of these conditions, but not for the most common cause of dementia, Alzheimer's disease. For this reason, Alzheimer's disease is considered a diagnosis of exclusion. Although some dementing diseases are treatable, many of our therapeutic strategies are inadequate. Thus, with most cases of dementia the clinician is faced with an incurable disease that affects not only the patient but the entire family unit. Assisting the family to deal with the practical problems of care for the patient at home is impeded by a fragmented, poorly coordinated health care delivery system that is difficult for the professional, let alone the family, to understand.

Societal Challenges

The major challenge to society juxtaposes the growing sense of dissatisfaction with our current health care delivery system, the recognition that dementia is the "epidemic of the century,"[4,7] and efforts to control costs of medical care. This growing problem of dementia is, in large part, due to the success of societies in improving health for their citizens. As life expectancy has increased, so has the number of individuals living in the period of maximum risk for the most common dementias. When Alzheimer described his first case, the average life expectancy in the United States and Western Europe was approximately 50; it is now approaching 80. The chance of suffering from dementia under the age of 50 is small; the chance of suffering from dementia after the age of 85 is perhaps as great as 50%.[3] The number of victims of Alzheimer's disease in the United States is projected to increase from approximately 2 to 4 million today to as many as 8 to 14 million by the middle of the next century.[12] This rapid growth reflects the aging of our population, particularly the increase in the number of those over age 85, who are most at risk for suffering from dementia.

Dementia is a worldwide problem currently felt most forcefully in countries with the oldest populations, like the United States, Western Europe, and Japan. In the future, third-world nations such as India and China will face an even more rapidly aging population than Western countries. How the stress imposed by the increasing number of dementia victims affects health care differs as the components and financial basis of the health care system vary in different countries. In most countries the quantity and quality of long-term care services, access to available services, and financing are common problems.

In the United States, reimbursement for health services focuses on hospitals and nursing homes. There is a growing recognition that more services for patients with dementia belong in the community, yet few reimbursement mechanisms exist for those services. The medical model, on which hospitals and nursing homes are based, is ill suited to deal with the chronic progressive diseases and the psychosocial problems from which the elderly suffer. A more integrated biomedical and psychosocial model valuing the contributions of different disciplines in the care of dementia victims and their families is needed. Regardless of which disciplines are involved in care, new emphasis needs to be placed on assessing the quality of care. In studying the quality of services, we need to be sure to demonstrate that an intervention is effective in improving the quality of life. Quality issues should drive reimbursement, not vice versa. From a sociologic perspective, dementia is a major challenge because of the difficulties in modifying an already complex and cumbersome health care delivery system.

OVERVIEW OF THE BOOK

To assist the clinician and scientist to meet the challenge of dementia, this book is divided into three major sections. Part I reviews the role of different disciplines — epidemiology, genetics, neuropsychology, clinical neurology, and neurobiology — in the study of dementia, addressing general principles as well as specific examples of particular approaches. The bulk of the book, Part II, reviews major categories of dementias by standard diagnostic groupings. Part III outlines principles of both biologic and nonbiologic aspects of the management of patients with dementia. A fourth section presents the challenges that lie ahead in research and care of patients with dementia.

The scope of this book is very broad, from molecular biology to the social aspects of health care. Such a perspective is necessary to assist the clinician with the challenges he or she will face in caring for patients with dementia. The authors were selected as the best in their respective fields; each chapter was designed to be an intensive review. The extensive reference lists allow further exploration, and the authors have tried to achieve a balance between classic and cutting-edge (but replicated) studies.

The challenge of dementia has grown to enormous proportions. Although one can admire the progress we have made in understanding the clinical state of dementia and dementing diseases over the past 150 years —especially over the last decade—the next century and a half promise, and require, even more. Let us be optimistic that our biologic research capabilities, clinical understanding, and societal concern have reached a point where we can accept this challenge with genuine hope of success.

PETER J. WHITEHOUSE, M.D., PH.D.

REFERENCES

1. Ackernecht EH (ed): Short History of Psychiatry. Hafner Publishing, New York, 1968.
2. Albert PC and Albert ML: History and scope of geriatric neurology. In Albert ML (ed): Clinical Neurology of Aging. Oxford University Press, New York, 1984, pp 3–8.
3. Evans DA, Funkenstein HH, Albert MS, et al: Prevalence of Alzheimer's disease in a community population of older persons. JAMA 262:2551–2556, 1989.
4. Katzman R: The prevalence and malignancy of Alzheimer disease: A major killer. Arch Neurol 33:217–218, 1976.
5. Lipowski ZJ: Organic mental disorders: Their history and classification with special reference to DSM-III. In Miller NE and Cohen GD (eds): Aging, Vol 15, Clinical Aspects of Alzheimer's Disease and Senile Dementia. Raven Press, New York, 1981, pp 37–45.
6. Meynert T: Psychiatry: A clinical treatise on diseases of the forebrain based upon its structure, function, and its nutrition. Bernard Sachs (trans). GP Putnam & Sons, New York, 1885.
7. Plum F: Dementia: An approaching epidemic. Nature 279:372–373, 1979.
8. Prichard JC: A Treatise on Insanity. Haswell, Barrington, and Haswell, Philadelphia, 1837.
9. Rafaelsen OJ: Thudichum: The founder of neurochemistry. In Rose FC and Bynum WF (eds): Historical Aspects of the Neurosciences. Raven Press, New York, 1982, pp 293–305.
10. Rowe JW and Khan R: Human aging: Usual versus successful. Science 237:143–149, 1987.
11. Thudichum JLW: A Treatise on the Chemical Constitution of the Brain Based Throughout upon Original Researches. Bailliere, Tindall and Cox, London, 1884.
12. US Congress, Office of Technology Assessment: Losing a Million Minds: Confronting the Tragedy of Alzheimer's Disease and Other Dementias. Publication OTA-BA-323. US Government Printing Office, Washington, DC, 1987.
13. Whitehouse PJ: Theodor Meynert: Foreshadowing modern concepts of neuropsychiatric pathophysiology. Neurology 35:389–391, 1985.

ACKNOWLEDGMENTS

The diversity of support that this book and its editor received mirror the breadth of its subject matter. Patients, families, scientists, clinicians, and policy makers are all struggling with the challenges that dementia poses, and individuals from all of these categories provided assistance and guidance in the development of this book. In an edited book, however, the first acknowledged debt must be to the contributing authors who gave their time and patience. A special thank-you is owed to two authors, Dr. Donald L. Price and particularly Dr. Fred Plum, who created the opportunity for me to edit the book in the first place. The staff at F.A. Davis was helpful in my education, and I particularly appreciate Bernice Wissler's well-organized campaign to bring the book to a close.

I was introduced to the field of dementia by Drs. Marshal Folstein, Peter V. Rabins, and Donald L. Price at Johns Hopkins University School of Medicine and appreciate their early support. I thank Dr. Robert B. Daroff, Chairman of Neurology at University Hospitals of Cleveland/Case Western Reserve University, for offering me the opportunity to develop our own Alzheimer program in Cleveland. I want to express my thanks to all members of the University Hospitals of Cleveland Alzheimer Center who contributed the ideas presented here. In this process my Staff Assistant, Cheryl Cowan, has been central and key to the success of developing several chapters and organizing the production schedule. Drs. Robert Butler, Joseph M. Foley, Sidney Katz, and Zaven S. Khachaturian have been particularly helpful over the last several years in developing my interest in dementia. I thank, too, Dr. Charles Wells, whose initial volume in this series helped stimulate my research career.

I am particularly grateful to the National Alzheimer's Association and its local chapter here in Cleveland for allowing me to participate in their activities and to my own patients and their families for challenging us to improve our care for patients affected by these devastating diseases.

More personal thanks are owed to my parents, who encouraged my career at all phases, and my wife, Catherine, and three children, Erin, Meghan, and Kirsten, who tolerate and support my multifaceted activities.

PETER J. WHITEHOUSE, M.D., PH.D.

CONTRIBUTORS

Mark J. Alberts, M.D.
Assistant Professor, Division of
  Neurology
Director, Neurology Intensive Care Unit
Duke University Medical Center
Durham, North Carolina

James Ashe, M.B., M.R.C.P.I.
Staff Member, Brain Sciences Center
Assistant Professor of Neurology
University of Minnesota
Minneapolis, Minnesota

Richard H. Civil, M.D.
Assistant Director
Clinical Neuroscience Division
Hoechst-Roussel Pharmaceuticals, Inc.
Somerville, New Jersey

Robert M. Cook-Deegan, M.D.
Director
Division of Biobehavioral Sciences
  and Mental Disorders
Institute of Medicine
National Academy of Sciences
Washington, D.C.

Suzanne Corkin, Ph.D.
Professor
Department of Brain and Cognitive
  Sciences
Massachusetts Institute of Technology
Cambridge, Massachusetts

Alice Cronin-Golomb, Ph.D.
Assistant Professor
Department of Psychology
Boston University
Boston, Massachusetts

Larry E. Davis, M.D., F.A.C.P.
Chief
Neurology Service
Albuquerque Veterans Administration
  Medical Center
Professor
Departments of Neurology and
  Microbiology
University of New Mexico School of
  Medicine
Albuquerque, New Mexico

Edward Feldmann, M.D.
Assistant Professor of Neurology
Brown University
Director, Vascular Laboratory
Rhode Island Hospital
Providence, Rhode Island

Norman L. Foster, M.D.
Associate Professor
Department of Neurology
University of Michigan Medical School
Ann Arbor, Michigan

John H. Growdon, M.D.
Associate Professor
Department of Neurology
Harvard Medical School
Massachusetts General Hospital
Boston, Massachusetts

Roland Hornbostel, M.Div., J.D.
State Long-Term Care Ombudsman
Ohio Department of Aging
Columbus, Ohio

Richard T. Johnson, M.D.
Professor and Director
Department of Neurology
Neurologist in Chief
The Johns Hopkins University Medical
    Center
Baltimore, Maryland

Edward H. Koo, M.D.
Assistant Professor
Department of Pathology
Brigham and Women's Hospital and
Harvard Medical School
Boston, Massachusetts

Douglas J. Lanska, M.D., M.S.
Assistant Professor
Departments of Neurology, Preventive
    Medicine, and Environmental Health
and the Sanders-Brown Center on
    Aging Albert B. Chandler Medical
    Center
University of Kentucky
Veterans Affairs Medical Center
Lexington, Kentucky

Nancy L. Mace, M.A.
Director
Alzheimer's Education Program
Consultant
California Pacific Medical Center and
    the Alzheimer's Association of the
    Greater Bay Area
San Francisco, California

John Marshall, M.D.
Emeritus Professor of Neurology
University of London
London, England

Richard Mayeux, M.D.
Gertrude H. Sergievsky Professor of
    Neurology and Psychiatry
Columbia University College of
    Physicians and Surgeons
New York, New York

**Justin C. McArthur, M.B., B.S.,
M.P.H.**
Associate Professor of Neurology and
    Gynecology
The Johns Hopkins University School
    of Medicine
Baltimore, Maryland

Mario F. Mendez, M.D., Ph.D.
Associate Professor
Department of Neurology
University of Minnesota Medical School
Attending Neurologist
St. Paul-Ramsey Medical Center
St. Paul, Minnesota

Godfrey D. Pearlson, M.B., B.S.
Associate Professor of Psychiatry
Department of Psychiatry and
    Behavioral Sciences
The Johns Hopkins University School
    of Medicine
Baltimore, Maryland

Margaret A. Pericak-Vance, Ph.D.
Associate Medical Research Professor
Division of Neurology
Duke University Medical Center
Durham, North Carolina

Fred Plum, M.D.
Chairman and Anne Parrish Titzell
    Professor of Neurology
Department of Neurology and
    Neuroscience
Cornell University Medical College
New York, New York

Donald L. Price, M.D.
Professor of Pathology, Neurology,
  and Neuroscience
Director, Neuropathology Laboratory
The Johns Hopkins University School
  of Medicine
Baltimore, Maryland

Peter V. Rabins, M.D., M.P.H.
Associate Professor of Psychiatry
Department of Psychiatry and
  Behavioral Sciences
The Johns Hopkins University School
  of Medicine
Baltimore, Maryland

Raymond P. Roos, M.D.
Professor
Department of Neurology
University of Chicago Medical Center
Chicago, Illinois

Steven A. Rosen, M.D.
South Shore Neurologic Association
Bay Shore, New York

T. John Rosen, Ph.D.
Research Scientist
Department of Neurology
Veterans Administration Medical
  Center
Boston, Massachusetts

Allen D. Roses, M.D.
Jefferson-Pilot Corporation Professor
  of Neurobiology and Neurology
Director, Joseph and Kathleen Bryan
  Alzheimer's Disease Research Center
Duke University Medical Center
Durham, North Carolina

Martin Rossor, M.D.
Professor of Neurology
The National Hospital
London, England

Bruce S. Schoenberg, M.D., Dr.P.H.
  (deceased)
Former Clinical Professor of Neurology
Uniformed Services University of the
  Health Sciences
Former Chief, Neuroepidemiology
  Branch
National Institute of Neurological
  Disorders and Stroke
Bethesda, Maryland

Kathleen A. Smyth, Ph.D.
Assistant Professor
Department of Epidemiology and
  Biostatistics
Case Western Reserve University
  School of Medicine
Alzheimer Center
University Hospitals of Cleveland
Cleveland, Ohio

Milton E. Strauss, Ph.D.
Professor
Departments of Psychology,
  Psychiatry, and Neurology
Case Western Reserve University
  School of Medicine
Cleveland, Ohio

Peter J. Whitehouse, M.D., Ph.D.
Associate Professor of Neurology
Case Western Reserve University
  School of Medicine
Director, Alzheimer Center and
  Division of Behavioral and Geriatric
  Neurology
University Hospitals of Cleveland
Cleveland, Ohio

CONTENTS

Part I

APPROACHES TO THE STUDY OF DEMENTIA

Chapter 1

THE EPIDEMIOLOGY OF DEMENTIA: METHODOLOGIC ISSUES AND APPROACHES

*Douglas J. Lanska, M.D., M.S., and Bruce S. Schoenberg, M.D., Dr.P.H.**

ISSUES IN THE EPIDEMIOLOGIC
   STUDY OF DEMENTIA
DESCRIPTIVE STUDIES: DISEASE
   MAGNITUDE AND DISTRIBUTION
ANALYTIC STUDIES: HYPOTHESIS
   TESTING

Dementia is a major cause of disability and death in developed countries and accounts for a disproportionate share of medical resource utilization and health care expenditures.[38,45,72] Unless cures or means of prevention are found for the common causes of dementia, the magnitude of the problem will continue to increase. The populations of most developed and developing countries are aging: The proportion of elderly persons in the populations is increasing, and the very elderly represent an increasing proportion of all elderly.[182] Because the prevalence of dementia rises steeply with increasing age, the number of demented individuals will increase in proportion to the increasing number of "at-risk" individuals in these older age groups.† In the United States, for example, the number of demented individuals in 1980 is expected to increase 33% by the year 2000 and double by the year 2025.[88,90] The increasing number of individuals with the AIDS-dementia complex will further compound this growing problem.[143,152]

ISSUES IN THE EPIDEMIOLOGIC STUDY OF DEMENTIA

Epidemiologic studies of dementia are needed to provide accurate data on the current economic, social, and medical impact of the disease, as well as projections for the future. Such information may help in organizing services and deploying limited resources. Epidemiologic studies may also provide estimates

---

*Deceased.
†References 38, 88, 90, 151, 159, 176, 182.

3

of an individual's risk of developing the condition, clarify the role of genetic factors, and produce a more accurate picture of the clinical spectrum, prognosis, and life expectancy than can be derived from clinical case series. In addition, field surveys, case-control studies, and longitudinal studies may identify risk factors, modification of which could potentially help prevent certain forms of dementia.

Diagnosis of Dementia

Dementia is a clinical state characterized by loss of function in multiple cognitive domains.* Diagnosis of dementia requires assessing an individual's current level of mental function and documenting a higher level of intellectual function in the past. Cognitive defects due to delirium, restricted brain lesions (e.g., aphasia), and psychiatric dysfunction (e.g., depression) must be distinguished and excluded. The term *dementia* does *not* necessarily imply irreversibility,[113] a progressive course, or any specific underlying cause.

There have been numerous attempts to develop valid and reliable operational criteria for the diagnosis of dementia.[4,5,62,166,196,202] Most criteria require that the patient is alert and attentive, that multiple domains of cognitive function are affected, and that the cognitive dysfunction is clinically significant. A clear sensorium is helpful in distinguishing dementia from an often reversible acute confusional state (delirium). Involvement of multiple domains of cognitive function helps distinguish the demented patient from a patient with a discrete focal lesion due, for example, to a tumor or a stroke. A clinically significant decline ensures that the change is not an artifact of the testing circumstances and helps to distinguish dementia from the relatively minor cognitive changes that occur with normal aging.

The most widely used criteria for dementia are those developed by the American Psychiatric Association for the *Diagnostic and Statistical Manual of Mental Disorders*. The first version to include specific criteria was the third edition, published in 1980 (*DSM-III*).[4] In a recent revision (*DSM-III-R*)[5] (Table 1–1), dementia is categorized with delirium as an "organic mental syndrome" but unlike delirium, the diagnosis of dementia is not made if symptoms occur *only* in the presence of reduced ability to maintain or shift attention (see Table 1–1D). To fulfill *DSM-III-R* diagnostic criteria for dementia, cognitive impairment must involve several domains and must include memory dysfunction (A and B); the cognitive disturbance must be clinically significant (C); and a specific etiologic organic factor must be identified, or in the absence of such a factor, nonorganic mental disorders such as depression must be excluded as possible explanations (E). How depression is to be excluded as a significant explanatory factor is not stated in the criteria, but in epidemiologic studies this has generally been done using either a nonstandardized physician assessment or one of several available depression rating scales.

Unfortunately, existing criteria, including those of *DSM-III-R*, are not fully operational:[5,129] they allow considerable latitude in judgment as to which cases fulfill the criteria.[99] There are still no uniform standards for determining how intellectual function is to be assessed, how intellectual decline is to be documented, or what degree of decline in intellectual function is sufficient for the diagnosis of dementia (Table 1–2).[129] In addition, *DSM-III-R* criteria[5] and others[11,79] include considerations such as "significantly interferes with work or usual social activities or relationships with others;"[5] however, occupations and life-styles vary in their tolerance of cognitive inefficiency, and some individuals may continue to function adequately and yet show a clear deterioration from their premorbid performance.

---

*References 4, 5, 37, 39, 53, 95, 129, 184, 202.

**Table 1 – 1 *DSM-III-R* DIAGNOSTIC CRITERIA
FOR DEMENTIA**

A. **Demonstrable evidence of impairment in short- and long-term memory.** Impairment in short-term memory (inability to learn new information) may be indicated by inability to remember three objects after 5 minutes. Long-term memory impairment (inability to remember information that was known in the past) may be indicated by inability to remember past personal information (e.g., what happened yesterday, birthplace, occupation) or facts of common knowledge (e.g., past presidents, well-known dates).

B. **At least one of the following:**
   1. **Impairment in abstract thinking**, as indicated by inability to find similarities and differences between related words, difficulty in defining words and concepts, and other similar tasks
   2. **Impaired judgment**, as indicated by inability to make reasonable plans to deal with interpersonal, family, and job-related problems and issues
   3. **Other disturbances of high cortical function**, such as aphasia (disorder of language), apraxia (inability to carry out motor activities despite intact comprehension and motor function), agnosia (failure to recognize or identify objects despite intact sensory function), and "constructional difficulty" (e.g., inability to copy three-dimensional figures, assemble blocks, or arrange sticks in specific designs)
   4. **Personality change**, that is, alteration or accentuation of premorbid traits

C. **The disturbance in A and B significantly interferes with work or usual social activities or relationships with others.**

D. **Not occurring exclusively during the course of Delirium.**

E. **Either (1) or (2):**
   1. **There is evidence from the history, physical examination, or laboratory tests of a specific organic factor (or factors) judged to be etiologically related to the disturbance.**
   2. **In the absence of such evidence, an etiologic organic factor can be presumed if the disturbance cannot be accounted for by any nonorganic mental disorder**, for example, Major Depression accounting for cognitive impairment.

Source: From American Psychiatric Association,[5] p. 107, with permission.

Identification of mild cases is especially difficult.[7,13,36,74,134,165,204] The commonly used screening tests for dementia are insensitive to mild cognitive dysfunction.[59,137] Diagnosis of mild dementia is further hampered by the lack of consistent, established values for what constitutes "normal" cognitive impairment associated with aging.[62,102,137] As a result, dementia is frequently unrecognized or its severity underestimated, particularly in older subjects.[62] Less intelligent or less educated individuals are more likely to be diagnosed as mildly demented,[6,64,140,156,211] particularly because performance on the screening tests is strongly influenced by education.[6,46,50,103,140] In addition, both depression[8,66,122,153,185,203] and delirium[27,122,185] are likely to be confused with mild dementia. Despite these difficulties, identification of mild cases of dementia is particularly important because treatment is likely to be most effective in mild cases (see Chapter 13).[139,165] In addition, early detection is essential to understand the natural his-

**Table 1 – 2 NINCDS-ADRDA CRITERIA
FOR DEMENTIA SYNDROME**

I. Decline in memory and other cognitive functions in comparison with the patient's previous level of functions as determined by
   1. A history of decline in performance
   2. Abnormalities noted on clinical examination
   3. Abnormalities noted on neuropsychological tests
II. Diagnosis of dementia cannot be made when consciousness is impaired by delirium, drowsiness, stupor, or coma or when other clinical abnormalities prevent adequate evaluation of mental status.

Source: Adapted from McKhann, et al,[129] p. 940.

tory of the disorder, avert crises, and maintain affected individuals within the community for as long as possible.[82]

Staging of Dementia Severity

Applying the label "dementia" or "dementia syndrome"[129,184] is not the final product of the diagnostic process. The statement that a patient is demented is strictly a phenomenologic diagnosis, saying nothing about the functional or anatomic extent of involvement, or the underlying pathologic process. Once a person is recognized as demented, it is necessary to determine which domains of cognitive function are impaired, to give some measure of the severity, and to identify the specific disease(s) underlying and causing the dementia.[179]

Diagnostic criteria for dementia have traditionally considered the syndrome categorically as present or absent. This approach accentuated problems of comparability between studies, insofar as various studies used different means of case identification and incorporated vastly different numbers of individuals with mild dementia. Furthermore, the care needs of affected individuals differ greatly as a function of severity. To deal with such problems, many studies have applied one set of criteria to establish the presence of dementia, and another set of criteria to establish the severity of dementia. Because newer dementia criteria like *DSM-III-R*[5] (Table 1–3) and the *International Classification of Diseases, Tenth Revision (ICD-10)* include their own staging systems for severity, separate staging instruments may be-

come less important in epidemiologic research.[88]

Because dementia is a clinical syndrome, it cannot be graded by the severity of a pathologic change, although measures of pathologic change may correlate with measures of impairment or disability.[17,206,207] Severity of dementia can be categorized in terms of impairment of cognitive function,[9,186,192] in terms of the disability resulting from the cognitive impairment,[20,35,49,55,92,93,192] or some combination of the two.[11,79,154,192,197] Earlier studies particularly tried to categorize dementia in terms of impairment by establishing various cutoff scores on lengthy psychometric tests; however, the groupings were generally arbitrary and unreliable. More recent studies have used overall scores or section scores from brief cognitive assessment scales.[9,186,192] Other investigators have assessed functional abilities or care needs using simple rating scales[15,20,35,49,55,92,93] or performance on functional measures.[119,168] Some of the instruments employed were developed as overall functional assessments for geriatric patients; as such, they do not concentrate on cognitive function but assess overall disability including that arising from other medical, social, and emotional problems. Data sources used in determining a patient's functional ability are not interchangeable; patients may overstate their abilities (especially early in the course), and family members may overstate or understate them, relative to assessments made by skilled nurses.[119,168]

The Washington University Clinical Dementia Rating (CDR) scale,[11,79]

Table 1–3 *DSM-III-R* CRITERIA FOR SEVERITY OF DEMENTIA

Mild: Although work or social activities are significantly impaired, the capacity for independent living remains, with adequate personal hygiene and relatively intact judgment.
Moderate: Independent living is hazardous, and some degree of supervision is necessary.
Severe: Activities of daily living are so impaired that continual supervision is required (e.g., unable to maintain minimal personal hygiene; largely incoherent or mute).

Source: From American Psychiatric Association,[5] p. 107, with permission.

which incorporates indices of impairment and disability, is probably the most widely used global dementia staging system in epidemiologic research.[88] It is also commonly employed in clinical studies and drug trials. It has good reliability when used by physicians[11,26] or clinical nurse specialists,[128] and the results correlate well with those of other dementia rating scales.[11] The current version (see Table 4–5) distinguishes five stages, ranging from not demented to severe dementia. Six cognitive or behavioral domains are assessed and rated independently: memory, orientation, judgment and problem solving, community affairs, home and hobbies, and personal care. The overall CDR is derived from these category ratings using a standard procedure, which considers memory as the primary category and gives it the greatest weight in assigning the stage. The scale has been criticized because it is felt to be cumbersome and because of the strong emphasis on memory,[88,167] particularly as cognitive functions with predictive utility such as language function[12] are not included.

Classification of Dementia

Several classification systems for dementia are currently in use, but none is entirely satisfactory.

DSM CLASSIFICATION

Initially published in 1952, the *Diagnostic and Statistical Manual of Mental Disorders* has undergone a number of revisions, including the influential third edition in 1980 (*DSM-III*)[4] and a subsequent revision in 1987 (*DSM-III-R*).[5] Although intended mainly for use in the United States, it has had considerable international influence, and versions have been translated into a number of languages other than English. The *DSM-III* classification and its diagnostic terms were included in the *International Classification of Diseases, Ninth Revision, Clinical Modification*

(*ICD-9-CM*),[198] which was published by the United States government for morbidity coding (see below). In addition, *DSM-III* diagnostic criteria have been adopted for inclusion in the mental disorders chapter of the upcoming *International Classification of Diseases, Tenth Revision (ICD-10)*.[5]

DSM-III-R employs a multiaxial coding system in which each axis corresponds to a different class of information; the dementing disorders are coded to Axis I (clinical syndromes), while the specific etiology, if known, is coded to Axis III (physical disorders and conditions). The codes for Axis III conditions are taken from *ICD-9* (or *ICD-9-CM*) and are not included in *DSM-III-R*.

In *DSM-III-R*, dementia is considered as an "organic mental syndrome," a group of psychological and behavioral signs and symptoms without regard to etiology. The dementia syndrome is a key element of a number of specific *DSM-III-R* "organic mental disorders," in which the etiology is known or presumed (Table 1–4): primary degenerative dementia of the Alzheimer type, multi-infarct dementia, dementia associated with alcoholism, and other or unspecified psychoactive substance dementia. Specific criteria are given for each disorder (see below).

When dementia is associated with an organic factor and cannot be classified as a specific *DSM-III-R* organic mental disorder, it is coded on Axis I as either senile or presenile dementia "not otherwise specified" (290.00 or 290.10) or as dementia associated with physical disorders or conditions, or whose etiology is unknown (294.10). The distinction between these residual categories is not sharp, and some disorders (e.g., dementia associated with brain tumor) may be classified arbitrarily to one or the other.[5]

ICD CLASSIFICATION

The World Health Organization's *International Classification of Diseases (ICD)* is a systematic classification that is widely used to classify mortality and

Table 1-4 *DSM-III-R* CLASSIFICATION OF DEMENTIA

I. Dementias arising in the senium and presenium
290.xx Primary degenerative dementia of the Alzheimer type
  1. Senile onset (after age 65)
    290.30 with delirium
    290.20 with delusions
    290.21 with depression
    290.00 uncomplicated
  2. Presenile onset (age 65 and below)
    290.11 with delirium
    290.12 with delusions
    290.13 with depression
    290.10 uncomplicated
290.4x Multi-infarct dementia
    290.41 with delirium
    290.42 with delusions
    290.43 with depression
    290.40 uncomplicated
290.00 Senile dementia Not Otherwise Specified
290.10 Presenile Dementia Not Otherwise Specified
II. Psychoactive Substance-induced Organic Mental Disorders
291.20 Dementia Associated with Alcoholism
292.82 Other or Unspecified Psychoactive Substance Dementia
III. Organic Mental Disorders Associated with Physical Disorders or Conditions, or Whose Etiology is Unknown
294.10 Dementia

Source: Adapted from American Psychiatric Association,[5] pp. 119–123, 133–134, 162.

morbidity information for statistical purposes, and to index hospital records by disease and operations. Revisions of the *ICD* system occur approximately every 10 years.

The ninth revision (*ICD-9*) is currently in use, along with several adaptations that have been developed for various purposes. The *ICD-9 Clinical Modification* (*ICD-9-CM*)[198] was developed by the United States National Center for Health Statistics to provide further detail for coding of hospital and morbidity data. *ICD-9-CM* is the basis for coding official morbidity and mortality statistics in the United States and is used widely for indexing hospital records. *ICD-9-CM* incorporates the *DSM-III* classification and terminology for organic mental disorders (see Table 1–4). Another adaptation is the *Application of the International Classification of Diseases to Neurology* (*ICD-NA*),[210] developed for trial purposes by the World Federation of Neurology to provide a more detailed classification for use in morbidity statistics, hospital record indexing, and research in the field of neurology. *ICD-9-CM* and *ICD-NA* are both fully compatible with the original *ICD-9* system, thus facilitating comparisons between statistics compiled using any of these versions.

All of the versions of *ICD-9* suffer from a number of inconsistencies and ambiguities that can make coding and retrieval of data on demented patients unreliable. For example, in ICD-9-CM, the categories 290.1 presenile dementia and 290.0 senile dementia do not describe the age of onset in affected individuals but instead describe the expected age of onset for the specific conditions comprising the categories. Presenile dementia is defined in this classification as "dementia occurring usually before the age of 65" in patients with Alzheimer's disease, Pick's disease, or Creutzfeldt-Jakob disease. Senile dementia is a residual category of dementia without specific pathology occurring usually after the age of 65. As a result, a person with the onset of Creutzfeldt-Jakob disease at age 80 would be coded by ICD-9-CM to 290.1 presenile dementia (rather than senile dementia), 046.1 Creutzfeldt-Jakob disease, or both.

The upcoming tenth revision (*ICD-10*) will have several advantages over previous ICD systems.[88] Two sets of diagnostic criteria for mental disorders will be provided (one for clinical use and one for research), along with a scale for rating the severity of dementia. Major inconsistencies in the classification have been removed. In addition, the categories correspond with current views on the frequency and importance of various dementias.[88]

Diagnostic Criteria

Because dementia is a prominent clinical manifestation of numerous diseases,[38,39,53,67,196] it may be extremely difficult (especially in the course of screening a large population) to identify patients with a specific dementia. Nevertheless, differentiation of the various dementing diseases is important because they occur with different frequency, have different risk factors, and will likely have different treatments. Of course, conditions currently considered as a single entity may represent a group of disorders with different causes and different potentials for benefit from specific therapies.[16,34,63,87,98,127]

Development and uniform application of explicit diagnostic criteria for specific dementing disorders will improve comparability between studies and may improve diagnostic accuracy. Criteria for AD and multi-infarct dementia (MID) are discussed below. Some criteria for other, less common, dementias have been developed,[4,5,65,126] but generally they have not been well validated, particularly in unselected populations.

DIAGNOSTIC CRITERIA FOR ALZHEIMER'S DISEASE

Despite the most sophisticated diagnostic techniques currently available, diagnosis of AD remains a probabilistic diagnosis of exclusion until the characteristic lesions can be documented on pathologic examination of the brain.[129] Although neuropathologic confirmation is generally considered the "gold standard" for validating the diagnosis of AD,[129] the histologic hallmarks of AD are not qualitatively specific for this diagnosis; qualitatively similar changes are present in "normal" aged brains. To date, there has been no agreement on the histopathologic criteria for the diagnosis of AD,[75,102,132,209] and many different histologic methods and criteria are employed.[209] Attempts are being made to standardize the histopathologic criteria.[102,132]

With the clinical diagnostic criteria available for AD, inclusion criteria are usually set broadly to identify individuals with dementia and to assure a high sensitivity. Because AD is the most common cause of dementia in most populations, a demented patient has a high a priori probability of having AD. To assure a high specificity, exclusion criteria are used to eliminate individuals with other diagnoses. Because the prevalence of AD is very low in those under age 40 and then rises exponentially with age,[88] incorporating a lower age cutoff in the diagnostic criteria[129] increases specificity and overall diagnostic accuracy. Exclusion of individuals with a sudden onset or stepwise deterioration[5,129] helps to eliminate cases of MID, another very common cause of dementia in the elderly. In addition, exclusion of individuals with any other identified dementia helps to further increase specificity and overall diagnostic accuracy, particularly because many of the other common causes of dementia are readily identified with clinical evaluations, laboratory studies, or brain imaging.

Current clinical criteria for AD achieve a reasonable degree of accuracy (usually but not universally better than 80%) when compared with neuropathologic findings.* The most widely used

---

*References 43, 86, 95, 108, 115, 125, 136, 155, 187, 193, 199.

**Table 1–5 *DSM-III-R* DIAGNOSTIC CRITERIA
FOR PRIMARY DEGENERATIVE DEMENTIA OF
THE ALZHEIMER TYPE**

A. Dementia (see Table 1–1)
B. Insidious onset with a generally progressive deteriorating course
C. Exclusion of all other specific causes of Dementia by history, physical examination, and laboratory tests

Source: From American Psychiatric Association,[5] p. 121, with permission.

criteria are those developed by the American Psychiatric Association (Table 1–5)[4,5] and those developed by the National Institute of Neurological and Communicative Disorders and Stroke-Alzheimer's Disease and Related Disorders Association (NINCDS-ADRDA) Work Group (Table 1–6).[129] In addition, several preliminary studies using strict inclusion and exclusion criteria combined with detailed clinical assessments have identified cases of early AD.[134,137,169] Diagnostic accuracy is maximized when medical history and physical examination are supplemented with psychological, laboratory, and radiologic tests.[95]

Although the approach used with clinical diagnostic criteria for AD has been demonstrably successful, it has inherent limitations. Sensitivity is limited by the difficulty of identifying individuals with mild dementia or atypical presentations; more sensitive criteria might identify a number of additional cases of AD, but such criteria would also likely have low specificity, allowing inclusion of large numbers of false-positive cases. In addition, whereas exclusions are very helpful in increasing specificity, some additional loss of sensitivity may result, particularly when individuals with prevalent conditions are excluded. For example, because stroke and AD are very common conditions in the elderly, these conditions frequently coexist;[133] excluding individuals with a sudden onset, a history of stepwise deterioration, focal neurologic findings, or imaging evidence of strokes will eliminate most individuals with MID but at the same time will exclude individuals with mixed dementia and some with atypical presentations of AD.[1,61,65,85,200] Further problems with existing criteria for AD include the following: the extensive evaluations used are not easily applied to large samples;[75] longitudinal assessment is often necessary to establish a decline;[14,137,169] differentiation from other degenerative dementias is very difficult or impossible;[65,115,155] and considerable latitude is available for individual interpretation of the criteria.[56,109,120]

DIAGNOSTIC CRITERIA FOR MULTI-INFARCT DEMENTIA

The size, number, and distribution of vascular lesions necessary to produce dementia remain uncertain.[24,51,194] Nevertheless, a significant volume of brain infarction is probably necessary to produce dementia.[194] Many studies, however, assume that vascular factors caused or contributed to the dementia if there is *any* clinical, radiologic, or pathologic evidence of stroke without regard to volume or location of infarcted brain. Because of this, MID is frequently overdiagnosed in clinical or pathologic studies and in epidemiologic studies using available criteria or "ischemic scores."

DSM-III-R uses a list of criteria for MID, each of which must be satisfied (Table 1–7).[5] These criteria have not been widely adopted because they are not well validated, they are vague and therefore likely to be unreliable, and they fail to distinguish MID from mixed dementia (AD and MID). In addition, although the criteria require a judgment that cerebrovascular disease was etio-

Table 1–6 NINCDS-ADRDA CRITERIA FOR CLINICAL DIAGNOSIS OF ALZHEIMER'S DISEASE

I. The criteria for the clinical diagnosis of *probable* Alzheimer's disease include:
  1. Dementia established by clinical examination and documented by the Mini-Mental State Test, Blessed Dementia Scale, or some similar examination, and confirmed by neuropsychological tests
  2. Deficits in two or more areas of cognition
  3. Progressive worsening of memory and other cognitive functions
  4. No disturbance of consciousness
  5. Onset between ages 40 and 90, most often after age 65
  6. Absence of systemic disorders or other brain diseases that in and of themselves could account for the progressive deficits in memory and cognition.
II. The diagnosis of *probable* Alzheimer's disease is supported by:
  1. Progressive deterioration of specific cognitive functions such as language (aphasia), motor skills (apraxia), and perception (agnosia)
  2. Impaired activities of daily living and altered patterns of behavior
  3. Family history of similar disorders, particularly if confirmed neuropathologically
  4. Laboratory results of:
    a. Normal lumbar puncture as evaluated by standard techniques
    b. Normal pattern or nonspecific changes in EEG, such as increased slow-wave activity
    c. Evidence of cerebral atrophy on CT with progression documented by serial observation
III. Other clinical features consistent with the diagnosis of *probable* Alzheimer's disease, after exclusion of causes of dementia other than Alzheimer's disease, include:
  1. Plateaus in the course of progression of the illness
  2. Associated symptoms of depression, insomnia, incontinence, delusions, illusions, hallucinations; catastrophic verbal, emotional, or physical outbursts; sexual disorders; and weight loss
  3. Other neurologic abnormalities in some patients, especially those with more advanced disease and including motor signs such as increased muscle tone, myoclonus, or gait disorder
  4. Seizures in advanced disease
  5. CT normal for age
IV. Features that make the diagnosis of *probable* Alzheimer's disease uncertain or unlikely include:
  1. Sudden, apoplectic onset
  2. Focal neurologic findings such as hemiparesis, sensory loss, visual field deficits, and incoordination early in the course of the illness
  3. Seizures or gait disturbances at the onset or very early in the course of the illness.
V. Clinical diagnosis of *possible* Alzheimer's disease:
  1. May be made on the basis of the dementia syndrome; in the absence of other neurologic, psychiatric, or systemic disorders sufficient to cause dementia; and in the presence of variations in the onset, presentation, or clinical course
  2. May be made in the presence of a second systemic or brain disorder sufficient to produce dementia, which is not considered to be the cause of the dementia
  3. Should be used in research studies when a single, gradually progressive, severe cognitive deficit is identified in the absence of other identifiable cause.
VI. Criteria for diagnosis of *definite* Alzheimer's disease are:
  1. The clinical criteria for probable Alzheimer's disease
  2. Histopathologic evidence obtained from a biopsy or autopsy
VII. Classification of Alzheimer's disease for research purposes should specify features that may differentiate subtypes of the disorder, such as:
  1. Familial occurrence
  2. Onset before age 65
  3. Presence of trisomy-21
  4. Coexistence of other relevant conditions such as Parkinson's disease.

Source: From American Psychiatric Association,[5] with permission.

logically related to the dementia, no rules are given for making this assessment; as a result, in practice *any* evidence of cerebrovascular disease is often interpreted as etiologically relevant.

The Hachinski Ischemic Score[68,69] and its modifications[118,164] rely on cutoff scores on scales incorporating a number of differently weighted items (Table 1–8). A low value on these scales does help to rule out MID, for it is un-

Table 1–7 *DSM-III-R* DIAGNOSTIC CRITERIA FOR MULTI-INFARCT DEMENTIA

A. Dementia (see Table 1–1)
B. Stepwise deteriorating course with "patchy" distribution of deficits (i.e., affecting some functions, but not others) early in the course
C. Focal neurologic signs and symptoms (e.g., exaggeration of deep tendon reflexes, extensor plantar response, pseudobulbar palsy, gait abnormalities, weakness of an extremity)
D. Evidence from history, physical examination, or laboratory tests of significant cerebrovascular disease that is judged to be etiologically related to the disturbance

Source: From American Psychiatric Association,[5] p. 123, with permission.

likely that vascular lesions could produce dementia and yet remain neurologically silent.[24,51,116] A high value supports the presence of vascular disease, but contrary to implicit assumptions, does not establish that the dementia is of vascular origin,[24,116] nor does it exclude the coexistence of other clinically important causes for dementia, such as AD.* Distinguishing AD, MID, and mixed AD/MID using clinical criteria will probably require a two-dimensional instrument, in which one score indicates the likelihood of AD and a separate score indicates the likelihood of MID.[65,75]

---

*References 24, 65, 101, 116, 118, 133, 164.

DESCRIPTIVE STUDIES: DISEASE MAGNITUDE AND DISTRIBUTION

A fundamental objective of epidemiologic studies of dementia is to describe the occurrence of dementia or dementia-related phenomena in populations, a process involving several steps (Table 1–9). The magnitude of the disease burden in the population is usually expressed in terms of the population at risk, using certain epidemiologic indices such as mortality, prevalence, and incidence (Table 1–10). The disease is further characterized in terms of the demographic, occupational, or personal features of the individuals who develop the disease, the particular lo-

Table 1–8 HACHINSKI ISCHEMIC SCORE AND MODIFIED ISCHEMIC SCORES

Feature	Hachinski[69]	Rosen[164]	Loeb[118]
Abrupt onset	2	2	2
Stepwise deterioration	1	1	
Fluctuating course	2		
Nocturnal confusion	1		
Relative preservation of personality	1	1*	
Depression	1		
Somatic complaints	1	1	
Emotional incontinence	1	1	
History of hypertension	1	1	
History of strokes	2	2	1
Evidence of associated atherosclerosis	1		
Focal neurologic symptoms	2	2	2
Focal neurologic signs	2	2	2
CT low-density areas			
Isolated			2
Multiple			3
Maximum Score	**18**	**13**	**12**

*Based on a different interpretation of the original paper by Rosen and colleagues,[164] this item is sometimes excluded, giving a maximum score of 12.

**Table 1–9 PROCEDURES FOR
DESCRIPTIVE EPIDEMIOLOGY**

1. Define boundaries of investigation according to population at risk and time interval of study.
2. Define disease or condition under investigation and specify operational criteria for its ascertainment.
3. Identify all cases within the boundaries of the investigation.
4. Calculate epidemiologic indices (e.g., mortality, prevalence, incidence).
5. Characterize the disease by
   —Person (e.g., age, sex, race, occupation)
   —Place (e.g., locality, urban/rural, geographic differences)
   —Time (e.g., seasonal, cyclic, trends).
6. Compare with known indices of disease.

Source: Adapted from Schoenberg,[173] p. 17.

cales in which the disease occurs, and the time period when the disease is most common. Comparison of disease patterns within and among populations often suggests etiologic hypotheses, which can then be tested using analytic epidemiologic studies.

Mortality

Mortality statistics, as derived from information reported on death certificates, are the only consistently available source of health data at national, state, and local levels. Many countries have long-standing systems for collecting such information in a centralized registry. Such data provide indices of the frequency of certain diseases in the population and have served as an inexpensive and convenient means of identifying potential etiologic factors (as, for example, in cancer epidemiology). Unfortunately, the level of accuracy of death certificate data for dementing illnesses is low.[88,124] Because medical certifications of death are made by medical practitioners of varying diagnostic abilities as well as by lay coroners, many reported diagnoses do not withstand rigorous clinical review. Dementia in general and AD in particular are frequently not recognized, and even when recognized are often not listed on death certificates.[88,124,147,148,205,208]

In addition, official tabulations of mortality data have generally reported only what is deemed the principal or underlying cause, that is, the starting point of the events that led to death. Reporting only a single underlying cause excludes information on intervening, contributory, and concurrent conditions. For chronic conditions such as dementia, the loss of information is par-

Table 1–10 COMMON EPIDEMIOLOGIC MEASURES

Mortality:	The frequency of deaths within a specific population. Often expressed as a death rate: deaths from a given disease per 100,000 persons at risk per year.
Prevalence:*	The frequency of all current cases of disease within a specific population. Usually expressed as a prevalence ratio: the number of persons with a given disease at a specified time per 100,000 persons capable of having the disease at that time
Incidence:*	The frequency of addition of new cases of a disease within a specific population, or the rapidity with which a disease occurs. Often expressed as an incidence rate: the number of new cases of a given disease during a specified time period (usually 1 year) per 100,000 persons at risk of having the disease for the first time that year.

*Prevalence and incidence are related to each other: prevalence approximately equals incidence multiplied by the average duration of the disease.

Source: Reprinted by permission from Schoenberg BS: *Seminars in Neurology*, Vol. 1, Thieme Medical Publishers, New York, 1981.

ticularly large. In fact, the number of death certificates on which dementia is mentioned is 15 times greater than the number of death certificates on which dementia is listed as the underlying cause of death.[30] Coding of multiple causes of death maximizes the use of available diagnostic information.[10,29,30,42,84]

Regardless of whether underlying-cause or multiple-cause mortality data are used, considerable spatial and temporal variation exists in the diagnosis of dementia and the reporting of dementia on death certificates.[28,52,88,89,124,145] As a result, assessment of geographic distribution and temporal trends of dementia mortality remains problematic. For example, death rates for AD and related conditions have been increasing rapidly in a number of countries over the past 20 to 30 years.[10,28,52,88,89,145] This is due largely to changes in diagnostic and reporting practices, with increased reporting of specific dementing conditions in preference to nonspecific labels such as "senility."[28,30,52,88,89,124] In addition, physician awareness of dementia as a significant cause of morbidity and mortality has been stimulated by professional admonitions,[94,151] increasing research activity and professional publications in the area, advocacy by active lay organizations, and growing public awareness and concern. Changes in the incidence or case fatality of dementia could also be contributing to these trends, but there is no evidence of parallel changes in these areas.[88,105,158]

Morbidity

DATA SOURCES

Morbidity data are much more difficult to obtain than mortality data because most countries do not have established systems for collecting this information. Several potential sources of morbidity data are shown in Table 1–11.[173,174] Because different procedures are used to acquire morbidity information, results must be compared carefully.

Some investigators have attempted to study a large number of patients coming to medical attention at particular medical institutions, but such patients may not be representative of all cases of the disease in the community. For example, socioeconomic status, family social problems, pre-illness levels of mental functioning, and whether people are living alone can significantly affect which demented individuals are brought for hospital care.[63] Also, geographic location, referral patterns, availability of specific services or facilities, hospital advertising, and other factors can influence which demented individuals receive care at a particular medical institution. Since hospital-based studies cannot precisely identify a population at risk, it is not possible to calculate rates, and generalization of the results is often unreliable.

Table 1–11 SOURCES OF MORBIDITY DATA FOR DEMENTING CONDITIONS

Hospital case series
Population-based registries
Tax-financed plans
Prepaid medical plans
Records-linkage systems
Special surveys
  Cross-sectional
  Longitudinal
Ad hoc studies of geographic isolates

Reprinted by permission from Schoenberg BS: *Seminars in Neurology*, Vol. 1, Thieme Medical Publishers, New York, 1981.

Data registries based on well-defined populations can be used in the epidemiologic study of dementia.[80,195] For example, Israel has established a registry for all residents of the country who are discharged from an Israeli hospital with any diagnosis related to a neurologic disorder.[2,91] This resource has provided important information about a number of neurologic conditions including dementia.[195] Unfortunately, this particular registry cannot identify individuals who are not hospitalized and those who do not seek medical care.

Because it is frequently prohibitively expensive and difficult to assemble records of representative population subsets, existing data registries of selected segments of the population might also be used to provide valuable information for studies of dementia. Such resources include medical records from tax-financed plans (e.g., the armed forces and Veterans Administration hospitals, Medicare, and Medicaid), prepaid medical plans, disability insurance groups, and so on.[97,173,174] In some of these programs it is possible to obtain relatively accurate and complete medical information, but the generalizability of the results may be limited because the patients in these programs are not representative of the general population. Some of these resources are accessible only to investigators affiliated with the organizations maintaining the data bases.

The application of a records-linkage system to a defined population provides another useful data resource, as exemplified by the medical records system maintained by the Mayo Clinic for residents of Olmstead County, Minnesota.[111,112] This system involves the cooperation of all medical facilities serving the area, including hospitals, clinics, nursing homes, state medical institutions, and private practitioners. Data concerning all medical contacts (i.e., outpatient records, inpatient records, physician house calls, emergency room visits, and so forth) are kept together in a single, computerized file.[111,112] Furthermore, the population has easy access to expertise in neurologic diagnosis, and this access is generally not limited by financial resources. Accurate population-based statistics on dementing conditions can therefore be obtained by applying defined diagnostic criteria to information available in this records-linkage system.[104,105,178]

Although not conducted routinely because of their high cost and methodologic and administrative difficulties, special surveys are occasionally carried out to obtain information on specific diseases. Most of these are cross-sectional studies that attempt to collect data on a population at one point in time or over a relatively brief period.[48,149,177] Longitudinal studies are less frequent because they are quite expensive and usually require extensive follow-up. Population-based longitudinal data resources for the study of dementing conditions include the Framingham Study[117] and the Lundby, Sweden Studies.[70,71,158] Other longitudinal data resources include the Duke Longitudinal Study,[27] the Baltimore Longitudinal Study,[171,183] and the Consortium to Establish a Registry for Alzheimer's Disease (CERAD).[135,204]

Ad hoc studies of small geographic isolates may yield associations or etiologic explanations that are not apparent in larger population groups.[110] Examples are the foci of kuru in New Guinea; and of parkinsonism-dementia complex in Guam, the other Mariana islands, and the Kii penisula of Japan.[110] The study of inbred and isolated populations may be particularly helpful in distinguishing genetic and nongenetic components of disease pathogenesis. In particular, the inbred Amish population of the United States has been suggested as a study population for distinguishing the effects of heredity in the development of AD.[102]

CASE IDENTIFICATION

Although it may be possible to examine an entire population for cases of a particular disease, in most instances this approach is impractical. Instead, one must use appropriate screening procedures and sampling techniques to choose a smaller but still representative subgroup of the population for intensive investigation.

Particularly in cross-sectional surveys, case identification generally proceeds in two stages.* The first stage is a screening process to identify persons whose level of cognitive function is low. This process may be applied to the entire study population or to some representative sample. In general, instruments are chosen that are brief, easily administered, and easily scored. Important limitations of currently available screening instruments include confounding by educational level and other socioeconomic factors,[46,50,103,140] and insensitivity to mild degrees of cognitive impairment.[59,99,137] Because of such limitations these instruments are inadequate for detecting the early stages of dementia in the general population. Screening large populations by in-person interviewing and administration of screening instruments is also very expensive and time consuming. For some applications, telephone-administered screening tests may provide a valid and economical alternative to traditional screening methods, particularly when the screening instruments involve verbal tasks rather than visuospatial tasks.[121,144]

The second stage of case identification involves more elaborate and specific tests for those individuals who have failed the screening test. It generally includes a historical component to determine whether deterioration of cognitive abilities has occurred. If a clear account of the person's past cannot be obtained, it may be necessary to observe the individual over time to determine whether the individual's abilities are, in fact, declining.[14,19,30,137,169,181] The second stage may also include examination by a neu-rologist,[177] and even hospital admission, to document the presence of dementia, rule out treatable causes, and establish the specific disease diagnosis. Occasionally, where medical information on the total population is available, it may be possible to obtain the necessary data by detailed examination of medical records.[105,178,193]

The two-stage approach provides a considerable increase in the efficiency of case finding but may produce considerable biases owing to the compounding effect of subject attrition at each stage.[54,75] In addition, it may not be feasible or appropriate to study rare conditions with this approach. For example, in order to derive accurate estimates of the prevalence of dementia among those under age 65, it may be necessary to study an enormous population just to document a few cases.[139,177] Indeed, in the Copiah County Study, Schoenberg and colleagues[177] screened 5489 individuals who were between the ages of 40 and 64 years to identify only three cases of severe dementia. Because few cases of severe dementia in this age category are likely to escape medical attention, it may be possible to obtain accurate estimates of prevalence in this group using disease registries[142,195] or records-linkage systems.

PREVALENCE STUDIES

There have been many surveys of the prevalence of dementia in elderly individuals.* Comparison of these prevalence studies is difficult since diagnostic criteria were not uniform, the populations studied varied in age distribution and severity, institutionalized individuals were not always included, and few studies attempted to differentiate the various dementing illnesses.† Differences in diagnostic criteria proba-

---

*References 48, 103, 149, 160, 175, 177, 211.

*References 38, 48, 88, 99, 104, 149, 159, 160, 211.

†References 38, 48, 62, 73, 88, 95, 104, 142, 149, 160, 211.

bly account for the greatest variation in prevalence estimates.[88,99,142] Fortunately, most studies conducted since 1980 have used standardized criteria,[4,5,129] dramatically reducing the variability between studies.[95] Variability in prevalence rates between studies also results from differing mechanisms of case identification.[38,88,142] For example, rates derived from hospital statistics are usually lower than those obtained from community surveys, because not all cases of dementia in the community are hospitalized.[177] Likewise, community studies based only on door-to-door inquiries produce lower rate estimates than studies that supplement door-to-door inquiries with an evaluation of residents in special medical facilities at the time of the survey (e.g., nursing homes, hospitals, special schools).[38,48,175,177]

Differences in the age distributions of the populations studied are another potential source of variability in the estimates of dementia prevalence.[142] Most prevalence surveys focus on dementia in the elderly because dementia is relatively common among these individuals; however, this group is certainly not homogeneous for risk of dementia. The prevalence of severe dementia rises steeply from less than 1% at ages 65 to 70, to over 25% by age 85.[38,191] Recent studies among community populations of older persons have suggested even higher rates.[48,144] When rates rise so steeply with age, it is meaningless to compare prevalence rates for the population "over 65" in two different populations because the age composition of populations over age 65 varies considerably;[62] instead, rates must be compared either within very narrow age ranges (age-specific rates), or after statistical procedures are carried out to remove the effect of differences in age composition (age-adjusted rates).[159] Substantial uncertainty about dementia prevalence still exists for mild or moderate dementia, the youngest and oldest age groups, ethnic and racial subgroups, nursing home populations, and subtypes of dementia.[196]

INCIDENCE STUDIES

Incidence studies of dementia focus on the development of this condition in a sample, or cohort, of nondemented individuals. The cohort is examined at the start of the study, and surviving members are reexamined at a later time to identify those who became demented during the interval. Information is also obtained on those who died during the interval, because some of these may have become demented and then died before they could be reexamined. Therefore, to obtain meaningful numbers with such studies, a sufficiently large population must be surveyed at least twice. Alternatively, incidence data may be obtained by continuous surveillance of a population.[105,178]

Incidence studies are extremely expensive, administratively difficult, and time consuming. Furthermore, in order to measure incidence (and survival), the onset of the dementia must be determined, a task that may be extremely difficult with a disorder that is insidious in onset and diverse in presentation; indeed, it is not atypical for the diagnosis of dementia to be made only in the advanced stages. Because of these difficulties, incidence studies of dementing illnesses in general population samples are rare compared with prevalence studies.*

ANALYTIC STUDIES: HYPOTHESIS TESTING

Different individuals are exposed to a variety of different factors or conditions, some of which may play an important role in the development of specific dementing illnesses. Analytic studies are used to identify these causal factors. Once risk factors have been identified, rational prevention programs can be established and tested. Two general approaches are used in

---

*References 70, 71, 96, 105, 146, 158, 159, 163, 178, 195.

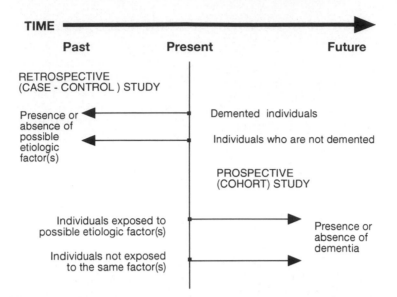

Figure 1–1. Format of the design of retrospective (case-control) and prospective (cohort) studies of dementia. In a case-control study, demented individuals (cases) are compared with persons who are not demented (controls). A retrospective case-control study compares past exposures of these groups to factors possibly related to the occurrence of dementia; a cross-sectional study measures present characteristics. In contrast, a prospective study starts with a group (cohort) of nondemented people with varying exposure to a proposed etiologic factor. The cohort is followed over time to determine differences in the rate at which dementia develops in relation to exposure to the factor. (Adapted from Schoenberg BS: Epidemiology of the inherited ataxias. In Kark P, Rosenberg R, and Schut L (eds): Advances in Neurology, Vol 21: The Inherited Ataxias: Biochemical, Viral, and Pathological Studies. Raven Press, New York, 1978, p. 211.)

analytic studies: case-control and prospective.

Case-Control Studies

In a case-control study, demented individuals (cases) are compared with persons who are not demented (controls) (Fig. 1–1). Present characteristics (in a cross-sectional study) or past exposures (in a retrospective study) of these groups are compared to identify factors possibly related to the occurrence of the disease.

Case-control studies have identified potential risk factors for several types of dementia. For example, risk factors identified for Creutzfeldt-Jakob disease include intraocular pressure testing; previous surgery; physical injury; and consumption of pork, lamb, processed meats, and animal brains.[40,41,107] Suggested risk factors for AD include de-

mentia or Down's syndrome in other family members,* older maternal age at the subject's birth,[3,88,158,159] and serious head injury.†

ADVANTAGES AND DISADVANTAGES

The major advantages and disadvantages of case-control studies are listed in Table 1–12. Case-control studies are particularly attractive because they can be carried out comparatively quickly and at relatively low cost.[83,100,172,173] They are well suited to studying rare dementing diseases, such as Creutzfeldt-Jacob disease,[18,40,41,107] or those with a long latency, such as AD.[3,22,31,77,180] To determine the past exposure history of

---

*References 3, 22, 77, 88, 157–159, 180.
†References 57, 60, 77, 88, 141, 157–159, 188.

Table 1–12 ADVANTAGES AND DISADVANTAGES OF CASE-CONTROL STUDIES

Advantages
1. Well suited to study of diseases with low incidence or long latency.
2. Relatively inexpensive and quick to execute.
3. Comparatively few subjects are required.
4. No risk to study subjects.
5. No follow-up necessary.
6. Multiple risk factors for a disease can be studied.

Disadvantages
1. Necessary information may not be available from routine records or may be inaccurately or incompletely recorded.
2. Demented individuals are not reliable sources of information on past exposures.
3. Differences in recall of past events between case and control groups may bias results.
4. Validation of information is difficult or impossible.
5. Selection of an appropriate control group may be difficult.
6. Rates of disease in exposed and unexposed individuals cannot be determined.
7. Presence of disease may influence factor being studied.
8. Control of extraneous variables may be incomplete.
9. Detailed study of disease pathogenesis is not possible.

Source: Adapted from Schoenberg,[173] p. 47 and Schlesselman,[172] p. 18.

an individual with regard to a specific factor, however, the investigator must rely on memory and past records, the accuracy of which may be uncertain, particularly in demented individuals.[161]

DESIGN AND IMPLEMENTATION

In the design and implementation of case-control studies of dementing illnesses, particular attention should be directed to selection of cases and controls, ascertainment of exposure status, and bias in data collection.[83,100,172]

Selection of Cases and Controls. The disease under study should be defined in specific, unambiguous terms by operational diagnostic criteria, as previously indicated. The goal of case definition is to specify a group of individuals who have a disease that is a homogeneous etiologic entity. Then, eligibility criteria are established to restrict the study to persons who were at risk of exposure. If individuals under study represent a mix of disease entities or if some of the individuals had no real chance of having had their disease caused by the exposure under study, a real association may be diluted or eliminated. Of course, diagnostic procedures and eligibility criteria must be applied equally to potential cases and controls.

Use of newly diagnosed or incident cases of dementia has several advantages: (1) recent diagnoses will be more uniform than those drawn from different time periods; (2) recall of past exposures may be more accurate; (3) the temporal sequence of etiologic-factor–then–disease can be established more reliably; and (4) the possibility of identifying factors associated with the course of the disease, but unrelated to an increased or decreased risk of developing the disease, will be minimized.

Individuals selected as controls should be free of the study disease and should be similar to cases in terms of potential for exposure during the period of risk under study.[172] If the controls differ from the cases in a number of factors, such as age, race, or gender, it may be these factors that are responsible for an observed association. Therefore, the control group should be comparable with the case group for all factors that might influence the outcome, except for the factors under study. For example, in case-control studies of environmental influences in diseases with genetic determinants, such as AD, groups of monozygotic twins discordant for dementia can be used to avoid confounding with genetic factors and to improve study power, because the cases and their matched controls carry the same genetic risk of developing AD. Such studies, however, are limited by greater cost and by the difficulty of finding a sufficient number of twin pairs for study.[21] When comparability cannot be fully achieved by selection (inclusion and exclusion criteria, matching, and so on), it may be partially accomplished during data analysis using statistical adjustment (stratification, multivariate analysis).

The source of controls is important, but there is no consensus on when family, hospital, population, or other controls should be used.[83,100,172] Each source of controls has specific advantages and disadvantages.[100,172] The choice of which control group to use depends largely on the source of the cases, the relative costs of obtaining the various possible control groups, and the facilities available to the investigator.[100] Some studies have used more than one control group to provide an internal measure of consistency, and to permit consideration of possible selection and recall bias.[3,40,41,141] Consistency of study findings using more than one control group strengthens confidence in the validity of the results, whereas inconsistency suggests biased selection.

Ascertainment of Exposure Status.
Because demented individuals are poor historians, the investigator is obligated to find another source of historical information for retrospective inquiries. Necessary information may not be available from routine records or may be inaccurately or incompletely recorded. Consequently, surrogate respondents have been used as one source of historical data for demented subjects.[22,32,77,161,162] For comparability, surrogate respondents must also be used for controls. The ability of surrogate respondents to provide useful information for a case-control study depends on a number of factors: question topic, degree of detail requested, race, gender, age, study area, length of time in which subject and surrogate respondent lived together, and frequency of contacts when living apart. The most important factor, however, is the relationship of the surrogate respondent to the individual: spouse and offspring are best able to describe events that occurred during adult life, whereas siblings best remember events of early life and characteristics of the family.* Next-of-kin respondents are generally well informed about the presence of chronic illnesses, prolonged use of medications, dietary habits, drinking, and smoking, but less knowledgeable about prior short-term, non–life-threatening disorders.† If cases and controls differ in the type of surrogate respondent, a potential bias might be introduced; hence, future studies should, if possible, match cases and controls for type of surrogate respondent available.[33,162]

Bias. Bias can be minimized if symmetry is maintained between comparison groups in all operational aspects of the study, including selection and exclusion criteria, history taking, recording of observations, staging, and so on.[170,172] There should be no major differences in either the quality or extent of information collected from the case and control groups. For example, to minimize bias in the collection of data for a case-control study of dementia, Chandra and colleagues[33] obtained surrogate respondents for both demented and nondemented individuals, used a structured interview, and blinded interviewers to the categorization of the respondent as surrogate for case or control. In addition, respondents were not even aware that the purpose of the study was to identify risk factors for AD. Similar methods have been used in other studies.[22] Nevertheless, sometimes subtle forms of bias may influ-

---

*References 44, 76, 81, 114, 123, 130, 150.
†References 44, 76, 77, 81, 106, 114, 123, 130, 161.

ence a study's results despite careful efforts to maintain symmetry between the two comparison groups. For example, selection bias may exist in some studies assessing family history of dementia as a risk factor, because families with more than one affected member are more likely to be included in studies based on a hospital case series.[157]

Recall bias is a particular concern in case-control studies. For questions such as the family history of dementia, the flow of family information about this condition is probably stimulated by a new case in the family.[157,170] Similarly, the next-of-kin of a demented individual may overreport adverse medical or surgical events in the patient's medical history in an effort to explain the individual's disease[170]; this phenomenon may explain the apparent association between head trauma and AD in case-control studies using interview data,[32,33,157,177] a finding that was not confirmed in a large, population-based study using prospectively collected data.[32] The problem of recall bias in case-control studies may be lessened by choosing a control group from among persons with other diseases that would similarly enhance recall of exposures. Ideally, study data should be validated (at least in a sample of the cases and controls) by obtaining information about exposure from independent sources unaffected by memory or by the flow of family information.[170] The use of "dummy hypotheses" may also indicate if these types of bias are occurring[73,180]; such hypotheses should be biologically improbable, yet credible to a lay person.[73]

Prospective Studies

A prospective study starts with a group of nondemented people (a cohort) with varying exposure to a proposed etiologic factor (see Figure 1–1). The cohort is followed over time to determine differences in the rate at which dementia develops in relation to exposure to the factor.

ADVANTAGES AND DISADVANTAGES

Prospective studies have several advantages compared with retrospective investigations (Table 1–13).[100,172,173] In principle, the prospective approach provides a complete description of events subsequent to exposure, including latency, rates of progression, staging of disease, and so on. The investiga-

Table 1–13 ADVANTAGES AND DISADVANTAGES OF
PROSPECTIVE STUDIES

Advantages
1. Can provide a complete description of experience following exposure.
2. Rates of disease in exposed and unexposed individuals can be calculated.
3. Less chance of misclassification of subjects by exposure, and less chance of bias in obtaining information.
4. Multiple effects of a given exposure can be studied.

Disadvantages
1. Relatively expensive and time-consuming.
2. Large numbers of subjects are required to study uncommon diseases.
3. Attrition of subjects is likely with prolonged follow-up.
4. Individuals who participate may not be representative of all individuals with disease.
5. The study itself may alter outcome.
6. Current practice may change, making findings irrelevant.
7. Incorporation of new knowledge into study protocol is difficult.
8. Control of extraneous variables may be incomplete.
9. Detailed study of disease pathogenesis is not possible.

Source: Adapted from Schoenberg,[173] p. 51 and Schlesselman,[172] p. 18.

tor has great flexibility in choosing the variables to be studied. Because exposure status is known from the outset and a uniform protocol is used, there is less risk of misclassification according to exposure and less subjective bias in obtaining information. It is unnecessary to rely on patients' or relatives' memories to gather this information.

Despite these advantages, prospective studies are expensive and generally unsuitable for investigating uncommon disorders. For example, dementia in those under age 65 would be extremely difficult to study with a prospective approach because of the rarity of the condition. Also, for conditions such as AD, the duration of follow-up may necessarily be many years. It is difficult to keep a large number of individuals under medical surveillance for this period; a substantial proportion of the original cohort may move away, lose interest in the study, or simply refuse to provide any required information.[183] Those who volunteer for a prospective study, and those of the initial volunteers who continue under medical surveillance, may not be representative of all individuals with the characteristic of interest,[170] particularly since "advantaged" persons (higher social status, better health, more active) are more likely than others to participate in such research studies.[27] Furthermore, while the study is ongoing, current practice may change or other information may come to light, making study findings irrelevant. Once a study protocol is established, it is difficult to incorporate new knowledge or tests later.[183]

NONCONCURRENT
PROSPECTIVE STUDIES

Most prospective studies begin in the present and continue into the future. Under certain circumstances, however, it may be possible to begin the point of observation at some time in the past and look at disease outcome in the present.[131] Such nonconcurrent prospective studies (or "historical cohort" studies) may greatly reduce the time and expense often associated with prospective studies. Furthermore, they are much more appropriate than "current cohort" studies when, as in the case of AD, there is a lack of information about risk factors and a resulting inability to choose high-risk populations for study.[183] Because of these considerations, the Epidemiology Commission of the Workshop-Conference on Alzheimer's Disease – Senile Dementia and Related Disorders urged the use of existing medically defined populations for nonconcurrent prospective studies of AD.[97] Although the commission recommended several potential data bases, it is unusual to find cohorts of individuals who have been examined, questioned, and observed in a standardized manner over a number of years.

Inferences from Analytic Epidemiology

If a statistically significant association is demonstrated in an analytic study of a dementing disease, chance alone is an unlikely explanation, but extraneous factors or systematic biases may account for the relationship and must be carefully considered as an explanation for an apparent association. It is possible to analyze data using statistical techniques that take into account, or control for, potentially confounding factors. It is difficult or impossible, however, to analyze the data in a way that controls for potential biases that may creep into a study. It is much better to prevent bias by careful study design and execution, maintaining symmetry between comparison groups in all operational aspects of the study. Finding the same association in several different studies provides some assurance that the association is not an artifact of the way a particular study was done or of an unusual group of study subjects.

A nonspurious association does not necessarily imply a cause-and-effect relationship, for the relationship may be indirect; the observed association may exist only because both the factor and the disease are related to some common underlying condition. Unfortunately, establishing a causal relationship in the absence of direct experiment is neither easy nor objective. Nevertheless, several criteria can be helpful in distinguishing causal and noncausal factors among associations identified by observational studies.[53,78,189,190,206,207]

First, the sequence of events must be consistent with a causal relationship, that is, the development of dementia should follow exposure to the factor presumed to cause it. The correct temporal sequence may be difficult to determine with certainty, however, because the onset of dementia is usually insidious, and affected individuals are often not recognized until late in the course of the disease. In addition, dementia itself may produce an increased frequency of some circumstances thought to cause dementia. For example, sorting out the correct temporal sequence of head injury and AD is particularly problematic, because dementia is an important risk factor for both serious falls[25,138] and motor vehicle accidents[58] even in the mild stages of the disease. Such problems are minimized with case-control studies using incident cases (see Selection of Cases and Controls, above) or, optimally, with longitudinal studies.

Other important considerations for establishing causality in observational studies include the strength of the association, the presence of a dose-response relationship, and the biologic plausibility of the presumed cause. The stronger the association between a suspected etiologic factor and a dementing illness, the more likely the association is to be causal; for a strong association to be spurious, the underlying factor that accounts for it must be even more strongly associated with the disease.[23] In addition, an increased frequency or degree of dementia with increased exposure to some presumed etiologic factor (dose-response relationship) is frequently an indication of a true causal relationship, although exceptions do occur.[201] Furthermore, if an association is consistent with the known facts concerning the development of the dementing illness being studied (biologic plausibility or coherence), it is more plausible as a cause-and-effect relationship. Other criteria have been proposed,[47,78,189,190,206,207] but many are difficult to apply or less valuable for assessing a cause-and-effect relationship. None of the criteria are sufficient for making a causal interpretation, and strict adherence to any one of them could result in incorrect conclusions.[78]

SUMMARY

Demographic projections suggest that the number of demented individuals will grow dramatically as the elderly segment of our population increases. Comparative studies of the incidence, prevalence, and duration of different forms of dementia using uniform methodologies are urgently needed. Such studies may provide important information for health care planning, settle theoretical questions, and suggest etiologic hypotheses that can be tested with well-designed analytic studies. This knowledge can then be used to develop rational programs for treating and preventing this major public health problem. The design and interpretation of studies of potential drug therapies are discussed in Chapter 13.

ACKNOWLEDGMENTS

The authors thank Dr. Mary Jo Lanska, Mrs. Devera Schoenberg, and Dr. Kathleen Smyth for editorial assistance and helpful suggestions. This work was supported in part by NIA Research Training Grant 1/T32/AG00144-01, NIA Alzheimer's Disease Research Center Program Project Grant P50-A6-05144-06, and NIH Clinical Investigator Development Award 1/K08/NSO 1549-01.

REFERENCES

1. Aikawa H, Suzuki K, Iwasaki Y, and Iizuka R: Atypical Alzheimer's disease with spastic paresis and ataxia. Ann Neurol 17:297–300, 1985.
2. Alter, M: Medical registers. In Schoenberg BS: Advances in Neurology, Vol 19, Neurologic Epidemiology: Principles and Clinical Applications. Raven Press, New York, 1978, pp 121–139.
3. Amaducci LA, Fratiglioni L, Rocca WA, et al: Risk factors for clinically diagnosed Alzheimer's disease: A case-control study of an Italian population. Neurology 36:922–931, 1986.
4. American Psychiatric Association: Diagnostic and Statistical Manual of Mental Disorders, ed 3 (DSM-III). American Psychiatric Association, Washington, DC, 1980.
5. American Psychiatric Association: Diagnostic and Statistical Manual of Mental Disorders, ed 3, rev. (DSM-III-R). American Psychiatric Association, Washington, DC, 1987.
6. Anthony JC, Niaz U, LeResche LA, Von Korff MR, and Folstein MF: Limits of the "Mini-Mental State" as a screening test for dementia and delirium among hospital patients. Psychol Med 12:397–408, 1982.
7. Arenberg D: Misclassification of "probable senile dementia—Alzheimer's type" in the Baltimore Longitudinal Study of Aging. J Clin Epidemiol 43:105–107, 1990.
8. Arie T: Pseudodementia. BMJ 286:1301–1302, 1983.
9. Ashford JW, Kolm P, Colliver JA, Bekian C, and Hsu L- N: Alzheimer patient evaluation and the Mini-Mental State: Item characteristic curve analysis. J Gerontol 44:P139–P146, 1989.
10. Aubert R, Parker R, Rothenberg R, and May D: Methodological issues in the reported prevalence of Alzheimer's disease on death certificates. In Data for an Aging Population: Proceedings of the 1987 Public Health Conference on Records and Statistics. US Department of Health and Human Services, Hyattsville, MD, 1987, pp 183–187.
11. Berg L: Clinical Dementia Rating (CDR). Psychopharmacol Bull 24:637–639, 1988.
12. Berg, L, Danziger, WL, Storandt, M, et al. Predictive features in mild senile dementia of the Alzheimer's type. Neurology 34:563–569, 1984.
13. Berg L, Hughes CP, Coben LA, Danziger WL, Martin RL and Knesevich J: Mild senile dementia of Alzheimer type: Research diagnostic criteria, recruitment, and description of a study population. J Neurol Neurosurg Psychiatry 45:962–968, 1982.
14. Berg L, Miller JP, Storandt M, et al. Mild senile dementia of the Alzheimer type: 2. Longitudinal assessment. Ann Neurol 23:477–484, 1988.
15. Berger EY: A system for rating the severity of senility. J Am Geriatr Soc 28:234–236, 1980.
16. Bird TD, Sumi SM, Nemens EJ, et al. Phenotypic heterogeneity in familial Alzheimer's disease: A study of 24 kindreds. Ann Neurol 25:12–25, 1989.
17. Blessed G, Tomlinson BE, and Roth M: The association between quantitative measures of dementia and of senile change in the cerebral grey matter of elderly subjects. Br J Psychiatry 114:797–811, 1968.
18. Bobowick AR, Brody JA, Matthews MR, Roos R, and Gajdusek DC: Creutzfeldt-Jakob disease: A case-control study. Am J Epidemiol 98: 381–394, 1973.
19. Botwinick J, Storandt M, and Berg L: A longitudinal, behavioral study of senile dementia of the Alzheimer type. Arch Neurol 43:1124–1127, 1986.
20. Branconnier RJ and Cole JO: The Impairment Index as a symptom-independent parameter of drug efficacy in geriatric psychopharmacology. J Gerontol 33:217–233, 1978.
21. Breitner JC, Murphy EA, and Woodbury MA: Case-control studies of environmental influences in diseases with genetic determinants, with an application to Alzheimer's disease. Am J Epidemiol 133:246–256, 1991.
22. Broe GA, Henderson AS, Creasey H, et al. A case-control study of Alzheimer's

disease in Australia. Neurology 40:1698–1707, 1990.

23. Bross ID: Spurious effects from an extraneous variable. J Chronic Dis 19: 637–647, 1966.

24. Brust JC: Vascular dementia — still overdiagnosed. Stroke 14:298–300, 1983.

25. Buchner DM and Larson EB: Falls and fractures in patients with Alzheimer-type dementia. JAMA 257: 1492–1495, 1987.

26. Burke WJ, Miller JP, Rubin EH, et al. Reliability of the Washington University Clinical Dementia Rating. Arch Neurol 45:31–32, 1988.

27. Busse EW: Duke Longitudinal Study I: Senescence and senility. In Katzman R, Terry RD, and Bick KL: Alzheimer's Disease: Senile Dementia and Related Disorders. Raven Press, New York, 1978, pp 59–68.

28. Centers for Disease Control: Mortality from Alzheimer disease — United States, 1979–1987. JAMA 265:313–314, 1991.

29. Chamblee RF and Evans MC: New dimensions in cause of death statistics. Am J Public Health 72:1265–1270, 1982.

30. Chandra V, Bharucha NE, and Schoenberg BS: Patterns of mortality from types of dementia in the United States, 1971 and 1973–1978. Neurology 36:204–208, 1986.

31. Chandra V, Bharucha NE, and Schoenberg BS: Conditions associated with Alzheimer's disease at death: Case-control study. Neurology 36:209–211, 1986.

32. Chandra V, Kokmen E, and Schoenberg BS: Head trauma with loss of consciousness as a risk factor for Alzheimer's disease using prospectively collected data. Neurology 37(Suppl 1):152, 1987.

33. Chandra V, Philipose V, Bell PA, Lazaroff A, and Schoenberg BS: Case-control study of late-onset "probable Alzheimer's disease." Neurology 37: 1295–1300, 1987.

34. Chui HC, Teng EL, Henderson VW, and Moy AC: Clinical subtypes of dementia of the Alzheimer type. Neurology 35:1544–1550, 1985.

35. Clark GS: Functional assessment in the elderly. In Williams TF: Rehabilitation in the Aging. Raven Press, New York, 1984, pp 111–123.

36. Cooper B and Bickel H: Population screening and early detection of dementing disorders in old age: A review. Psychol Med 14:81–95, 1984.

37. Council on Scientific Affairs: Dementia. JAMA 256:2234–2238, 1986.

38. Cross PS and Gurland GJ: The epidemiology of dementing disorders. Contract report prepared for the Office of Technology Assessment, US Congress, 1986.

39. Cummings JL and Benson DF: Dementia: A clinical approach. Butterworths, London, 1983.

40. Davanipour Z, Alter M, Sobel E, Ascher DM, and Gajdusek DK: Creutzfeldt-Jakob disease: Possible medical risk factors. Neurology 35:1483–1486, 1985.

41. Davanipour Z, Alter M, Sobel E, Ascher DM, and Gajdusek DK: A case-control study of Creutzfeldt-Jakob disease: Dietary risk factors. Am J Epidemiol 122:443–451, 1985.

42. Dorn HF and Moriyama IM: Uses and significance of multiple cause tabulations for mortality statistics. Am J Public Health 54:400–406, 1964.

43. Eisdorfer C and Cohen D: Diagnostic criteria for primary neuronal degeneration of the Alzheimer's type. J Fam Pract 11:553–557, 1980.

44. Enterline PE and Capt KG: A validation of information provided by household respondents in health surveys. Am J Public Health 49:205–212, 1959.

45. Erkinjuntti T, Wikström J, Palo J, and Autio L: Dementia among medical inpatients: Evaluation of 2000 consecutive admissions. Arch Intern Med 146: 1923–1926, 1986.

46. Escobar JI, Burnam A, Karno M, Forsythe A, Landsverk J, and Golding JM: Use of the Mini-Mental State Examination (MMSE) in a community population of mixed ethnicity. J Nerv Ment Dis 174:607–614, 1986.

47. Evans AS: Causation and disease: A chronological journey. Am J Epidemiol 108:249–258, 1978.

48. Evans DA, Funkenstein H, Albert MS, et al.: Prevalence of Alzheimer's disease in a community population of older persons: Higher than previously reported. JAMA 262:2551–2556, 1989.

49. Fillenbaum GG: Screening the elderly: A brief instrumental activities of daily living measure. J Am Geriatr Soc 33:698–706, 1985.

50. Fillenbaum G, Heyman A, Williams K, Prosnitz B, and Burchett B: Sensitivity and specificity of standardized screens of cognitive impairment and dementia among elderly black and white community residents. J Clin Epidemiol 43:651–660, 1990.

51. Fisher CM: Dementia in cerebral vascular disease. In Seikert R and Whisnant J: Cerebral Vascular Disease, 6th Conference. Grune and Stratton, New York, 1968, pp 232–236.

52. Flaten TP: Mortality from dementia in Norway, 1969–1983. J Epidemiol Community Health 43:285–289, 1989.

53. Foley JM, Cassel CK, Eastman P, et al.: Differential diagnosis of dementing diseases. JAMA 258:3411–3416, 1987.

54. Folstein M, Romanoski A, Nestadt G, et al.: Diagnosis of dementia in Eastern Baltimore. NINCDS Final Report. Johns Hopkins University, Baltimore, 1986.

55. Ford AB, Folmar SJ, Salmon RB, Medalie JH, Roy AW, and Galazka SS: Health and function in the old and very old. J Am Geriatr Soc 36:187–197, 1988.

56. Forette F, Henry JF, Orgogozo JM, et al.: Reliability of criteria for the diagnosis of dementia: A longitudinal multicenter study. Arch Neurol 46:646–648, 1989.

57. French LR, Schuman LM, Mortimer JA, Hutton JT, Boatman RA, and Christians B: A case-control study of dementia of the Alzheimer type. Am J Epidemiol 121:414–421, 1985.

58. Friedland RP, Koss E, Kumar A, et al.: Motor vehicle crashes in dementia of the Alzheimer type. Ann Neurol 24:782–786, 1988.

59. Galasko D, Klauber MR, Hofstetter CR, Salmon DP, Lasker B, and Thal LJ: The Mini-Mental State Examination in the early diagnosis of Alzheimer's disease. Arch Neurol 47:49–52, 1990.

60. Graves AB, White E, Koepsell T, and Reifler B: A case-control study of Alzheimer's disease. Am J Epidemiol 126:754, 1987.

61. Green J, Morris JC, Sandson J, McKeel DW, Jr., and Miller JW: Progressive aphasia: A precursor of global dementia? Neurology 40:423–429, 1990.

62. Gruenberg EM: Epidemiology of senile dementia. In Schoenberg BS: Advances in Neurology, Vol 19, Neurologic Epidemiology: Principles and Clinical Applications. Raven Press, New York, 1978, pp 437–457.

63. Grufferman S: Alzheimer's disease and senile dementia: One disease or two? In Katzman R and Terry RD: Alzheimer's Disease: Senile Dementia and Related Disorders. Raven Press, New York, 1978, pp 35–45.

64. Gurland BJ, Dean LL, Copeland J, Gurland R, and Golden R: Criteria for the diagnosis of dementia in the community elderly. Gerontologist 22:180–186, 1982.

65. Gustafson F and Nilsson L: Differential diagnosis of presenile dementia on clinical grounds. Acta Psychiatr Scand 65:194–209, 1982.

66. Gustafson L: Differential diagnosis with special reference to treatable dementias and pseudodementia conditions. Dan Med Bull 32(Suppl 1):55–60, 1985.

67. Haase GR: Diseases presenting as dementia. In Wells CE: Dementia, ed 2. FA Davis, Philadelphia, 1977, pp 27–67.

68. Hachinski VC: Differential diagnosis of Alzheimer's disease: Multi-infarct dementia. In Reisberg, B: Alzheimer's Disease: The Standard Reference. Free Press, New York, 1983, pp 188–192.

69. Hachinski V, Iliff L, Zilhka E, et al.: Cerebral blood flow in dementia. Arch Neurol 32:632–637, 1975.

70. Hagnell O, Lanke J, Rorsman B, and Öjesjö L: Does the incidence of age psychosis decrease? A prospective, longitudinal study of a complete population investigated during the 25-year period 1947–1972: The Lundby study. Neuropsychobiology 7:201–211, 1981.

71. Hagnell O, Lanke J, Rorsman B, Öhman R, and Öjesjö L: Current trends in the incidence of senile and multi-infarct dementia. Archiv für Psychiatrie und Nervenkrenk heiten 233:423–438, 1983.

72. Hay JW and Ernst RL: The economic costs of Alzheimer's disease. Am J Public Health 77:1169–1175, 1987.

73. Henderson AS: The epidemiology of Alzheimer's disease. Br Med Bull 42:3–10, 1986.

74. Henderson AS and Huppert FA: Editorial: The problem of mild dementia. Psychol Med 14:5–11, 1984.

75. Henderson AS and Jorm AF: Is case-ascertainment of Alzheimer's disease in field surveys practicable? Psychol Med 17:549–555, 1987.

76. Herrmann N: Retrospective information from questionnaires: I. Comparability of primary respondents and their next-of-kin. Am J Epidemiol 121:937–947, 1985.

77. Heyman A, Wilkinson WE, Stafford JA, Helms MJ, Sigmon AH, and Weinberg T: Alzheimer's disease: A study of epidemiological aspects. Ann Neurol 15:335–341, 1984.

78. Hill AB: Principles of Medical Statistics, ed 9. Oxford University Press, London, 1971.

79. Hughes CP, Berg L, Danziger W, Coben LA, and Martin RL: A new clinical scale for the staging of dementia. Br J Psychiatry 140:566–572, 1982.

80. Hughes JP, van Belle G, Kukull W, Larson EB, and Teri L: On the uses of registries for Alzheimer's disease. Technical report no. 87. University of Washington, Seattle, 1988.

81. Humble CG, Samet JM, and Skipper BE: Comparison of self- and surrogate-reported dietary information. Am J Epidemiol 119:86–98, 1984.

82. Huppert FA and Tym E: Clinical and neuropsychological assessment of dementia. Br Med Bull 42:11–18, 1986.

83. Ibrahim MA: The case-control study: Consensus and controversy. J Chronic Dis 32:1–144, 1979.

84. Israel RA, Rosenberg HM, and Curtin LR: Analytic potential for multiple cause-of-death data. Am J Epidemiol 124:161–179, 1986.

85. Jagust WJ, Davies P, Tiller-Borcich JK, and Reed BR: Focal Alzheimer's disease. Neurology 40:14–19, 1990.

86. Joachim CL, Morris JH, and Selkoe DJ: Clinically diagnosed Alzheimer's disease: Autopsy results in 150 cases. Ann Neurol 24:50–56, 1988.

87. Jorm AF: Subtypes of Alzheimer's dementia: A conceptual analysis and critical review. Psychol Med 15:543–553, 1985.

88. Jorm AF: The Epidemiology of Alzheimer's Disease and Related Disorders. Chapman & Hall, London, 1990.

89. Jorm AF, Henderson AS, and Jacomb PA: Regional differences in mortality from dementia in Australia: An analysis of death certificate data. Acta Psychiatr Scand 79:179–185, 1989.

90. Jorm AF, Korten AE, and Jacomb PA: Projected increases in the number of dementia cases for 29 developed countries: Application of a new method for making projections. Acta Psychiatr Scand 78:493–500, 1988.

91. Kahana E, Leibowitz Y, Schoenberg BS, and Alter M: Israeli National Neurologic Disease Register. Neuroepidemiology 1:239–248, 1982.

92. Katz S: NIA Conference on Assessment. Assessing self-maintenance: Activities of daily living, mobility, and instrumental activities of daily living. J Am Geriatr Soc 31:721–727, 1983.

93. Katz S, Ford AB, Moskowitz RW, Jackson BA, and Jaffe MW: Studies of illness in the aged. The Index of ADL: A standardized measure of biological and psycho social function. JAMA 185:914–919, 1963.

94. Katzman R: The prevalence and malignancy of Alzheimer's disease: A

major killer. Arch Neurol 33:217–218, 1976.

95. Katzman R: Alzheimer's disease. N Engl J Med 314:964–973, 1986.

96. Katzman R, Aronson M, Fuld P, et al.: Development of dementing illnesses in an 80-year-old volunteer cohort. Ann Neurol 25:317–324, 1989.

97. Katzman R, Terry RD, and Bick KL: Recommendations of the Nosology, Epidemiology, and Etiology and Pathophysiology Commissions of the Workshop-Conference on Alzheimer's Disease–Senile Dementia and Related Disorders. In Katzman R, Terry RD, and Bick KL: Alzheimer's Disease: Senile Dementia and Related Disorders. Raven Press, New York, 1978, pp 579–585.

98. Kay DW: Heterogeneity in Alzheimer's disease: Epidemiological and family studies. Trends Neurosci 10:194–195, 1987.

99. Kay DW, Henderson AS, Scott R, Wilson J, Rickwood D, and Grayson DA: Dementia and depression among the elderly living in the Hobart community: The effect of the diagnostic criteria on prevalence rates. Psychol Med 15:771–778, 1985.

100. Kelsey JL, Thompson WD, and Evans AS: Methods in Observational Epidemiology. Oxford University Press, New York, 1986.

101. Kenny RA, Stevens S, and Hodkinson HM: Hachinski Ischemic Score in demented elderly patients. Journal of Clinical and Experimental Gerontology 6:63–74, 1984.

102. Khachaturian ZS: Diagnosis of Alzheimer's disease. Arch Neurol 42:1097–1105, 1985.

103. Kittner SJ, White LR, Farmer ME, et al.: Methodological issues in screening for dementia: The problem of education adjustment. J Chronic Dis 39:163–170, 1986.

104. Kokmen E, Beard CM, Offord KP, and Kurland LT: Prevalence of medically diagnosed dementia in a defined United States population: Rochester, Minnesota, January 1, 1975. Neurology 39:773–776, 1989.

105. Kokmen E, Chandra V, and Schoen-berg BS: Trends in incidence of dementing illness in Rochester, Minnesota, in three quinquennial periods, 1960–1974. Neurology 38:975–980, 1988.

106. Kolonel LN, Hirohata T, and Nomura AM: Adequacy of survey data collected from substitute respondents. Am J Epidemiol 106:476–484, 1977.

107. Kondo K and Kuroiwa Y: A case-control study of Creutzfeldt-Jakob disease: Association with physical injuries. Ann Neurol 11:377–381, 1981.

108. Kukull WA, Larson EB, Reifler BV, Lampe TH, Yerby MS, and Hughes JP: The validity of 3 clinical diagnostic criteria for Alzheimer's disease. Neurology 40:1364–1369, 1990.

109. Kukull WA, Larson EB, Reifler BV, Lampe TH, Yerby M, and Hughes J: Interrater reliability of Alzheimer's disease diagnosis. Neurology 40:257–260, 1990.

110. Kurland LT: Geographic isolates: Their role in neuroepidemiology. In Schoenberg, BS: Advances in Neurology, Vol 19, Neurologic Epidemiology: Principles and Clinical Applications. Raven Press, New York, 1978, pp 69–82.

111. Kurland LT and Brian DD: Contributions to neurology from records linkage in Olmsted County, Minnesota. In Schoenberg BS: Advances in Neurology, Vol 19, Neurologic Epidemiology: Principles and Clinical Applications. Raven Press, New York, 1978, pp 93–105.

112. Kurland LT, Molgaard CA, and Schoenberg BS: Mayo Clinic records-linkage: Contributions to neuroepidemiology. Neuroepidemiology 1:102–114, 1982.

113. Larson EB, Reifler BV, Featherstone HJ, and English DR: Dementia in elderly outpatients: A prospective study. Ann Intern Med 100:417–423, 1984.

114. Lerchen ML and Samet JM: An assessment of the validity of questionnaire responses provided by a surviving spouse. Am J Epidemiol 123:481–489, 1986.

115. Liss L: How accurate is the clinical diagnosis of Alzheimer's disease? J

Neuropathol Exp Neurol 49:271, 1990.

116. Liston EH and La Rue A: Clinical differentiation of primary degenerative and multi-infarct dementia: A critical review of the evidence. Part II: Pathological studies. Biol Psychiatry 18: 1467–1484, 1983.

117. Liu IY, LaCroix AZ, White LR, Kittner SJ, and Wolf PA: Cognitive impairment and mortality: A study of possible confounders. Am J Epidemiol 132:136–143, 1990.

118. Loeb C and Gandolfo C: Diagnostic evaluation of degenerative and vascular dementia. Stroke 14:399–401, 1983.

119. Loewenstein DA, Amigo E, Duara R, et al.: A new scale for the assessment of functional status in Alzheimer's disease and related disorders. J Gerontol 44:P114–P121, 1989.

120. Lopez OL, Swihart AA, Becker JT, et al. Reliability of NINCDS-ADRDA clinical criteria for the diagnosis of Alzheimer's disease. Neurology 40: 1517–1522, 1990.

121. Magruder-Habib K, Breitner JC, and Welsh K: Performance characteristics of the telephone interview for cognitive status. Am J Epidemiol 132:788, 1990.

122. Marsden CD and Harrison MJ: Outcome of investigation of patients with presenile dementia. BMJ 2:249–252, 1972.

123. Marshall J, Priore R, Haughey B, Rzepka T, and Graham S: Spouse-subject interviews and the reliability of diet studies. Am J Epidemiol 112:675–683, 1980.

124. Martin CN and Pippard EC: Usefulness of mortality data in determining the geography and time trends of dementia. J Epidemiol Community Health 42:134–137, 1988.

125. Martin EM, Wilson RS, Penn RD, Fox JH, Clasen RA, and Savoy SM: Cortical biopsy results in Alzheimer's disease: Correlation with cognitive deficits. Neurology 37:1201–1204, 1987.

126. Masters CL, Harris JO, Gajdusek C, Gibbs CJ, Jr, Bernoulli C, and Asher DM: Creutzfeldt-Jakob disease: Patterns of worldwide occurrence and the significance of familial and sporadic clustering. Ann Neurol 5:177–188, 1979.

127. Mayeux R, Stern Y, and Spanton S: Heterogeneity in dementia of the Alzheimer type: Evidence of subgroups. Neurology 35:453–461, 1985.

128. McCulla MM, Coats M, Van Fleet N, Duchek J, Grant E, and Morris JC: Reliability of clinical nurse specialists in the staging of dementia. Arch Neurol 46:1210–1211, 1989.

129. McKhann G, Drachman D, Folstein M, Katzman R, Price D, and Stadlan EM: Clinical diagnosis of Alzheimer's disease: Report of the NINCDS-ADRDA Work Group under the auspices of the Department of Health and Human Services Task Force on Alzheimer's Disease. Neurology 34:939–944, 1984.

130. McLaughlin JK, Dietz MS, Mehl ES, and Blot WJ: Reliability of surrogate information on cigarette smoking by type of informant. Am J Epidemiol 126:144–164, 1987.

131. Mikkelsen S: A cohort study of disability pension and death among painters with special regard to disabling presenile dementia as an occupational disease. Scand J Soc Med 16(Suppl):34–43, 1980.

132. Mirra SS, Heyman A, McKeel D, et al. The Consortium to Establish a Registry for Alzheimer's Disease (CERAD). Part II. Standardization of the neuropathologic assessment of Alzheimer's disease. Neurology 41: 479–486, 1991.

133. Molsa PK, Paljarvi L, Rinne JO, Rinne UK, and Sako E: Validity of clinical diagnosis in dementia: A prospective clinicopathological study. J Neurol Neurosurg Psychiatry 48: 1085–1090, 1985.

134. Morris JC and Fulling K: Early Alzheimer's disease: Diagnostic considerations. Arch Neurol 45:345–349, 1988.

135. Morris JC, Heyman A, Mohs RC, et al.: The Consortium to Establish a Registry for Alzheimer's Disease (CERAD). Part I. Clinical and neuropsychological

assessment of Alzheimer's disease. Neurology 39:1159–1165, 1989.

136. Morris JC, McKeel DW, Jr, Fulling K, Torack RM, and Berg L: Validation of clinical diagnostic criteria for Alzheimer's disease. Ann Neurol 24:17–22, 1988.

137. Morris JC, McKeel DW, Jr, Storandt M, et al.: Very mild Alzheimer's disease: Informant-based clinical, psychometric, and pathologic distinction from normal aging. Neurology 41:469–478, 1991.

138. Morris JC, Rubin EH, Morris EJ, and Mandel SA: Senile dementia of the Alzheimer's type: An important risk factor for serious falls. J Gerontol 42:412–417, 1987.

139. Mortimer JA; Epidemiological aspects of Alzheimer's disease. In Perogyols FG and Maletta GJ (eds): The Aging Nervous System. Oxford University Press, New York, 1980, pp 307–332.

140. Mortimer JA: Do psychosocial risk factors contribute to Alzheimer's disease? In Henderson AS and Henderson JH: Etiology of Dementia of Alzheimer's Type. John Wiley & Sons, New York, 1988, pp 39–52.

141. Mortimer JA, French R, Hutton JT, and Schuman LM: Head injury as a risk factor for Alzheimer's disease. Neurology 35:264–267, 1985.

142. Mortimer JA, Schuman LM, and French LR: Epidemiology of dementing illness. In Mortimer JA and Schuman LM (eds): The Epidemiology of Dementia. Oxford University Press, New York, 1981, pp 3–23.

143. Navia BA, Jordan BD, and Price RW: The AIDS dementia complex: I. Clinical features. Ann Neurol 19:517–524, 1986.

144. Nesselroade JR, Pedersen NL, McClearn GE, Plomin R, and Bergeman CS: Factorial and criterion validities of telephone-assessed cognitive ability measures. Research on Aging 10:220–234, 1988.

145. Newman SC and Bland RC: Canadian trends in mortality from mental disorders, 1965–1983. Acta Psychiatr Scand 76:1–7, 1987.

146. Nilsson LV: Incidence of severe dementia from 70 to 79 years of age. Acta Psychiatr Scand 70:478–486, 1984.

147. O'Connor DW, Pollitt PA, Hyde JB, Brook CP, Reiss BB, and Roth M: Do general practitioners miss dementia in elderly patients? BMJ 297:1107–1110, 1988.

148. Parsons PL: Mental health in Swansea's old folk. Br J Prev Soc Med 19:43–47, 1965.

149. Pfeffer RI, Afifi AA, and Chance JM: Prevalence of Alzheimer's disease in a retirement community. Am J Epidemiol 125:420–436, 1987.

150. Pickle LW, Brown LM, and Blot WJ: Information available from surrogate respondents in case-control interview studies. Am J Epidemiol 118:99–108, 1983.

151. Plum F: Dementia: An approaching epidemic. Nature 279:372–373, 1979.

152. Price RW, Brew B, Sidtis J, Rosenblum M, Scheck AC, and Cleary P: The brain in AIDS: Central nervous system HIV-1 infection and AIDS dementia complex. Science 239:573–579, 1988.

153. Reifler BV, Larson E, and Hanley R: Coexistence of cognitive impairment and depression in geriatric outpatients. Am J Psychiatry 139:623–626, 1982.

154. Reisberg B, Ferris SH, De Leon MJ, and Crook T: The Global Deterioration Scale for assessment of primary degenerative dementia. Am J Psychiatry 139:1136–1139, 1982.

155. Risse SC, Raskind MA, Nochlin D, et al.: Neuropathological findings in patients with clinical diagnoses of probable Alzheimer's disease. Am J Psychiatry 147:168–172, 1990.

156. Roca RP, Klein LE, Kirby SM, et al.: Recognition of dementia among medical inpatients. Arch Intern Med 144:73–75, 1984.

157. Rocca WA: The etiology of Alzheimer's disease: epidemiologic contributions with emphasis on the genetic hypothesis. J Neural Transm Suppl 24:3–12, 1987.

158. Rocca WA and Amaducci L: Epidemiology of Alzheimer's disease. In Anderson DW: Neuroepidemiology: A

Tribute to Bruce Schoenberg. CRC Press, Boca Raton, FL, 1991, pp 55–96.

159. Rocca WA, Amaducci LA, and Schoenberg BS: Epidemiology of clinically diagnosed Alzheimer's disease. Ann Neurol 19:415–424, 1986.

160. Rocca WA, Bonainto S, Lippi A, et al.: Prevalence of clinically diagnosed Alzheimer's disease and other dementing disorders: A door-to-door survey in Appignano, Macerata Province, Italy. Neurology 40:626–631, 1990.

161. Rocca WA, Fratiglioni A, Bracco L, Pedone D, Groppi C, and Schoenberg BS: The use of surrogate respondents to obtain questionnaire data in case-control studies of neurologic diseases. J Chronic Dis 39:907–912, 1986.

162. Rocca WA, Fratiglioni L, Bracco L, Grigoletto F, Amaducci L, and Schoenberg BS: Italian multicenter case-control study of clinically diagnosed Alzheimer disease: Strategies and instruments for data collection. Ital J Neurol Sci 8:97–108, 1987.

163. Rorsman B, Hagnell O, and Lanke J: Prevalence and incidence of senile and multi-infarct dementia in the Lundby Study: A comparison between the time periods 1947–1957 and 1957–1972. Neuropsychobiology 15:122–129, 1986.

164. Rosen WG, Terry RD, Fuld PA, Katzman R, and Peck A: Pathological verification of Ischemic Score in differentiation of dementias. Ann Neurol 7:486–488, 1980.

165. Roth M: Some strategies for tackling the problems of senile dementia and related disorders within the next decade. Dan Med Bull 32(Suppl 1):92–111, 1985.

166. Roth M: The natural history of mental disorders in old age. J Ment Sci 101:281–301, 1955.

167. Roth M, Tym E, Mountjoy CQ, et al.: CAMDEX: A standardized instrument for the diagnosis of mental disorder in the elderly with special reference to the early detection of dementia. Br J Psychiatry 149:698–709, 1986.

168. Rubenstein LZ, Schairer C, Wieland GD, and Kane R: Systematic biases in functional status of elderly adults: Effects of different data sources. J Gerontol 39:686–691, 1984.

169. Rubin EH, Morris JC, Grant EA, and Vandegna T: Very mild senile dementia of the Alzheimer type. I. Clinical assessment. Arch Neurol 46:379–382, 1989.

170. Sackett DL: Bias in analytic research. J Chronic Dis 32:51–63, 1979.

171. Sayetta RB: Rates of senile dementia-Alzheimer's type in Baltimore longitudinal study. J Chronic Dis 36:271–286, 1986.

172. Schlesselman JJ: Case-control studies: Design, conduct, analysis. Oxford University Press, New York, 1982.

173. Schoenberg BS: Principles of neurologic epidemiology. In Schoenberg, BS: Advances in Neurology, Vol 19: Neurological Epidemiology: Principles and Clinical Applications. Raven Press, New York, 1978, pp 11–54.

174. Schoenberg BS: Neuroepidemiologic considerations in studies of Alzheimer's disease–senile dementia. In Katzman R, Terry RD, and Bick KL: Alzheimer's disease: Senile Dementia and Related Disorders. Raven Press, New York, 1978, pp 327–335.

175. Schoenberg BS: Clinical neuroepidemiology in developing countries: Neurology with few neurologists. Neuroepidemiology 1:137–142, 1982.

176. Schoenberg BS: Epidemiology of Alzheimer's disease and other dementing illnesses. J Chronic Dis 39:1095–1104, 1986.

177. Schoenberg BS, Anderson DW, and Haerer AF: Severe dementia: Prevalence and clinical features in a biracial US population. Arch Neurol 42:740–743, 1985.

178. Schoenberg BS, Kokmen E, and Okazaki H: Alzheimer's disease and other dementing illnesses in a defined U.S. population: Incidence rates and clinical features. Ann Neurol 22:724–729, 1987.

179. Seltzer B and Sherwin I: "Organic brain syndromes": An empirical study and critical review. Am J Psychiatry 135:13–21, 1978.

180. Shalat SL, Seltzer B, Pidcock C, and Baker EL: Risk factors for Alzheimer's

disease: A case-control study. Neurology 37:1630–1633, 1987.

181. Shore D, Overman CA, and Wyatt RJ: Improving accuracy in the diagnosis of Alzheimer's disease. J Clin Psychiatry 44:207–212, 1983.

182. Siegel JS: Recent and prospective demographic trends for the elderly population and some implications for health care. In Haynes SG and Feinleib M: Second Conference on the Epidemiology of Aging. US Government Printing Office, Washington, DC, 1980, pp 289–315.

183. Sluss TK, Gruenberg EM, and Kramer M: The use of longitudinal studies in the investigation of risk factors for senile dementia–Alzheimer type. In Mortimer JA and Schuman LM: The Epidemiology of Dementia. Oxford University Press, New York, 1981, pp 132–153.

184. Small GW and Jarvik LF: The dementia syndrome. Lancet ii:1443–1446, 1982.

185. Smith JS and Kiloh LG: The investigation of dementia: Results in 200 consecutive admissions. Lancet i: 824–827, 1981.

186. Stern Y, Hesdorffer D, Sano M, and Mayeux R: Measurement and prediction of functional capacity in Alzheimer's disease. Neurology 40:8–14, 1990.

187. Sulkava R, Haltia M, Paetau A, Wikström J, and Palo J: Accuracy of clinical diagnosis in primary degenerative dementia: Correlation with neuropathological findings. J Neurol Neurosurg Psychiatry 46:9–13, 1983.

188. Sullivan P, Petitti D, and Barbaccia J: Head trauma and age of onset of dementia of the Alzheimer type. JAMA 257:2289, 1987.

189. Susser M: What is a cause and how do we know one? A grammar for pragmatic epidemiology. Am J Epidemiol 133:635–648, 1991.

190. Susser M: Falsification, verification, and causal inference in epidemiology: Reconsiderations in light of Sir Karl Popper's philosophy. In Rothman KJ: Causal Inference. Epidemiology Resources, Chestnut Hill, MA, 1988, pp 33–57.

191. Terry RD and Katzman R: Senile dementia of the Alzheimer type. Ann Neurol 14:497–506, 1983.

192. Teunisse S, Derix MM, and van Crevel H: Assessing the severity of dementia: Patient and caregiver. Arch Neurol 48:274–277, 1991.

193. Tierney MC, Fisher RH, Lewis AJ, et al. The NINCDS-ADRDA Workgroup criteria for the clinical diagnosis of probable Alzheimer's disease: A clinicopathologic study of 57 cases. Neurology 38:359–364, 1988.

194. Tomlinson BE, Blessed G, and Roth M: Observations on the brains of demented old people. J Neurol Sci 11:205–242, 1970.

195. Treves T, Korczyn AD, Zilber N, et al.: Presenile dementia in Israel. Arch Neurol 43:26–29, 1986.

196. US Congress, Office of Technology Assessment: Losing a Million Minds: Confronting the Tragedy of Alzheimer's Disease and Other Dementias, OTA-BA-323. US Government Printing Office, Washington, DC, April 1987.

197. US Department of Health and Human Services: Disability evaluation under social security. SSA Pub. No. 05-10089. US Government Printing Office, Washington, DC, 1986.

198. US Department of Health and Human Services: The International Classification of Diseases, 9th Revision, Clinical Modification: ICD-9-CM, ed 3. DHHS Pub. No. (PHS) 89-1260. US Government Printing Office, Washington, DC, 1989.

199. Wade JPH, Mirsen TR, Hachinski VC, Fisman M, Lau C, and Merskey H: The clinical diagnosis of Alzheimer's disease. Arch Neurol 44:24–29, 1987.

200. Wechsler AF: Presenile dementia presenting as aphasia. J Neurol Neurosurg Psychiatry 40:303–305, 1977.

201. Weiss NS: Inferring causal relationships. Elaboration of the criterion of "dose-response." Am J Epidemiol 113:487–490, 1981.

202. Wells CE: Dementia: Definition and

description. In Wells, CE (ed): Dementia, ed 2. FA Davis, Philadelphia, 1977, pp 1–11.

203. Wells CE: Pseudodementia. Am J Psychiatry 136:895–900, 1979.

204. Welsh K, Butters N, Hughes J, Mohs R, and Heyman A: Detection of abnormal memory decline in mild cases of Alzheimer's disease using CERAD neuropsychological measures. Arch Neurol 48:278–281, 1991.

205. Wyerer S: Mental disorders among the elderly. True prevalence and use of medical services. Arch Gerontol Geriatr 2:11–22, 1983.

206. Whitehouse PJ, Tabaton M, and Lanska DJ: Pathological and chemical correlates of dementia. In Nebes, RD and Corkin, SH: Handbook of Neuropsychology, Vol 4. Elsevier, New York, 1990, pp 29–37.

207. Whitehouse PJ, Unnerstal JR, Tabaton M, and Lanska DJ: Neurochemistry of dementia: Clinical patho-

logical relationships. In Bergener M and Reisberg B: Diagnosis and Treatment of Senile Dementia. Springer-Verlag, Berlin, 1989, pp 54–59.

208. Williamson J, Stockoe IH, Gray S, et al.: Old people at home: Their unreported needs. Lancet i:1117–1120, 1964.

209. Wisniewski HM, Rabe A, Zigman W, and Silverman W: Neuropathological diagnosis of Alzheimer's disease. J Neuropathol Exp Neurol 48:606–609, 1989.

210. World Health Organization: Mental disorders: Glossary and guide to their classification in accordance with the Ninth Revision of the International Classification of Diseases. World Health Organization, Geneva, 1978.

211. Zhang M, Katzman R, Salmon D, et al.: The prevalence of dementia and Alzheimer's disease in Shanghai, China: Impact of age, gender, and education. Ann Neurol 27:428–437, 1990.

Chapter 2

THE GENETICS OF DEMENTIA

Mark J. Alberts, M.D.,
Margaret A. Pericak-Vance,
  Ph.D.,
and Allen D. Roses, M.D.

CLINICAL GENETICS
MOLECULAR GENETICS
APPLICATIONS TO THE STUDY OF
  DEMENTIA
FUTURE ISSUES

This chapter reviews the clinical genetics of several dementing illnesses, then focuses on the current techniques such as genetic epidemiology and molecular genetics that are being used to study these dementias. The last section applies this knowledge to analysis of the pathogenesis of, and potential therapies for, these disorders. Because an understanding of the nomenclature of recombinant DNA and molecular genetics will help clinicians to understand future developments in the field, a glossary of commonly used terms is included at the end of this chapter.

For discussion of the relationships between genetics and neurobiology, see Chapter 3; for other aspects of clinical genetics, see Chapter 6.

CLINICAL GENETICS

Many common dementing disorders have important genetic components. The classic genetic dementia is Hunt-ington's disease (HD), which is inherited as an autosomal dominant trait with age-dependent penetrance.[10,32] The gene responsible for HD has been mapped to the distal short arm of chromosome 4, but the disease gene has not been specifically defined.[24] Alzheimer's disease (AD), the most common cause of dementia in the elderly,[73] also appears to have a major genetic component.[27,28,31,60] (See also Chapter 6.) Recent studies have shown that in some cases AD is familial and is inherited as an autosomal dominant trait with variable age of onset.[7,27] The AD gene may not be fully expressed until age 90 years, which may explain the increasing prevalence of AD as the population lives longer.[7] Studies have linked familial AD to loci on chromosomes 19 and 21.[52,61]

Multiple cerebral infarcts are a leading cause of dementia.[34] (See Chapter 7.) The factors responsible for atherosclerosis and stroke are multiple, with genetic and environmental factors having a major role. The role of platelet-derived growth factor, which has striking similarities to an oncogene, may be important.[2] The complex interactions between different lipid species suggests that the control of atherosclerosis may be multigenic.[8,85] Less common inherited diseases such as homocysteinuria, antithrombin III deficiency, and protein S and protein C deficiency have also been associated with stroke.[13,22,25,43]

In other dementing illnesses such as Parkinson's disease and Pick's disease, the role of genetic factors remains to be determined.[9,26] Although there are several documented cases of familial Parkinson's disease, large epidemiologic studies and twin studies have not shown a significant genetic risk.[80] In some cases, Pick's disease may be inherited as an autosomal dominant trait.[66] Familial Creutzfeldt-Jakob disease and Gerstmann-Sträussler syndrome (GSS) have been linked to the prion protein gene on chromosome 20.[20,49,56,68] Specific mutations in the gene have been associated with these dementing illnesses. For example, the ataxic form of GSS has been associated with proline-to-leucine substitution in the prion protein caused by a cytosine-to-thymidine mutation at codon 102.[20] Linkage studies have confirmed this chromosome-20 localization for GSS.[30,69] When this mutated form of prion protein (PRP) is transmitted to a mouse, a lethal spongiform degeneration occurs.[67] This transmissible disease can then be bred through multiple generations of mice. (See also Chapters 3 and 8.) The importance of genetic factors in the etiology of many dementing diseases has focused laboratory research toward molecular and epidemiologic genetics.

MOLECULAR GENETICS

The advent and wide application of recombinant DNA technology has revolutionized research in genetic disorders, especially the neurodegenerative diseases.[59] The goal of such molecular genetic research is to determine the underlying genetic defect causing a disease, so that effective therapeutic strategies may be developed. We will provide an overview of genetic techniques, their applications and limitations in the study of the dementias.

Any of several different molecular genetic approaches may be applicable, depending on whether an abnormal protein has been identified for a disease. Figures 2–1 and 2–2 outline two useful approaches. In the first example (Fig. 2–1), molecular genetic techniques are used to study a disease with a known protein abnormality. The amino acid sequence of the defective protein is determined, and a DNA probe is then synthesized in vitro. The DNA probe is used to identify and isolate the actual gene that codes for the abnormal protein. The size, chromosomal location, and DNA sequence of the entire abnormal gene is determined and compared with the normal gene. In this manner the DNA abnormalities causing diseases such as sickle cell anemia and hemophilia have been determined.[87]

The second approach (Fig. 2–2) is useful when a disease has an unknown protein defect, as is true for most of the hereditary dementias. Linkage analysis (see below) is performed using DNA probes with both known and unknown chromosomal localizations. The purpose of linkage studies is to identify a probe that is close to the gene causing the disease. If there were a candidate gene or protein (such as cerebral amyloid for AD), it would receive priority for linkage testing. Once a closely linked probe is found, physical methods of chromosomal mapping, such as chromosomal walking and hopping, can be used to locate the abnormal gene. Once the gene is identified, it is sequenced and compared with known genes to determine whether any similarities exist. The gene can also be put into an expression system that will produce the gene product (usually a protein) for further study. By using this approach, previously unknown proteins can be identified, isolated, and studied. This general approach was applied by Kunkel and colleagues to isolate and characterize the genetic and protein defect responsible for Duchenne's muscular dystrophy.[29,37] More recently the gene for neurofibromatosis was defined using similar techniques.[12,79] These

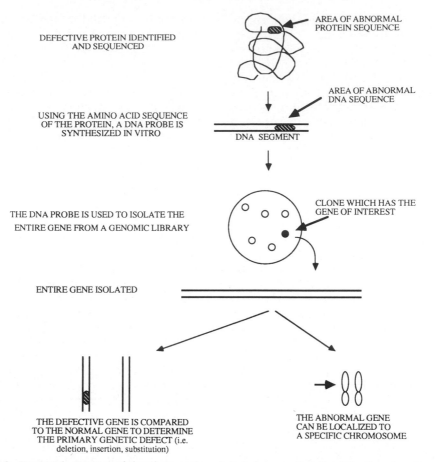

DEFECTIVE PROTEIN IDENTIFIED AND SEQUENCED

AREA OF ABNORMAL PROTEIN SEQUENCE

USING THE AMINO ACID SEQUENCE OF THE PROTEIN, A DNA PROBE IS SYNTHESIZED IN VITRO

AREA OF ABNORMAL DNA SEQUENCE

DNA SEGMENT

THE DNA PROBE IS USED TO ISOLATE THE ENTIRE GENE FROM A GENOMIC LIBRARY

CLONE WHICH HAS THE GENE OF INTEREST

ENTIRE GENE ISOLATED

THE DEFECTIVE GENE IS COMPARED TO THE NORMAL GENE TO DETERMINE THE PRIMARY GENETIC DEFECT (i.e. deletion, insertion, substitution)

THE ABNORMAL GENE CAN BE LOCALIZED TO A SPECIFIC CHROMOSOME

Figure 2–1. Research strategy if the abnormal protein is known, but the defective gene is unknown.

techniques have now been successful in a growing list of genetic disorders. In cases where the gene is entirely unknown and no convincing candidate genes exist, one could use subtraction or differential hybridization of complementary DNA (cDNA) libraries to generate new candidate genes (see below).

Genetic Epidemiology

The use of linkage studies has revolutionized the study of genetic disorders of unknown etiology. Genetic linkage is established when two genes or other DNA markers are located so closely together on the same chromosome that they do not segregate independently. In the absence of recombination, linked loci are transmitted as a unit to the same gamete during meiosis. The probability of crossing over (recombination) or exchange of chromosomal material (thereby causing the two loci to become separated) depends on the distance between the two loci. The probability of crossing over increases as the distance between the two loci increases. The distance between loci is expressed as centimorgans (cM). When the recombination fraction (θ) is small, it approximates the genetic map distance in cM. Thus, $\theta = 0.1$ is approximately equal to a distance of 10 cM. One cM is approximately 1 million bases. A value of $\theta = 0.5$ represents free recombination, or a distance too great to detect linkage.[14]

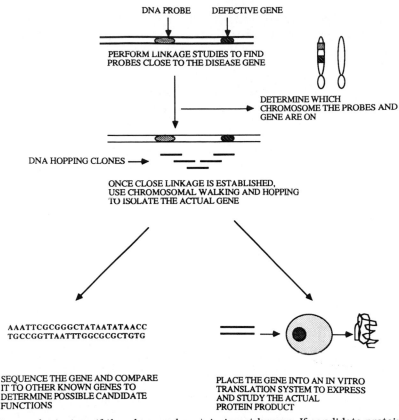

Figure 2–2. Research strategy if the abnormal protein is not known. If candidate proteins or genes exist, linkage studies can begin with an appropriate DNA probe. Otherwise, probes spaced throughout the genome can be used to look for linkage.

Family linkage studies are widely used to map genes to chromosomes and to identify disease loci. These studies are also useful for measuring distances between loci. Pedigree analysis involves the use of likelihood calculations. The likelihood of observing a particular combination of traits in a family given free recombination (i.e., no linkage) is calculated and compared with the likelihood of observing the same traits in the family over a selected range of recombination fractions ($\theta = 0.0$ to $\theta = 0.5$). The logarithm of the ratio of these likelihoods is referred to as a Lod score (log of the odds of linkage), z. Thus with z = Lod score and L = likelihood:

$$z = \log_{10} \frac{L \text{ (family given } \phi = 0.0 \text{ to } 0.5)}{L \text{ (family given } \phi = 0.5)}$$

Lod scores can be added over families. Sums of Lod scores $> +3$ (1000:1 odds for linkage) are generally considered significant evidence of linkage, and sums < -2 (100:1 odds against linkage) are indicative of nonlinkage.[46] Intermediate values require additional family data before a conclusion can be made. The calculation of Lod scores is facilitated by computerized linkage programs.[48]

The investigation of linkage through family studies for a particular disease requires comparing the disease locus with a common polymorphic locus. A polymorphism is the occurrence together in a population of two or more genotypically determined phenotypes or genotypes, neither of which is rare (frequency of more than 0.01). Marker loci can include blood group polymorphisms, isoenzymes, and genotypic DNA polymorphisms (see below). Many phenotypic systems have been identified and linked to a number of genetic disorders. The major limitation of this form of gene mapping is the lack of highly polymorphic marker systems. Less than 5% of the human genome had been mapped prior to the advent of recombinant DNA technology. The National Institutes of Health and the Department of Energy are cosponsoring a program to sequence and map the entire human genome.

Recombinant DNA technology has provided a new type of marker, the restriction fragment length polymorphism (RFLP).[5] RFLPs are differences in the DNA sequence that can be recognized by the pattern of DNA fragments produced after cleavage by a restriction enzyme (Fig. 2–3). Because many RFLPs segregate as Mendelian codominant traits, each one can be considered a unique locus and can be tested for genetic linkage in human pedigrees. Many RFLPs are ideal for linkage studies because they are highly polymorphic, thereby increasing the number of informative matings in a family.[5] An informative individual is someone who is heterozygous at both of the markers under consideration. By determining the number of recombinant and nonrecombinant offspring of an informative mating, the probability of linkage can be calculated. Therefore, the information a particular family contributes to linkage analysis is based on several factors such as the number of people tested, the number of informative matings, and the extent of the polymorphism. Because RFLPs have been identified at random sites throughout the entire human genome, the means exist for the chromosomal localization of many genetic disorders once appropriate family data and DNA have been obtained.[5,14,59] Thousands of polymor-

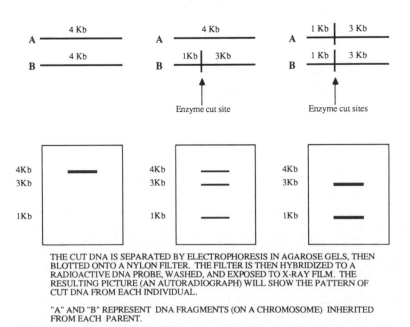

RESTRICTION FRAGMENT LENGTH POLYMORPHISMS
(RFLPs)

THE CUT DNA IS SEPARATED BY ELECTROPHORESIS IN AGAROSE GELS, THEN BLOTTED ONTO A NYLON FILTER. THE FILTER IS THEN HYBRIDIZED TO A RADIOACTIVE DNA PROBE, WASHED, AND EXPOSED TO X-RAY FILM. THE RESULTING PICTURE (AN AUTORADIOGRAPH) WILL SHOW THE PATTERN OF CUT DNA FROM EACH INDIVIDUAL.

"A" AND "B" REPRESENT DNA FRAGMENTS (ON A CHROMOSOME) INHERITED FROM EACH PARENT.

Figure 2–3. Examples of restriction fragment length polymorphism (RFLP) patterns that can be seen after enzyme digestion and gel electrophoresis of genomic DNA. The presence or absence of enzyme cut sites in homozygous or heterozygous forms is a trait that can be tracked through families and used for linkage analysis.

phisms have been reported for loci throughout the human genome.[87] The DNA for these linkage studies can be obtained from white blood cells, fibroblasts, muscle, brain, or other tissue. Cultures of white blood cells or fibroblasts can be grown for years after a patient dies, thereby providing a source of DNA for future studies.

Highly polymorphic repeating sequences have proven very useful in increasing the amount of informative data available from pedigrees, as compared with using RFLPs. An example is the use of repeating cytosine adenosine (CA) motifs, (CA)n, which can be different on each allele.[82] Thus, all four parental alleles are likely to be different, making every meiotic event (sibling) highly informative. As additional informative, highly variable polymorphisms are discovered throughout the genome, rapid and thorough linkage searches become a reality. Fascioscapulo-humeral muscular dystrophy and autosomal dominant limb-girdle muscular dystrophy were two diseases that had been screened with RFLPs for several years but were linked by (CA)n screening in less than 6 weeks.[82,84]

The aim of linkage studies is to identify probes that are tightly linked to the disease locus. By knowing the chromosomal location of a linked probe, the disease gene can also be assigned to a chromosome. This approach has been used successfully to link HD to a probe on chromosome 4 and familial AD to chromosomes 19 and 21.[24,52,61] Even tightly linked probes may be several million bases away from the actual disease locus, however. In such cases, genomic mapping of chromosomes with large overlapping cloned DNA can be used to traverse the area between a tightly linked probe and the actual disease gene (see below).

Gene Isolation

Once a tightly linked probe is identified, the techniques of molecular genetics can be used to isolate and characterize the disease gene. Early techniques involved chromosomal walking or hopping.[37,45] In the case of chromosomal walking, overlapping pieces of DNA are cloned and used to detect adjacent overlapping pieces of DNA. By repeating the procedure, it is possible to slowly "walk" along a chromosome from a tightly linked probe to the disease gene (Fig. 2–2). A more rapid technique is chromosomal hopping, in which much larger pieces of DNA are cut by restriction enzymes that have infrequent cut sites (i.e., they will cut DNA approximately once every 100,000 to 500,000 bases). By cloning these larger pieces of DNA and detecting overlapping sequences, it is possible to take larger "steps" along the chromosome and reach the disease gene more rapidly.[15,45] Cosmid contig (see Glossary) mapping of chromosomes 16 and 19 by the National Laboratories at Los Alamos and Lawrence Livermore has demonstrated new, rapid genomic mapping potential,[6,11] as has the use of yeast artificial chromosomes for mapping.

The goal of chromosome analysis is to detect a clone that is so close to the disease gene that no crossovers occur. Once such a clone is identified, it can be further tested as a candidate gene for the disease. The first test would be to demonstrate that the clone is a gene that is expressed in the tissue of interest (i.e., the brain in dementia). This can be done using Northern blots, which are made by electrophoresing messenger RNA (mRNA) on a gel that separates the different mRNAs based on size.[57] The particular collection of mRNAs found in a tissue represents all the genes expressed in that tissue. Once the mRNA is electrophoresed, it can be blotted onto a nylon filter, then hybridized to the probe of interest, which has been made radioactive. If that probe did represent a gene (or part of the gene) expressed in that tissue, a radioactive band would be detected when the blot is exposed to x-ray paper.

The DNA probe might not represent the entire gene, however. One way of isolating the entire gene involves screening a cDNA library with the probe of interest. A cDNA library is a collection of all the genes expressed in a given tissue or organ. It is made as follows: the mRNAs expressed in the tissue are isolated, and DNA is synthesized using the mRNA as a template, thus creating cDNA. Working with DNA rather than RNA is preferred because the latter is highly labile and can be degraded by ubiquitous RNAses. The cDNA can then be placed in a vector (usually a bacteriophage or plasmid), amplified, and stored.[42] Once a candidate probe or gene is found, it can be used to screen a cDNA library and extract a clone that has the full-length cDNA and represents the transcribed gene.

Whereas the cDNA clone represents the portion of the gene that is transcribed, it may not represent the entire gene of interest, as certain areas of a gene such as regulatory sequences and intervening sequences (introns) may not be transcribed. To isolate the entire gene, the cDNA clone can be used to screen a genomic DNA library. The genomic DNA library consists of the DNA from one tissue (usually lymphoblasts), which can be isolated in fairly large quantities.[16] Because the DNA content is the same in each cell of a particular organism or individual, the genomic DNA library will contain all of the genes found in that organism. A cDNA clone can then be used to screen the genomic library and identify those clones that contain the complete gene of interest. Certain DNA landmarks such as transcription sequences, initiation codons, and termination codons can be used to identify the extent of some genes.

Once the complete gene is isolated, it can be further analyzed by doing DNA sequencing, to determine the exact order of each base. The sequence can then be compared with known genes to look for evidence of deletions, insertions, or other mutations that could account for abnormalities in gene expression or function.[63]

A new type of gene mutation, triplet repeats, has recently been found to cause several diseases including the fragile X syndrome (characterized by mental retardation) and myotonic dys-trophy.[11a] In these conditions, triplet repeats of specific nucleotides (i.e., GCT in myotonic dystrophy) expands in successive generations, causing earlier symptom onset and more severe disease. Different types of mutations can produce the same disease phenotype. For example, Gaucher disease can be caused by point mutations, insertions, and deletions within the glucocerebrosidase gene.[4a] If the gene has no close homology to previously described genes, it can be placed in an expression vector that would permit the gene to be transcribed and translated so the protein produced could be isolated and characterized.[51] Using the above techniques, it is possible to investigate a hereditary disease and systematically ascertain its etiology at both the gene and protein level. Once the abnormal gene is identified and characterized, genetic counseling and therapy can be planned.

Another molecular genetic technique is subtraction hybridization, which can be used to compare gene expression between two organs or tissues of interest. For example, one might wish to know if differences exist in the genes expressed in specific brain regions from AD patients compared with controls. If such differences were detected, they may represent genes that have a role in the etiology or pathogenesis of AD. The first step in performing subtraction hybridization is the isolation of high-quality mRNA from the tissue of interest. Complementary DNA (cDNA) is then made by the enzyme reverse transcriptase, which uses the mRNA as a template. The cDNAs from the disease and control organs are then hybridized to each other. Those cDNAs that are overexpressed, underexpressed, or absent in one tissue will not fully hybridize and can be isolated, amplified, and studied.[74] The subtracted clones that are located within or near areas where linkage has been established can then be studied as candidate genes. This technique may also lead to the characterization of previously unknown genes and their products.

Finally, the polymerase chain reaction (PCR) has revolutionized much of the work in molecular biology and molecular genetics. It uses a thermostable enzyme, Taq polymerase, and DNA primers to amplify specific segments of DNA in vitro over a millionfold in only a few hours.[46a,62a] In the laboratory, PCR is used routinely to amplify cloned DNA sequences, screen for new genes, and detect various genetic abnormalities such as deletions and point mutations, which makes it useful for genetic diagnosis. PCR is technically easy to set up, requiring only basic components and a computer-controlled thermocycler. Various modifications in the PCR procedure allow it to be used for amplification of DNA from fresh or archival material, as well as for DNA sequencing, genomic mapping, forensic science, and other applications.[43a]

APPLICATIONS TO THE STUDY OF DEMENTIA

All of the above techniques have been applied to the study of dementia. In 1983, Gusella and colleagues used random DNA probes and performed linkage studies on a large Venezuelan family with hundreds of members having HD. These studies found linkage for HD to the probe G8 on the short arm of chromosome 4.[24] Since then probes closer to the HD gene have been identified and studied.[81] A reliable means of carrier detection is now available with 99% accuracy in informative families.[44] In the case of early-onset AD (EOAD), several investigators considered β-amyloid a candidate protein. Using the published amino acid sequence for β-amyloid, a small DNA probe was constructed and used to isolate the β-amyloid gene from a genomic DNA library.[21] The gene was found to be on chromosome 21, which is interesting because of the association between AD and Down's syndrome. Several studies have found an increased incidence of Down's syndrome in families with familial AD.[27] St. George-Hyslop[61] then used chromosome 21 probes in four families with EOAD to determine linkage to a region that was near the β-amyloid gene on chromosome 21. Further studies found crossovers between the β-amyloid gene and the familial AD gene, indicating that the β-amyloid gene was not responsible for AD in most of those families.[72] Ongoing studies are attempting to find chromosome 21 probes that are closer to the familial EOAD locus. An initial report described duplication of the β-amyloid gene in patients with familial AD and in karyotypically normal patients with Down's syndrome,[17] but this report has since been refuted.[55,71] Further details about the cell biology and metabolism of β-amyloid and its precursor protein can be found in a recent review.[37a]

Although most of the larger EOAD families demonstrated recombination events between the FAD locus and the amyloid locus, several families did not. Following the finding that hereditary cerebral hemorrhages with amyloidosis (Dutch-type; HCHWA-D) were associated with a mutation of codon 693 in the amyloid precursor protein (APP),[40,76] Goate and colleagues[18] applied the same methodology to a large early-onset familial Alzheimer's disease (FAD) family in which no crossovers with amyloid were present. A point mutation at codon 717 was present in this European family and in a family from North Carolina. Another nearby polymorphism demonstrated that these two families were of different genetic lineage. Subsequently, several more AD families with the APP 717 mutations were described.[12a,46b,47,78] These mutations affect the valine at position 717 and cause a change to either isoleucine, phenylalanine, or glycine.[12a,18,46b] The phenotypic spectrum of diseases with APP mutations appears to include a vascular amyloidopathy as well as EOAD. Additional mutations of APP have been found in controls.[50a] The "causative" nature of these mutations or their relationships to the pathogenetic mechanism of disease expression is not yet understood. Thus there appears to be a rare form of an uncommon disease, EOAD, associated with a mutation at APP 717, whereas a locus for the vast majority of EOAD families is more centromeric on chromosome 21[19,62] or another chromosome.[19,65]

The first questions have already been raised by finding a mutation in the APP gene, which, when present in one copy, is associated with an early-onset form of AD. Does the altered APP cause AD? Does an APP 717 mutation change the age of onset of an otherwise later-presenting disease trait? Are various pathogenetic processes accelerated in the presence of an altered APP metabolic product? Is APP 717 the only mutation resulting in EOAD?[50a] Many testable, imaginative questions can now be asked.

It is difficult to determine whether or not the APP-717 is "causative," that is, sufficient for the accelerated development of AD. This rare mutation in a rare disease (early-onset AD) is certainly not a *necessary* condition for AD. Identification of additional mutations at other loci or in APP should shed more light on the molecular basis for disease expression. Elucidation of other mutations associated with familial AD may describe a family of proteins or a pathogenetic pathway that leads to the phenotype. It is conceivable that late-onset neurogenetic diseases such as AD, amyotrophic lateral sclerosis, Parkinson's disease, and others may have similar pathogenetic mechanisms, with the clinical and pathologic specificity resulting from the selection of affected neurons or families of neurons.

Recent studies have shown that late-onset AD (LOAD) may also be familial, with a pattern consistent with autosomal dominant inheritance.[7,31] Pericak-Vance and associates,[54] using a combination of EOAD and LOAD families, failed to establish linkage using the same probes linked in the EOAD families studied by St. George-Hyslop. Schellenberg and co-workers[65] also failed to detect linkage to chromosome 21 using their FAD pedigrees. The failure to detect linkage of autosomal domi-

nant LOAD to the region of chromosome 21 where the EOAD gene was reportedly localized suggests that there is genetic heterogeneity for familial AD.

In 1990, Roses and colleagues[58] presented preliminary evidence for linkage of LOAD to chromosome 19. They used a nonparametric method of linkage analysis developed by Weeks and Lange,[83] called the affected pedigree members (APM) method. This method was especially useful in the study of LOAD because the family members who are alive and informative for the disease are usually in a single, older generation. Two probes located on the proximal long arm of chromosome 19 gave a significant test statistic for AD linkage when analyzed with the APM method. These probes were then tested using the standard likelihood Lod score linkage methods. Linkage data for these chromosome 19 probes using multipoint analysis are shown in Figure 2–4.[52,53] The probe order and approximate distances are known. Multipoint linkage analysis allows the disease locus to be "moved" through the previously established chromosome map (D19S13-ATP1A3-BCL3-telomere). The data generated when the affected individuals in each pedigree are used in the analysis (at-risk individuals, i.e., spouses, are coded as unknown with respect to AD status) results in a Lod score of 4.2 for all families and 4.6 for only LOAD families.[52] Three families with EOAD are included in the series of 32 families. These EOAD families were negative for chromosome 19 probes, but slightly positive for chromosome 21 probes (Fig. 2–5). Due to limitations of family size and data on EOAD families, there were insufficient data for the heterogeneity test to reach statistical significance. St. George-Hyslop and co-workers[60] reported evidence for heterogeneity (chromosome 21 and some other loci) in a large combined analysis. Preliminary results combining the data from several series for an analysis, which includes both chromosome 19 and chromosome 21 probes, strengthen the conclusion that some

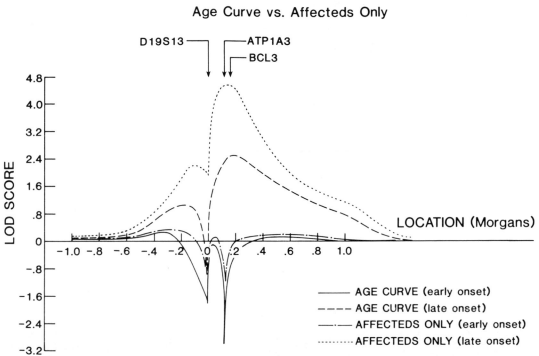

Figure 2-4. Multipoint linkage analysis of three chromosome 19 (CH 19) markers. Three chromosome 19 markers of known order and distance are used in this analysis of 32 AD families (early and late onset). Multipoint analysis of late-onset Alzheimer's disease (AD) families produces a peak LOD score of 4.60 for affecteds only and 2.48 for age-adjusted analysis. The results are negative or noninformative for early-onset families with the chromosome 19 markers. At-risk but clinically normal individuals and spouses are coded as unknown with respect to AD status. (From Alberts MJ and Roses AD: Alzheimer's disease: Etiology and therapy. In Appel, SH [ed]: Current Neurology, Vol 11. Chicago, Mosby-Year Book, p. 156, with permission.)

families with EOAD may be linked to a chromosome 21 locus other than APP 717, and some families with LOAD are linked to a chromosome 19 locus. Formal testing of the combined data will determine the significance of this heterogeneity and may suggest the existence of additional loci. Linkage of LOAD to chromosome 19 has been confirmed in an independent series of families.[57a]

The study of HD and AD show how modern molecular genetic techniques can be applied to determine the chromosomal localization of two common hereditary dementing illnesses. One experimental strategy used random probes to screen for gene location be-

cause no candidate genes or proteins were known. The second strategy was influenced by the known location of a candidate protein, β-amyloid. Additional research focusing on identifying the genes responsible for these diseases will provide information on pathogenesis and potential therapies.

FUTURE ISSUES

Genetic Counseling

There are three major areas for future advances in the genetic study of the dementias. One is the improved ability to

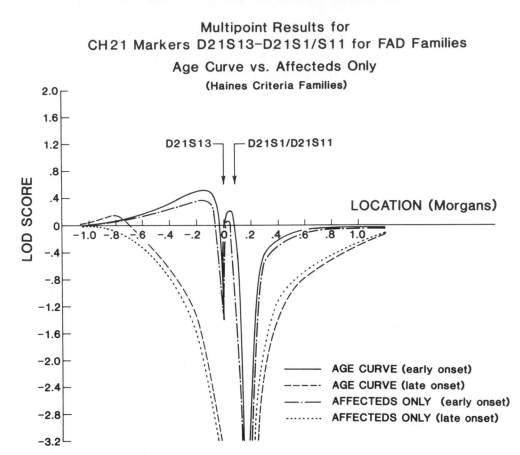

Figure 2–5. Multipoint linkage analysis of two chromosome 21 (CH 21) markers. Late-onset families show very negative LOD scores for linkage to these markers. The three early-onset families showed small positive scores with chromosome 21 markers, supporting other published data[18,61] and emphasizing the need for heterogeneity testing using collaborative data for chromosome 19 and 21.

diagnose accurately patients who carry the gene for a disease and are at risk for developing the disease. This type of genetic counseling is already available for selected diseases such as HD, inasmuch as probes for HD are sufficiently close to the gene to allow highly accurate determination whether a person carries the HD gene. Adults at risk for HD can be determined with 99% accuracy. In the case of HD, genetic counseling surrounding a pregnancy almost always will rely on accurate determination of the parental genotype. Whereas it had been suggested that presymptomatic patients may be reluctant to learn that they carry a gene for an untreatable disease, a recent study found that concern to be overstated.[44] By using amniocen-

tesis or chorionic villus biopsy, it is possible to diagnose affected fetuses. As more closely linked probes are identified for other diseases, it will be possible to provide even more accurate prenatal and postnatal counseling about whether a person at risk carries the gene for a disease.

Since the description of well-documented families with an autosomal dominant form of familial AD,[18,19,52,61,65] the issue of genetic counseling for members of AD families has been raised. For members of pathologically proven AD families with an autosomal dominant pattern of inheritance, it is reasonable to inform at-risk individuals of a 50% chance of inheriting the gene, emphasizing the variable age of expression. The use of linked probes for more accurate counseling in AD families (as is done with HD) must await resolution of disease heterogeneity, however. Even using the APP 717 mutation in unaffected family members in the few identified pedigrees presents problems. Whether to disclose a presymptomatic diagnosis in the absence of effective therapy is a particularly difficult ethical issue. On the other hand, when effective therapy does become a reality, accurate presymptomatic diagnosis may allow treatment to prevent disease expression.

New Genes and Proteins

The second major advance will be the discovery and characterization of the causative gene(s) for specific dementias. Various types of pathophysiologic abnormalities have been hypothesized to occur, including defective structural proteins, abnormal regulation of protein or gene expression, and abnormal metabolism of a normal protein.[38] In Duchenne's muscular dystrophy, reverse genetic methods have led to the discovery and characterization of the gene for dystrophin, a previously unknown muscle protein that is deficient in patients with this disorder.[29,45] As these techniques are applied to the dementing illnesses, it is reasonable to anticipate that similar novel genes and proteins in the brain will be discovered. Once the defective proteins are identified, not only will the pathophysiology of the disease be clarified, but much will be learned about how the brain functions normally.

Gene Therapy

Third, the determination of the genes or family of genes that are associated with the expression of a disease may provide insight into therapeutic options. Interdiction of the pathogenetic process producing neuronal death or other processes necessary for the disease to become clinically apparent may be a realistic therapy. If the pertinent processes underlying disease pathogenesis can be identified, then rational therapy aimed at stopping disease progression may be a reasonable goal.

In AD there may be multiple genotypes with similar phenotypes. Understanding the multiple genes that could be affected may provide an understanding of the disease processes leading to accelerated cell death in specific brain regions. Therapeutic opportunities based on manipulation of critical pathogenetic steps may well prevent disease expression and thus become the pharmacology of the 21st century. Our own view is that the relevant genetic traits associated with a disease presenting as AD will illuminate the pathologic processes and provide insight into appropriate pharmacologic interventions aimed at controlling disease expression.[57b,58a]

THERAPEUTIC OPTIONS

Once a defective gene is identified, gene therapy can be considered. The ultimate goal of therapy would be to prevent the disease from developing, although symptomatic treatments may be easier to develop. The treatment strategy for preventing a genetic disease from developing may involve systemic therapy designed to compensate for the genetic defect, correction of an abnormal process, or substitution of a normal gene.[39] For example, if a disease were found to be due to the abnormal accumulation of a metabolite, medications might be given to increase the metabolism of the metabolite, or perhaps changes in diet would decrease the accumulation of the excess metabolite. Gene therapy might attempt to replace the missing or defective enzyme by introducing a normal gene into those cells found to be defective.[70]

In planning genetic therapy for a disease, the problems of specificity, expression, and regulation need to be considered. For some diseases a gene or gene product may be introduced into a specific cell or population of cells. The dementing illnesses such as AD and HD pose a problem, inasmuch as current evidence suggests a primary defect involving brain cells. Pharmacologic or genetic therapy might have to cross the blood-brain barrier (BBB) to be effective. Lipid-coated vesicles called liposomes may be able to cross the BBB and deliver undegraded proteins or DNA into the brain.

Several techniques have been developed to introduce DNA into cells. Transfection is the chemical process by which cells exposed to calcium phosphate will absorb small amounts of DNA. Transfection is inefficient, in that only 1 in 100,000 cells will integrate the DNA into its chromosomes.[64] Microinjection involves the direct injection of DNA into the nucleus of a cell. Although efficient, it is laborious and can be used to treat only a limited number of cells.[39] Viral-mediated gene transfer involves placing pieces of RNA into a virus (most commonly a retrovirus).[3] When the virus infects a cell, the RNA is changed into DNA and the DNA is then incorporated into the host cell's chromosomes.[77] This process, though highly efficient, is nonspecific and has a risk of causing malignant transformation of cells.[36,64]

Gene expression and regulation are best considered together. Not all genes are expressed at all times. The expression of certain genes depends upon the presence of promoters (which begin transcription), polyadenylation sites (which direct the attachment of a poly A tail to messenger RNA [mRNA]), splice signals (which help form the final mRNA before translation), and translation signals (which begin and end the synthesis of proteins from mRNA). All of these steps are regulated by different factors such as the specific organ and needs of the cells. Expression vectors are being designed that incorporate these features and allow for the expression and regulation of certain genes in specific tissues.[35]

Despite these problems, experiments are under way to introduce genes into live animals. The most practical approach involves retroviral modification of specific cell types. To be successful, such a modification would have to be targeted at cells that undergo mitosis, a necessary step to integrate the retroviral DNA. Unfortunately, mature neurons do not undergo mitosis and therefore would not be candidates for such therapy. Glial cells and endothelial cells in the central nervous system do divide, however, and thus could be potential targets.[86]

In broad terms, potential cell targets for gene therapy can be divided into those cells that ordinarily produce the defective protein, or heterologous cells that can be used as vehicles to introduce the correct protein into the organism. In the first case, bone marrow stem cells[50] have been used successfully to introduce several genes, including those for adenosine deaminase,[41] hypoxanthine phosphoribosyl transferase,[23] and β-globin.[4] An example of heterologous cells that are genetically altered and placed into the organ to be treated is genetically altered fibroblast containing the gene for beta nerve growth factor (β-NGF). These cells have been injected into the brain and have been shown to express the NGF protein, resulting in the functional improvement of animals following lesions of the cholinergic septal tract.[75] Additional technical aspects and clinical protocols for gene therapy can be found in a recent review article.[1]

These preliminary studies will obviously require close follow-up to ensure the stability of the genetically altered cells and to obtain long-term data on the potential risk for neoplastic transformation of these genetically altered cells. In addition, because this genetic therapy is unlikely to affect the germ cells, the treated individual would still pass on the gene defect to future generations, unless adequate genetic counseling is undertaken.

Germ cell therapy is aimed at altering the genes within either sperm or ovum. For practical purposes, only the ovum or early stem cells would be treated, because treatment of sperm would require altering millions of cells. The introduction of genes into mouse embryos has been accomplished using either microinjection or transformation with retroviruses. The resulting transgenic mice can transmit these genetic changes to their progeny.[33,70] Although seemingly promising, these techniques have serious problems. The introduction of genes into germ cells or embryos is frequently associated with the development of insertional mutations, which may cause developmental malformations. Exogenous DNA can increase the risk of nondisjunction during meiosis, thereby increasing the risk of genetic defects in progeny. Finally, because there is no realistic way of diagnosing a genetic defect at the germ cell or embryonic stage, such therapy would needlessly endanger potentially normal offspring.[39]

Despite these problems, recombinant DNA techniques still hold the best hope for identifying relevant genes, preventing genetic disease through accurate counseling, and treating such diseases by gene manipulation or by somatic therapy.

SUMMARY

Many of the dementias, including some forms of AD, are associated with genetic abnormalities. The use of recombinant DNA techniques has greatly accelerated the pace of research in the genetic dementias and has led to the chromosomal localization of the genes responsible for several dementias. Ongoing research using these approaches will lead to the isolation of the defective genes, accurate genetic counseling, and the initiation of specific somatic or gene therapies.

ACKNOWLEDGMENTS

The authors wish to thank Ms. Susan Howard Alberts for her assistance in preparing the figures.

Some of the research reported in this chapter is supported by the Joseph and Kathleen Bryan Alzheimer Disease Research Center grant (AG05128), a grant from the Denver Foundation for Health and Research, a grant from the Alzheimer's Association, and grants NS19999 and NS23008 from the National Institutes of Neurological and Communicative Disorders and Stroke. Dr. Alberts is a recipient of a Clinical Investigator Development Award (NS01241) for research in Alzheimer's disease, and Dr. Roses is a recipient of a Leadership and Excellence in Alzheimer's Disease Award (AG07922) from the National Institute on Aging.

REFERENCES

1. Anderson WF: Human gene therapy. Science 256:808–813, 1992.
2. Barrett TB and Benditt EP: Platelet-derived growth factor gene expression in human atherosclerotic plaques and normal artery wall. Proc Natl Acad Sci U S A 85:2810–2814, 1988.
3. Belmont J, Tigges J, Chang S, et al: Expression of human adenosine deaminase in murine haematopoietic progenitor cells following retroviral transfer. Nature 322:385–387, 1986.
4. Bender MA, Gelinas RE, and Miller AD: A majority of mice show longterm expression of a human beta-globin gene after retrovirus transfer into hematopoietic stem cells. Mol Cell Biol 9:1426–1434, 1989.
4a. Beutler E: Gaucher disease: New molecular approaches to diagnoses and treatment. Science 256:794–799, 1992.
5. Botstein D, White RL, Skolnick M, and Davis RW: Construction of a genetic linkage map in man using restriction fragment length polymorphisms. Am J Hum Genet 32:314–331, 1980.
6. Branscomb E, Slezak T, Pae R, Galas D, Carrano AV, and Waterman M: Optimizing restriction fragment fingerprinting methods for ordering larger genetic libraries. Genomics 8(2): 351–366, 1990.

7. Breitner JCS, Silverman JM, Mohs RC, and Davis KL: Familial aggregation in Alzheimer's disease: Comparison of risks among relatives of early- and late-onset cases, and among male and female relatives in successive generations. Neurology 38:207–212, 1988.

8. Breslow JL: Human apolipoprotein molecular biology and genetic variation. Annu Rev Biochem 54:699–727, 1985.

9. Brown RG and Marsden CD: How common is dementia in Parkinson's disease? Lancet 2:1262–1265, 1984.

10. Burch PRJ: Huntington's disease: Types, frequency, and progression. In Chase TN, Wexler NS, and Barbeau A (eds): Huntington's Disease. Adv Neurol 23:43–57, 1979.

11. Carrano AV, de Jong PJ, Branscomb E, Slezak T, and Watkins BW: Constructing chromosome- and region-specific cosmid maps of the human genome. Genome 31(2):1059–1065, 1989.

11a. Caskey CT, Pizzuti A, Fu Y-H, Fenwick RG, and Nelson DL: Triplet repeat mutations in human disease. Science 256:784–789, 1992.

12. Cawthon RM, Weiss R, Xu G, et al: A major segment of the neurofibromatosis type 1 gene: cDNA sequence, genomic structure, and point mutations. Cell 62:193–201, 1990.

12a. Chartier-Harlin M-C, Crawford F, Houlden H, et al.: Early-onset Alzheimer's disease caused by mutations at codon 717 of the β-amyloid precursor protein gene. Nature 353:844–846, 1991.

13. Comp PC and Esmon CT: Recurrent venous thromboembolism in patient with a partial deficiency of protein S. N Engl J Med 311:1525–1528, 1984.

14. Conneally PM and Rivas ML: Linkage analysis in man. In Harris H and Hirschhorn K (eds): Advances in Human Genetics, Vol 10. Plenum, New York, 1980, pp 209–266.

15. C-T Ton C, Collins F, Weil MM, et al: Chromosome jumping: Application in the search for the Wilms tumor/aniridia loci within human chromosome 11 band p13 (abstr). Am J Hum Genet 41:A189, 1987.

16. Dahl HH, Flavell RA, and Grosveld FG: The use of genomic libraries for the isolation and study of eukaryotic genes. In Williamson R (ed): Genetic Engineering, vol 2. Academic Press, London, 1981, pp 49–127.

17. Delabar J, Goldgaber D, Lamour Y, et al: β-amyloid gene duplication in Alzheimer's disease and karyotypically normal Down syndrome. Science 235:1390–1392, 1987.

18. Goate AM, Chartier-Harlin MC, Mullan M, et al: Segregation of a missense mutation in the amyloid precursor protein gene with familial Alzheimer's disease. Nature 349:704–706, 1991.

19. Goate AM, Haynes AR, Owen MJ, et al: Predisposing locus for Alzheimer's disease on chromosome 21. Lancet 1:352–355, 1989.

20. Goldgaber D, Goldfarb L, Brown P, Asher DM, Brown WT, and Lin S: Mutations in familial Creutzfeldt-Jakob disease and Gerstmann-Sträussler-Scheinker syndrome. Exp Neurol 106:204–206, 1989.

21. Goldgaber D, Lerman MI, McBride OW, Saffiotti U, and Gajdusek DC. Characterization and chromosomal localization of a cDNA encoding brain amyloid of Alzheimer's disease. Science 235:877–880, 1987.

22. Griffin JH, Evatt B, Zimmerman TS, Kleiss AJ, and Wideman C: Deficiency of protein C in congenital thrombotic disease. J Clin Invest 68:1370–1373, 1981.

23. Gruber HE, Finley KD, Luchtman LA, et al: Insertion of hypoanthine phosphoribosyltransferase cDNA into human bone marrow cells by a retrovirus. Adv Exp Med Biol 195(a):171–175, 1986.

24. Gusella JF, Wexler NS, Conneally PM, et al: A polymorphic DNA marker genetically linked to Huntington's disease. Nature 306:234–238, 1983.

25. Harker LA, Slichter S, Scott CR, and Ross R: Homocystinemia: vascular injury and arterial thrombosis. N Engl J Med 291:537–543, 1974.

26. Heston LL: The clinical genetics of

Pick's disease. Acta Psychiatr Scand 57:202–206, 1978.

27. Heston LL, Mastri AR, Anderson VE, and White J: Dementia of the Alzheimer's type. Clinical genetics, natural history and associated conditions. Arch Gen Psychiatry 38:1085–1090, 1981.

28. Heyman A, Wilkinson WE, Hurwitz BJ, et al: Alzheimer's disease: Genetic aspects and associated clinical disorders. Ann Neurol 14:507–515, 1983.

29. Hoffman EP, Fischbeck KH, Brown RH, et al: Characterization of dystrophin in muscle-biopsy specimens from patients with Duchenne's or Becker's muscular dystrophy. N Engl J Med 318:1363–1368, 1988.

30. Hsiao K, Baker HF, Crow TJ, et al: Linkage of a prion protein missense variant to Gerstmann-Sträussler syndrome. Nature 338(6213):342–345, 1989.

31. Huff FJ, Auerbach J, Chakravarti A, and Boller F: Risk of dementia in relatives of patients with Alzheimer's disease. Neurology 38:786–790, 1988.

32. Huntington G: On chorea. Med Surg Reporter 26:317, 1872.

33. Jahner D, Haase K, Mulligan R, and Jaenisch R: Insertion of the bacterial gpt gene into the germ line of mice by retroviral infection. Proc Natl Acad Sci U S A 82:6927–6931, 1985.

34. Katzman R: Vascular disease and dementia. In Yahr MD (ed): H Houston Merritt Memorial Volume. Raven Press, New York, 1983, pp 153–176.

35. Kelly JH and Darlington GJ: Hybrid genes: Molecular approaches to tissue specific gene regulation. Annu Rev Genet 19:273, 1985.

36. King W, Patel MD, and Lobel LI: Insertion mutagenesis of embryonal carcinoma cells by retroviruses. Science 228:554, 1985.

37. Koenig M, Hoffman EP, Bertelson CJ, Monaco AP, Feener C, and Kunkel LM: Complete cloning of the Duchenne muscular dystrophy (DMD) cDNA and preliminary genomic organization of the DMD gene in normal and affected individuals. Cell 50:509–517, 1987.

37a. Kosik KS: Alzheimer's disease: A cell biological perspective. Science 256:780–783, 1992.

38. Ledley FD: Somatic gene therapy for human disease: Background and prospects. Part I. J Pediatrics 110:1–8, 1987.

39. Ledley FD: Somatic gene therapy for human disease: Background and prospects. Part II. J Pediatrics 110:167–174, 1987.

40. Levy E, Carman MD, Fernandez-Madrid IJ, et al: Mutation of the Alzheimer's disease amyloid gene in hereditary cerebral hemorrhage with amylodosis of Dutch type. Science 248:1124–1126, 1990.

41. Lim B, Williams DA, and Orkin S: Retrovirus-mediated transfer of human adenosine deaminase: Expression of functional enzyme in murine hematopoietic stem cells in vivo. Mol Cell Biol 7:3456–3459, 1987.

42. Maniatis T, Kee SG, Efstratiadis A, and Kafatos FC: Amplification and characterization of a β-globin gene synthesized in vitro. Cell 8:163–182, 1976.

43. Marciniak E, Farley CH, and DeSimone PA: Familial thrombosis due to anti-thrombin III deficiency. Blood 43:219–231, 1974.

43a. McPherson M, Quirke P, and Taylor G: PCR: A Practical Approach. In Rickwood D, and Hames BD (eds): Gel Electrophoresis of Nucleic Acids. Oxford University Press, Oxford, 1991.

44. Meissen GJ, Myers RH, Mastromauro CA, et al: Predictive testing for Huntington's disease with use of a linked DNA marker. N Engl J Med 318:535–542, 1988.

45. Monaco AP, Neve RL, Colletti-Feener C, Bertelson CJ, Kurnit DM, and Kunkel, LM: Isolation of candidate cDNAs for portions of the Duchenne muscular dystrophy gene. Nature 323:646–650, 1986.

46. Morton NE: Detection and estimation of linkage between genes for elliptocytosis and Rh blood type. Am J Hum Genet 8:80–96, 1956.

46a. Mullis K and Faloona F: Specific synthesis of DNA in vitro via a polymerase catalysed chain reaction. In WU R: Methods in Enzymology. Academic Press, San Diego, 1987, pp 335–350.

46b. Murrell J, Farlau M, Ghetti B, and Benson MD: A mutation in the amyloid precursor protein associated with hereditary Alzheimer's disease. Science 254:97–99, 1991.

47. Naruse S, Igarashi S, Aoki K, et al: Missense mutation Val–Ile in exon 17 of amyloid precursor protein gene in Japanese familial Alzheimer's disease. Lancet 337:978–979, 1991.

48. Ott J: Estimation of the recombination fraction in human pedigrees: Efficient computation of the likelihood for human linkage studies. Am J Hum Genet 26:588–597, 1974.

49. Owen F, Poulter M, Shah T, et al: An in-frame insertion in the prion protein gene in familial Creutzfeldt-Jakob disease. Brain Res Mol Brain Res 7:273–276, 1990.

50. Parkman R: The application of bone marrow transplantation to the treatment of genetic disease. Science 232:137, 1986.

50a. Peacock ML, Warren JT, Jr, Roses AD, and Fink JK: Novel polymorphism in A4-region of amyloid precursor protein without Alzheimer's disease. Neurology, in press.

51. Pelham HRB and Jackson RJ: An efficient mRNA dependent translation system from reticulocyte lysates. Eur J Biochem 67:247–256, 1976.

52. Pericak-Vance MA, Bebout JL, Gaskell PC, et al: Linkage studies in familial Alzheimer's disease: Evidence for chromosome 19 linkage. Am J Hum Genet 48(6):1034–1050, 1991.

53. Pericak-Vance MA, Bebout JL, Yamaoka LH, et al: Linkage studies in familial Alzheimer's disease: Application of the Affected Pedigree Member (APM) method of linkage analysis. Proceedings of the International Symposium on Dementia: Molecular Biology and Genetics of Alzheimer's Disease. Excerpta Medica International Congree Series, Elsevier, 1990, pp. 215–228.

54. Pericak-Vance MA, Yamaoka LH, Haynes CS, et al: Genetic linkage studies in Alzheimer's disease families. Exp Neurol 102:271–279, 1988.

55. Podlisny MB, Lee G, and Selkow DJ: Gene dosage of the amyloid β precursor protein in Alzheimer's disease. Science 238:669–671, 1987.

56. Prusiner SB: Creutzfeldt-Jakob disease and scrapie prions. Alzheimer Dis Assoc Disord 3:52–78, 1989.

57. Rickwood D and Hames BD (eds): Gel Electrophoresis of Nucleic Acids. IRL Press, London, 1982.

57a. Ropers HH, Pericak-Vance MA, Siciliano M, and Mohrenweiser H: Report on the 2nd International Workshop on Human Chromosome 19. Cytogenet Cell Genet, in press.

57b. Roses AD: Current status of genetics and Alzheimer's disease. Comments in Toxicology, in press.

58. Roses AD, Bebout J, Yamaoka L, et al: Linkage studies in familial Alzheimer's disease (FAD): Application of the affected pedigree member (APM) method. Neurology (Suppl 1)40:275, 1990.

58a. Roses A, Pericak-Vance M, Alberts M, et al.: Locus heterogeneity of Alzheimer's disease. In Cristen Y, et al. (eds): The Genetics of Alzheimer's Disease. Elsevier, in press.

59. Roses AD, Pericak-Vance MA, and Yamaoka LH: Recombinant DNA strategies in genetic neurological diseases. Muscle Nerve 6:339–355, 1983.

60. St George-Hyslop P, Haines J, Farrer L, et al: Genetic linkage studies suggest that Alzheimer's disease is not a single homogenous disorder. Nature 347:194–197, 1990.

61. St George-Hyslop P, Tanzi R, Polinsky R, et al: The genetic defect causing familial Alzheimer's disease maps on chromosome 21. Science 235:885–890, 1987.

62. St George-Hyslop P, Tanzi R, Polinsky R, et al: Molecular genetic markers in sporadic and familial Alzheimer's disease (abstr). Neurology (Suppl 1)38:264, 1988.

62a. Saiki R, Gelfand D, Stoffel S, et al: Primer-directed enzymatic amplification of DNA with a thermostable DNA polymerase. Science 239:487–491, 1988.

63. Sanger F: Determination of nucleotide sequences in DNA. Science 214: 1205–1210, 1981.

64. Scangos G and Ruddle FH: Mechanisms and applications of DNA mediated gene transfer in mammalian cells: A review. Gene 14:1, 1981.

65. Schellenberg GD, Bird TD, Wijsman EM, et al: Absence of linkage of chromosome 21q21 markers to familial Alzheimer's disease. Science 241: 1507–1510, 1988.

66. Schenk VWD: Re-examination of a family with Pick's disease. Ann Hum Genet 23:325–333, 1959.

67. Scott M, Foster D, Mirenda C, et al: Transgenic mice expressing hamster prion protein produce species-specific scrapie infectivity and amyloid plaques. Cell 59:847–857, 1989.

68. Seitelberger F: Spinocerebellar ataxia with dementia and plaque-like deposits (Straussler's disease). In Vinken P and Bruyn G (eds): Handbook of Clinical Neurology. North-Holland, Amsterdam, 1981, pp 182–183.

69. Speer M, Goldgaber D, Goldfarb L, et al: Support of linkage of Gerstmann-Sträussler-Scheinker's syndrome to the prion protein gene on chromosome 20p12-pter. Genomics 9:366–368, 1991.

70. Tabin CJ, Hoffman JN, Goff SP, and Weinberg RA: Adaptation of a retrovirus as a eukaryotic vector transmitting the herpes simplex virus thymidine kinase gene. Mol Cell Biol 2:426, 1982.

71. Tanzi RE, Bird ED, Latt SA, and Neve RL: The amyloid β protein gene is not duplicated in brains from patients with Alzheimer's disease. Science 238:666–669, 1987.

72. Tanzi RE, St. George-Hyslop PH, Haines JL, et al: The genetic defect in familial Alzheimer's disease is not tightly linked to the amyloid beta protein gene. Nature 329:156, 1987.

73. Terry RD and Katzman R: Senile dementia of the Alzheimer type. Ann Neurol 14:497, 1983.

74. Travis GH and Sutcliffe JG: Phenol emulsion-enhanced DNA-driven subtractive cDNA cloning: Isolation of low-abidance monkey cortex-specific mRNAs. Proc Natl Acad Sci U S A 85:1696, 1988.

75. Tuszynski MH, Jinnah HA, and Gage FH: Delivery of neuroactive compounds to the brain: Potential utility of genetically modified cells. Neurobiol Aging 10:644–645, 1989.

76. Van Broeckhoven C, Haan J, Bakker B, et al: Amyloid β protein precursor gene and hereditary cerebral hemorrhage with amyloidosis (Dutch). Science 248:1120–1122, 1990.

77. Van der Patten H, Botteri FM, Miller AD, et al: Efficient insertion of genes into mouse germ line via retrovirus infection. Proc Natl Acad Sci U S A 82:6148, 1985.

78. Van Duijn CM, Hendriks L, Cruts M, Hardy, JA, Hofman A, and Van Broeckhoven C: Amyloid precursor protein gene mutation in early-onset Alzheimer's disease. Lancet 337:978, 1991.

79. Wallace MR, Marchuk DA, Andersen LB, et al: Type 1 neurofibromatosis gene: Identification of a large transcript disrupted in three NF1 patients. Science 249:181–186, 1990.

80. Ward CD, Duvoisin RC, Ince SE, Nutt JD, Eldridge R, and Calne DB: Parkinson's disease in 65 pairs of twins and in a set of quadruplets. Neurology 33:815–824, 1983.

81. Wasmuth JJ, Hewitt J, Smith B, et al: A highly polymorphic locus very tightly linked to the Huntington's disease gene. Nature 332:734–738, 1988.

82. Weber JL: Informativeness of human (dC-dA)n polymorphisms. Genomics 7(4):524–530, 1990.

83. Weeks DE and Lange K: The affected-pedigree-member method of linkage analysis. Am J Hum Genet 42:315–326, 1988.

84. Wijmenga C, Frants RR, Brouwer OF, Moerer P, Weber, JL, and Padberg GW: Location of facioscapulohumeral muscular dystrophy gene on chromosome 4. Lancet 336:651–653, 1990.

85. Zannis VI and Breslow JL: Genetic

mutations affecting human lipopro-
tein metabolism. In Harris H and
Hirschhorn K (eds): Advances in
Human Genetics, Vol 14. Plenum,
New York, 1985, pp 125–215.

86. Zwiebel JA, Freeman SM, Newman K,
Dichek D, Ryan US, and Anderson
WF: Drug delivery by genetically engineered cell implants. Ann NY Acad Sci
618:394–404, 1991.

87. Tenth International Workshop on
Human Gene Mapping (HGM 10). Cytogenet Cell Genet 51:11–17, 1989.

GLOSSARY OF MOLECULAR AND GENETIC TERMS

allele: One of two or more different forms of a gene containing specific inheritable characteristics that occupy corresponding positions (loci) on paired chromosomes.

blotting: Procedure in which pieces of DNA or mRNA are transferred to a membrane (usually made of nitrocellulose or nylon) by capillary action. The DNA or mRNA can then be easily manipulated and used for hybridization to various probes.

cDNA: Complementary DNA, synthesized from mRNA obtained from a tissue or cell of interest.

centromere: The area of a chromosome to which microtubules attach for chromosomal movement during meiosis. Typically, centromeres are located near the middle of a chromosome. The region above the centromere is termed the short arm or "p" (for petite) arm; the region below the centromere is the "q" (long) arm.

chromosome hopping: Cloning large segments of DNA (several hundred thousand bases) and detecting overlapping sequences in order to move from one point to another on a chromosome (such as from a tightly linked probe to the disease gene) by hopping over intervening fragments. The larger DNA segments are cut by restriction enzymes that have infrequent cut sites. Faster than chromosome walking, but may be less exact because bigger steps are made with each hop (see *chromosome walking*).

chromosome walking: Cloning overlapping pieces of DNA to detect adjacent pieces of DNA. By repeating the procedure, it is possible to "walk" slowly from one point to another point on a chromosome, such as from a tightly linked probe to the disease gene. Tedious, because all the intervening sequences must be cloned and walked before the actual gene is reached (see *cosmid contig*).

clone: See *molecular cloning.*

cM: Centimorgan; the unit of distance between loci on a chromosome. One cM is approximately 1 million bases.

codominant inheritance: The existence at a particular locus of several alleles that can be distinguished from each other (i.e., heterozygotes can be differentiated from homozygotes).

codon: One of the fundamental buildimg blocks of the genetic code. It consists of three consecutive nucleotides that code for an amino acid. For example, the nucleotide sequence "G-C-U" codes for alanine, and "A-G-C" codes for serine. Mutation of a gene that results in an insertion, deletion, or change of a single nucleotide may alter the sequence or composition of codons, leading to the incorporation of an incorrect amino acid into a protein, thereby producing an abnormal protein.

cosmid: A DNA vector that can be grown in bacteria, not unlike plasmids, and isolated using common molecular genetic techniques. Cosmids can be used to clone relatively large pieces of genomic DNA ($\approx$40 kb) (see *cosmid contig*).

cosmid contig: Large numbers of cosmids that are contiguous (and continuous), representing a long genomic distance. For example, a cosmid contig may be created by cloning human DNA into cosmids and selecting continuous overlapping pieces. This genomic distance may be defined by flanking markers for a disease locus, thus defining the region within which a disease gene is located. Projects are under way to map several complete chromosomes with thousands of cosmid contigs.

expressivity: The phenotype produced by a gene. A gene that has variable expressivity will produce different phenotypes in different individuals.

hybridization: The binding of one nucleic acid to another owing to high degrees of complementation in their base pair sequences. Various hybridization combinations include DNA to DNA, DNA to RNA, or RNA to RNA. Typically one of the pieces of nucleic acid (usually the probe) is made radioactive by using a radiolabeled nucleotide. Thus, when the probe is hybridized to a blot, it will preferentially bind to a piece of DNA or RNA with a complementary base sequence. This will form a unique banding pattern of radioactivity that can be detected by exposing the hybridized blot to x-ray film.

informative: Useful in providing information; for example, if all alleles of both parents at a locus are the same genotype (AA × AA), then one specific allele cannot be followed through meiosis and is noninformative. If all alleles are different (AB × CD), then each can be distinguished for linkage to another genetic marker, and is highly informative.

library: A collection of cloning vectors, each containing an original piece of DNA from a particular organism or tissue. Commonly used types of libraries include:

cDNA library: A representation of all the genes expressed in a given tissue. It consists of pieces of DNA synthesized from mRNA obtained from the tissue of interest (e.g., a brain cDNA library would represent all of the mRNAs expressed in the brain). The enzyme reverse transcriptase is used to synthesize cDNA from the mRNA. (The mRNA is not used for the library because DNA is more stable and less susceptible to degradation.) Such a library can be used to determine which genes are expressed, and can be compared to libraries from diseased tissues to look for differences in gene expression.

genomic DNA library: The DNA extracted directly from one tissue (usually lymphoblasts), which can be isolated in fairly large quantities, cut into fragments, and cloned into a vector for amplification. Useful for isolating particular genes or segments of DNA, since they are available in discrete fragments and can be amplified.

chromosome-specific DNA library: A library prepared from the DNA of a particular chromosome, such as a chromosome-21-specific DNA library. Useful for producing chromosome-specific probes.

linkage: Finding that two loci are close enough together on the same chromosome that they do not segregate independently during meiosis.

Lod score: Log of the odds of linkage of a combination of markers or traits.

molecular cloning: The process of isolating, characterizing, modifying, producing, and replicating segments of DNA. For example, a particular segment of DNA can be inserted into a vector such as a plasmid or phage (a virus), which is placed inside living cells (i.e., bacteria such as *E. coli*). As the bacteria multiply, so will the plasmid and the inserted piece of DNA. The plasmid can then be isolated and the cloned piece of DNA removed for further study. Pieces of DNA ranging from 10 to 200,000 bases can be cloned successfully. This technique allows the production of almost unlimited quantities of very small or rare pieces of DNA.

Northern blot: The electrophoresis of mRNA on a gel that separates the different mRNAs based on size. Blotting and hybridization can then be performed. Because mRNA is used, any transcripts detected represent genes expressed in that particular tissue (see *Southern blot*).

penetrance: Whether a gene is expressed in all or some of the individuals who have the gene. A completely penetrant gene is expressed in all individuals who have the gene, whereas an incompletely penetrant gene is expressed only in some.

polymerase chain reaction (PCR): An enzymatic reaction used to amplify a specific segment of DNA. The reaction consists of multiple steps of denaturation of the DNA template, annealing of specific primers to the template, and synthesis of the new DNA strands. This is an extremely powerful technique, allowing a segment of DNA to be amplified over a millionfold in just a few hours.

polymorphism: The occurrence together in a population of two or more genotypically determined phenotypes or genotypes, neither of which is rare. An example of a common expressed polymorphism is the ABO blood types: several phenotypes are recognized as the expression of differences at a single locus. RFLPs are DNA-based genetic differences that can be detected using laboratory techniques. Variable repeated motifs or sequences at specific loci are another source of genetic variation that can be recognized and mapped with laboratory techniques.

recombinant DNA: Specific pieces of DNA selectively isolated or amplified for use in research, using various means such as cutting, ligation, cloning, and so on. Sometimes used as a generic term to describe many current techniques in molecular biology and molecular genetics.

recombination: The crossing over or exchange of chromosomal material.

recombination fraction (θ): A statistical measure of the distance between two loci.

restriction enzymes: Enzymes that cleave nucleic acids, mostly DNA, at very specific locations determined by a particular nucleic acid sequence. There are several hundred restriction enzymes that recognize different DNA sequences. For example, the restriction enzyme Eco RI recognizes the DNA sequence "GAATTC" and will cut it between the "G" and "A." Another enzyme, HIND III, recognizes "AAGCTT" and cuts only between the two "A's." By cutting DNA at very specific base sequences, researchers can manipulate DNA and determine where specific DNA sequences occur (see *restriction fragment length polymorphisms* [RFLPs]).

restriction fragment length polymorphisms (RFLPs): Differences in the DNA sequence that can be detected by enzymes (restriction enzymes) that cut DNA. RFLPs have provided the basis for almost all linkage studies performed after 1980. Because these differences in DNA sequence are sometimes inherited as a Mendelian trait, they can be tested for genetic linkage using pedigrees.

Southern blot: The transfer of DNA from a gel to a membrane. The DNA is first separated (based on size) by electrophoresis through a gel. Then it is transferred (by capillary, electrical, or vacuum techniques) onto a special membrane, which is stable and can be used for various hybridization experiments. Numerous samples can be run simultaneously on a single gel and blotted.

subtraction hybridization: The process used to isolate genes that are overexpressed or underexpressed in one tissue compared with another. By hybridizing and then subtracting genes that are expressed equally in both tissues, differentially expressed genes can be isolated and characterized.

telomere: The end of a chromosome. This portion of DNA appears to have a special structure and specific DNA sequence that help to seal and stabilize the end of a chromosome.

translation: Process by which messenger RNA is used as a template to synthesize into a particular sequence of amino acids (e.g., peptide or protein).

transcription: Process by which DNA is used as a template for the synthesis of RNA.

Chapter 3

THE NEUROBIOLOGY OF DEMENTIA

Edward H. Koo, M.D., and
Donald L. Price, M.D.

ALZHEIMER'S DISEASE
PARKINSON'S DISEASE
HUNTINGTON'S DISEASE
CREUTZFELDT-JAKOB DISEASE

The dementing disorders[111] are associated with a multiplicity of structural, chemical, and functional abnormalities involving different brain regions and different populations of nerve cells. Dysfunction and death of these neurons lead to impairments in thought, memory, language, visuospatial skills, behavior, and personality. Recent investigations, taking advantage of approaches derived from a variety of disciplines, have substantially enhanced our understanding of the mechanisms that lead to brain abnormalities in several human disorders. In this chapter we demonstrate how some of these approaches have clarified the biologic substrates of four types of dementia — Alzheimer's disease (AD), Parkinson's disease (PD), Huntington's disease (HD), and Creutzfeldt-Jakob disease (CJD). After briefly introducing each of these disorders, we discuss investigations of structural or chemical abnormalities of brain and studies of animal models. Further information concerning epidemiology, etiology, and clinical features of the first three disorders can be found in Chapter 6 and more information on CJD appears in

Chapter 8. Table 3–1 presents a list of abbreviations used in this chapter.

ALZHEIMER'S DISEASE

AD, characterized by progressive impairments in memory and cognition,[199] is the most common type of dementia occurring in late life. Unfortunately, present laboratory tests cannot establish an unequivocal antemortem diagnosis of AD,[199] which can only be ascertained by quantitative assessment of the number of neurofibrillary tangles (NFT) and senile plaques in brain tissue obtained at biopsy or at postmortem examination[146] (Table 3–2). The accuracy of clinical diagnosis is increased by laboratory examinations or imaging studies (e.g., cerebrospinal fluid [CSF] examinations, computed tomography [CT], and magnetic resonance imaging [MRI]) that demonstrate other causes of dementia (e.g., subdural hematoma, intracranial tumor, infection, brain infarction) or that disclose patterns consistent with, but not diagnostic of, AD.[199] Although many of these changes are nonspecific, one report suggests that the A68 protein, originally identified with a monoclonal antibody termed Alz-50, may be selectively enriched in CSF and brains of subjects with AD.[326,327] Based on Alz-50, an assay was developed to screen for "Alzheimer

55

Table 3–1 ABBREVIATIONS

AChE	acetylcholinesterase
ACT	α_1-antichymotrypsin
AD	Alzheimer's disease
APP	amyloid precursor protein(s)
β/A4	β-amyloid protein
cDNA	complementary deoxyribonucleic acid(s)
ChAT	choline acetyltransferase
CJD	Creutzfeldt-Jakob disease
CRF	corticotropin-releasing factor
CRH	corticotropin-releasing hormone
CSF	cerebrospinal fluid
CT	computed tomography
DAB	diaminobenzidine
GABA	γ-aminobutyric acid
GSS	Gerstmann-Sträussler syndrome
GVD	granulovacuolar degeneration
HD	Huntington's disease
kD	kilodalton(s)
MAP	microtubule-associated protein(s)
MPP+	1-methyl-4-phenylpyridinium
MPTP	1-methyl-4-phenyl-1,2,3,6,tetrahydropyridine
MRI	magnetic resonance imaging
mRNA	messenger ribonucleic acid(s)
NFT	neurofibrillary tangle(s)
NGF	nerve growth factor
NMDA	N-methyl-D-aspartate
PD	Parkinson's disease
PHF	paired helical filament(s)
PN-I	protease nexin I
PN-II	protease nexin II
PrP	prion protein
SNpc	substantia nigra, pars compacta

disease associated proteins'' (ADAP) in postmortem brain tissue.[91] ADAP was readily detected in AD brains but was undetectable in control or neurologically abnormal cases. Whether this assay can be extended to premortem testing from, for example, CSF, remains to be established. More recently, levels of amyloid precursor protein (APP) in CSF have been reported to be altered in subjects with AD, although the results so far have been inconsistent.[150,221,238] Further studies of the neurobiology of AD and other dementias will likely lead to better premortem diagnostic tools.

Brain Abnormalities

NEOCORTEX

The brains of individuals with AD show diffuse atrophy, and brain weight may be reduced approximately 20% as compared with controls. Cortical atrophy is usually most prominent in the frontal and temporal lobes, with variable involvement of the anterior portion of the parietal lobe. Although the gray matter is generally affected, the white matter may at times be quite atrophic.[40]

Cortical atrophy is accompanied by neuronal loss (loss of synapses and astrogliosis). The latter tends to be most severe in layers III and V. NFT and senile plaques are consistently observed in neocortex.* Affected neurons include pyramidal cells that use excitatory amino acids[75,116] as well as cortical interneurons, some of which use corticotropin-releasing factor (CRF) or somatostatin as transmitters.† Moreover,

---

*References 115, 144, 182, 207, 223, 284.
†References 20, 21, 27, 62, 70, 79, 247, 252, 315.

Table 3-2 NEUROBIOLOGIC APPROACHES TO THE STUDY OF ALZHEIMER'S DISEASE

Biologic Measures	Methods	Examples
Brain metabolism	In vivo imaging studies	Reduced glucose utilization in neocortex, esp. parietal and temporal areas
Histology of brain	Histochemistry, immunocytochemistry	β/A4 immunoreactive plaques in neocortex and hippocampus
Quantitation of pathology	Morphometric methods	Reduced number of neurons in basal forebrain cholinergic system
Neuron size and shape	Golgi stains	Abnormal dendritic arborizations
Ultrastructure	Electron microscopy, immunocytochemistry	PHF in NFT and β/A4 fibrils in plaques
Transmitters and enzymes	Assays of markers	Reduced levels of ChAT, somatostatin, and CRF in cortex
Receptors	Binding assays, in vitro autoradiography	Reduced cortical somatostatin receptors and increased cortical CRF receptors
Proteins in abnormal organelles	Purification of constituents, analyses of proteins and other components, immunocytochemistry, freeze-fracture/deep-etch	Decoration of PHF with antineurofilament and antitau antibodies; tubulinlike immunoreactivity in GVD; actin in Hirano bodies; β/A4 in plaque cores and congo philic angiopathy
Proteins and their modifications	Immunoblots, immunocytochemistry, in vitro incorporation of amino acids	Phosphorylated 200-kD neurofilament A68 and tau associated with NFT; aberrant processing of APP and PrP amyloid
RNAs	Hybridization on gels and in situ; measurements of mRNAs and enzymes acting on RNAs	Reduced mRNA in some cells; PrP and APP mRNA present in neurons
Genes	Recombinant DNA technology	Anonymous marker on chromosome 21 linked to familial AD; APP gene localized to chromosome 21

these intrinsic cortical peptidergic systems contribute neurites to senile plaques.

HIPPOCAMPUS AND HIPPOCAMPAL-ASSOCIATED CIRCUITS

Pyramidal neurons in hippocampus and medial temporal lobe develop NFT, Hirano bodies, and granulovacuolar degeneration (GVD),[144] but involvement is not equal in all hippocampal zones.[14,16,290] For example, NFT and loss of pyramidal neurons appear to be greatest in CA1, CA2, and entorhinal cortex.[129,144] The formation of NFT and loss of neurons in the entorhinal cortex may contribute to memory impairments (see below). Moreover, quantitative morphometric studies have suggested that the dementia seen in AD may be attributable to histopathologic changes in the hippocampus, even in the absence of neocortical lesions.[15] Although preliminary, these studies implicate the importance of hippocampal circuitry in the clinical manifestations of AD. NFT and plaques are also consistently present in the amygdala. Loss of neurons has also been documented, particularly in central and medial nuclei of the amygdala.[144,145]

BASAL FOREBRAIN CHOLINERGIC SYSTEM

Cholinergic neurons, located in the medial septum, diagonal band of Broca, and nucleus basalis of Meynert, provide the principal cholinergic innervation of amygdala, hippocampus, and neocortex. The basal forebrain cholinergic system shows consistent neuronal loss of varying degrees.[8,84,274,313] The remaining neurons commonly develop NFT,[44] and immunocytochemical studies have demonstrated that distal axons/nerve terminals of these cells form neurites in some cortical plaques.[9] As these neurons degenerate, cholinergic markers are reduced in distal fields in amygdala, hippocampus, and neocortex.[34,63,84,143,311,312]

These cholinergic cells express nerve growth factor (NGF) receptors[258,278] and respond to NGF. NGF is synthesized in target fields[12,267,317] and taken up by NGF receptors in nerve terminals, and the NGF-receptor complex is then retrogradely transported to cell bodies of neurons[262] to enhance the viability of these nerve cells. Initial studies in cases of AD have not demonstrated a decrease in either NGF mRNA or protein in hippocampus, a target field of basal forebrain neurons.[96] One recent report does suggest that NGF receptor gene expression may be decreased in the basal forebrain.[119] Several experimental models have shown the ability of NGF to enhance survival of basal forebrain cholinergic neurons in adult animals following injury, however. In rats and monkeys, transection of the fimbria-fornix leads to atrophy and degeneration of medial septal cholinergic neurons.[85,157,169,318] Reductions in cell size and in choline acetyltransferase (ChAT) immunoreactivity accompany this axotomy reaction. Treatment of lesioned rats and monkeys with NGF substantially reduces the severity of degenerative changes of these cholinergic neurons, suggesting that NGF may be able to rescue these neurons following injury.[85,158,159,169,291] The availability of recombinant human NGF and of genetically engineered cells designed to deliver NGF by intracerebal grafting provides exciting opportunities in altering the behavior of these cholinergic neurons. Although there is no evidence yet to suggest that alterations of NGF underlie the degeneration of basal forebrain cholinergic neurons in AD, NGF may be useful in enhancing the survival of these neurons.[231,232]

BRAINSTEM MONOAMINERGIC SYSTEMS

Involvement of these systems is more variable: neurons of the locus ceruleus frequently contain NFT; noradrenergic axons/terminals may be abnormally enlarged and form neurites in plaques; the number of nerve cells may be reduced; and noradrenergic markers may be decreased in cortex.[32,59,61,226,290,331] Several studies suggest that reductions in numbers of neurons of the locus ceruleus may be related to the presence of depression in individuals with AD.[334,336] Serotonergic neurons of the raphe complex show NFT, numbers of cells may be reduced, and changes may also occur in serotonergic markers in target fields.[60]

Neurochemical Alterations

Alterations in neurotransmitter markers have been described in AD. The most consistent abnormality is the loss of cholinergic markers. In the cerebral cortices of individuals with AD, ChAT is reduced 40% to 90%.[34,63,84,225] Other measurements of cholinergic function, such as acetylcholinesterase (AChE) activity and acetylcholine levels, parallel reductions in ChAT activity.[225] These neurochemical deficits have been attributed to dysfunction and death of cholinergic neurons. The re-

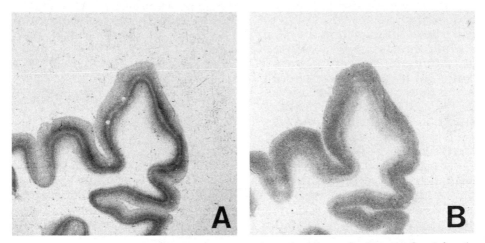

Figure 3-1. Bright-field x-ray images of in vitro receptor autoradiography from the frontal cortex of an adult rhesus monkey. (A) Distribution of the M2 muscarinic receptor subtype is represented by [³H]oxy-tremorine binding. There is a distinct laminar pattern with increased binding in the deeper cortical layers. (B) Distribution of the M1 muscarinic receptor subtype is represented by binding to [³H]pirenze-pine. In contrast to M2 receptor, a relatively homogeneous pattern is seen in the cortex. (Courtesy of Dr. M. V. Wagster.)

sults of cholinergic receptor studies have been less consistent. Of the muscarinic receptors, M1 and M2 subtypes have been studied most extensively. M1 receptors appear to be postsynaptic sites represented by pirenzepine binding, whereas M2 represents presynaptic receptors (Fig. 3-1). There is no clear consensus concerning the status of muscarinic receptors in AD, in part because of nonselective ligands, and in part owing to the existence of at least five muscarinic receptor subtypes defined on the genetic level.[33] At present, it appears that M2 binding may be decreased up to 60% in cortices of individuals with AD but that M1 binding may be unaltered.[64,143, 190,225] The densities of nicotinic receptors is decreased in cortical and hippocampal regions in the brains of patients.[7,311,312] Alterations of synaptic function systems may also be caused by more than binding of agonist and antagonist to receptors.[83] For example, signal transduction involving receptor coupling to effector systems, as well as the actions of second messengers, may play important roles during disease states. A recent study[269] has suggested that in AD, cortical M1 mus-

carinic receptors may be partially uncoupled from G proteins. Future studies may provide valuable insight into signal transduction systems in AD and correlate the synaptic changes seen microscopically to alterations in neurotransmitter markers.

Some cases of AD show abnormalities of adrenergic and serotonergic systems. Levels of adrenaline are decreased in the cerebral cortices of individuals with AD, and the activity of dopamine β-hydroxylase, a marker for adrenergic neurons, is also reduced.[253] Decreased concentration of α-2 binding sites[140a] and increased binding of β-2 sites[140b] have been reported in cortex. As described above, cell loss in the locus ceruleus, a source of noradrenergic innervation of neocortex and hippocampus, may be related to the presence of depression in some patients with AD.[334,336] Similar changes have been described in the serotonergic system; levels of 5-hydroxytryptamine and its metabolite as well as the density of 5-hydroxytryptamine binding sites are reduced in cortex.[253]

In cortex, reductions in levels of γ-aminobutyric acid (GABAergic) markers have been described, particularly in temporal cortex, in some cases of AD.[64] The integrity of glutamatergic system neurons has been assessed by uptake of excitatory amino acids; there appears to be a reduction in glutaminergic terminals owing to pyramidal cell deafferentation.[55,75,116] Several cortical peptidergic systems are affected in this disorder. Levels of somatostatin immunoreactivity are consistently reduced (up to 75%) in the cerebral cortex.[62,253] Corticotropin-releasing hormone (CRH) immunoreactivity is decreased in cortex; CRF receptors are increased in affected cortical areas.[70,315] This finding suggests that there is a corresponding up-regulation of CRH receptors in response to the decrement in presynaptic CRH activity. Fibers of a variety of peptidergic neurons are associated with neurites of some senile plaques.[154–156,273,299,301] Levels of a variety of other peptides do not show consistent alterations in neocortex,[79] although some of these peptidergic systems, which do not show reductions by radioimmunoassays, do contribute neurites to plaques.[48,49,171,172,275]

Cellular Pathology

NEUROFIBRILLARY TANGLES (NFT)

NFT are readily visualized by silver stains such as the Bielschowsky method and appear as fibrillary structures within perikarya (Fig. 3–2). NFT-containing neurons eventually die, leaving extracellular "ghosts" or "tombstones" at sites of affected nerve cells. Although NFT are a major histopathologic hallmark of AD, they are not specific to AD. Other conditions that exhibit variable degrees of NFT formation include normal aging, aged individuals with Down's syndrome, dementia pugilistica, the parkinsonian-dementia

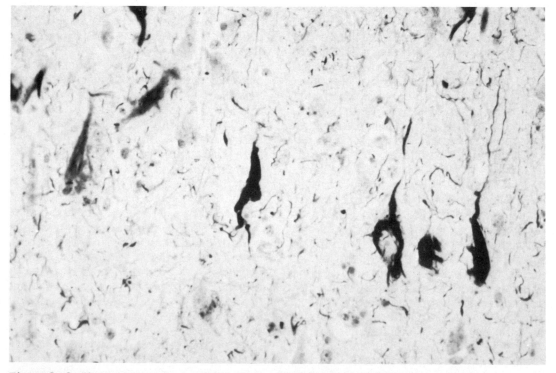

Figure 3–2. Photomicrograph of a cluster of neurofibrillary tangles (NFT) in the amygdala of a patient with Alzheimer's disease (Bielschowsky stain, magnification ×450).

complex of Guam, postencephalitic parkinsonism, and subacute sclerosing panencephalitis.[325] Ultrastructurally, NFT are composed of 15-nm straight filaments and 10-nm paired helical filaments (PHF).[147,283,322] PHF are seen in perikarya, within neurites that surround senile plaques, and in extracellular spaces, presumably following neuronal death. X-ray diffraction studies of PHF suggest a β-pleated conformation, a property that contributes to the insolubility of the material. Indeed, the insolubility of PHF has frustrated numerous attempts at purification, and unequivocal identification of the chemical components has been elusive. Nevertheless, recent evidence suggests that NFT represent sites of cytoskeletal disruption. Immunocytochemical studies have identified several cellular constituents within NFT, including microtubule-associated proteins (MAP2 and tau), A68 (a 68-kiloDalton [kd] protein enriched in AD brains), neurofilaments (particularly phosphorylated epitopes of the 200-kD protein), ubiquitin, and the β-amyloid protein (β/A4).* As described above, A68 is a protein that appears enriched in the CSF and brains of individuals with AD. The identity of A68 is unclear, although recent evidence strongly points to this protein being a highly modified form of tau protein.[170,178] In addition, the presence of the A68 epitope may antedate other cytoskeletal abnormalities and may be a marker for neurons vulnerable to the subsequent development of AD-type abnormalities.[72] It is controversial whether PHF may be composed of β/A4 protein, the principal component of amyloid in senile plaques. Because NFT have properties of amyloid (e.g., birefringerence under polarized light), it has been suggested that NFT are similar to the amyloid fibrils found in the cores of senile plaques. Additional evidence was obtained by showing cross-reactivity of β/A4 antibodies with PHF and, subsequently, by sequencing the putative amino terminus of PHF.[108,192] A recent study using highly purified samples showed significant differences in amino acid composition between PHF and amyloid cores.[250] Finally, consistent with immunocytochemical data, tau has been isolated from PHF,[97,166,320] but it is not clear that this microtubule-associated protein is within the core of PHF.[319] Thus the components of PHF remain to be clarified.

The pathogenesis of NFT, and whether these structures are primary or secondary to neuronal injury, is unknown. The possibility that PHF and the β/A4 protein are derived from a common precursor or from similar cellular processes is under active investigation. Regardless of the actual specificity of NFT for AD, it is likely that NFT formation contributes to the dementia of AD. An example of this clinical-pathologic correlation is seen in neurons of the entorhinal cortex, whose projections along the perforant pathway form the major cortical input into hippocampus. In the brains of individuals with AD, NFT are consistently observed in these neurons, and their terminal zones in hippocampus contain numerous senile plaques. Thus the hippocampus is effectively disconnected from its associated cortices, thereby contributing to the memory impairment seen in the disease.[129,145,294] Another example is the presence of dystrophic neurites, also called neuropil threads or curly fibers,[198,287] in neocortex. In addition to tau, these structures contain NFT and PHF and represent sites of major cytoskeletal disruption both in the neuropil and within neurites of mature senile plaques in the cortices of individuals with AD.[6,35] It is hypothesized that these abnormal neurites are related to the altered cortical synaptic architecture, thus contributing to the dementia.

SENILE PLAQUES

Occurring in high frequency in amygdala, hippocampus, and neocortex,

*References 5, 37, 53, 90, 107, 138, 165, 166, 193, 227, 229, 230, 319, 320, 326.

these spherical structures (up to 200 μm in diameter) have two principal components: enlarged nerve processes (dystrophic neurites), and a central core of extracellular deposits of amyloid[145,286,323] (Fig. 3–3). Astrocytes are frequently present in the periphery of plaques, whereas microglial cells are occasionally seen at the periphery and within the plaque core.

Neurites surrounding senile plaques are readily visualized by silver stains and consist of axons, nerve terminals, and dendrites.[103,147,283] By ultrastructure, neurites contain PHF, 15-nm straight filaments, neurofilaments, and various organelles including mitochondria and synaptic vesicles.[323] Not surprisingly, immunocytochemical studies have documented the presence of phosphorylated epitopes of neurofilaments, tau, PHF, and A68 antigens.* Neurites are thought to represent sites of abnormal synaptic interactions. Consistent with this hypothesis is the observation that markers for a variety of neurotransmitters are present in neurites of senile plaques. Thus, neurites appear to be derived from a number of transmitter systems, and it is clear that in a single plaque, neurites arise from more than one neuron.[299]

In the center of the plaque is a core of amyloid which is readily stained by thioflavin S or Congo red.[324] By electron microscopy, the amyloid core consists of 10-nm straight filaments deposited in the extracellular space. A laminar distribution of senile plaques in the cortex can often be observed.[36,57,243] Occasionally, senile plaques are adjacent to walls of blood vessels that may contain a variable amount of amyloid.[204] The presence of amyloid within walls of blood vessels (congophilic angiopathy) is seen in the majority of cases of AD, although instances of cerebrovascular amyloid in the absence of features of AD is not uncommon in elderly individuals.[296]

Amyloid fibrils in plaques and congophilic angiopathy are composed principally of a unique $\approx$ 4-kd β-protein or A4 peptide (β/A4).[94,192,194] Other constituents identified within the amyloid core include α_1-antichymotrypsin (ACT),[1] sulfated glycosaminoglycans,[270] and, possibly, aluminosilicates.[74] The full-length peptide consists of 42 to 43 amino acid residues.[141] A hydrophobic region of 14 residues (positions 29 to 42) in the C-terminal renders the peptide insoluble.[46] In vitro studies using synthetic peptides have shown that β/A4 spontaneously assembles into amyloid fibrils with a cross-β conformation.[47,148] In particular, a sequence of only 14 residues (positions 15 to 28) is sufficient for assembly and to confer the typical fibrillar configuration and x-ray diffraction pattern.[46]

Molecular cloning studies have determined that β/A4 peptide is a truncated form of a much larger amyloid precursor protein (APP), a membrane-associated glycoprotein.[73,141,305] The β/A4 peptide encompasses 14 amino acids of the putative transmembrane domain and 28 amino acids of the adjacent extracellular domain of APP.[141] The APP gene is located on chromosome 21, in the region of 21q21.[100,141,246,280] A report suggesting a duplication of the APP gene in sporadic AD,[67] as occurs in Down's syndrome, has not been confirmed.[234,255,279,304] In addition, initial mapping studies showed that the APP gene is not linked to the putative familial AD locus.[280] Recently, however, a conservative missense mutation within the APP gene has been shown to segregate with the disease in three families.[95,210] This change resulted in a valine-to-isoleucine substitution at a residue within the transmembrane segment (position 640 of the APP-695 sequence,[141] two residues beyond the putative C-terminus of the β/A4 protein. Coincidently, an unrelated mutation was identified in the β/A4 region (a glutamine–to–glutamic acid substitution at position 618), associated with the Dutch type of hereditary cerebral amyloid angiopathy.[179] In concert,

*References 5, 37, 53, 90, 107, 165, 166, 168, 227, 229, 230, 326.

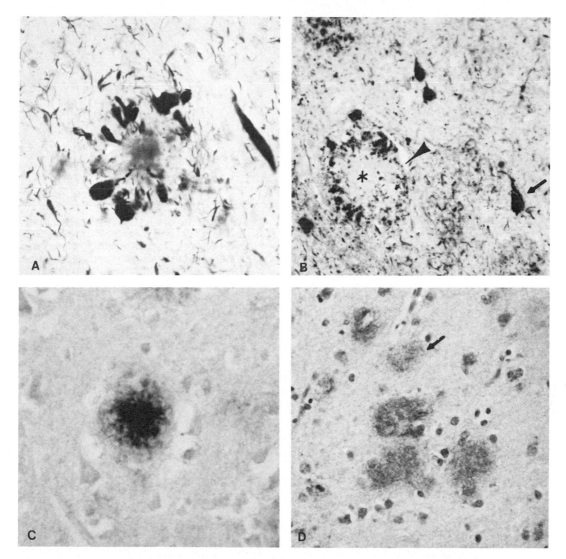

Figure 3–3. Senile plaques in Alzheimer's disease brains stained by various methods. (*A*) A "mature" senile plaque visualized by silver staining. Dystrophic neurites appear as darkly stained distended structures surrounding the amyloid core (Bielschowsky stain, magnification ×500). (*B*) A68 immunoreactivity of neurites of a senile plaque (*arrowhead*), and neurofibrillary tangle (*arrow*) detected by Alz-50 monoclonal antibody. Note that the amyloid core (*asterisk*) is not immunoreactive (diaminobenzidine [DAB], magnification ×250). (*C*) The amyloid core of a "mature" senile plaque is immunostained by an antibody directed to the β/A4 peptide (DAB, magnification ×400). (*D*) Several "diffuse" plaques are seen in the cortex of this individual using a β/A4-specific antisera. Note that these plaques are less well defined and lack a dense core. One plaque is seen juxtaposed to a capillary (*arrow*) (DAB, with hematoxylin counterstain, magnification ×400).

these findings offer evidence that, in some cases, abnormalities of APP may underlie AD as well as the formation of amyloid in the brain. A further description of the molecular genetics of AD can be found in Chapter 2.

At least four APP messenger ribonu-

cleic acids (mRNA), encoding 563, 695, 751, and 770 amino acids respectively, have been identified.[68,141,149,235,281] The APP-751 and APP-770 molecules are identical to APP-695 except that they contain a domain that shares homology with the Kunitz class of serine protease

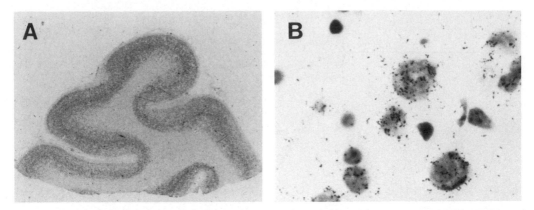

Figure 3–4. Bright field in situ hybridization images of amyloid precursor protein (APP) mRNA in the frontal cortex of an adult rhesus monkey. A 30-mer synthetic oligonucleotide probe specific to APP-695 was used. (*A*) A laminar pattern of hybridization to the radiolabeled probe can be seen in the neocortex after exposure to x-ray film. (*B*) After exposing to nuclear track emulsion, the signal seen in (*A*) corresponds primarily to neurons, especially large pyramidal neurons in the deep cortical layers. Note that glial cells within the microscopic field show few, if any, detectable grains (Nissl stain, magnification ×800).

inhibitors.[149,235,281] APP-695 mRNA is expressed predominantly in the nervous system (Fig. 3–4), whereas APP-751 and APP-770 transcripts are expressed both in brain tissue and systemic organs.[211,235,281] Currently, little is known about the shortest APP transcript (APP-563), which lacks the membrane domain.[68] The differential expression of the transmembrane APP transcripts in brain is regulated developmentally.[162] Whether there is a selective change in APP expression in AD is a source of continuing controversy. Studies[139,212,219] using in situ hybridization methodologies have reported selective increases in the levels of APP-695, APP-751, and APP-563 mRNA in the brains of individuals with AD. Using somewhat different approaches, other studies[98,140,160,162,211] show either a decrease in APP-695 mRNA in the brains of patients with AD, or no difference between those with AD and controls, so the relationship between the expression of APP mRNA and amyloid deposition in the brain remains unclear.

The physiologic roles of APP are not known. APP isoforms are glycosylated and sulfated molecules that, in cultured systems, have a short intracellular half-life and appear transiently on the cell surface.[259,305] APP molecules lacking the cytoplasmic C-terminal domain are secreted into the media. The presence of C-terminal truncated forms in human CSF indicates that a similar process is likely to occur in vivo.[220,305] A trophic or autocrine property of APP has been suggested by recent studies using in vitro systems.[256,316] This hypothesis is in accord with the recent discovery that APP is identical to protease nexin II (PN-II).[216,295] The protease nexins are a class of molecules that modulate the actions of certain proteases, including one (PN-I) that stimulates neurite outgrowth. In addition, PN-II is a potent inhibitor of chymotrypsin and forms inhibitory complexes with the β-subunit of NGF.[295] At present, the biochemical events that result in the cleavage of β/A4 from APP, leading to the deposition of amyloid, are unclear.[208] Because β/A4 includes parts of both the predicted extramembrane region and the transmembrane domain, the generation of β/A4 from the precursor molecule must require at least two (or more) proteolytic cleavages. Two recent reports[78,268] have determined that, in cultured systems, a physiologic cleavage occurs near the middle of the β/A4 domain during secretion (lysine at position 16 of the β/A4 peptide). This finding suggests that normal constitutive processing of APP precludes the formation of an intact amyloidogenic β/A4 fragment. As a result, amyloidogenesis must presumably require the absence of this normal cleavage event. At present, the actual proteolytic events that result in the β/A4 peptide, hypothesized to involve various proteases and protease inhibitors, remain to be defined.

The origin of β/A4 in deposits of amyloid in plaques and in the walls of blood vessels is controversial. Two prevailing hypotheses, not mutually exclusive, argue for neuronal[192,194] and vascular[94,264] origins of β/A4. Evidence for a neuronal origin centers on five principal findings: (1) the topographic distribution of senile plaques within gray matter; (2) the neuronal localization of APP mRNA, including high levels of expression of the brain-enriched transcript (APP-695)[118,162,180,211]; (3) the transport of APP in axons[161]; (4) the localization of the N- and C-terminus of APP in neurites surrounding amyloid deposits[58,130,134]; and (5) the finding of β/A4 deposits adjacent to neurites in plaques.[189] The vascular hypothesis implicates serum sources or cells related to blood vessels. Evidence for the latter includes the proximity of blood vessels to senile plaques[204,205]; deposits of amyloid in meningeal vessels outside the brain parenchyma and in vascular malformations[94,117]; the presence of full-length APP molecules in platelets[43,52]; the presence of serum components (serum amyloid P and complement factors) in amyloid; the possible increased permeability of the blood-brain barrier (BBB) in aging; and the presence of β/A4 immunoreactivity in the skin of individuals with AD.[135] These two hypotheses do not exclude the possibility that the deposition of amyloid in brain parenchyma and in walls of blood vessels may be the result of two independent processes that arise from different compartments of the brain. Nevertheless, regardless of the ultimate origin of APP, proteolytic

events that liberate the amyloidogenic β/A4 fragment are likely to occur in proximity to sites of amyloid deposition. Several lines of evidence support this view. First, immunocytochemical studies have documented the presence of APP epitopes, which exclude the β/A4 domain, from both N- and C-terminals within amyloid deposits.[58,130,134,228,263] Second, the in vitro assembly of β/A4 is inhibited by membrane association, but β/A4 unassociated with the membrane is highly insoluble.[192,208]

Although senile plaques are a pathologic hallmark of AD, they are seen in normal aged subjects as well as in aged individuals with Down's syndrome. The numbers of senile plaques in the cortices of cases of AD far exceeds those seen in age-matched controls, however. A diagnosis of AD in individuals >75 years of age requires the finding of >15 plaques in a ×200 microscopic field, an amount that is rarely, if ever, seen in nondemented individuals.[146] As with NFT, the severity of dementia has also been correlated to the number of plaques seen on postmortem examination.[288]

Finally, recent studies have suggested that senile plaques may evolve in stages. Using antibodies directed against the β/A4 peptide or modifications of traditional silver stains, a less compact form (designated as "preamyloid" or "diffuse" plaques) is seen in cerebrum and cerebellum.[137,277,328] These fluffy structures, when present, are patchy in distribution and may be circular or irregularly shaped. Diffuse plaques are more common in molecular layers of the cortex and cerebellum and possibly in the spinal cord as well.[215] A recent report indicated that similar deposits may be present in the dermis of the skin in individuals with AD.[135] Amyloid in these diffuse plaques is apparently not in a fibrillar or compacted form, and thus is not detected by either Congo red or thioflavin-S stains.[329,330] Moreover, dystrophic neurites are not observed around these diffuse plaques. It has been suggested that these structures represent a very early form of senile plaque. In this scenario the neuritic component and amyloid deposited in a β-conformation would appear later to form a "classic" or "mature" plaque. In time the neuritic component may become less prominent, leaving only a solid amyloid core or "burnt out" plaque.[321]

HIRANO BODIES AND GRANULOVACUOLAR DEGENERATION (GVD)

Hirano bodies are rod-shaped eosinophilic inclusions that are common in pyramidal cells of the hippocampus.[88,89] Composed of microfilaments arranged in paracrystalline arrays, Hirano bodies contain actin and a variety of other proteins, including tropomyosin, β-actinin, vinculin, and tau. Hippocampal neurons also develop GVD, structures consisting of a basophilic granule inside a small vacuole within the cytoplasm.[14,290] By electron microscopy the granules appear as electron-dense material within a membrane-lined vacuole. Recently, tubulin immunoreactivity was demonstrated in these granules.[237] Like the other pathologic alterations seen in AD, Hirano bodies and GVD are not specific for AD and may be seen in brains of normal aged individuals.

Animal Models: Nonhuman Primates

Until relatively recently, a satisfactory model for AD has not been available, but it is now known that aged rhesus monkeys may show age-associated cognitive deficits, neurochemical alterations, and AD-type pathology.

BEHAVIORAL STUDIES

Rhesus monkeys have a potential life span of over 35 years. Monkeys older than 25 years of age may be impaired in a variety of tasks, including visual recognition memory, direct-delayed spatial learning, habit formation, and visuo-spatial orientation.[10,18,19,24,236,302] As expected, significant interanimal variability has been found in the performance of different tasks, but age-related impairments were observed in nearly all test categories. Spatial abilities are noted to decline in the late teens, but the other skills are not affected until early in the third decade of life. Because these deficits are similar to recent memory deficits seen in aged humans, these animals can provide a useful model for investigations of age-associated impairments of memory.

NEUROPATHOLOGIC-NEUROCHEMICAL STUDIES

The brains of aged monkeys exhibit in a variety of structural abnormalities similar to those occurring in older humans, and there are differences in the distributions and severities of these lesions in different animals of the same age.

Nerve cells develop a variety of structural alterations. Some cortical neurons become atrophic, as occurs in human subjects.[282] A number of cortical neurons exhibit abnormal immunoreactivity (e.g., some cells show A68 immunoreactivity). Significantly, one old rhesus monkey (34 years of age) had NFT visualized with silver stains and immunocytochemistry.[54] Abnormalities of axons, not associated with deposits of amyloid, can be detected in neocortex at the end of the second decade of life (equivalent to 50 to 60 years of age in humans). Neurites in plaques appear at approximately the same time, and it has been speculated that these abnormalities are an early stage in the formation of plaques. Neurites are derived from a variety of transmitter-specific populations of neurons, including cells that show immunoreactivities for ChAT,[154] somatostatin,[273] catecholamines,[155] glutamic acid decarboxylase,[301] neuropeptide Y,[299] or serotonin.[156] Furthermore, in individual plaques, neurites may be derived from two or more systems.[299] Neurotransmitter studies have demonstrated that monoaminergic and cholinergic markers may decline in some regions of cortex in older animals.[102,298,303,306] Thus, in both monkeys and humans, a variety of neuronal systems show age-associated alterations.

Senile plaques, morphologically similar to those seen in humans, appear in the cortices of aged monkeys at the end of the second decade.* Amyloid deposited in plaques and in walls of blood vessels is antigenically similar to that occurring in individuals with AD.[2,265,300] The monkey APP-695 complementary deoxyribonucleic acid (cDNA) has been identified, and the predicted amino acid sequence is 100% homologous to the human form.[233] Thus the $\beta/A4$ sequence in monkey and human is identical. In addition, APP transcripts containing the protease inhibitor domains APP-751 and APP-770 are also expressed in monkey, although there are four amino acid substitutions in this sequence (E. H. Koo, S. S. Sisodia, and D. L. Price, personal communication, 1991). The cellular distribution of APP transcripts in monkey brain is similar to that seen in humans.[162] Recent studies[162] suggest that the deposition of amyloid in the brains of aged monkeys is not accompanied by any changes in the differential expression of APP mRNAs. As in humans, deposits of

---

*References 265, 272, 276, 299, 300, 323.

amyloid in monkey coexist with ACT[2] and glycosaminoglycans.

PARKINSON'S DISEASE

Classical paralysis agitans, or PD, one of the most common degenerative neurologic diseases, occurs in 1% of individuals over 65 years of age. This disorder is characterized by slowness of voluntary movement (bradykinesia), rigidity, tremor, and postural instability.[184,224] Some patients develop impairments of cognition and memory.[29,181,195,196] Some correlations exist between the presence of cognitive abnormalities (particularly of visuospatial skills and psychomotor speed) and the severity of PD-related motor signs.[197,206,333] (See also Chapter 6.)

Brain Abnormalities

DOPAMINERGIC NEURONS OF THE SUBSTANTIA NIGRA, PARS COMPACTA

The number of pigmented nerve cells in the substantia nigra, pars compacta (SNpc), especially in the lateral portions, is decreased[82,133,184] (Table 3–3). A feature diagnostic of idiopathic PD is the Lewy body, a spherical eosinophilic intracytoplasmic inclusion. Lewy

Table 3–3 NEUROBIOLOGIC APPROACHES TO THE STUDY OF PARKINSON'S DISEASE

Biologic Measures	Methods	Examples
Brain metabolism	In vivo imaging studies	Alterations in striatal dopamine receptors
Histology of brain	Histochemistry, immunocytochemistry	Neurofilament antigens in Lewy bodies
Quantitation of pathology	Morphometric methods	Reduced number of neurons in SNpc
Transmitters and enzymes	Assays of markers	In PD and MPTP model, decreased dopamine in striatum
Proteins in abnormal organelles	Purification of constituents, analyses of proteins and other components, immunocytochemistry, freeze-fracture/deep-etch	Neurofilament epitopes associated with Lewy bodies

bodies are commonly seen in the SNpc, but they are also seen in neurons of the nucleus basalis, locus ceruleus, and dorsal motor nucleus of the vagus. Using immunocytochemical methods, neurofilament antigens have been demonstrated in the Lewy body.[101] In classical PD, nerve cells in the SNpc rarely contain NFT; this pathology is more commonly observed in postencephalitic parkinsonism.[82] Abnormalities of SNpc are associated with reductions (80% to 95%) in dopaminergic markers in the striatum.[123,245] Dopaminergic deafferentation is associated with an increased number of dopamine receptors in striatum.

OTHER BRAINSTEM MONOAMINERGIC SYSTEMS

In some cases, pathology occurs in nonnigral catecholaminergic pathways. The number of dopaminergic neurons in the ventral tegmental area is decreased,[132,293] and dopaminergic markers are reduced in mesolimbic and mesocortical target fields.[122,132,257] The number of neurons in the locus ceruleus may be diminished,[82] with decreased (50%) noradrenergic markers in cortex.[3,257] Finally, serotonergic markers, reflecting innervation from neurons located in the raphe complex, may also be reduced in subcortical and cortical regions.[257]

OTHER NEURONAL SYSTEMS

Other transmitter systems may be affected in PD. In the basal ganglia, changes have been documented in markers of several cell populations, including neurons using γ-aminobutyric acid (GABA), met-enkephalin, leu-enkephalin, substance P, and bombesin as neurotransmitters.[3,26] Neurotensin receptors, believed to be located on SNpc neurons,[218] are reduced in the SNpc.[292] Some patients show reductions in nerve cells in the basal forebrain cholinergic system[8,44,209,310] and decreases in cortical cholinergic markers.[254] Loss of neurons occurs in the pedunculopontine nucleus, pars

compacta.[335] Somatostatinlike immunoreactivity may be decreased in hippocampus and neocortex,[77] and cortical levels of CRF may be reduced in some patients.[315] In PD these abnormalities are sometimes, but necessarily, associated with typical features of AD (e.g., senile plaques and NFT in amygdala, hippocampus, and neocortex).[4,29,114,209,242] The overlap between AD and PD is discussed further in Chapter 6.

Animal Model: Intoxication with MPTP

In monkeys (as in human intravenous drug users), systemic administration of 1-methyl-4-phenyl-1,2,3,6-tetrahydropyridine (MPTP) produces akinesia, rigidity, flexed posture, and postural tremors by preferentially damaging the nigrostriatal dopaminergic system.[42,153,176] These abnormalities can be reversed by treatment with L-dopa.* After gaining access to brain, MPTP binds to monoamine oxidase B, an enzyme enriched in certain regions of the central nervous system (including the striatum),[222] and is converted to the toxic metabolite 1-methyl-4-phenylpyridinium (MPP+),[177] which is taken up by high-affinity dopamine uptake systems located on terminals of SNpc nerve cells.[131] At high doses MPTP selectively destroys SNpc neurons, with secondary reductions in dopaminergic markers in the striatum. At lower doses, some nigral neurons degenerate, but other SNpc neurons suffer damage to distal axons.[153] In time some injured neurons die, but others recover, and their axons/terminals may reinnervate the striatum. This process may account for some of the restoration of motor functions occurring in certain animals. The neurotoxic effects of MPTP can be blocked by administration of inhibitors of monoamine oxidase B activity and dopamine uptake.[131,163,177,271] On the

---

*References 13, 42, 65, 163, 175, 177, 271.

basis of these studies, monoamine oxidase B inhibitors have been used to retard the progression of parkinsonian symptoms and signs in human subjects.[285]

MPTP intoxication[163] provides a model for examining the evolution of changes in presynaptic and postsynaptic markers in basal ganglia, the physiology of dopamine-denervated circuits of the basal ganglia, the mechanisms of toxic injury of neurons, and the repair of processes in motor circuits; and for the development and testing of new pharmacologic and therapeutic approaches, including neural grafts.

HUNTINGTON'S DISEASE

HD is an autosomal-dominant disorder characterized by involuntary movements (choreoathetosis), dementia, and psychosis. HD usually begins in the fourth decade, with variations occurring among kindreds. Movements and behavioral changes are usually the initial manifestations of the illness, and, over years, patients develop the classical syndrome of HD.[185,187] Mental abnormalities consist of cognitive impairments, memory loss, personality changes, and a variety of psychological symptoms, including irritability and depression.[41,80,81] (See also Chapter 6.)

HD provides an excellent example of the application of molecular genetics to human neurologic disease. Linkage has been demonstrated between the HD locus and DNA markers located on chromosome 4.[109,110,186,309] Anonymous DNA markers, located in the distal region of the short arm of chromosome 4, are linked to HD.[93] Using this approach, presumptive testing of vulnerable individuals is now possible.

Brain Abnormalities

BASAL GANGLIA

The striatum is atrophic[173,174] (Table 3–4). The earliest damage takes place in medial caudate, dorsal putamen, and tail of the caudate.[167] A system for grading the severity of the neuropathology of HD has been established, and the grade correlates with the extent of clinical disability.[297] Several types of abnormalities have been detected in striatal neurons in specific populations of nerve cells that appear to be affected in the striatum, including spiny I and II neurons (GABAergic, enkephalinergic, and substance P nerve cells) and larger intrinsic spiny II cholinergic neurons.[25,76,87,185] Alterations have been documented in the sizes, shapes, and densities of spines of medium-sized

Table 3–4 NEUROBIOLOGIC APPROACHES TO THE STUDY OF HUNTINGTON'S DISEASE

Biologic Measures	Methods	Examples
Brain metabolism	Imaging studies	Decreased volume and glucose metabolism of caudate
Histology of brain	Histochemistry, immunocytochemistry	Decreased substance-P fibers in nigra
Quantitation of pathology	Morphometric methods	Decreased number of neurons in striatum
Neuron size and shape	Golgi stains	Abnormal dendritic arborizations
Transmitters and enzymes	Assays of markers	Decreased GABAergic and substance-P markers in striatum and its targets
Receptors	Binding assays, in vitro autoradiography	Reduced levels of NMDA receptors in putamen
Genes	Recombinant DNA technology	HD gene linked to DNA locus D4S43 present on chromosome 4

spiny neurons.[104] Aspiny I somato-statin/neuropeptide-Y neurons (dia-phorase positive) in the striatum are spared.[11,69,167] Loss of striatal efferents to targets in basal ganglia is associated with reductions in GABA, met-enkeph-alin, substance P, and CRF markers in substantia nigra and globus pal-lidus.[69,76,87] Enkephalin-containing neurons projecting to external pallidum are more affected than substance-P–containing neurons projecting to ven-tral pallidum; substance-P–containing neurons projecting to SNpc are more af-fected than substance P neurons pro-jecting to SNpc.[244] In striatum, reductions occur in GABA, benzodiaze-pine, dopaminergic, and muscarinic cholinergic receptors; the density of do-paminergic terminals and concentra-tions of dopamine are increased in this region.[25] Binding of N-methyl-D-aspar-tate (NMDA) receptors is greatly de-creased (93%) in striatum.[105,322] This decrease could be the result of an excess of an endogenous neurotoxin (such as quinolinic acid), a genetic defect in NMDA receptors, or, secondarily, de-generation of a subset of striatal neurons expressing this receptor.[332] In the latter case, locally liberated neuro-toxins could exacerbate the disease pro-cess. In the GABA-denervated globus pallidus and substantia nigra, GABA and benzodiazepine receptors are in-creased, presumably owing to denerva-tion supersensitivity.[314]

CEREBRAL CORTEX

The thickness of the cerebral cortex, particularly in the frontal regions, is often reduced.[174] In frontal and parietal lobes, the number of neurons is reduced in layers III, V, and VI. Some of these neurons may be part of the cortical-striatal system, which may use excit-atory amino acids or as-yet-unknown peptides as transmitters. Levels of so-matostatin and neuropeptide Y are in-creased in frontal cortex, whereas levels of substance P are reduced.[185] The number of benzodiazepine recep-tors also is increased in frontal cor-tex.[314]

Animal Model: Excitotoxic Damage to Striatal Neurons

An inherited animal disorder resem-bling HD has not yet been identified. Eventually, identification of the HD gene on chromosome 4 should allow molecular neurobiologists to create more satisfactory models of HD. Studies over the last few years have suggested that NMDA-receptor–mediated toxicity may play a role in the pathology of HD.[51,249,332] Some neurons in the stria-tum can be damaged by direct injection of excitotoxins.[56,249] This procedure de-stroys some neurons whose perikarya are located in striatum, but spares fibers of passage. When the excitatory quinolinic acid, a tryptophan metabo-lite that acts on NMDA receptors, is in-jected into the striatum, GABA and sub-stance P markers are reduced, whereas somatostatin and neuropeptide Y are preserved.[142] In cases of HD, the activity of the enzyme that synthesizes quino-linic acid[260] is elevated in striatum, but it is not clear whether this event is pri-mary or secondary to gliosis. The obser-vation that excitotoxic damage to stria-tum reproduces some of the HD-type neurochemical deficits lends credence to the idea that presynaptic or postsyn-aptic dysfunction of NMDA-receptor–mediated mechanisms may play a role in the pathogenesis of HD. Drug thera-pies designed to prevent excitatory amino acid damage may be helpful in the disease.

CREUTZFELDT-JAKOB DISEASE

CJD is a progressive dementia asso-ciated with myoclonus and motor dys-function.[86,191,239,251] In addition, ataxia and visual disturbances may occur in some patients. Although a diagnosis may be suspected during life, definitive diagnosis requires pathologic examination of the tissue or animal transmission.

The disease belongs to the group of slow, transmissible spongiform encephalopathies. These disorders are chronic, progressive, and invariably fatal diseases of the central nervous system characterized by the presence of vacuolation within neuronal processes.[22,23,289] Other diseases of this type include kuru (occurring in Fore tribesman of New Guinea) and Gerstmann-Sträussler-Scheinker syndrome (GSS) in humans, as well as scrapie and transmissible mink encephalopathy in animals.[86,239] The etiologic agent of these unusual disorders is unknown but is hypothesized to be an "unconventional virus" or "prion" (proteinaceous infectious agent) (PrP).[71,86,121] The latter term was introduced to emphasize the apparent lack of nucleic acid in the transmissible agent. In this section we have tried to emphasize the pathology as well as the newer neurobiologic studies of this group of disorders. A more detailed discussion of the clinical aspects of this disease appears in Chapter 8.

Brain Abnormalities

CJD is confined to the central nervous system.[22,23,289] The gray matter in a variety of brain regions may be affected, including the neocortex, subcortical nuclei (e.g., striatum, thalamus), hippocampus, cerebellum, and brainstem (Table 3–5). Less frequently, the white matter may be involved. The pathologic features of the disease are spongiform change, neuronal loss, and gliosis,[193] but depending on the chronicity of the disease, the severity of these changes can be quite variable.[191,193] Spongiform change, the hallmark of CJD, consists of microvacuolation of the neuropil. These vacuoles are fine, round-to-ovoid structures, which, by electron microscopy, appear to involve dendrites, axons, neuronal perikarya and, to a lesser extent, astrocytes. The spongiform change is most prominent in cases of relatively short duration (less than 6 months) and can be diagnostic of CJD. Neuronal loss and gliosis may be quite minimal in these early stages of the disease. In cases of longer duration, however, neuronal loss and gliosis coexist with severe spongy degeneration, a pathologic state termed *status spongiosus*. Notable negative findings include the absence of inflammatory response, microglial nodules, viral particles, and inclusion bodies.

In approximately 10% of cases of CJD, amyloid plaques (kuru plaques) are present in the cerebellum.[151,152,289] These plaques consist of a central dense

Table 3–5 NEUROBIOLOGIC APPROACHES TO THE STUDY OF CREUTZFELDT-JAKOB DISEASE

Biologic Measures	Methods	Examples
Histology of brain	Histochemistry, immunocytochemistry	Spongiform abnormalities in cortex and PrP immunoreactivity in plaques
Ultrastructure	Electron microscopy, immunocytochemistry	Presence of PrP fibrils
Proteins in abnormal organelles	Purification of constituents, analyses of proteins and other components, immunocytochemistry, freeze-fracture/deep-etch	PrP in scrapie plaques
Proteins and their modifications	Immunoblots, immunocytochemistry, in vitro incorporation of amino acids	Aberrant processing of APP and PrP amyloid

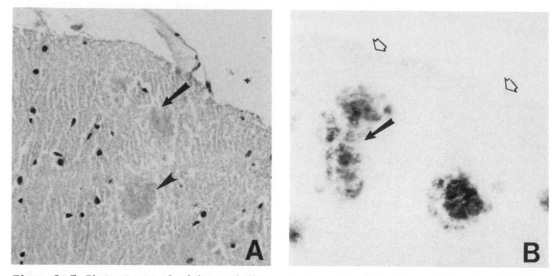

Figure 3–5. Photomicrograph of the cerebellar cortex in a case of Gerstmann-Sträussler-Scheinker syndrome. (*A*) Amyloid plaques appear as poorly defined aggregates within the molecular layer when seen with routine hematoxylin and eosin stains. Two forms are often seen in this disorder: solitary plaques (*arrowhead*) and multicentric plaques (*arrow*) (magnification ×300). (*B*) Plaques in the molecular layer are immunostained by an anti-PrP antibody. Multicentric plaques (*arrow*) appear as multiple cores in aggregates (open arrows indicate the pial surface of the molecular layer (diamenobenzidine [DAB], magnification ×350).

core of amyloid surrounded by a halo of fine, radiating fibrils in the periphery. In contrast to the classic senile plaques of AD, there is no surrounding neuritic component. In GSS cases these amyloid plaques are much more prominent and extensive, occurring in both cerebrum and cerebellum and forming coalescing, or multicentric, structures ("GSS plaques") (Fig. 3–5). Immunostaining of the amyloid in kuru and GSS plaques with anti-PrP antibodies,[151,152,248] (see below) but not with anti-β/A4 antisera, further distinguishes these plaques from those of AD. Indeed, using PrP-specific antibodies, familial cases of dementia previously diagnosed as AD have now been reclassified as variants of GSS.[92,213]

Animal Model: Scrapie

Scrapie, occurring in sheep and goats, is the prototype for this type of slow infection.[112,307] Animals develop ataxia, wasting, and pruritus; the name

comes from their tendency to scrape their fleece, presumably due to unusual cutaneous sensations. These animals also exhibit behavioral changes (hyperexcitability or somnolence), grinding of teeth, and rapid movements of lips and tongue. Usually afebrile, sheep become progressively ataxic and debilitated; death ensues in weeks to months.

In the central nervous system of scrapie-infected animals, the pathology is similar to that occurring in CJD.[17,22,23,112] Many neurons are vacuolated, and some cortical neurons show varicosities and decreased numbers of dendritic spines.[120] Gliosis is most conspicuous in the gray matter of the cerebellar cortex, pontine nuclei, midbrain, and diencephalon. PrP-immunoreactive amyloid plaques may develop in the cerebellum of infected sheep. These plaques also develop in the brains of mice and hamsters after inoculation of scrapie-infected tissue.[66,321] The scrapie and CJD agents are thought to be very similar.[71,86,121,307] Both infected scrapie or CJD tissue can be transmitted into primates and rodents. In the brains, both of patients with CJD and scrapie-infected animals, characteristic 10 to 20-nm fibrils (also termed scrapie-associated fibrils) have been identified by ultrastructural analysis.[200–202] Further studies have demonstrated that scrapie-associated fibril concentrations correlate with infectivity titers, and they are not present in control tissues. These fibrils can also be distinguished from PHF and amyloid fibrils that occur in AD. Whether the scrapie-associated fibril is identical to PrP remains controversial.[71] PrP 27-30, a protein with an apparent molecular weight of 27 to 30 kd, was initially isolated from scrapie-infected hamster brains and copurified with the infectious agent.[30,240] Subsequently, PrP 27-30 has been identified as a sialoglycoprotein,[31] derived by limited proteolysis from a larger precursor protein, PrP 33-35.[203] The native protein (PrP 33-35^c) is a normal cellular protein encoded by a gene on chromosome 20.[50,214,246] PrP 27-30 can be detected in brain tissue during infection.[28,66] This material may also aggregate into fibrils to form the kuru or GSS plaque, consistent with in vitro studies showing that highly purified PrP 27-30 assembles into rod-shaped structures that somewhat resemble scrapie-associated fibrils.[241] The presence of PrP 27-30 in the brains of affected individuals has now been used to diagnose CJD on the basis of immunoblotting of frozen brain tissue with antibodies directed against PrP 27-30.[38,266]

Although the precise identity of the scrapie/CJD agent remains unclear, this agent is notable for its resistance to conventional methods used to destroy infectious agents, such as high temperature, formaldehyde fixation, denaturation, and ultraviolet irradiation. Moreover, albeit controversial, purified fractions of tissue homogenates containing PrP and retaining infectivity apparently lack nucleic acids. At present, whether PrP 27-30 is a by-product of infection or the etiologic agent remains unclear.[183] Recent genetic evidence strongly supports the concept that the abnormal PrP may be causal to the disease and suggests a novel host-pathogen interaction.[45] In rodents the incubation period of scrapie infection appears to be genetically determined at or near the prion locus.[307] For example, substitutions of two amino acid residues at codons 108 and 189 correlate with incubation times in mice infected with scrapie.[308] In addition, when transgenic mice expressing hamster PrP are inoculated with hamster prion, the rodents develop scrapie with a time course and pathology characteristic of scrapie infection in hamsters, not mice.[261] In human prion diseases, it has been known that most cases of GSS and a minority of cases of CJD are familial. Recent studies[125] suggest that a number of mutations in the PrP gene may be associated with these familial cases. A mutation in the PrP gene, resulting in a proline-to-leucine substitution at codon 102, was first linked to affected members of two families with GSS.[124] Subsequently, various mutations, including insertions, have been discovered at multiple sites of the PrP gene in familial CJD and GSS.[39,99,126,128,217] A pattern emerges from these studies, suggesting that specific PrP mutations are associated with different clinical manifestations of these familial cases. In other words, familial CJD and GSS may be allelic variants of PrP. In summary, these findings provide strong evidence that the familial condition is both inherited and infectious. Furthermore, the results imply that these mutations are likely to result in alterations of the structure of PrP as well as susceptibility to the disease. Recent direct and dramatic evidence of this concept was obtained when spontaneous spongiform degeneration developed in transgenic mice expressing mouse PrP transgenes with the proline-to-leucine substitution at codon 102 of familial GSS.[127] The brains of the animals contained low concentrations of protease-resistant PrP, however, and transmission of infectivity to other animals by direct inoculation has not been obtained. Moreover, the result leaves unresolved the mechanism by which the mutated prion causes the disease. Understanding the pathogenesis of this slow, transmissible encephalopathy remains a fascinating problem in the study of neurodegenerative diseases.

SUMMARY AND CONCLUSIONS

New concepts and approaches to the biology of neurologic diseases have substantially enhanced our understanding of several types of dementia. In particular, the past few years have been associated with extraordinary advances in our knowledge of AD, PD, HD, and spongiform encephalopathy. Critical issues that remain to be classified in these disorders include the mechanism of selective vulnerability (particularly in AD, PD, and HD); processes that lead to perturbation of the neuronal cytoskeleton (AD and PD); the pathogenesis of amyloid genes (in AD and spongiform encephalopathy); the role of genetic abnormalities in the expression of disease (AD, HD, and spongiform encephalopathy); and the contribution of age and environmental factors to the development of disease (AD and PD). In the future, clinical and basic science, particularly cellular and molecular biology, will continue to create new opportunities to explore ways in which these diseases cause dysfunction and death of neural cells in animal models and affected humans. Finally, we believe that the next decade will see great advances in the therapies of disease, such as the use of specific enzyme inhibitors (e.g., monoamine oxidase B antagonists in PD), the use of NMDA receptor blockers in disorders associated with excitotoxins, and the use of trophic factors for degenerative processes that affect specific neuronal circuits.

ACKNOWLEDGMENTS

The authors thank Drs. Linda C. Cork, Lary C. Walker, Cheryl A. Kitt, Sangram S. Sisodia, Juan C. Troncoso, Gary L. Wenk, Molly V. Wagster, and Peter J. Whitehouse for helpful discussions. This work was supported by grants from the U.S. Public Health Service (NIH AG 03359, NS 20471, AG 05146, NS 07179) and grants from The Robert L. & Clara G. Patterson Trust, the American Health Assistance Foundation, and The Metropolitan Life Foundation. Dr. Price is the recipient of a Javits Neuroscience Investigator Award (NIH NS 10580). Drs. Price and Koo are recipients of a Leadership and Excellence in Alzheimer's Disease (LEAD) award (NIA AG 07914).

REFERENCES

1. Abraham CR, Selkoe DJ, and Potter H; Immunocytochemical identification of the serine protease inhibitor, α_1-antichymotrypsin, in the brain amyloid deposits of Alzheimer's disease. Cell 52:487–501, 1988.
2. Abraham CR, Selkoe DJ, Potter H, Price DL, and Cork LC: α_1-Antichymotrypsin is present together with the β-protein in monkey brain amyloid deposits. Neuroscience 32:715–720, 1989.
3. Agid Y and Javoy-Agid F: Peptides and Parkinson's disease. Trends Neurosci 8:30–35, 1985.
4. Alvord EC Jr, Forno LS, Kusske JA, Kauffman RJ, Rhodes JS, and Goetowski CR: The pathology of parkinsonism: A comparison of degenerations in cerebral cortex and brainstem. In McDowell FH, and Barbeau A (eds): Second Canadian-American Conference on Parkinson's Disease. Advances in Neurology, Vol 5. Raven Press, New York, 1974, pp 175–193.
5. Anderton BH, Breinburg D, Downes MJ, et al: Monoclonal antibodies show that neurofibrillary tangles and neurofilaments share antigenic determinants. Nature 298:84–86, 1982.
6. Arai H, Lee VM-Y, Otvos L Jr, et al: Defined neurofilament τ- and β-amyloid precursor protein epitopes dis-

tinguish Alzheimer from non-Alzheimer senile plaques. Proc Natl
Acad Sci U S A 87:2249–2253,
1990.

7. Araujo DM, Lapchak PA, Robitaille
Y, Gauthier S, and Quirion R: Differential alteration of various cholinergic markers in cortical and subcortical regions of human brain in
Alzheimer's disease. J Neurochem
50:1914–1923, 1988.

8. Arendt T, Bigl V, Arendt A, and
Tennstedt A: Loss of neurons in the
nucleus basalis of Meynert in Alzheimer's disease, paralysis agitans,
and Korsakoff's disease. Acta Neuropathol (Berl) 61:101–108, 1983.

9. Armstrong DM, Bruce G, Hersh LB,
and Terry RD: Choline acetyltransferase immunoreactivity in neuritic
plaques of Alzheimer brain. Neurosci
Lett 71:229–234, 1986.

10. Arnsten AFT and Goldman-Rakic
PS: α_2-Adrenergic mechanisms in
prefrontal cortex associated with
cognitive decline in aged nonhuman
primates. Science 230:1273–1276,
1985.

11. Aronin N, Cooper PE, Lorenz LJ, et
al: Somatostatin is increased in the
basal ganglia in Huntington disease.
Ann Neurol 13:519–526, 1983.

12. Ayer-LeLievre C, Olson L, Ebendal T,
Seiger Å, and Persson H: Expression
of the β-nerve growth factor gene
in hippocampal neurons. Science
240:1339–1341, 1988.

13. Ballard PA, Tetrud JW, and Langston JW: Permanent human parkinsonism due to 1-methyl-4-phenyl-
1,2,3,6,tetrahydropyridine (MPTP):
Seven cases. Neurology 35:949–
956, 1985.

14. Ball MJ: Neuronal loss, neurofibrillary tangles and granulovaculor degeneration in the hippocampus with
ageing and dementia. A qualitative
study. Acta Neuropathol (Berl) 37:
111–118, 1977.

15. Ball MJ, Fisman M, Hachinski V, et
al: A new definition of Alzheimer's
disease: A hippocampal dementia.
Lancet 1:14–16, 1985.

16. Ball MJ, Merskey H, Fisman M, et al:
Hippocampal morphometry in Alz-

heimer dementia: Implications for
neurochemical hypotheses. Biological Aspects of Alzheimer's Disease.
Banbury Report 15:45–64, 1983.

17. Baringer JR and Prusiner SB: Experimental scrapie in mice: Ultrastructural observations. Ann Neurol 4:
205–211, 1978.

18. Bartus RT, Dean RL III, Beer B, and
Lippa AS: The cholinergic hypoth-
esis of geriatric memory dysfunction.
Science 217:408–417, 1982.

19. Bartus RT, Fleming D, and Johnson
HR: Aging in the rhesus monkey: Debilitating effects on short-term memory. J Gerontol 33:858–871, 1978.

20. Beal MF, Mazurek MF, Chattha GK,
Svendsen CN, Bird ED, and Martin
JB: Neuropeptide Y immunoreactiv-
ity is reduced in cerebral cortex in
Alzheimer's disease. Ann Neurol
20:282–288, 1986.

21. Beal MF, Mazurek MF, Tran VT,
Chattha G, Bird ED, and Martin JB:
Reduced numbers of somatostatin
receptors in the cerebral cortex in
Alzheimer's disease. Science 229:
289–291, 1985.

22. Beck E and Daniel PM: Kuru and
Creutzfeldt-Jakob disease: Neuro-
pathological lesions and their signifi-
cance. In Prusiner SB, and Hadlow
WJ (eds): Clinical, Epidemiological,
Genetic, and Pathological Aspects of
the Spongiform Encephalopathies.
Slow Transmissible Diseases of the
Nervous System, Vol 1. Academic
Press, New York, 1979, pp 253–270.

23. Beck E, Daniel PM, Matthews WB, et
al: Creutzfeldt-Jakob disease: The
neuropathology of a transmission experiment. Brain 92:699–716, 1969.

24. Becker PE: Atrophia musculorum
spinalis pseudomyopathica. Heredi-
taire neurogene proximale Amyotro-
phie von Kugelberg und Welander.
Z. menschl. Vereb. u Konstit-Lehre
37:193–220, 1964.

25. Bird ED: Chemical pathology of
Huntington's disease. Annu Rev
Pharmacol Toxicol 20:533–551,
1980.

26. Bissette G, Nemeroff CB, Decker MW,
Kizer JS, Agid Y, and Javoy-Agid F:
Alterations in regional brain concen-

trations of neurotensin and bombesin in Parkinson's disease. Ann Neurol 17:324–328, 1985.

27. Bissette G, Reynolds GP, Kilts CD, Widerlöv E, and Nemeroff CB: Corticotropin-releasing factor (CRF)-like immunoreactivity in senile dementia of the Alzheimer type. JAMA 254: 3067–3069, 1985.

28. Bockman JM, Kingsbury DT, McKinley MP, Bendheim PE, and Prusiner SB: Creutzfeldt-Jakob disease prion proteins in human brains. N Engl J Med 312:73–78, 1985.

29. Boller F, Mizutani T, Roessmann U, and Gambetti P: Parkinson disease, dementia, and Alzheimer disease: Clinicopathological correlations. Ann Neurol 7:329–335, 1980.

30. Bolton DC, McKinley MP, and Prusiner SB: Identification of a protein that purifies with the scrapie prion. Science 218:1309–1311, 1982.

31. Bolton DC, Meyer RK, and Prusiner SB: Scrapie PrP 27-30 is a sialoglycoprotein. J Virol 53:596–606, 1985.

32. Bondareff W, Mountjoy CQ, and Roth M: Loss of neurons or origin of the adrenergic projection to cerebral cortex (nucleus locus ceruleus) in senile dementia. Neurology 32:164–168, 1982.

33. Bonner TI: New subtypes of muscarinic acetylcholine receptors. Trends Pharmacol Sci 10:11–15, 1989.

34. Bowen DM, Smith CB, White P, and Davison AN: Neurotransmitter-related enzymes and indices of hypoxia in senile dementia and other abiotrophies. Brain 99:459–496, 1976.

35. Braak H, Braak E, Grundke-Iqbal I, and Iqbal K: Occurrence of neuropil threads in the senile human brain and in Alzheimer's disease: A third location of paired helical filaments outside of neurofibrillary tangles and neuritic plaques. Neurosci Lett 65: 351–355, 1986.

36. Braak H, Braak E, and Kalus P: Alzheimer's disease: Areal and laminar pathology in the occipital isocortex. Acta Neuropathol (Berl) 77:494–506, 1989.

37. Brion JP, van den Bosch de Aguilar P, and Flament-Durand J: Senile dementia of the Alzheimer type: Morphological and immunocytochemical studies. In Traber J, and Gispen WH (eds): Senile Dementia of the Alzheimer Type. Springer-Verlag, Berlin, 1985, pp 164–174.

38. Brown P, Coker-Vann M, Pomeroy K, et al: Diagnosis of Creutzfeldt-Jakob disease by Western blot identification of marker protein in human brain tissue. N Engl J Med 314:547–551, 1986.

39. Brown P, Goldfarb LG, Brown WT, et al: Clinical and molecular genetic study of a large German kindred with Gerstmann - Sträussler - Scheinker syndrome. Neurology 41:375–379, 1991.

40. Brun A and Englund E: A white matter disorder in dementia of the Alzheimer type: A pathoanatomical study. Ann Neurol 19:253–262, 1986.

41. Bruyn GW: Huntington's chorea: Historical, clinical and laboratory synopsis. In Vinken PJ, and Bruyn GW (eds): Diseases of the Basal Ganglia. Handbook of Clinical Neurology, Vol 6. North-Holland, Amsterdam, 1968, pp 298–378.

42. Burns RS, Chiueh CC, Markey SP, Ebert MH, Jacobowitz DM, and Kopin IJ: A primate model of parkinsonism: Selective destruction of dopaminergic neurons in the pars compacta of the substantia nigra by N-methyl-4-phenyl-1,2,3,6-tetrahydropyridine. Proc Natl Acad Sci U S A 80:4546–4550, 1983.

43. Bush AI, Martins RN, Rumble B, et al: The amyloid precursor protein of Alzheimer's disease is released by human platelets. J Biol Chem 265: 15977–15983, 1990.

44. Candy JM, Perry RH, Perry EK, et al: Pathological changes in the nucleus of Meynert in Alzheimer's and Parkinson's diseases. J Neurol Sci 59: 277–289, 1983.

45. Carlson GA, Hsiao K, Oesch B, Westaway D, and Prusiner SB: Genetics of prion infections. Trends Genet 7:61–65, 1991.

46. Castaño EM and Frangione B: Biol-

ogy of disease: Human amyloidosis, Alzheimer disease and related disorders. Lab Invest 58:122–132, 1988.

47. Castaño EM, Ghiso J, Prelli, Gorevic PD, Migheli A, and Frangione B: In vitro formation of amyloid fibrils from two synthetic peptides of different lengths homologous to Alzheimer's disease β-protein. Biochem Biophys Res Commun 141:782–789, 1986.

48. Chan-Palay V, Köhler C, Haesler U, Lang W, and Yasargil G: Distribution of neurons and axons immunoreactive with antisera against neuropeptide Y in the normal human hippocampus. J Comp Neurol 248:360–375, 1986.

49. Chan-Palay V, Lang W, Haesler U, Köhler C, and Yasargil G: Distribution of altered hippocampal neurons and axons immunoreactive with antisera against neuropeptide Y in Alzheimer's-type dementia. J Comp Neurol 248:376–394, 1986.

50. Chesebro B, Race R, Wehrly K, et al: Identification of scrapie prion protein-specific mRNA in scrapie-infected and uninfected brain. Nature 315:331–333, 1985.

51. Choi DW: Glutamate neurotoxicity and diseases of the nervous system. Neuron 1:623–634, 1988.

52. Cole GM, Galasko D, Shapiro IP, and Saitoh T: Stimulated platelets release amyloid β-protein precursor. Biochem Biophys Res Commun 170:288–295, 1990.

53. Cork LC, Sternberger NH, Sternberger LA, Casanova MF, Struble RG, and Price DL: Phosphorylated neurofilament antigens in neurofibrillary tangles in Alzheimer's disease. J Neuropathol Exp Neurol 45:56–64, 1986.

54. Cork LC, Walker LC, and Price DL: Neurofibrillary tangles and senile plaques in a cognitively impaired, aged nonhuman primate. J Neuropathol Exp Neurol 48:378, 1989.

55. Cowburn RF, Hardy JA, Briggs RS, and Roberts PJ: Characterisation, density, and distribution of kainate receptors in normal and Alzheimer's diseased human brain. J Neurochem 52:140–147, 1989.

56. Coyle JT and Schwarcz R: Model for Huntington's chorea: Lesion of striatal neurons with kainic acid. Nature 263:244–246, 1976.

57. Crain BJ and Burger PC: The laminar distribution of neuritic plaques in the fascia dentata of patients with Alzheimer's disease. Acta Neuropathol (Berl) 76:87–93, 1988.

58. Cras P, Kawai M, Siedlak S, et al: Neuronal and microglial involvement in β-amyloid protein deposition in Alzheimer's disease. Am J Pathol 137:241–246, 1990.

59. Cross AJ, Crow TJ, Perry EK, Perry RH, Blessed G, and Tomlinson BE: Reduced dopamine-beta-hydroxylase activity in Alzheimer's disease. BMJ 282:93–94, 1981.

60. Curcio CA and Kemper T: Nucleus raphe dorsalis in dementia of the Alzheimer type: Neurofibrillary changes and neuronal packing density. J Neuropathol Exp Neurol 43:359–368, 1984.

61. D'Amato RJ, Zweig RM, Whitehouse PJ, et al: Aminergic systems in Alzheimer's disease and Parkinson's disease. Ann Neurol 22:229–236, 1987.

62. Davies P, Katzman R, and Terry RD: Reduced somatostatin-like immunoreactivity in cerebral cortex from cases of Alzheimer disease and Alzheimer senile dementia. Nature 288:279–280, 1980.

63. Davies P and Maloney AJF: Selective loss of central cholinergic neurons in Alzheimer senile dementia. Nature 288:279–280, 1976.

64. Davies P and Wolozin BL: Recent advances in the neurochemistry of Alzheimer's disease. J Clin Psychiatry (Suppl)48:23–30, 1987.

65. Davis GC, Williams AC, Markey SP, et al: Chronic parkinsonism secondary to intravenous injection of meperidine analogues. Psychiatry Res 1:249–254, 1979.

66. DeArmond SJ, McKinley MP, Barry RA, Braunfeld MB, McColloch JR, and Prusiner SB: Identification of prion amyloid filaments in scrapie-

infected brain. Cell 41:221–235, 1985.

67. Delabar J-M, Goldgaber D, Lamour Y, et al: β-amyloid gene duplication in Alzheimer's disease and karyotypically normal Down syndrome. Science 235:1390–1392, 1987.

68. de Sauvage F and Octave J-N: A novel mRNA of the A4 amyloid precursor gene coding for a possibly secreted protein. Science 245:651–653, 1989.

69. De Souza EB, Whitehouse PJ, Folstein SE, Price DL, and Vale WW: Corticotropin-releasing hormone (CRH) is decreased in the basal ganglia in Huntington's disease. Brain Res 437:355–359, 1987.

70. De Souza EB, Whitehouse PJ, Kuhar MJ, Price DL, and Vale WW: Reciprocal changes in corticotropin-releasing factor (CRF)-like immunoreactivity and CRF receptors in cerebral cortex of Alzheimer's disease. Nature 319:593–595, 1986.

71. Diener TO: PrP and the nature of the scrapie agent. Cell 49:719–721, 1987.

72. Doebler JA, Markesbery WR, Anthony A, Davies P, Scheff SW, and Rhoads RE: Neuronal RNA in relation to Alz-50 immunoreactivity in Alzheimer's disease. Ann Neurol 23:20–24, 1988.

73. Dyrks T, Weidemann A, Multhaup G, et al: Identification, transmembrane orientation and biogenesis of the amyloid A4 precursor of Alzheimer's disease. EMBO J 7:949–957, 1988.

74. Edwardson JA, Klinowski J, Oakley AE, Perry RH, and Candy JM: Aluminusilicates and the aging brain: Implications for the pathogenesis of Alzheimer's disease. Ciba Found Symp 121:160–179, 1986.

75. Ellison DW, Beal MF, Mazurek MF, Bird ED, and Martin JB: A postmortem study of amino acid neurotransmitters in Alzheimer's disease. Ann Neurol 20:616–621, 1986.

76. Emson PC, Arregui A, Clement-Jones V, Sandberg BEB, and Rossor M: Regional distribution of methionine-enkephalin and substance P-like immunoreactivity in normal human brain and in Huntington's disease. Brain Res 199:147–160, 1980.

77. Epelbaum J, Ruberg M, Moyse E, Javoy-Agid F, Dubois B, and Agid Y: Somatostatin and dementia in Parkinson's disease. Brain Res 278:376–379, 1983.

78. Esch FS, Keim PS, Beattie EC, et al: Cleavage of amyloid peptide during constitutive processing of its precursor. Science 248:1122–1124, 1990.

79. Ferrier IN, Cross AJ, Johnson JA, et al: Neuropeptides in Alzheimer type dementia. J Neurol Sci 62:159–170, 1983.

80. Folstein M, Anthony JC, Parhad I, Duffy B, and Gruenberg EM: The meaning of cognitive impairment in the elderly. J Am Geriatr Soc 33:228–235, 1985.

81. Folstein SE and Folstein MF: Psychiatric features of Huntington disease: recent approaches and findings. Psychiatr Dev 2:193–206, 1983.

82. Forno LS: Pathology of Parkinson's disease. In Marsden CD, and Fahn S (eds): Movement Disorders, Neurology, Vol 2. Butterworth & Co, London, 1982, pp 25–40.

83. Fowler CJ, O'Neill C, Garlind A, and Cowburn RF: Alzheimer's disease: Is there a problem beyond recognition? Trends Pharmacol Sci 11:183–184, 1990.

84. Francis PT, Palmer AM, Sims NR, et al: Neurochemical studies of early-onset Alzheimer's disease. Possible influence on treatment. N Engl J Med 313:7–11, 1985.

85. Gage FH, Armstrong DM, Williams DR, and Varon S: Morphological response of axotomized septal neurons to nerve growth factor. J Comp Neurol 269:147–155, 1988.

86. Gajdusek DC: Unconventional viruses causing subacute spongiform encephalopathies. In Fields BN, et al (eds): Virology. Raven Press, New York, 1985, pp 1519–1557.

87. Gale JS, Bird ED, Spokes EG, Iversen LL, and Jessell T: Human brain substance P: Distribution in controls and

Huntington's chorea. J Neurochem 30:633–634, 1978.

88. Galloway PG, Perry G, and Gambetti P: Hirano body filaments contain actin and actin-associated proteins. J Neuropathol Exp Neurol 46:185–199, 1987.

89. Galloway PG, Perry G, Kosik KS, and Gambetti P: Hirano bodies contain tau protein. Brain Res 403:337–340, 1987.

90. Gambetti P, Autilio-Gambetti L, Manetto V, and Perry G: Composition of paired helical filaments of Alzheimer's disease as determined by specific probes. Banbury Report 27:309–320, 1987.

91. Ghanbari HA, Miller BE, Haigler HJ, et al: Biochemical assay of Alzheimer's disease—associated protein(s) in human brain tissue. A clinical study. JAMA 263:2907–2910, 1990.

92. Ghetti B, Tagliavini F, Masters CL, et al: Gerstmann-Sträussler-Scheinker disease. II. Neurofibrillary tangles and plaques with PrP-amyloid coexist in an affected family. Neurology 39:1453–1461, 1989.

93. Gilliam TC, Bucan M, MacDonald ME, et al: A DNA segment encoding two genes very tightly linked to Huntington's disease. Science 238:950–952, 1987.

94. Glenner GG and Wong CW: Alzheimer's disease: Initial report of the purification and characterization of a novel cerebrovascular amyloid protein. Biochem Biophys Res Commun 120:885–890, 1984.

95. Goate A, Chartier-Harlin M-C, Mullan M, et al: Segregation of a missense mutation in the amyloid precursor protein gene with familial Alzheimer's disease. Nature 349:704–706, 1991.

96. Goedert M, Fine A, Hunt SP, and Ullrich A: Nerve growth factor mRNA in peripheral and central rat tissues and in the human central nervous system: Lesion effects in the rat brain and levels in Alzheimer's disease. Molecular Brain Research 1:85–92, 1986.

97. Goedert M, Wischik CM, Crowther RA, Walker JE, and Klug A: Cloning and sequencing of the cDNA encoding a core protein of the paired helical filament of Alzheimer disease: Identification as the microtubule-associated protein tau. Proc Natl Acad Sci U S A 85:4051–4055, 1988.

98. Golde TE, Estus S, Usiak M, Younkin LH, and Younkin SG: Expression of β-amyloid protein precursor mRNAs: Recognition of a novel alternatively spliced form and quantitation in Alzheimer's disease using PCR. Neuron 4:253–267, 1990.

99. Goldgaber D, Goldfarb LG, Brown P, et al: Mutations in familial Creutzfeldt-Jakob disease and Gerstmann-Sträussler-Scheinker's syndrome. Exp Neurol 106:204–206, 1989.

100. Goldgaber D, Lerman MI, McBride OW, Saffiotti U, and Gajdusek DC: Characterization and chromosomal localization of a cDNA encoding brain amyloid of Alzheimer's disease. Science 235:877–880, 1987.

101. Goldman JE: The association of actin with Hirano bodies. J Neuropathol Exp Neurol 42:146–152, 1983.

102. Goldman-Rakic PS and Brown RM: Regional changes of monamines in cerebral cortex and subcortical structures of aging rhesus monkeys. Neuroscience 6:177–187, 1981.

103. Gonatas NK, Anderson W, and Evangelista I: The contribution of altered synapses in the senile plaque: An electron microscopic study in Alzheimer's dementia. J Neuropathol Exp Neurol 26:25–39, 1967.

104. Graveland GA, Williams RS, and DiFiglia M: Evidence for degenerative and regenerative changes in neostriatal spiny neurons in Huntington's disease. Science 227:770–773, 1985.

105. Greenamyre JT, Penney JB, Young AB, D'Amato CJ, Hicks SP, and Shoulson I: Alterations in L-glutamate binding in Alzheimer's and Huntington's diseases. Science 227:1496–1499, 1985.

106. Grimes AM, Grady CL, Foster NL, Sunderland T, and Patronas NJ:

Central auditory function in Alzheimer's disease. Neurology 35:352–358, 1985.

107. Grundke-Iqbal I, Iqbal K, Quinlan M, Tung Y-C, Zaidi MS, and Wisniewski HM: Microtubule-associated protein tau. A component of Alzheimer paired helical filaments. J Biol Chem 261:6084–6089, 1986.

108. Guiroy DC, Miyazaki M, Multhaup G, et al: Amyloid of neurofibrillary tangles of Guamanian parkinsonism-dementia and Alzheimer disease share identical amino acid sequence. Proc Natl Acad Sci U S A 84:2073–2077, 1987.

109. Gusella JF, Tanzi RE, Anderson MA, et al: DNA markers for nervous system diseases. In Abelson PH, Butz E, and Snyder SH (eds): Neuroscience. American Association for the Advancement of Science, Washington, DC, 1985, pp 184–196.

110. Gusella JF, Wexler NS, Conneally PM, et al: A polymorphic DNA marker genetically linked to Huntington's disease. Nature 306:234–238, 1983.

111. Haase GR: Diseases presenting as dementia. In Wells CE (ed): Dementia, Ed 2. FA Davis, Philadelphia, 1977, pp 27–67.

112. Hadlow WJ: Scrapie and kuru. Lancet 2:289–290, 1959.

113. Hadlow WJ, Race RE, Kennedy RC, and Eklund CM: Natural infection of sheep with scrapie virus. In Prusiner SB and Hadlow WJ (eds): Pathogenesis, Immunology, Virology, and Molecular Biology of the Spongiform Encephalopathies: Slow Transmissible Diseases of the Nervous System, Vol 2. Academic Press, New York, 1979, pp 3–12.

114. Hakim AM and Mathieson G: Dementia in Parkinson disease: A neuropathologic study. Neurology 29:1209–1214, 1979.

115. Hansen LA, DeTeresa R, Davies P, and Terry RD: Neocortical morphometry, lesion counts, and choline acetyltransferase levels in the age spectrum of Alzheimer's disease. Neurology 38:48–54, 1988.

116. Hardy J, Cowburn R, Barton A, et al: Region-specific loss of glutamate innervation in Alzheimer's disease. Neurosci Lett 73:77–80, 1987.

117. Hart MN, Merz P, Bennett-Gray J, et al: β-Amyloid protein of Alzheimer's disease is found in cerebral and spinal cord of vascular malformations. Am J Pathol 132:167–172, 1988.

118. Higgins GA, Lewis DA, Bahmanyar S, et al: Differential regulation of amyloid-β-protein mRNA expression within hippocampal neuronal subpopulations in Alzheimer disease. Proc Natl Acad Sci U S A 85:1297–1301, 1988.

119. Higgins GA and Mufson EJ: NGF receptor gene expression is decreased in the nucleus basalis in Alzheimer's disease. Exp Neurol 106:222–236, 1989.

120. Hogan RN, Baringer JR, and Prusiner SB: Scrapie infection diminishes spines and increases varicosities of dendrites in hamsters: A quantitative Golgi analysis. J Neuropathol Exp Neurol 46:461–473, 1987.

121. Hope J and Kimberlin RH: The molecular biology of scrapie: The last two years. Trends Neurosci 10:149–151, 1987.

122. Hornykiewicz O: Brain neurotransmitter changes in Parkinson's disease. In Marsden CD and Fahn S (eds): Movement Disorders, Neurology, Vol 2. Butterworth & Co, London, 1982, pp 41–58.

123. Hornykiewicz O and Kish SJ: Biochemical pathophysiology of Parkinson's disease. In Yahr MD and Bergmann KJ (eds): Parkinson's Disease. Advances in Neurology, Vol 45. Raven Press, New York, 1986, pp 19–34.

124. Hsiao K, Baker HF, Crow TJ, et al: Linkage of a prion protein missense variant to Gerstmann-Sträussler syndrome. Nature 338:342–345, 1989.

125. Hsiao KK, Cass C, Schellenberg GD, et al: A prion protein variant in a family with the telencephalic form of Gerstmann-Sträussler-Scheinker

syndrome. Neurology 41:681–684, 1991.

126. Hsiao KK, Meiner Z, Kahana E, et al: Mutation of the prion protein in Libyan Jews with Creutzfeldt-Jakob disease. N Engl J Med 324:1091–1097, 1991.

127. Hsaio KK and Prusiner SB: Inherited human prion diseases. Neurology 40:1820–1827, 1990.

128. Hsiao KK, Scott M, Foster D, Groth DF, DeArmond SJ, and Prusiner SB: Spontaneous neurodegeneration in transgenic mice with mutant prion protein. Science 250:1587–1590, 1990.

129. Hyman BT, Van Hoesen GW, Kromer LJ, and Damasio AR: Perforant pathway changes and the memory impairment of Alzheimer's disease. Ann Neurol 20:472–481, 1986.

130. Ishii T, Kametani F, Haga S, and Sato M: The immunohistochemical demonstration of subsequences of the precursor of the amyloid A4 protein in senile plaques in Alzheimer's disease. Neuropathol Appl Neurobiol 15:135–147, 1989.

131. Javitch JA, D'Amato RJ, Strittmatter SM, and Snyder SH: Parkinsonism-inducing neurotoxin, N-methyl-4-phenyl-1, 2, 3, 6-tetrahydropyridine: Uptake of the metabolite N-methyl-4-phenylpyridine by dopamine neurons explains selective toxicity. Proc Natl Acad Sci U S A 82:2173–2177, 1985.

132. Javoy-Agid F and Agid Y: Is the mesocortical dopaminergic system involved in Parkinson's disease? Neurology 30:1326–1330, 1980.

133. Jellinger K: Overview of morphological changes in Parkinson's disease. In Yahr MD and Bergmann KJ (eds): Parkinson's Disease. Advances in Neurology, Vol 45. Raven Press, New York, 1986, pp 1–18.

134. Joachim C, Games D, Morris J, Ward P, Frenkel D, and Selkoe D: Antibodies to non-beta regions of the beta-amyloid precursor protein detect a subset of senile plaques. Am J Pathol 138:373–384, 1991.

135. Joachim CL, Mori H, and Selkoe DJ: Amyloid β-protein deposition in tissues other than brain in Alzheimer's disease. Nature 341:226–230, 1989.

136. Joachim CL, Morris JH, and Selkoe DJ: Clinically diagnosed Alzheimer's disease: Autopsy results in 150 cases. Ann Neurol 24:50–56, 1988.

137. Joachim CL, Morris JH, and Selkoe DJ: Diffuse senile plaques occur commonly in the cerebellum in Alzheimer's disease. Am J Pathol 135:309–319, 1989.

138. Joachim CL, Morris JH, Selkoe DJ, and Kosik KS: Tau epitopes are incorporated into a range of lesions in Alzheimer's disease. J Neuropathol Exp Neurol 46:611–622, 1987.

139. Johnson SA, McNeill T, Cordell B, and Finch CE: Relation of neuronal APP-751/APP-695 mRNA ratio and neuritic plaque density in Alzheimer's disease. Science 248:854–857, 1990.

140. Johnson SA, Pasinetti GM, May PC, Ponte PA, Cordell B, and Finch CE: Selective reduction of mRNA for the β-amyloid-precursor protein that lacks a Kunitz-type protease inhibitor motif in cortex for Alzheimer brains. Exp Neurol 102:264–268, 1988.

140a. Kalaria RN and Andorn AC: Adrenergic receptors in aging and Alzheimer's disease: Decreased α-2 receptors demonstrated by [³H] p-aminoclonidine binding in prefrontal cortex. Neurobiol Aging 12:131–136, 1991.

140b. Kalaria RN, Andorn AC, Tabaton M, Whitehouse PJ, Harik SI, and Unnerstall JR: Adrenergic receptors in aging and Alzheimer's disease: Increased β-2 receptors in prefrontal cortex and hippocampus. J Neurochem 53:1772–1781, 1989.

141. Kang J, Lemaire H-G, Unterbeck A, et al: The precursor of Alzheimer's disease amyloid A4 protein resembles a cell-surface receptor. Nature 325:733–736, 1987.

142. Karp HR: Effects of aging. In Asbury AK, McKhann GM, and McDonald WI (eds): Diseases of the Nervous Sys-

tem, Vol 1. WB Saunders, Philadelphia, 1986, pp 736–745.

143. Kellar KJ, Whitehouse PJ, Martino-Barrows AM, Marcus K, and Price DL: Muscarinic and nicotinic cholinergic binding sites in Alzheimer's disease cerebral cortex. Brain Res 436:62–68, 1987.

144. Kemper TL: Organization of the neuropathology of the amygdala in Alzheimer's disease. Biological Aspects of Alzheimer's Disease. Banbury Report 15:31–35, 1983.

145. Kemper T: Neuroanatomical and neuropathological changes in normal aging and in dementia. In Albert ML (ed): Clinical Neurology of Aging. Oxford University Press, New York, 1984, pp 9–52.

146. Khachaturian ZS: Diagnosis of Alzheimer's disease. Arch Neurol 42: 1097–1105, 1985.

147. Kidd M: Alzheimer's disease—an electron microscopical study. Brain 897:307–320, 1964.

148. Kirschner DA, Inouye H, Duffy LK, Sinclair A, Lind M, and Selkoe DJ: Synthetic peptide homologous to β protein from Alzheimer disease forms amyloid-like fibrils in vitro. Proc Natl Acad Sci U S A 84:6953–6957, 1987.

149. Kitaguchi N, Takahashi Y, Tokushima Y, Shiojiri S, and Ito H: Novel precursor of Alzheimer's disease amyloid protein shows protease inhibitory activity. Nature 311:530–532, 1988.

150. Kitaguchi N, Tokushima Y, Oishi K, et al: Determination of amyloid β protein precursors harboring active form of proteinase inhibitor domains in cerebrospinal fluid of Alzheimer's disease patients by trypsin-antibody sandwich ELISA. Biochem Biophys Res Commun 166:1453–1459, 1990.

151. Kitamoto T, Tateishi J, and Sato Y: Immunohistochemical verification of senile and kuru plaques in Creutzfeldt-Jakob disease and the allied disease. Ann Neurol 24:537–542, 1988.

152. Kitamoto T, Tateishi J, Tashima T, et

al: Amyloid plaques in Creutzfeldt-Jakob disease stain with prion protein antibodies. Ann Neurol 20:204–208, 1986.

153. Kitt CA, Cork LC, Eidelberg E, Joh TH, and Price DL: Injury of nigral neurons exposed to 1-methyl-4-phenyl-1,2,3,6-tetrahydropyridine: A tyrosine hydroxylase immunocytochemical study in monkey. Neuroscience 17:1089–1103, 1986.

154. Kitt CA, Price DL, Struble RG, et al: Evidence for cholinergic neurites in senile plaques. Science 226:1443–1445, 1984.

155. Kitt CA, Struble RG, Cork LC, et al: Catecholaminergic neurites in senile plaques in prefrontal cortex of aged nonhuman primates. Neuroscience 16:691–699, 1985.

156. Kitt CA, Walker LC, Molliver ME, and Price DL: Serotonergic neurites in senile plaque of aged nonhuman primates. Anat Rec 211:98A, 1985.

157. Koliatsos VE, Applegate MD, Kitt CA, Walker LC, DeLong MR, and Price DL: Aberrant phosphorylation of neurofilaments accompanies transmitter-related changes in rat septal neurons following transection of the fimbria-fornix. Brain Res 482:205–218, 1989.

158. Koliatsos VE, Clatterbuck RE, Nauta HJW, et al: Human nerve growth factor prevents degeneration of basal forebrain cholinergic neurons in primates. Ann Neurol 30:831–840, 1991.

159. Koliatsos VE, Nauta HJW, Clatterbuck RE, Holtzman DM, Mobley WC, and Price DL: Mouse nerve growth factor prevents degeneration of axotomized basal forebrain cholinergic neurons in the monkey. J Neurosci 10:3801–3813, 1990.

160. König G, Salbaum JM, Wiestler O, et al: Alternative splicing of the β/A4 amyloid gene of Alzheimer's disease in cortex of control and Alzheimer's disease patients. Molecular Brain Research 9:259–262, 1991.

161. Koo EH, Sisodia SS, Archer DR, et al: Precursor of amyloid protein in Alzheimer disease undergoes fast ante-

rograde axonal transport. Proc Natl Acad Sci U S A 87:1561–1565, 1990.

162. Koo EH, Sisodia SS, Cork LC, Unterbeck A, Bayney RM, and Price DL: Differential expression of amyloid precursor protein mRNAs in cases of Alzheimer's disease and in aged nonhuman primates. Neuron 2:97–104, 1990.

163. Kopin IJ and Markey SP: MPTP toxicity: Implications for research in Parkinson's disease. Annu Rev Neurosci 11:81–96, 1988.

164. Kosik KS: The molecular and cellular pathology of Alzheimer neurofibrillary lesions. J Gerontol Biol Sci 44:B55–B58, 1989.

165. Kosik KS, Duffy LK, Dowling MM, Abraham C, McCluskey A, and Selkoe DJ: Microtubule-associated protein 2: Monoclonal antibodies demonstrate the selective incorporation of certain epitopes into Alzheimer neurofibrillary tangles. Proc Natl Acad Sci U S A 81:7941–7945, 1984.

166. Kosik KS, Joachim CL, and Selkoe DJ: Microtubule-associated protein (tau) is a major antigenic component of paired helical filaments in Alzheimer disease. Proc Natl Acad Sci U S A 83:4044–4048, 1986.

167. Kowall NW, Ferrante RJ, and Martin JB: Patterns of cell loss in Huntington's disease. Trends Neurosci 10:24–29, 1987.

168. Kowall NW and Kosik KS: Axonal disruption and aberrant localization of tau protein characterize the neuropil pathology of Alzheimer's disease. Ann Neurol 22:639–643, 1987

169. Kromer LF: Nerve growth factor treatment after brain injury prevents neuronal death. Science 235:214–216, 1987.

170. Ksiezak-Reding H, Binder LI, and Yen S-H: Immunochemical and biochemical characterization of proteins in normal and Alzheimer's disease brains with Alz 50 and Tau-1. J Biol Chem 263:7948–7953, 1988.

171. Kulmala HK: Immunocytochemical localization of enkephalin-like immunoreactivity in neurons of human hippocampal formation: Effects of aging and Alzheimer's disease. Neuropathol Appl Neurobiol 11:105–115, 1985a.

172. Kulmala HK: Some enkephalin- or VIP-immunoreactive hippocampal pyramidal cells contain neurofibrillary tangles in the brains of aged humans and persons with Alzheimer's disease. Neurochem Pathol 3:41–51, 1985b.

173. Lange H, Thorner G, Hopf A, and Schroder KF: Morphometric studies in the neuropathological changes in choreatic diseases. J Neurol Sci 28:401–425, 1976.

174. Lange HW: Quantitative changes of telencephalon, diencephalon, and parkinsonism. Vehr Anat Ges 75:923–925, 1981.

175. Langston JW: MPTP and Parkinson's disease. Trends Neurosci 8:79–83, 1985.

176. Langston JW, Forno LS, Rebert CS, and Irwin I: Selective nigral toxicity after systemic administration of 1-methyl-4-phenyl-1, 2, 5, 6-tetrahydropyrine (MPTP) in the squirrel monkey. Brain Res 292:390–394, 1984.

177. Langston JW, Irwin I, Langston EB, and Forno LS: 1-Methyl-4-phenylpyridinium ion (MPP+): Identification of a metabolite of MPTP, a toxin selective to the substantia nigra. Neurosci Lett 48:87–92, 1984.

178. Lee VM-Y, Balin BJ, Otvos L Jr, and Trojanowski JQ: A68: A major subunit of paired helical filaments and derivatized forms of normal tau. Science 251:675–678, 1991.

179. Levy E, Carman MD, Fernandez-Madrid IJ, et al: Mutation of the Alzheimer's disease amyloid gene in hereditary cerebral hemorrhage, Dutch type. Science 248:1124–1126, 1990.

180. Lewis DA, Higgins GA, Young WG, et al: Distribution of precursor amyloid-β-protein messenger RNA in human cerebral cortex: Relationship to neurofibrillary tangles and neuritic

plaques. Proc Natl Acad Sci U S A 85:1691–1695, 1988.

181. Lieberman A, Dziatolowsky M, Kupersmith M, et al: Dementia in Parkinson disease. Ann Neurol 6:355–359, 1979.

182. Mann DMA, Yates PO, and Marcyniuk B: Some morphometric observations on the cerebral cortex and hippocampus in presenile Alzheimer's disease, senile dementia of Alzheimer type and Down's syndrome in middle age. J Neurol Sci 69:139–159, 1985.

183. Manuelidis L, Sklaviadis T, and Manuelidis EE: Evidence suggesting that PrP is not the infectious agent in Creutzfeldt-Jakob disease. EMBO J 6:341–347, 1987.

184. Marsden CD: Neurotransmitters and CNS disease. Lancet 2:1141–1146, 1982.

185. Martin JB: Huntington's disease: New approaches to an old problem. Neurology 34:1059–1072, 1984.

186. Martin JB: Molecular genetics: Applications to the clinical neurosciences. Science 238:765–772, 1987.

187. Martin JB and Gusella JF: Huntington's disease. Pathogenesis and management. N Engl J Med 315:1267–1276, 1986.

188. Martin LJ, Cork LC, Koo EH, et al: Localization of amyloid precursor protein (APP) in brains of young and aged monkeys. Society for Neuroscience Abstracts 15:23, 1989.

189. Martin LJ, Sisodia SS, Koo EH, et al: Amyloid precursor protein in aged nonhuman primates. Proc Natl Acad Sci U S A 88:1461–1465, 1991.

190. Mash DC, Flynn DD, and Potter LT: Loss of M2 muscarine receptors in the cerebral cortex in Alzheimer's disease and experimental cholinergic denervation. Science 228:1115–1117, 1985.

191. Masters CL and Gajdusek DC: The spectrum of Creutzfeldt-Jakob disease and the virus-induced subacute spongiform encephalopathies. In Smith WT and Cavanagh JB (eds): Recent Advances in Neurology, Vol 2.

Churchill Livingstone, Edinburgh, 1982, pp 139–163.

192. Masters CL, Multhaup G, Simms G, Pottgiesser J, Martins RN, and Beyreuther K: Neuronal origin of a cerebral amyloid: Neurofibrillary tangles of Alzheimer's disease contain the same protein as the amyloid of plaque cores and blood vessels. EMBO J 4:2757–2763, 1985.

193. Masters CL and Richardson EP Jr: Subacute spongiform encephalopathy (Creutzfeldt-Jakob disease). The nature and progression of spongiform change. Brain 101:333–344, 1978.

194. Masters CL, Simms G, Weinman NA, Multhaup G, McDonald BL, and Beyreuther K: Amyloid plaque core protein in Alzheimer disease and Down Syndrome. Proc Natl Acad Sci U S A 82:4245–4249, 1985.

195. Mayeux R: Depression and dementia in Parkinson's disease. In Marsden CD and Fahn S (eds): Movement Disorders, Neurology, Vol 2. Butterworth & Co, London, 1982, pp 75–95.

196. Mayeux R and Stern Y: Intellectual dysfunction and dementia in Parkinson disease. In Mayeux R and Rosen WG (eds): The Dementias. Advances in Neurology, Vol 38. Raven Press, New York, 1983, pp 211–227.

197. Mayeux R, Stern Y, and Spanton S: Heterogeneity in dementia of the Alzheimer type: Evidence of subgroups. Neurology 35:453–461, 1985.

198. McKee AC, Kosik KS, and Kowall NW: Dystrophic neurites in the neocortex are the critical neuropathological correlate of dementia in Alzheimer's disease. J Neuropathol Exp Neurol 49:649, 1990.

199. McKhann G, Drachman D, Folstein M, Katzman R, Price D, and Stadlan EM: Clinical diagnosis of Alzheimer's disease: Report of the NINCDS-ADRDA Work Group under the auspices of Department of Health and Human Services Task Force on Alzheimer's Disease. Neurology 34:939–944, 1984.

200. Merz PA, Rohwer RG, Kascsak R, et

al: Infection-specific particle from the unconventional slow virus diseases. Science 225:437–440, 1984.

201. Merz PA, Somerville RA, Wisniewski HM, and Iqbal K: Abnormal fibrils from scrapie-infected brain. Acta Neuropathol (Berl) 54:63–74, 1981.

202. Merz PA, Somerville RA, Wisniewski HM, Manuelidis L, and Manuelidis EE: Scrapie-associated fibrils in Creutzfeldt-Jakob disease. Nature 306:474–476, 1983.

203. Meyer RK, McKinley MP, Bowman KA, Braunfeld MB, Barry RA, and Prusiner SB: Separation and properties of cellular and scrapie prion proteins. Proc Natl Acad Sci U S A 83:2310–2314, 1986.

204. Miyakawa T, Katsuragi S, Watanabe K, Shimoji A, and Ikeuchi Y: Ultrastructural studies of amyloid fibrils and senile plaques in human brain. Acta Neuropathol (Berl) 70:202–208, 1986.

205. Miyakawa T, Shimoji A, Kuramoto R, and Higuchi Y: The relationship between senile plaques and cerebral blood vessels in Alzheimer's disease and senile dementia. Morphological mechanism of senile plaque production. Virchows Arch [B] 40:121–129, 1982.

206. Mortimer JA, Pirozzolo FJ, Hansch EC, and Webster DD: Relationship of motor symptoms to intellectual deficits in Parkinson disease. Neurology 32:133–137, 1982.

207. Mountjoy CQ, Roth M, Evans NJR, and Evans HM: Cortical neuronal counts in normal elderly controls and demented patients. Neurobiol Aging 4:1–11, 1983.

208. Müller-Hill B and Beyreuther K: Molecular biology of Alzheimer's disease. Annu Rev Biochem 58:287–307, 1989.

209. Nakano I and Hirano A: Parkinson's disease: Neuron loss in the nucleus basalis without concomitant Alzheimer's disease. Ann Neurol 15:415–418, 1984.

210. Naruse S, Igarashi S, Aoki K, et al: Mis-sense mutation Val-Ile in exon 17 of amyloid precursor protein gene in Japanese familial Alzheimer's disease. Lancet 337:978–979, 1991.

211. Neve RL, Finch EA, and Dawes LR: Expression of the Alzheimer amyloid precursor gene transcripts in the human brain. Neuron 1:669–677, 1988.

212. Neve RL, Rogers J, and Higgins GA: The Alzheimer amyloid precursor-related transcript lacking the β/A4 sequence is specifically increased in Alzheimer's disease brain. Neuron 5:329–338, 1990.

213. Nochlin D, Sumi SM, Bird TD, et al: Familial dementia with PrP-positive amyloid plaques: A variant of Gerstmann-Sträussler syndrome. Neurology 39:910–918, 1989.

214. Oesch B, Westaway D, Wälchli M, et al: A cellular gene encodes scrapie PrP 27-30 protein. Cell 40:735–746, 1985.

215. Ogomori K, Kitamoto T, Tateishi J, Sato Y, Suetsugu M, and Abe M: β-Protein amyloid is widely distributed in the central nervous system of patients with Alzheimer's disease. Am J Pathol 134:243–251, 1989.

216. Oltersdorf T, Fritz LC, Schenk DB, et al: The secreted form of the Alzheimer's amyloid precursor protein with the Kunitz domain is protease nexin-II. Nature 341:144–147, 1989.

217. Owen F, Poulter M, Lofthouse R, et al: Insertion in prion protein gene in familial Creutzfeldt-Jakob disease. Lancet 1:51–52, 1989.

218. Palacios JM and Kuhar MJ: Neurotensin receptors are located on dopamine-containing neurones in rat midbrain. Nature 294:587–589, 1981.

219. Palmert MR, Golde TE, Cohen ML, et al: Amyloid protein precursor messenger RNAs: Differential expression in Alzheimer's disease. Science 241:1080–1084, 1988.

220. Palmert MR, Podlisny MB, Witker DS, et al: The β-amyloid protein precursor of Alzheimer disease has soluble derivatives found in human brain and cerebrospinal fluid. Proc Natl

Acad Sci U S A 86:6338–6342, 1989.

221. Palmert MR, Usiak M, Mayeux R, Raskind M, Tourtellotte WW, and Younkin SG: Soluble derivatives of the β-amyloid protein precursor in cerebrospinal fluid: Alterations in normal aging and in Alzheimer's disease. Neurology 40:1028–1034, 1990.

222. Parson B and Rainbow TC: High-affinity binding sites for [³H]MPTP may correspond to monamine oxidase. Eur J Pharmacol 102:375–377, 1984.

223. Pearson RCA, Esiri MM, Hiorns RW, Wilcock GK, and Powell TPS: Anatomical correlates of the distribution of the pathological changes in the neocortex in Alzheimer disease. Proc Natl Acad Sci U S A 82:4531–4534, 1985.

224. Penney JB Jr and Young AB: Speculations on the functional anatomy of basal ganglia disorders. Annu Rev Neurosci 6:73–94, 1983.

225. Perry EK: The cholinergic hypothesis —ten years on. Br Med Bull 42:63–69, 1986.

226. Perry EK, Tomlinson BE, Blessed G, et al: Neuropathological and biochemical observations on the noradrenergic system in Alzheimer's disease. J Neurol Sci 51:279–287, 1981.

227. Perry G, Friedman R, Shaw G, and Chau V: Ubiquitin is detected in neurofibrillary tangles and senile plaque neurites of Alzheimer disease brains. Proc Natl Acad Sci U S A 84:3033–3036, 1987.

228. Perry G, Lipphardt S, Kancherla M, et al: Amyloid precursor protein in senile plaques of Alzheimer's disease. Lancet 2:746, 1988.

229. Perry G, Mulvihill P, Manetto V, Autilio-Gambetti L, and Gambetti P: Immunocytochemical properties of Alzheimer straight filaments. J Neurosci 7:3736–3738, 1987.

230. Perry G, Rizzuto N, Autilio-Gambetti L, and Gambetti P: Paired helical filaments from Alzheimer disease patients contain cytoskeletal compo-

nents. Proc Natl Acad Sci U S A 82:3916–3920, 1985.

231. Phelps CH, Gage FH, Growdon JH, et al: (Ad hoc working group on nerve growth factor and Alzheimer's disease): Potential use of nerve growth factor to treat Alzheimer's disease. Science 243:11, 1989.

232. Phelps CH, Gage FH, Growdon JH, et al: Potential use of nerve growth factor to treat Alzheimer's disease. Neurobiol Aging 10:205–207, 1989.

233. Podlisny MB, Gronbeck A, Tolan D, Oltersdorf T, and Selkoe D: Studies of the processing of β-amyloid precursor protein (β-APP) in human, monkey and rodent brain and in cDNA-transfected cells. J Neuropathol Exp Neurol 48:353, 1989.

234. Podlisny MB, Lee G, and Selkoe DJ: Gene dosage of the amyloid β precursor protein in Alzheimer's disease. Science 238:669–671, 1987.

235. Ponte P, Gonzalez-DeWhitt P, Schilling J, et al: A new A4 amyloid mRNA contains a domain homologous to serine proteinase inhibitors. Nature 331: 525–527, 1988.

236. Presty SK, Bachevalier J, Walker LC, et al: Age differences in recognition memory of the rhesus monkey (Macaca mulatta). Neurobiol Aging 8: 435–440, 1987.

237. Price DL, Altschuler RJ, Struble RG, Casanova MF, Cork LC, and Murphy DB: Sequestration of tubulin in neurons in Alzheimer's disease. Brain Res 385:305–310, 1986.

238. Prior R, Mönning U, Schreiter-Gasser U, et al: Quantitative changes in the amyloid β/A4 precursor protein in Alzheimer cerebrospinal fluid. Neurosci Lett 124:69–73, 1991.

239. Prusiner SB and DeArmond SJ: Biology of disease. Prions causing nervous system degeneration. Lab Invest 56: 349–363, 1987.

240. Prusiner SB, Groth DF, Bolton DC, Kent SB, and Hood LE: Purification and structural studies of a major scrapie prion protein. Cell 38:127–134, 1984.

241. Prusiner SB, McKinley MP, Bowman KA, et al: Scrapie prions aggregate to form amyloid-like birefringent rods. Cell 35:349–358, 1983.

242. Quinn NP, Rossor MJ, and Marsden CD: Dementia and Parkinson's disease—pathological and neurochemical considerations. Br Med Bull 42:86–90, 1986.

243. Rafalowska J, Barcikowska M, Wen GY, and Wisniewski HM: Laminar distribution of neuritic plaques in normal aging, Alzheimer's disease and Down's syndrome. Acta Neuropathol (Berl) 77:21–25, 1988.

244. Reiner A, Albin RL, Anderson KD, D'Amato CJ, Penney JB, and Young AB: Differential loss of striatal projection neurons in Huntington disease. Proc Natl Acad Sci U S A 85:5733–5737, 1988.

245. Riederer P and Wuketich St: Time course of nigrostriatal degeneration in Parkinson's disease. A detailed study of influential factors in human brain amine analysis. J Neural Transm Park Dis Dement Sect 38:277–301, 1976.

246. Robakis NK, Sawh PR, Wolfe GC, Rubenstein R, Carp RI, and Innis MA: Isolation of a cDNA clone encoding the leader peptide of prion protein and expression of the homologous gene in various tissues. Proc Natl Acad Sci U S A 83:6377–6381, 1986.

247. Roberts GW, Crow TJ, and Polak JM: Location of neuronal tangles in somatostatin neurones in Alzheimer's disease. Nature 314:92–94, 1985.

248. Roberts GW, Lofthouse R, Allsop D, et al: CNS amyloid proteins in neurodegenerative diseases. Neurology 38:1534–1540, 1988.

249. Robinson MB and Coyle JT: Glutamate and related acidic excitatory neurotransmitters: From basic science to clinical application. FASEB J 1:446–455, 1987.

250. Roher AE, Palmer KC, Chau V, and Ball MJ: Isolation and chemical characterization of Alzheimer's disease paired helical filament cytoskeletons: Differentiation from amyloid plaque core protein. J Cell Biol 107:2703–2716, 1988.

251. Roos R, Gajdusek DC, and Gibbs CJ Jr: The clinical characteristics of transmissible Creutzfeldt-Jakob disease. Brain 96:1–20, 1973.

252. Rossor MN, Emson PC, Mountjoy CQ, Roth M, and Iversen LL: Reduced amounts of immunoreactive somatostatin in the temporal cortex in senile dementia of Alzheimer type. Neurosci Lett 20:373–377, 1980.

253. Rossor MN and Iversen LL: Non-cholinergic neurotransmitter abnormalities in Alzheimer's disease. Br Med Bull 42:70–74, 1986.

254. Ruberg M, Ploska A, Javoy-Agid F, and Agid Y: Muscarinic binding and choline acetyltransferase activity in parkinsonian subjects with reference to dementia. Brain Res 232:129–139, 1982.

255. St George-Hyslop PH, Tanzi RE, Polinsky RJ, et al: Absence of duplication of chromosome 21 genes in familial and sporadic Alzheimer's disease. Science 238:664–666, 1987.

256. Saitoh T, Sundsmo M, Roch J-M, et al: Secreted form of amyloid β protein precursor is involved in the growth regulation of fibroblasts. Cell 58:615–622, 1989.

257. Scatton B, Javoy-Agid F, Rouquier L, Dubois B, and Agid Y: Reduction of cortical dopamine, noradrenaline, serotonin and their metabolites in Parkinson's disease. Brain Res 275:321–328, 1983.

258. Schatteman GC, Gibbs L, Lanahan AA, Claude P, and Bothwell M: Expression of NGF receptor in the developing and adult primate central nervous system. J Neurosci 8:860–873, 1988.

259. Schubert D, LaCorbiere M, Saitoh T, and Cole G: Characterization of an amyloid β precursor protein that binds heparin and contains tyrosine sulfate. Proc Natl Acad Sci U S A 86:2066–2069, 1989.

260. Schwarcz R, Okuno E, White RJ, Bird ED, and Whetsell WO Jr: 3-Hydroxyanthranilate oxygenase activ-

ity is increased in the brains of Huntington disease victims. Proc Natl Acad Sci U S A 85:4079–4081, 1988.

261. Scott M, Foster D, Mirenda C, et al: Transgenic mice expressing hamster prion protein produce species-specific scrapie infectivity and amyloid plaques. Cell 59:847–857, 1989.

262. Seiler M and Schwab ME: Specific retrograde transport of nerve growth factor (NGF) from neocortex to nucleus basalis in the rat. Brain Res 300:33–39, 1984.

263. Selkoe DJ: Biochemistry of altered brain proteins in Alzheimer's disease. Annu Rev Neurosci 12:463–490, 1989.

264. Selkoe DJ: Molecular pathology of amyloidogenic proteins and the role of vascular amyloidosis in Alzheimer's disease. Neurobiol Aging 10:387–395, 1989.

265. Selkoe DJ, Bell DS, Podlisny MB, Price DL, and Cork LC: Conservation of brain amyloid proteins in aged mammals and humans with Alzheimer's disease. Science 235:873–877, 1987.

266. Serban D, Taraboulos A, DeArmond SJ, and Prusiner SB: Rapid detection of Creutzfeldt-Jakob disease and scrapie prion proteins. Neurology 40:110–117, 1990.

267. Shelton DL and Reichardt LF: Studies on the expression of the nerve growth factor (NGF) gene in the central nervous system: Level and regional distribution of NGF mRNA suggest that NGF functions as a trophic factor for several distinct populations of neurons. Proc Natl Acad Sci U S A 83:2714–2718, 1986.

268. Sisodia SS, Koo EH, Beyreuther K, Unterbeck A, and Price DL: Evidence that β-amyloid protein in Alzheimer's disease is not derived by normal processing. Science 248:492–495, 1990.

269. Smith CJ, Perry EK, Perry RH, Fairbairn AF, and Birdsall NJM: Guanine nucleotide modulation of muscarinic cholinergic receptor binding in postmortem human brain—a prelimi-

nary study in Alzheimer's disease. Neurosci Lett 92:227–232, 1987.

270. Snow AD, Willmer JP, and Kisilevsky R: Sulfated glycosaminoglycans in Alzheimer's disease. Hum Pathol 18: 506–510, 1987.

271. Snyder SH and D'Amato RJ: MPTP: A neurotoxin relevant to the pathophysiology of Parkinson's disease. The 1985 George C Cotzias Lecture. Neurology 36:250–258, 1986.

272. Struble RG, Cork LC, Whitehouse PJ, and Price DL: Cholinergic innervation in neuritic plaques. Science 216:413–415, 1982.

273. Struble RG, Hedreen JC, Cork LC, and Price DL: Acetylcholinesterase activity in senile plaques of aged macaques. Neurobiol Aging 5:191–198, 1984.

274. Struble RG, Lehmann J, Mitchell SJ, et al: Basal forebrain neurons provide major cholinergic innervation of primate neocortex. Neurosci Lett 66: 215–220, 1986.

275. Struble RG, Powers RE, Casanova MF, Kitt CA, Brown EC, and Price DL: Neuropeptidergic systems in plaques of Alzheimer's disease. J Neuropathol Exp Neurol 46:567–584, 1987.

276. Struble RG, Price RL Jr, Cork LC, and Price DL: Senile plaques in cortex of aged normal monkeys. Brain Res 361:267–275, 1985.

277. Tagliavini F, Giaccone G, Frangione B, and Bugiani O: Preamyloid deposits in the cerebral cortex of patients with Alzheimer's disease and nondemented individuals. Neurosci Lett 93:191–196, 1988.

278. Taniuchi M, Schweitzer JB, and Johnson EM Jr: Nerve growth factor receptor molecules in rat brain. Proc Natl Acad Sci U S A 83:1950–1954, 1986.

279. Tanzi RE, Bird ED, Latt SA, and Neve RL: The amyloid β protein gene is not duplicated in brains from patients with Alzheimer's disease. Science 238:666–669, 1987.

280. Tanzi RE, Gusella JF, Watkins PC, et al: Amyloid β protein gene: cDNA, mRNA distribution, and genetic link-

age near the Alzheimer locus. Science 235:880–884, 1987.

281. Tanzi RE, McClatchey AI, Lampert ED, Villa-Komaroff L, Gusella JF, and Neve RL: Protease inhibitor domain encoded by an amyloid protein precursor mRNA associated with Alzheimer's disease. Nature 311: 528–530, 1988.

282. Terry RD, DeTeresa R, and Hansen LA: Neocortical cell counts in normal human adult aging. Ann Neurol 21:530–539, 1987.

283. Terry RD, Gonatas NK, and Weiss M: Ultrastructural studies in Alzheimer's presenile dementia. Am J Pathol 44:269–297, 1964.

284. Terry RD, Peck A, DeTeresa R, Schechter R, and Horoupian DS: Some morphometric aspects of the brain in senile dementia of the Alzheimer type. Ann Neurol 10:184–192, 1981.

285. Tetrud JW and Langston JW: The effect of deprenyl (Selegiline) on the natural history of Parkinson's disease. Science 245:519–522, 1989.

286. Tomlinson BE: The pathology of dementia. In Wells CE (ed): Dementia, Ed 2. FA Davis, Philadelphia, 1977, pp 113–153.

287. Tomlinson BE: The neuropathology of Alzheimer's disease—issues in need of resolution. Second Dorothy S Russell Memorial Lecture. Neuropathol Appl Neurobiol 15:491–512, 1989.

288. Tomlinson BE, Blessed G, and Roth M: Observations on the brains of non-demented old people. J Neurol Sci 7:331–356, 1968.

289. Tomlinson BE and Corsellis JAN: Aging and the dementias. In Adams JH, Corsellis JAN, and Duchen LW (eds): Greenfield's Neuropathology, Ed 4. John Wiley & Sons, New York, 1984, pp 951–1025.

290. Tomlinson BE, Irving D, and Blessed G: Cell loss in the locus coeruleus in senile dementia of Alzheimer type. J Neurol Sci 49:419–428, 1981.

291. Tuszynski MH, U HS, Amaral DG, and Gage FH: Nerve growth factor infusion in the primate brain reduces lesion-induced cholinergic neuronal degeneration. J Neurosci 10:3604–3614, 1990.

292. Uhl GR, Hackney GO, Javitch J, et al: Receptors in substantia nigra in normal humans and persons with Parkinson's disease. Ann Neurol 16: 128, 1984.

293. Uhl GR, Hedreen JC, and Price DL: Parkinson's disease: Loss of neurons from the ventral tegmental area contralateral to therapeutic surgical lesions. Neurology 35:1215–1218, 1985.

294. Van Hoesen GW and Damasio AR: Neural correlates of cognitive impairment in Alzheimer's disease. In Mountcastle VB (ed): Handbook of Physiology, Section 1: The Nervous System, Vol V, Higher Functions of the Brain, Part 2. American Physiological Society, Bethesda, MD, 1987, pp 871–898.

295. Van Nostrand WE, Wagner SL, Suzuki M, et al: Protease nexin-II, a potent antichymotrypsin, shows identity to amyloid β-protein precursor. Nature 341:546–549, 1989

296. Vinters HV: Cerebral amyloid angiopathy. A critical review. Stroke 18:311–324, 1987.

297. Vonsattel J-P, Myers RH, Stevens TJ, Ferrante RJ, Bird ED, and Richardson EP Jr: Neuropathological classification of Huntington's disease. J Neuropathol Exp Neurol 44: 559–577, 1985.

298. Wagster MV, Whitehouse PJ, Walker LC, Kellar KJ, and Price DL: Laminar organization and age-related loss of cholinergic receptors in temporal neocortex of rhesus monkey. J Neurosci 10:2879–2885, 1990.

299. Walker LC, Kitt CA, Cork LC, Struble RG, Dellovade TL, and Price DL: Multiple transmitter systems contribute neurites to individual senile plaques. J Neuropathol Exp Neurol 47:138–144, 1988.

300. Walker LC, Kitt CA, Schwam E, et al: Senile plaques in aged squirrel monkeys. Neurobiol Aging 8:291–296, 1987.

301. Walker LC, Kitt CA, Struble RG, et al:

Glutamic acid decarboxylase-like immunoreactive neurites in senile plaques. Neurosci Lett 59:165–169, 1985.

302. Walker LC, Kitt CA, Struble RG, Wagster MV, Price DL, and Cork LC: The neural basis of memory decline in aged monkeys. Neurobiol Aging 9:657–666, 1988.

303. Walker LC, Koliatsos VE, Kitt CA, Richardson RT, Rökaeus Å, and Price DL: Peptidergic neurons in the basal forebrain magnocellular complex of the rhesus monkey. J Comp Neurol 280:272–282, 1989.

304. Warren AC, Robakis NK, Ramakrishna N, et al: β-Amyloid gene is not present in three copies in autopsy-validated Alzheimer's disease. Genomics 1:307–312, 1987.

305. Weidemann A, König G, Bunke D, et al: Identification, biogenesis, and localization of precursors of Alzheimer's disease A4 amyloid protein. Cell 57:115–126, 1989.

306. Wenk GL, Pierce DJ, Struble RG, Price DL, and Cork LC: Age-related changes in multiple neurotransmitter systems in the monkey brain. Neurobiol Aging 10:11–19, 1989.

307. Westaway D, Carlson GA, and Prusiner SB: Unraveling prion diseases through molecular genetics. Trends Neurosci 12:221–227, 1989.

308. Westaway D, Goodman PA, Mirenda CA, McKinley MP, Carlson GA, and Prusiner SB: Distinct prion proteins in short and long scrapie incubation period mice. Cell 51:651–662, 1987.

309. Wexler NS, Conneally PM, Housman D, and Gusella JF: A DNA polymorphism for Huntington's disease marks the future. Arch Neurol 42:20–24, 1985.

310. Whitehouse PJ, Hedreen JC, White CL III, and Price DL: Basal forebrain neurons in the dementia of Parkinson's disease. Ann Neurol 13:243–248, 1983.

311. Whitehouse PJ, Martino AM, Antuono PG, et al: Nicotinic acetycholine binding sites in Alzheimer's disease. Brain Res 371:146–151, 1986.

312. Whitehouse PJ, Martino AM, Wagster MV, et al: Reductions in [³H]nicotinic acetylcholine binding in Alzheimer's disease and Parkinson's disease: An autoradiographic study. Neurology 38:720–723, 1988.

313. Whitehouse PJ, Price DL, Struble RG, Clark AW, Coyle JT, and DeLong MR: Alzheimer's disease and senile dementia: Loss of neurons in the basal forebrain. Science 215:1237–1239, 1982.

314. Whitehouse PJ, Trifiletti RR, Jones BE, et al: Neurotransmitter receptor alterations in Huntington's disease: Autoradiographic and homogenate studies with special reference to benzodiazepine receptor complexes. Ann Neurol 18:202–210, 1985.

315. Whitehouse PJ, Vale WW, Zweig RM, et al: Reductions in corticotropin releasing factor–like immunoreactivity in cerebral cortex in Alzheimer's disease, Parkinson's disease, and progressive supranuclear palsy. Neurology 37:905–909, 1987.

316. Whitson JS, Selkoe DJ, and Cotman CW: Amyloid β protein enhances the survival of hippocampal neurons in vitro. Science 243:1488–1490, 1989.

317. Whittemore SR, Ebendal T, Lärkfors L, et al: Developmental and regional expression of nerve growth factor messenger RNA and protein in the rat central nervous system. Proc Natl Acad Sci U S A 83:817–821, 1986.

318. Will B and Hefti F: Behavioural and neurochemical effects of chronic intraventricular injections of nerve growth factor in adult rats with fimbria lesions. Behav Brain Res 17:17–24, 1985.

319. Wischik CM, Novak M, Edwards PC, Klug A, Tichelaar W, and Crowther RA: Structural characterization of the core of the paired helical filament of Alzheimer disease. Proc Natl Acad Sci U S A 85:4884–4888, 1988.

320. Wischik CM, Novak M, Thogersen HC, et al: Isolation of a fragment of tau derived from the core of the paired helical filament of Alzheimer disease. Proc Natl Acad Sci U S A 85:4506–4510, 1988.

321. Wisniewski HM, Moretz RC, and Lossinsky AS: Evidence for induction of localized amyloid deposits and neuritic plaques by an infectious agent. Ann Neurol 10:517–522, 1981.

322. Wisniewski HM, Narang HK, and Terry RD: Neurofibrillary tangles of paired helical filaments. J Neurol Sci 27:173–181, 1976.

323. Wisniewski HM and Terry RD: Reexamination of the pathogenesis of the senile plaque. In Zimmerman HM (ed): Progress in Neuropathology, Vol II. Grune & Stratton, New York, 1973, pp 1–26.

324. Wisniewski HM, Wen GY, and Kim KS: Comparison of four staining methods on the detection of neuritic plaques. Acta Neuropathol (Berl) 78:22–27, 1989.

325. Wisniewski K, Jervis GA, Moretz RC, and Wisniewski HM: Alzheimer neurofibrillary tangles in diseases other than senile and presenile dementia. Ann Neurol 5:288–294, 1979.

326. Wolozin BL and Davies P: Alzheimer-related neuronal protein A68: Specificity and distribution. Ann Neurol 22:521–526, 1987.

327. Wolozin BL, Pruchnicki A, Dickson DW, and Davies P: A neuronal antigen in the brains of Alzheimer patients. Science 232:648–650, 1986.

328. Yamaguchi H, Hirai S, Morimatsu M, Shoji M, and Harigaya Y: Diffuse type of senile plaques in the brains of Alzheimer-type dementia. Acta Neuropathol (Berl) 77:113–119, 1988.

329. Yamaguchi H, Nakazato Y, Hirai S, and Shoji M: Immunoelectron microscopic localization of amyloid β protein in the diffuse plaques of Alzheimer-type dementia. Brain Res 508:320–324, 1990.

330. Yamaguchi H, Nakazato Y, Hirai S, Shoji M, and Harigaya Y: Electron micrograph of diffuse plaques. Initial stage of senile plaque formation in the Alzheimer brain. Am J Pathol 135:593–597, 1989.

331. Yates CM, Simpson J, Gordon A, et al: Catecholamines and cholinergic enzymes in pre-senile and senile Alzheimer-type dementia and Down's syndrome. Brain Res 280:119–126, 1983.

332. Young AB, Greenamyre JT, Hollingsworth Z, et al: NMDA receptor losses in putamen from patients with Huntington's disease. Science 241:981–983, 1988.

333. Zetusky WJ, Jankovic J, and Pirozzolo FJ: The heterogeneity of Parkinson's disease: Clinical and Prognostic implications. Neurology 35:522–526, 1985.

334. Zubenko GS and Moossy J: Major depression in primary dementia: Clinical and neuropathologic correlates. Arch Neurol 45:1182–1186, 1988.

335. Zweig RM, Jankel WR, Hedreen JC, Mayeux R, and Price DL: The pedunculopontine nucleus in Parkinson's disease. Ann Neurol 26:41–46, 1989.

336. Zweig RM, Ross CA, Hedreen JC, et al: The neuropathology of aminergic nuclei in Alzheimer's disease. Ann Neurol 24:233–242, 1988.

Chapter 4

THE CLINICAL EVALUATION OF PATIENTS WITH DEMENTIA

*Richard Mayeux, M.D.,
Norman L. Foster, M.D.,
Martin Rossor, M.D., and
Peter J. Whitehouse, M.D.,
Ph.D.*

**DIAGNOSTIC CRITERIA
DEMENTIA AND AGING
ELEMENTS OF THE CLINICAL
EVALUATION**

The diagnosis and evaluation of patients with dementia is a major concern for many professionals, particularly neurologists. In 1982 in the United States, Kurtzke[133] showed that one out of every 50 neurologic consultations was for the assessment of dementia, and that a neurologist might expect to see one patient with dementia for every two patients with stroke. In the future, physicians will be evaluating and caring for more patients with dementia, because the world population is aging and both the prevalence and incidence of dementia rise dramatically with age. For example, in the United States, early studies showed that dementia affects 5% to 10% of those over age 60, but more than 20% of those over age 80.[124,125,191] A more recent epidemiologic study in East Boston demonstrated that almost 50% of those over age 85 were demented.[65] The number of younger people with dementia will also rise as a consequence of infection with the human immunodeficiency virus.[42] (See Chapters 1 and 8.)

Although dementia has a number of causes, as listed in Table 4–1, the most common cause, by far, is Alzheimer's disease (AD), which accounts for at least 70% of the patients identified in community, hospital, or clinic surveys of dementia.[124,125,150,205] Multi-infarct dementia (MID) and mixed AD/MID cause dementia in another large proportion (20%) of elderly patients. An additional 5% to 10% of patients have potentially "reversible" causes, such as hypothyroidism.

Determining the cause of dementia requires not only a history and physical examination, but also laboratory screening tests for potentially reversible disorders that cause dementia. Such screening tests include blood tests and structural brain imaging, that is, computed tomography (CT) or magnetic resonance imaging (MRI). The clinical use of neuropsychologic tests has increased, and new diagnostic methods that include computerized neurophysiologic techniques, such as electroencephalogram (EEG) spectral analysis, and functional brain imaging studies, are under development. In this era of

Table 4 – 1 CONDITIONS CAUSING DEMENTIA

DEGENERATIVE DISORDERS OF THE CENTRAL NERVOUS SYSTEM (Chapter 6)

Alzheimer's disease
Pick's disease
Huntington's disease
Parkinson's disease
Progressive supranuclear palsy
Hallervorden-Spatz syndrome
Spinocerebellar degenerations
Progressive myoclonic epilepsy
Progressive subcortical gliosis
Amyotrophic lateral sclerosis (ALS)
ALS-parkinsonism-dementia complex
Frontal lobe degeneration of the non-Alzheimer type

METABOLIC ENDOCRINE DISORDERS (Chapter 10)

Hypothyroidism
Wilson's disease
Hepatic encephalopathy
Prolonged hypoglycemia
Hypoxia
Cushing's syndrome
Hypopituitarism
Uremia

CEREBROVASCULAR DISEASE (Chapter 7)

Multiple cortical strokes
Multiple subcortical strokes (lacunar state)
Cortical and subcortical strokes
Binswanger's multifocal leukoencephalopathy
(Multiple etiologies, see Table 4 – 2)

DEFICIENCY DISORDERS (Chapter 10)

Alcohol-related syndromes
Pellagra
Marchiafava-Bignami disease
Combined systems disease or B_{12} deficiency

TOXINS/DRUGS (Chapter 10)

Heavy metals
Carbon monoxide
Medication

BRAIN TUMORS (Chapter 11)

Direct effect
Paraneoplastic effects

TRAUMA (Chapter 11)

Sequelae of both open and closed head injury

INFECTIONS (Chapters 8, 9)

Brain abscess
Bacterial, fungal, tuberculosis, and other forms of meningitis
Postviral encephalitic syndromes
Progressive multifocal leukoencephalopathy
Behçet's syndrome
Syphilis
Human immunodeficiency virus

PRION DISEASES (Chapter 8)

Creutzfeldt-Jakob disease
Gerstmann-Sträussler syndrome
Kuru

(continued)

Table 4 – 1 — *Continued*

PSYCHIATRIC SYNDROMES (Chapter 12)

Affective disorders
Schizophrenic disorders
Hysterical disorders

OTHER (Chapters 6, 11)

Multiple sclerosis
Muscular dystrophy
Whipple's disease
Storage diseases, such as Kufs' disease
Obstructive hydrocephalus (referred to later in the text)
Normal pressure hydrocephalus (referred to later in the text)
Sequela of subarachnoid hemorrhage, intracerebral hemorrhage (or intracranial hemorrhage)
Electrical injury
Hereditary dysphasic dementia (referred to later in the text)

escalating medical costs, however, the cost-effectiveness of these new approaches, as well as that of the standard diagnostic workup, has been questioned.[136,137]

The intent of this chapter is to guide the clinician through the differential diagnosis of dementia. We will discuss current clinical criteria and methods used to establish the diagnosis of some specific forms of dementia.

DIAGNOSTIC CRITERIA

According to the revised, third edition of the *Diagnostic and Statistical Manual of Mental Disorders* (*DSM-III-R*),[5] criteria for the diagnosis of dementia include the presence of impaired memory and (1) a disturbance in abstract thought, judgment, language, praxis, recognition, or perception; or (2) a personality change. These impairments must "significantly" interfere with work, social functions, or relationships with others. The magnitude of cognitive impairment necessary to alter work performance and life-style to a noticeable degree will depend, of course, on the nature of the job and premorbid social activities. The criteria for the dementia syndrome include a cognitive decline from a previous usual baseline.[40] This loss may be apparent in the performance of household chores and work-related activities or may only be apparent subjectively to the patient. Most often, however, the immediate family is the first to raise concern about failing abilities. All criteria must be met during a normal state of consciousness, that is, in the absence of delirium. (See also Chapter 1.)

Delirium, often misdiagnosed as dementia, is common in the same population of patients affected by dementia.[146] Among 2000 medical inpatients, only 5.3% had dementia, whereas 15% had delirium as their diagnosis.[63] Delirium is usually a more florid state characterized by reduced, often fluctuating, attention; disordered thought content; and incoherent speech. The onset is often acute with perceptual disturbances, altered sleep and psychomotor activity, disorientation, and in some a reduced level of consciousness.[5,146] Demented patients are predisposed to delirium; as many as 25% of demented patients experience delirium at some time during their illness. The diagnosis of dementia can only be made with certainty in the absence of delirium.[5,63]

Criteria for specific types of dementing illnesses have also been established. Several sets of criteria have been proposed for AD. (See Chapter 1.) For example, the term Primary Degenerative Dementia of the Alzheimer Type[5,56] is used in *DSM-III-R*. A combined effort by the National Institute of Neurological

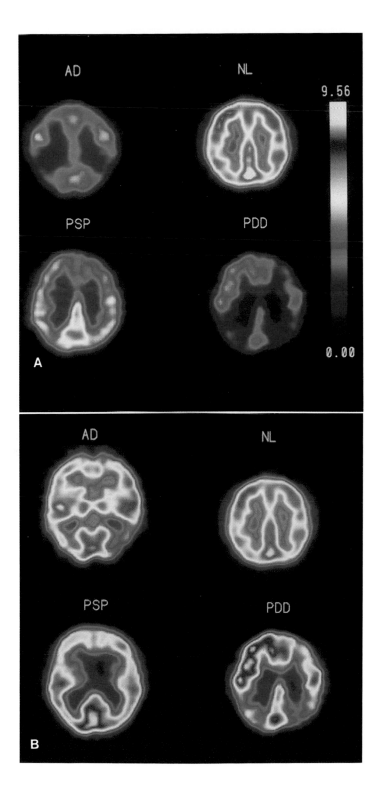

Figure 4-5. PET images following injection of ^{18}F-2-fluoro-2-deoxy-D-glucose in patients with dementia due to a variety of disorders. Horizontal images of the brain are displayed in colors that correspond to a value calculated for each part of the brain. As shown by the color bar, the highest calculated values are represented in red and the lowest in blue. In (A), colors represent local rates of glucose utilization in mg/100 g per minute. Patients with dementia due to Alzheimer's disease, progressive supranuclear palsy, and Parkinson's disease, demonstrate hypometabolism relative to a normal subject of similar age. In (B), when all images are normalized so that the colors represent glucose metabolic rates relative to the mean for that image, predominant posterior temporoparietal hypometabolism is most apparent in the patients with Alzheimer's disease and Parkinson's disease, whereas frontal hypometabolism predominates in the patient with progressive supranuclear palsy. (Studies performed in collaboration with Dr. Sid Gilman, Dr. David E. Kuhl, and other members of the Department of Neurology and the Division of Nuclear Medicine at the University of Michigan.)

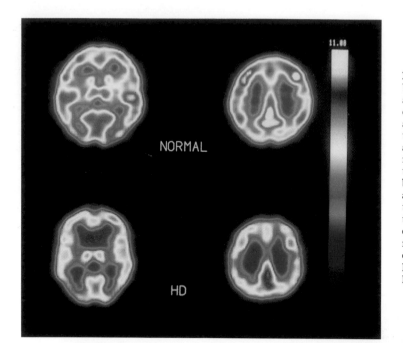

Figure 4-6. Comparisons between a normal subject and a patient with Huntington's disease. Images on the left are horizontal slices through the level of the basal ganglia and thalamus; on the right, images are through the centrum semiovale. Similar cerebral glucose metabolic rates are seen in both subjects, but the patient with Huntington's disease shows a striking decline in caudate and putamenal metabolism. (Courtesy of Dr. Anne B. Young and collaborators, the University of Michigan.)

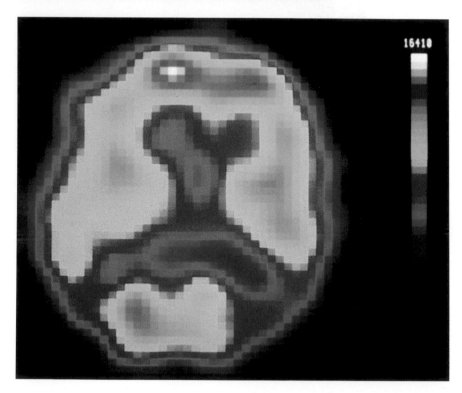

Figure 4-7. SPECT scan of an Alzheimer disease patient following the injection of ^{125}I-Iodoamphetamine. The relative hypoperfusion in bilateral posterior temporoparietal regions is similar to the changes in glucose meta-bolism seen in Figure 4-5. The color bar indicates the number of counts per pixel. (Image obtained in collaboration with Dr. James M. Mountz, Dr. David E. Kuhl, and others in the Division of Nuclear Medicine, the University of Michigan.)

Disorders and Stroke and the Alzheimer's Association led to diagnoses of AD graded by certainty of assignment: possible, probable, and definite.[148,159,169,222] These criteria also include suggested laboratory and neuropsychological studies that may assist diagnosis (See Table 1 – 7.)

There are many causes of "vascular dementia."[147,217] (See Table 4 – 2 and Chapter 7.) Criteria for dementia associated with cerebrovascular disease, specifically, MID, have also been published[5,93] (see Table 1 – 8); these include a stuttering course associated with focal neurologic signs or symptoms of a prior cerebrovascular accident. MID may start abruptly, followed by a brief period of partial recovery or slight improvement.[124,125,150,205] Clinicians often differentiate MID from AD by a historical review of the onset and progression and on the basis of risk factors related to cerebrovascular disease. The Hachinski Ischemic Score[93] formalizes this approach (see Table 1 – 9); Rosen and colleagues[197] validated a shortened version of this instrument in a clinicopathologic study. Scores on such scales need to be combined with radiologic evidence of stroke in identifying cerebrovascular dementia.[197] The presence of a stroke does not necessarily mean that cerebrovascular disease is the cause of dementia, however, because AD and strokes are both common in the elderly and "mixed" dementia is not infrequent.[229]

Criteria-based diagnoses for other less common causes of dementia are rarely specified. The American Psychiatric Association[5] recommends using the same criteria for Primary Degenerative Dementia, but with an attempt to specify the etiology. A drug overdose usually presents as delirium but with chronic exposure — for example, to benzodiazepines — an overdose or adverse side effects to medication can mimic dementia (Table 4 – 3).

The characterization of dementia in association with alcoholism is difficult. Postmortem examination of alleged alcoholic dementia often reveals a variety of pathologic changes including those of the Wernicke-Korsakoff syndrome, subdural hematomas and other evidence of hemorrhage or trauma, AD, or cortical atrophy without specific stigmata.[31,227] No specific pattern of memory loss or cognitive dysfunction occurs with alcoholic dementia associated with alcoholism. The amnestic disorder of the Wernicke-Korsakoff syndrome is

---

Table 4 – 2 CEREBROVASCULAR DISORDERS ASSOCIATED WITH DEMENTIA*

Multiple emboli
  Septic
  Decompression disease
  Atrial fibrillation
  Cardiac and valvular thrombus
Multiple infarcts
Lacunae or état lacunaire (lacunar state)
Watershed or zone infarctions
Anoxia and hypoxia
Aortic and supra-aortic vessel diseases
Inflammatory disease of blood vessels:
  Lupus erythematosus
  Thromboangiitis obliterans
  Anticardiolipin antibody syndromes
Binswanger's disease
Arteriovenous malformations, aneurysms and subarachnoid hemorrhage after rupture of intracranial
  aneurysms
Subdural hematoma
Moya moya disease

*See also Chapter 7.
Source: Adapted from Loeb,[147] p. 90.

**Table 4–3 MEDICATIONS THAT MIGHT IMPAIR
MENTAL FUNCTION IN THE ELDERLY**

Antibiotics, e.g., penicillin
Cardiac glycosides, e.g., digitalis
Antihypertensive agents
  Clonidine
  Alpha methyldopa
  Propranolol
  Reserpine
Autonomic agents
  Anticholinergics
  Benzhexine
  Cholinesterase inhibitors
  Sympathomimetics
  Metoclopramide
  Antihistamines (e.g., Benadryl)
Psychotropic agents
  Antipsychotics (e.g., haloperidol, chlorpromazine)
  Anxiolytics (e.g., benzodiazepines)
  Lithium salts
  Antidepressants
Antiparkinsonian drugs
  Anticholinergics
  Dopamine agonists
Anticonvulsants
Analgesics/antipyretics
  Salicylates
  Indomethacin
  Opioids, morphine, pentazocine, meperidine
Steroids
Antidiabetic agents
  Insulin
  Oral hypoglycemic agents (e.g., sulfonylureas)
  Drugs that mimic hypoglycemic agents, e.g., ethyl alcohol, salicylates
Cancer chemotherapeutic agents
  Ethyl alcohol

Source: Adapted from Cummings and Benson,[40] p. 200.

characterized by impairment in recent and remote memory in the absence of dementia.[227] (See Chapter 10.)

Posttraumatic dementia has no specific criteria but is suspected when there is a history of head injury with loss of consciousness associated with both retrograde and anterograde amnesia or with cognitive impairment dating from the injury. (See Chapter 11.) CT may reveal evidence of coup or contrecoup injury. Dementia pugilistica occurs after repeated episodes of head injury such as those that occur to professional boxers. After a delay of several years, a progressive dementia, often associated with other neurologic symptoms, begins insidiously. Neurofibrillary tangles, and amyloid plaques, are found at autopsy.

Criteria for Creutzfeldt-Jakob disease (CJD) include a rapidly evolving dementia (less than 6 months) associated with: (1) pyramidal-frontal motor signs, (2) occipitoparietal signs with prominent disturbances in vision, or (3) diffuse motor signs including basal ganglia, cerebellar, or spinal cord involvement.[193] Myoclonic jerks especially in response to startle and a periodic pattern of activity in the EEG support this diagnosis. (See Chapter 8.)

Other degenerative disorders are difficult to differentiate from AD unless accompanied by other neurologic signs in addition to dementia. (See Chapter 6.) In Pick's disease, although rare and difficult to establish as an antemortem diagnosis, patients often present with disinhibited behavior and language difficulty but with relatively intact memory and construction ability.[41] Radiologically, preferential frontotemporal atrophy, often asymmetric, is present.[156] Dementia in a patient with Huntington's disease (HD) can occur before the onset of chorea and is often associated with affective or personality disorders.[151] In Parkinson's disease (PD), dementia is found in 10% to 40% of patients.[154] "Subcortical dementia" was a popular term used to describe dementia in patients with movement disorders such as PD and HD. Originally applied to demented patients with progressive supranuclear palsy, the concept was then generalized to disorders in which pathologic changes were felt to be primarily located outside the cerebral cortex, but this distinction does not assist the clinician in formulating a diagnosis, treatment plan, or prognosis.[152,235]

A dementia syndrome can occur with depression or other major psychopathology. (See Chapter 12.) A history of antecedent mental disorder should raise suspicion of a link between the dementia and a psychiatric illness. A family history of unipolar or bipolar illness may aid diagnosis.[178] Weingartner and associates[199] observed a diminished capacity to recall certain types of information in patients with major depression. The cognitive impairment occurs with or after the onset of depression, evolves and fluctuates with the mood disturbance, and is associated with other evidence of depression such as loss of appetite, sleep disturbance, and other vegetative signs. Affective illnesses may coexist with dementing illnesses, particularly early in the course.[22,129] Patients with depression often complain of memory trouble out of proportion to the degree of impairment, whereas the patient with a dementia complains relatively less; instead, the family complains.

Schizophrenia may be associated with cognitive impairment, but is not usually confused with other dementing illnesses. Many demented patients are psychotic, but the onset of delusions or hallucinations most often occurs after intellectual function is affected.[177] The onset of schizophrenia is also relatively infrequent in individuals over age 65.

Illiteracy, a low level of education, and mental retardation pose problems in making a diagnosis of dementia. Performance on formal and "bedside" mental status examinations can be heavily influenced by education, language, and culture.[226] Thus caution must be used when the diagnosis is based on mental status examination alone; performance in activities of daily life and other functions assist in the estimation of intellectual capacity. Similarly, it is difficult to diagnose dementia in a person with mental retardation, and measuring decline from a previously impaired baseline may be difficult. A history of developmental delay, difficulty in school, or a need for "special education" may be a clue to the preexistent cognitive deficit. Comparison of performance on standardized neuropsychological tests over time may be helpful. Of course, mental retardation and dementia can coexist, as in the case of Down's syndrome. Individuals with trisomy 21 invariably develop AD-type pathologic changes and not infrequently manifest clinical dementia in their 30s and 40s. (See Chapters 2 and 6.)

The Diagnostic Interview Schedule was adapted by Robins and colleagues[190] for clinical diagnoses listed in *DSM-III-R*.[5] Other schedules[56,182,196] can assist in the interview of a demented patient. Clinicians may enhance their interview skills by reviewing these schedules, but they are not essential to the diagnosis of dementia in practice.

DEMENTIA AND AGING

In common with other biologic functions, certain cognitive functions decline with age, although there is marked variability among individuals.[1,119,126,127] The distinction between cognitive impairment in old age and that found in early dementia may be difficult. "Benign senescent forgetfulness"[127] was originally used to describe normal, mild, relatively nonprogressive memory loss. Because it is a poorly defined term, it is now being replaced by less loosely formulated concepts such as "age-associated memory impairment" (AAMI). AAMI is defined as mild memory loss occurring in the elderly unassociated with other cognitive deficits or with any identifiable illness that may be causing memory difficulty. Specific criteria for this condition have been developed for use in drug studies (Table 4–4).

One of the difficulties in comparing cognitive problems in early dementing illnesses with those of old age is the choice of appropriate comparison groups. Old age is associated with an increased probability of ill health, which in itself may influence cognitive function. Distinctions have been drawn between "normal" aging and "successful" aging, although various formulations of these distinctions have been proposed.[198] "Normal aging" can be used to refer to a statistical average; most older individuals have one or more chronic conditions, some of which may affect cognition. On the other hand, "normal" can be used to indicate the rarer state of disease-free aging. The term "successful aging" has also been used to denote an ideal, relatively disease-free state that is not the statistical norm or to indicate a state of good adaptation to chronic disease. All reports of changes in cognition with age emphasize the variability among individuals. In general, however, it is found that tasks undertaken with time constraints are performed less well by the elderly than by the young, and this difference is heightened by increasing task complexity. The moderately or severely demented patient can be confidently differentiated from the person who is aging normally. The clinical problem is to differentiate healthy individuals from those with dementing illness in which the earliest changes are found only in memory and speed of performance. The psychometric testing can, however, help to distinguish between benign and more malignant conditions.[69,170]

The indistinct boundaries between dementing conditions and old age are not confined to neuropsychologic func-

Table 4–4 DIAGNOSTIC CRITERIA FOR AGE-ASSOCIATED MEMORY IMPAIRMENT (AAMI)

- Modest decline in sensory memory, minimal impairments in primary (short-term or immediate) memory, and minimal impairment in tertiary (remote) memory, with substantial age-related deficits in secondary (recent or long-term) memory
- Adults at least 50 years of age
- Gradual onset of memory loss without sudden worsening in recent months
- Memory test performance at least one standard deviation below the mean established for young adults on a standardized test of secondary (recent) memory with adequate normative data
- Adequate intellectual function determined by Wechsler Adult Intelligence Scale Vocabulary subtest score of at least 9 (raw score of at least 32)
- Absence of dementia as determined by a score of 24 or higher on the Mini-Mental State Examination
- No history of any neurologic or medical disorder that could produce cognitive deterioration
- No evidence of delirium, confusion, or other disturbances of consciousness
- No history of brain infection or inflammatory disease
- No evidence of significant cerebral vascular pathology as determined by a Hachinski Ischemia Score of 4 or more or by neuroradiologic examination
- No history of repeated head injury (e.g., boxing) or of unconsciousness for 1 hour or more
- No current psychiatric disorder according to *DSM-III* criteria, including depression, mania, or any major psychiatric disorder
- No evidence of depression as determined by a Hamilton Depression Rating Scale* score of 13 or more
- Use of any psychotropic drug or any other drug that may significantly affect cognitive function during the month prior to psychometric testing

*Hamilton M: A rating scale for depression. J Neurol Neurosurg Psychiatry 23:56–62, 1960.
Source: Adapted from age-associated memory impairment: Measures of clinical change—a report of a National Institute of Mental Health Work Group. Developmental Neuropsychology 2(4):261–276, 1986.

tion. For example, widespread senile plaques and neurofibrillary tangles throughout the cerebral neocortex permit a confident postmortem diagnosis of AD in a patient who has been diagnosed clinically as demented. More difficult to interpret are the same histologic features confined to the hippocampus, and it is rare indeed to find a patient who has died of old age without some evidence of tangle and plaque formation.[223] Similarly, neurochemical differentiation of normal aging from dementing diseases may be difficult. A reduction in choline acetyltransferase activity in the cerebral cortex is consistently seen in AD, but can occur, although to a lesser extent, in aged, intellectually normal individuals.[13,181] There is no qualitative distinction between the clinical and pathologic features of AD and aging, and all of the features of AD increase linearly in the aging population.[21]

These observations often prompt the statement that AD is merely an exaggeration of aging. As long as the underlying mechanisms of aging and AD are unknown, statements concerning the fundamental relationships between the two will be of limited value. It is entirely possible, however, that the markers currently used for AD (senile plaques, neurofibrillary tangles, and cell loss within a setting of dementia) are end-stage markers of diverse pathologic processes. Such theoretical arguments aside, the pragmatic distinction between a normal elderly subject and a patient with dementia remains clinically important,[200] indeed essential, if one is to diagnose and successfully manage these patients.

ELEMENTS OF THE CLINICAL EVALUATION

The Neuropsychiatric History

Forgetting the names of objects or people and mismanaging financial or work-related activities are frequent early complaints in patients with dementia. Losing track of time, getting lost in familiar places, and being unable to learn new skills also occur. In the early stages, language, perception, and motor skills such as those involved in driving may be preserved, but with disease progression these abilities also deteriorate. In the early stages of dementia, it may be impossible to distinguish the memory loss from that which occurs "normally" as individuals age (AAMI). Memory failure that leads to personal harm or that appears to be rapidly progressive is of particular concern.

Depression, anxiety, or a change in personality or in the level of depression or anxiety are often minor, and occasionally major, features of dementia.[22,129] Inability to express one's emotions, or comprehend the emotions of others, may be interpreted by the family as "depression." Many patients develop delusions and hallucinations during the illness, which can have profound effects on disability and management.[177] The most common delusion is that someone is stealing from the patient. Such a fixed belief (if false) is probably due to a combination of the memory deficit and personality changes.

Other psychiatric manifestations, such as compulsive behaviors, restlessness, agitation, wandering, and sleep-wake disturbances, can occur in dementia. New rating scales are being developed to assess these noncognitive manifestations. For example, the BEHAV-AD is a general screening instrument,[187] whereas the Cornell Scale for Depression in Dementia[2] assesses primarily affective features.

The patient's medical history must be queried to consider past illnesses that could contribute to the current dementia. A history of strokes, seizures, head injury, infections, drug abuse, risk factors for AIDS, endocrine dysfunction, anemia, vitamin deficiencies, and cancer should be sought. Prescribed medications, particularly sedatives, anxiolytics, and antidepressants with potent anticholinergic activity, impair intellectual acuity and should be inventoried and their use evaluated.[166] Over-the-counter drug use should also be considered.

Activities of Daily Living

Some criteria for dementia require demonstration of a decline in "social or occupational function." Families often bring a patient to medical attention when activities of daily living (ADL) are affected. Instrumental ADLs[138] such as managing finances, transportation, and communication are impaired before basic ADLs such as toileting, bathing, and mobility.[6,116] (See Table 14 – 1.) Although measurement of ADLs in general elderly populations is used widely to predict the need for services, few ADL scales are designed specifically to evaluate the effects of dementia on functional abilities. Some commonly used scales incorporate cognitive and ADL assessment in an abbreviated fashion. The dementia rating scale of Blessed, Tomlinson, and Roth,[19] for example, measures ADLs such as the ability to perform household chores, manage money, move about in familiar places, dress, eat, and toilet. The Alzheimer's Disease Assessment Scale[196] also measures some functional activities. Hughes and associates[108] developed the Clinical Dementia Rating Scale (Table 4 – 5), which has proven to have high interrater reliability and to determine the severity of dementia. Such scales are a practical way of observing the course of dementia.

Family History

Many dementias are familial, although specific genetic mechanisms of inheritance are not known for most. (See Chapters 2 and 6.) In AD, several compelling observations point to the importance of genetic mechanisms. Several large kindreds of patients with AD show a clear autosomal dominant pattern of inheritance.[17,18,71,90,172,201] Twin studies,[38,173,185] the association between Down's syndrome and AD,[99,135,159] and epidemiologic studies[3,23,100,107,239] suggest that genetic factors play an important but ill-defined role in other forms of AD. HD, a degenerative disease with dementia, always follows autosomal dominant inheritance. Many other forms of dementia may be familial or have family aggregates, such as Gerstmann-Sträussler syndrome, Pick's disease, and CJD.

Several assessment procedures are available for family history taking. At a minimum, the ages and causes of death for the first-degree relatives (siblings and parents) should be recorded. Interviews with informants other than the spouse, such as siblings of the proband, will often help clarify the pedigree.

The Neurologic Examination

GAIT AND POSTURE

With aging itself and age-associated illnesses such as degenerative arthritis and sensory impairments, gait may become slower and more unsteady in a nonspecific way. Most elderly individuals can perform the Romberg test with little difficulty, but if asked to stand for several minutes, swaying may occur. The healthy elderly person may also have difficulty tandem walking.[241] Particular changes in gait and posture may suggest a specific illness associated with dementia. A stooped posture with a shuffling gait may indicate PD. A wide-based stance or gait and difficulty turning implicate cerebellar disease or posterior column damage such as that due to vitamin B_{12} deficiency. A "magnetic gait" can be associated with normal-pressure hydrocephalus. (See Chapter 11.) In AD, gait is usually normal until it becomes slowed and uncoordinated in later stages.

CRANIAL NERVES

Impairments of the sensory and motor aspects of cranial nerve function occur with aging.[10,37,96,184] Special attention to vision and hearing is an important part of the evaluation of cognitive impairment. Slowed pupillary response, diminished smooth pursuit, and decreased saccadic frequency are frequently noted in patients with AD.[68,134] Diminished upward gaze is present in 20% of healthy elderly people,[184] but when limited downward and horizontal gaze also occurs, the diagnosis of progressive supranuclear palsy is suggested. Disorders of smell and taste may be related to medications, although Doty and colleagues[50,51] found impaired recognition of odors as an early manifestation of AD and PD.

MOTOR SYSTEM

Motor strength diminishes 60% to 80% in late life.[218] The loss is not a particular feature of dementia. In contrast, muscle tone, elicited by passive movement of the limbs or the neck, may be abnormal in certain conditions. Paratonia, or "gegenhalten," is an apparent inability to relax voluntarily; the level of resistance generally increases with the pressure applied by the examiner. In dementia, paratonia occurs in the later stages; its pathogenesis is unknown. Rigidity, a plasticlike resistance to passive movement (often associated with cogwheeling, a ratchetlike movement), occurs in many patients with extrapyramidal disorders and in some patients with AD.[155]

SENSATION

Preserved or slightly reduced pain and tactile perception and position sense in the elderly are the rule, but vibratory sense is almost always reduced at the feet and, to a degree, at the ankles.[202] Dementia with more prominent sensory loss can be a manifestation of a systemic disease such as lupus erythematosus or vitamin B_{12} deficiency, in which peripheral neuropathy or myelopathy can occur.

REFLEXES

Stretch reflexes may become more difficult to elicit, but most remain symmetrical and intact in the older patient except for the ankle jerk, which may be diminished. Primitive "release" re-flexes such as glabellar, snout, rooting, or sucking responses are present in some normal individuals, particularly when anxious, but are also more prominent in degenerative disorders of the central nervous system.[225] Palmomental, grasp, and plantar grasp responses may also be present in some elderly individuals, but their implications in otherwise normal people are unclear.

Cognitive Testing

At present, neuropsychological evaluation is the best tool for establishing the presence of dementia, particularly in early stages.[192] Most neuropsychological tests measure performance for a specific cognitive function, such as memory, language, or perception; poor performance on a particular test implies specific areas of brain dysfunction. Factors such as age, education, and socioeconomic background affect performance and scores on these tests. Dementia may be overdiagnosed when the patient is assessed with an instrument in his or her secondary language. Although neuropsychological studies can identify patients with dementia with great sensitivity, their specificity for different forms of dementia is less well established.[61,211,222] (See also Chapter 5 for discussions of patterns of impairment seen in different dementias.)

One goal of cognitive assessment in dementia is to determine whether performance reflects a decline from previous ability. To establish that a change has occurred, an estimate of premorbid abilities is needed. Wilson and associates[236] use occupational level, ethnic group, sex, and age to estimate a premorbid IQ. Certain abilities are retained much longer than others; patients with mild and even moderate dementia perform well on tests that depend on previously overlearned material such as vocabulary. These relatively preserved functions can be used to estimate premorbid function. In cases of mild cognitive dysfunction, particularly if limited

Table 4–5 CLINICAL DEMENTIA RATING SCALE

	Healthy CDR 0	Questionable Dementia CDR 0.5	Mild Dementia CDR 1	Moderate Dementia CDR 2	Severe Dementia CDR 3
Memory	No memory loss or slight inconstant forgetfulness	Mild consistent forgetfulness; partial recollection of events; "benign" forgetfulness	Moderate memory loss, more marked for recent events; defect interferes with everyday activities	Severe memory loss; only highly learned material retained; new material rapidly lost	Severe memory loss; only fragments remain
Orientation	Fully oriented		Some difficulty with time relationships; oriented for place and person at examination, but may have geographic disorientation	Usually disoriented in time, often to place	Orientation to person only
Judgment and problem solving	Solves everyday problems well; judgment good in relation to past performance	Only doubtful impairment in solving problems, similarities/ differences	Moderate difficulty in handling complex problems; social judgment usually maintained	Severely impaired in handling problems, similarities/ differences; social judgment usually impaired	Unable to attempt judgment or problem solving
Community affairs	Independent function at usual level in job, shopping, business and financial affairs, volunteer and social groups	Only doubtful or mild impairment, if any, in these activities	Unable to function independently at these activities, though may still be engaged in some; may still appear normal to casual inspection	No pretense of independent function outside home	

Home and hobbies	Life at home, hobbies, intellectual interests well maintained	Life at home, hobbies, intellectual interests well maintained or only slightly impaired	Mild but definite impairment of function at home; more difficult chores abandoned; more complicated hobbies and interests abandoned	Only simple chores preserved; very restricted interests, poorly sustained	No significant function in home outside of own room
Personal care	Fully capable of self-care		Needs occasional prompting	Requires assistance in dressing, hygiene, keeping of personal effects	Requires much help with personal care; often incontinent

Score 0.5, 1, 2, 3 only if impairment is due to cognitive loss.

Although rules for assigning CDR stages beyond CDR 3 have not been established, the following have been proposed to distinguish additional levels of impairment in advanced dementia:

Profound (CDR 4): Speech usually unintelligible or irrelevant; unable to follow simple instructions or comprehend commands; occasionally recognizes spouse or caregiver. Uses fingers more than utensils, requires much assistance. Frequently incontinent despite assistance or training. Able to walk a few steps with help; usually chair-bound; rarely out of home or residence; purposeless movements often present.

Terminal (CDR 5): No response or comprehension. No recognition. Needs to be fed, may have nasogastric tube and/or swallowing difficulties. Total incontinence. Bedridden, unable to sit or stand, contractures.

Source: Adapted from Hughes et al,[108] p. 568. See also references 16, 168.

to memory or speed of processing, the presence of dementia may be hard to differentiate from poor premorbid functioning or normal age-related changes (AAMI). In such cases, serial examinations to look for deterioration are essential.

In addition to diagnosing early dementia, there are several other situations in which a neuropsychological evaluation (see Chapter 5) is particularly useful in patient assessment. The contribution of psychological factors (e.g., affective or hysterical features) can be assessed. When dementia is suspected in the presence of stroke, the diagnostic process is complicated because the cognitive change may be the result of the focal effect of the stroke or of a more generalized dementia. Stroke may also complicate the course of AD, however, resulting in a mixed pattern of impairment.[30] Finally, the pattern of cognitive impairment found on testing can be used to counsel the caregiver about how to build on preserved skills and to avoid situations that tax failing abilities. (See Chapter 14.)

Neuropsychological tests should be chosen based on established reliability, validity, sensitivity, specificity, appropriateness for a demented population, and to examine a variety of cognitive skills including memory. Selected examples of commonly used instruments will be reviewed here; more detailed discussion of instruments designed to test specific areas of cognitive function are included in Chapter 5.

MENTAL STATUS INSTRUMENTS

Brief mental status instruments are useful to screen for the presence of cognitive impairment and to observe a patient longitudinally to assess change. Several reliable instruments include the "Mini-Mental State Examination" (MMSE)[70] (Table 4–6), and the Blessed Information-Memory-Concentration Test.[19] Modified versions of both also exist,[117,153] and other tests are available that are similar in structure

and design.[92,113,182] These tests have limitations owing to their brevity: they do not cover all cognitive abilities equally and adequately, they may not be sensitive to early dementia, and they may overdiagnose dementia in patients with limited education. Some authors suggest education-specific norms to optimize the MMSE.[226]

THE WECHSLER ADULT INTELLIGENCE SCALE (WAIS)

The WAIS, in either the original or revised version (WAIS-R),[231] is frequently used to assess present level of intellectual function. The WAIS yields an IQ score, standardized such that 100 is the mean expected value at any age, with a standard deviation of 15. Verbal and Performance IQs are also obtained and use the same scale.

The WAIS consists of 11 subtests, 6 for Verbal and 5 for Performance IQ. Each yields a scaled score that ranges from 1 to 19 with a mean of 10 and a standard deviation of 3, so that normal subtest scaled scores range from 7 to 13. Scaled scores are not age corrected; they are based on the entire normative population for the WAIS or WAIS-R. Age-adjusted scaled scores can be calculated to compare the patient's performance to that expected of his or her age group. Because the WAIS subtests are often included in a neuropsychological report, they are briefly described in Table 4–7. The "scatter" of subtest scores represents the strengths and weaknesses in the patient's performance in different areas of intellectual activity.

In dementia the performance IQ is usually significantly lower than the verbal IQ. Timed visuospatial tests, such as Block Design and Digit Symbol Substitution, typically yield the lowest scores. Subtests tapping "old stores" of knowledge, such as Vocabulary, usually yield the highest age-scaled scores; tests of abstract reasoning, such as Similarities, are performed at a lower level.

Table 4–6 MINI-MENTAL STATE EXAMINATION

Maximum Score	Score	
		ORIENTATION
5	( )	What is the (*year*) (*season*) (*date*) (*day*) (*month*)?
5	( )	Where are we: (*state*) (*county*) (*town*) (*hospital*) (*floor*)?
		REGISTRATION
3	( )	Name three objects, one second to say each, then ask the patient to repeat all three after you have said them. Give one point for each correct answer. Continue repeating all three objects until the patient learns all three. Count trials and record.
		ATTENTION AND CALCULATION
5	( )	Serial 7's. One point for each correct response. Stop after five answers. Alternatively, spell "world" backward.
		RECALL
3	( )	Ask for the three objects named in *Registration*. Give one point for each correct answer.
		LANGUAGE
2	( )	Name a pencil and watch.
1	( )	Repeat the following "No ifs, ands, or buts."
3	( )	Follow a 3-stage command: "Take paper in your right hand, fold it in half, and put it on the floor."
1	( )	Read and obey the following: CLOSE YOUR EYES.
1	( )	Write a sentence.
1	( )	Copy a design.
30		

Assess level of consciousness along a continuum

Alert	Drowsy	Stupor	Coma

Source: From Folstein et al,[70] pp. 196–197, with permission.

VISUOSPATIAL TESTS

Decline in visuospatial function can be seen on the Block Design subtest of the WAIS or on other drawing tasks such as the Rosen Drawing Test,[195] which consists of 15 drawings that the patient is asked to copy. The drawings range in difficulty from simple shapes to complex three-dimensional figures. Having the patient draw a clock can provide information about visuospatial ability and about severity of dementia in evaluating the presence of irrelevant figures, absence of numbers, irrelevant spatial arrangement, counterclock rotation, and placing of hands.[212] In the study of Wolf-Klein and colleagues,[240] this test had high sensitivity and specificity.

THE WECHSLER MEMORY SCALE (WMS)

The WMS[230] is commonly used to assess memory and yields a "memory quotient" (MQ), which theoretically should parallel the patient's IQ. Three subtests are particularly useful. Logical Memory consists of two paragraphs that the patient listens to and then attempts to recall. In the Visual Reproduction subtest, the patient has 10 seconds to study designs and then must draw them from memory. The Paired Associates subtest consists of 10 word

Table 4−7 DESCRIPTION OF WAIS-R SUBTESTS

VERBAL

Information	29 general information items, e.g., "Who wrote Hamlet?" Assess "old stores" of information.
Digit Span	Standardized assessment of digits forward and backward. Primarily assesses attention.
Vocabulary	Defining 30 words. Typically represents "premorbid" level of ability.
Arithmetic	14 verbal arithmetic problems
Comprehension	16 items assessing appreciation of social norms and standards and proverb interpretation
Similarities	Deriving relevant superordinate category or similarity for 14 word pairs; e.g., "How are coat and suit alike?" Assesses abstract reasoning.

PERFORMANCE

Picture Completion	Determining the missing feature in 20 pictures
Picture Arrangement	Arranging sets of comic-strip pictures so that they tell a coherent story. Ten items.
Block Design	Arranging blocks with red, white and half-red and half-white sides to form nine designs. A complex visuospatial task.
Object Assembly	Assembling four jigsaw puzzles
Digit Symbol	Using a table of nine digit-symbol pairs to fill in the proper symbols for a series of numbers. Taps new learning, visuospatial abilities and speeded performance

pairs. Six are "easy" associates, such as North-South, and four are "hard," such as Cabbage-Pen. The patient has three trials to learn these word pairs and supply the second word of the pair when given the first. Also included in the WMS are subtests assessing personal and current information and orientation to time and place.

THE SELECTIVE REMINDING TEST

The Selective Reminding Test,[28] another commonly used test of memory function in which the patient listens to a list of words and then attempts to recall them, is often used to aid diagnosis. The patient is reminded of the words forgotten and asked to attempt to recall the entire list again. This process continues for 6 to 12 trials, and summary scores describe performance in terms of total number of words recalled and those recalled without reminding.

A standard part of memory testing is to assess recall of test material at some time after the original administration. Typically delays of 15 to 30 minutes are employed. In dementia, there is typically a marked increase in impairment with greater delays.

THE BOSTON DIAGNOSTIC APHASIA EVALUATION AND THE BOSTON NAMING TEST

Many aspects of language function usually remain intact in early dementia; patients can maintain conversation, with good comprehension and adherence to social aspects of communication (pragmatics). Selected subtests from the Boston Diagnostic Aphasia Evaluation[87] can be used to assess repetition, comprehension, and simple reading. Word-finding difficulty, particularly for low-frequency words, often occurs early and can be appreciated by listening for circumlocution or empty speech. Confrontational naming can be assessed with the Boston Naming Test,[115] which consists of 60 line drawings. If pictures cannot be named spontaneously, semantic cues are given first (the general category of the object) and then phonemic cues (the first sound of the word) to assess the magnitude and nature of the naming difficulty.

THE CONTROLLED WORD ASSOCIATION TEST

Also typically affected early in dementia is the ability to generate words by letter or category, referred to as verbal fluency, which can be assessed with the Controlled Word Association Test.[14,194] In this test the patient is given a minute to recite words beginning with a particular letter (usually *F*, *A*, or *S*). Age-, education-, and sex-adjusted norms are available to derive percentile scores.

PRAXIS TESTING

Evaluation of skilled motor activity is a necessary part of the diagnosis of dementia. Patients may not be able to imitate hand positions or perform motor commands. For example, when asked to use an imaginary hammer to hit an imaginary nail, they may substitute body part (fist) for object (imaginary hammer). Patients sometimes have difficulty learning or accurately carrying out diadokinetic (rapid double-alternating) movements. Sensory testing, such as double simultaneous stimulation in the tactile, auditory, or visual modality, is typically within normal limits. Early on, right-left orientation is usually intact, but sometimes the patient has trouble reversing this orientation, as when pointing out right and left on the examiner.

Laboratory Studies

For many years a standardized evaluation of blood and cerebrospinal fluid (CSF) has been considered part of the examination of demented patients. Recent studies, however, have questioned the need for extensive metabolic screens, which are used primarily to exclude potentially reversible forms of dementia.[136,137] Although only a few conditions recognizable by a blood examination cause dementia, they are important because some are correctable. (See Chapter 10.) The clinical interview and neurologic examination should identify patients at risk for the metabolic causes of dementia recognized by these laboratory studies, allowing for more selective use of laboratory tests to confirm clinical impressions.

SCREENING BLOOD TESTS

A recent National Institute of Health Consensus Conference has suggested the following screening laboratory tests: (1) complete blood cell count; (2) electrolyte panel; (3) screening metabolic panel; (4) thyroid gland function tests; (5) vitamin B_{12} and folate levels; (6) tests for syphilis and, depending on history, for human immunodeficiency antibodies; (7) urinalysis; (8) electrocardiogram; and (9) chest roentgenogram.[174] Larson and co-workers[137] found most of these studies to be normal in their clinic population, so they recommended the routine use of only the complete blood count, thyroid function tests, and the chemistry panel. Folate or cyanocobalamin would be investigated in patients with anemia with or without macrocytosis. This procedure agrees with another study,[145] which found only a single patient with dementia as the sole manifestation of B_{12} deficiency. The difference in cost per patient is several hundred dollars when the modified battery is employed, with selected use of other tests.

The likelihood of missing reversible causes of dementia is minimal if a careful history and physical examination are performed in addition to these screening examinations. The number of patients with so-called "reversible dementia" ranges from 3% to 10%, raising questions about the need for extensive screening laboratory investigations.[12,158] Antibody titers to human immunodeficiency virus should be included as part of the examination of any individual with dementia who is engaged in high-risk activities such as promiscuous sexual behavior or intravenous drug use. Sedimentation rate should be determined and screens for connective tissue disease (such as anti-nuclear antibodies and rheumatoid factor) performed if the clinical picture suggests evidence of vasculitis or arthritis.

LUMBAR PUNCTURE

The lumbar puncture is important in the investigation of dementia accompanied by a history suggestive of an infectious process, but the routine examination of CSF in dementia is probably not necessary.[95] (See Chapters 8 and 9.) In the degenerative disorders, attempts have been made to find specific markers of the disease process in CSF. Variable patterns of neurotransmitter changes have been reported in different dementing illnesses. In PD and in AD with extrapyramidal signs, reduced content of the dopamine metabolite homovanillic acid may be observed,[120] but this has little diagnostic utility. Variable changes are found in the cholinesterase activities and somatostatin levels of lumbar CSF in patients with AD.[7,213] The lack of consistent changes makes these tests useless in clinical practice.[88]

Wolozin and Davies[242] identified immunoreactivity with a monoclonal antibody, Alz-50, which reacts with a 68-kd protein in AD brain in the CSF of patients with AD; its specificity and sensitivity as a diagnostic test are currently being investigated. Other components of the cytoskeletal pathology in AD, such as the amyloid precursor protein, are found in CSF, but their diagnostic utility is not clear.[175]

ELECTROENCEPHALOGRAPHY

The usefulness of the EEG in the diagnosis and management of dementia is limited in part by overlap with normal age-related changes. The mean alpha rhythm for young adults is approximately 10 to 10.5 Hz, but for an older person, for example, 70 to 80 years of age, it slows to between 8.5 and 9 Hz.[179] Activities normally infrequent in the EEG of the young adult, such as theta and delta rhythm, are commonly re-ported over temporal regions, particularly on the left in people over age 60.[228] Typically, this is either rhythmic or polymorphic in type, and no discernible etiology has been established. Changes in the EEG also occur during sleep; total sleep time and length of stage 3 and 4 sleep diminish in aging.

Abnormalities on EEG correlate to the severity of dementia and may have some predictive utility, especially if done serially.[35,54,98,180,186] The EEG in AD, PD (with or without dementia), and HD shows a reduction in the posterior dominant alpha rhythm.[179] As the severity of dementia increases, mild and intermittent reduction in the posterior rhythm to 7 Hz and then to theta and delta rhythms occurs. Generalized slowing of all cerebral activity occurs with progression of the illness. Pick's disease, in contrast, is usually accompanied by a normal EEG until late in the disorder. Dementia associated with vascular disease may also be accompanied by focal or lateralized slow activity over the area of the infarction. The EEG is most useful in identifying CJD, where, in addition to generalized slowing, a distinctive pattern of periodic complexes with a frequency of 1 Hz generally accompanies the onset of myoclonus (Fig. 4–1). As the disease progresses, the periodic pattern will persist, and the background activity may completely disappear or be of extremely low amplitude. Metabolic disorders such as hypothyroidism and B_{12} deficiency, or toxic disorders such as those resulting from overdosage of medications, may slow the EEG patterns considerably.

Computer-assisted spectral analysis of EEG activity quantitates frequencies and permits colorful displays of the regional electrical activity. Regional changes have been found[25,54] similar to those seen with positron emission tomography in AD and other forms of dementia. The ability to discriminate correctly between AD and vascular forms of dementia has been reported to be quite high.[143] Although specific changes have been reported to occur in dementia and to correlate with severity

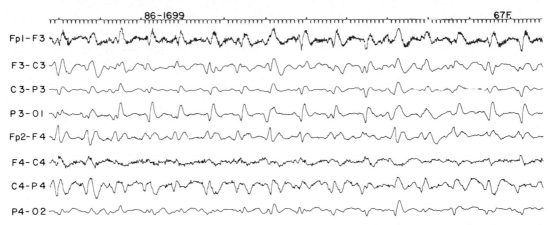

Figure 4 – 1. An electroencephalogram of a patient with Creutzfeldt-Jakob disease, revealing the typical periodicity. (Courtesy of Timothy Pedley, M.D., Columbia University.)

of disease,[24,206] the added value of this approach over traditional EEG has not been established.[4]

EVOKED POTENTIALS

Evoked potentials measure brain activity triggered by a particular event or stimulus provided by the examiner. The early portions of the evoked potential waveform are considered to be related to sensory aspects of the stimuli, and the late components to information processing. The P300 wave (a late event – related brain potential) may reflect a physiologic measure of mental processing speed and selective attention.[208,214] Several changes in this waveform, including absence, delay, or decreased amplitude, may be related to cognitive change. In patients with dementia, the size and latency of the P300 wave can be affected. Although evoked potentials may be able to distinguish demented patients from healthy and depressed patients of a similar age, the specificity and sensitivity of this technique is currently less than that required for diagnostic use.[176]

Brain Imaging

The availability of methods to image brain structure has significantly improved the accuracy of diagnosis in pa-

tients with dementia. Focal brain lesions can be readily detected and, as a result, brain imaging has become widely accepted as part of the routine evaluation of dementia. A variety of radiographic and radioisotopic imaging techniques are now available to assist the physician. Additional methods are being developed that permit imaging of brain chemistry and are likely in the future to improve diagnosis and further define the pathophysiology of dementing disorders.

RADIOGRAPHIC IMAGING

Standard Radiographic Techniques. Routine skull films are not indicated in the evaluation of dementia. Most brain diseases produce no change in the skull, and appropriate selection of CT image views and windowing can provide superior information when there is evidence of sinus or bone disease. Likewise, pneumoencephalography has been made obsolete by CT, MRI, and isotope cisternography.

Cerebral angiography plays a limited role in the evaluation of patients suspected of having dementia due to cerebrovascular disease. Narrowing or "beading" of intracranial vessels due to focal inflammatory lesions can be seen in patients with vasculitis,[67] and the nature and severity of vascular lesions can be delineated when the etiology of stroke is unclear. Angiography cannot detect congophilic angiopathy, which may accompany AD.

Computed Tomography. CT provides an image that reflects three-dimensional structure and recognizes small differences in brain x-ray attenuation. Contrast agents can exaggerate these small differences, test the integrity of the BBB and, to a limited extent, permit examination of intracranial vessels and cerebral perfusion.[122,245]

Focal brain diseases that cause dementia, such as tumor, abscess, infarction, hemorrhage, and demyelinating disease, are well visualized by CT, particularly when contrast media are used. Although CT is quite sensitive, it is not infallible. The site and size of a lesion are critical to its detection, and the resolution limits of individual CT scanners must be kept in mind. The posterior fossa is particularly difficult to visualize with CT because of beam-hardening artifact,[27] so that MR scanning is preferred when lesions in this location are suspected. Timing of the CT examination may also be critical; x-ray absorption varies during the evolution of subdural hematomas and stroke. Acute subdural hematomas have attenuation values higher than normal brain tissue, but later they can become isodense with surrounding brain tissue,[203] and, particularly when bilateral, can be overlooked when contrast agents are not used.[224] Ischemic stroke also undergoes changes in radiodensity with time. Recent infarcts may cause no detectable change in attenuation. Improved identification of lesions is possible, especially between 7 and 21 days, by use of contrast agents.[233,238] Finally, hypodensity and substance loss without contrast enhancement become apparent if the infarct is of sufficient size.

Enlargement of intracranial spaces due to disorders causing loss of brain substance or obstruction of CSF flow is also easily seen by CT. AD causes reduced brain weight, widening of sulci, and ventricular enlargement,[104,219] but the diagnosis of AD cannot be based on CT findings alone.[105] Because there is a strong correlation between age and atrophy, a patient's age must be considered in determining the significance of enlarged ventricles and sulci.[26,109] In addition, radiographic atrophy is reversible in several conditions, including alcoholism, nutritional deficiency, renal disease, and steroid use.[15,29,30,123,128]

Neither visual inspection of CT scans nor linear measurement of ventricular or sulcal size is sufficient to predict the presence of AD.[83,142,237] Careful computer-assisted measurement of the volume of CSF-containing spaces does appear to correlate with patient symptomatology, however.[64,81,243] Because there is considerable overlap with normals, this technique still cannot be used to establish the presence of AD in an individual, but when serial scans are available, progressive ventricular and sulcal enlargement is considered supportive of the diagnosis.[82,149,171] (Fig. 4–2).

Enlargement of the ventricular system without corresponding widening of the sulci in a patient with appropriate clinical features suggests normal pressure hydrocephalus (NPH).[80,244] Low attenuation in periventricular regions, thought to represent increased transependymal flow of CSF, can also be seen,[244] but neither feature is predictive of response to shunting. Isolated lobar atrophy may be seen in Pick's disease,[41,156] progressive aphasia with or without dementia,[121,161] AD,[216] hereditary dysphasic dementia,[167] and also as a normal variant. The sensitivity and reliability of this finding in each of these disorders has not been established.

White-matter changes on CT scanning have also been described in demented patients. These changes are discussed below since they are even more frequently observed with MRI.

Magnetic Resonance Imaging. MRI uses the response to radiowave pulses of magnetic properties of tissue to visualize the brain. Differences in radiofrequency pulse durations and se-

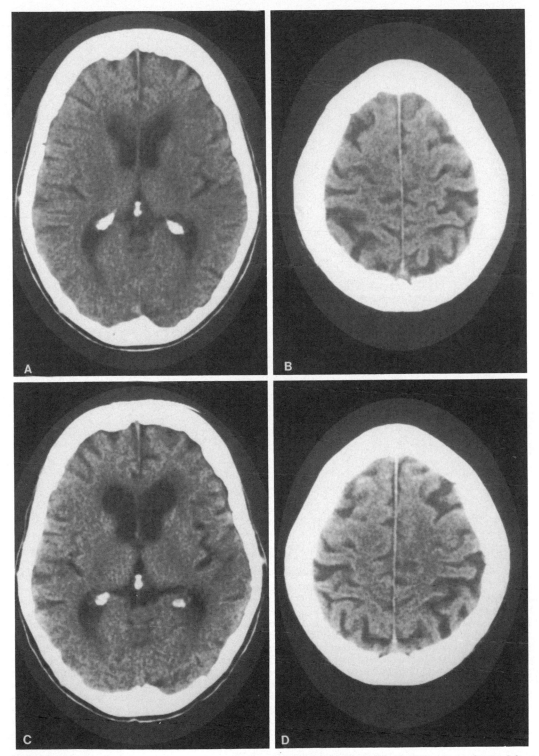

Figure 4–2. CT images obtained in a patient with Alzheimer's disease. (*A, B*) At the time of initial diagnosis, there is diffuse, symmetric enlargement of sulci and ventricles. (*C, D*) Similar images obtained 2 years later with the same scanner demonstrate progressive ventricular and sulcal enlargement.

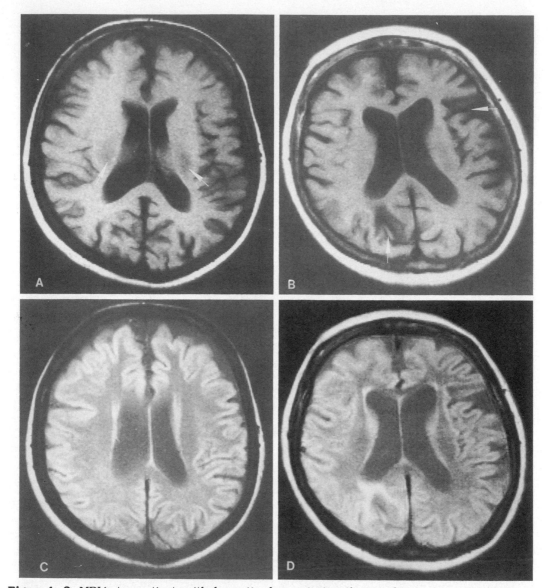

Figure 4–3. MRI in two patients with dementia, demonstrating the use of T_1- and T_2-weighted images to differentiate atrophy from stroke. The images on the left (A, C, E) are from a patient with clinically diagnosed Alzheimer's disease; those on the right (B, D, F) are from a patient with cerebral infarction. The images have progressively greater T_2 and progressively less T_1 weighting from the top (A, B) to the bottom (E, F). In (A) and (B), predominantly T_1-weighted images (TR 500, TE 30) demonstrate widening of the sulci and ventricular enlargement in both patients. Although atrophic changes are seen diffusely in both patients, decreased signal is seen in the white matter in the AD patient (*arrows*), and areas of focally pronounced sulcal widening (*arrows*) are noted in the other patient, of thus far uncertain significance. In (C) and (D), greater T_2 weighting (TR 2000, TE 60), cerebrospinal fluid produces an intermediate signal and gray matter is seen more distinctly. In the Alzheimer disease patient (C), the increased periventricular signal indicates the caudate nucleus; no abnormalities are seen in the white matter, indicating that the suspicious areas in (A) are normal and probably represent the most superior aspects of the subcortical nuclei. In (D), the cortical ribbon is normal in the suspicious, focally atrophic sylvian fissure, but there is loss of the gray-white junction in the contralateral occipital lobe, with an extensive area of increased signal in the white matter extending to the ventricle.

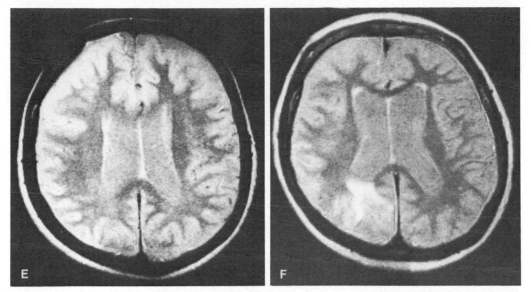

Figure 4–3 *Continued* (*E*) and (*F*) provide the greatest T_2 weighting (TR 2000, TE 30), which intensifies the occipital white-matter lesion in (*F*) but indicates no additional lesions in either subject. The two areas of focal atrophy indicated in (*B*) therefore are different. The atrophy in the occipital cortex almost certainly represents a stroke, but the atrophy in the sylvian fissure could represent an old nonischemic injury, a distant infarct, or a degenerative process.

quences can be used to highlight different aspects of brain structure. Echo time refers to the time between pulses. Spin-spin relaxation time (T_1) weighted images (short relaxation time [TR], long echo time [TE]) maximize gray-white differentiation and are best at imaging structural features such as ventricular and sulcal size. Conversely, spin-lattice relaxation time (T_2) weighted images (long TR, short TE) usually increase the contrast between pathologic and normal brain tissue, and thus are best at demonstrating white-matter lesions, edematous and inflammatory lesions, and infarcts. Therefore, both T_1- and T_2-weighted images should be obtained in patients with dementia (Fig. 4–3).

MRI allows one to visualize brain in three planes and seems to be the most sensitive imaging technique for demonstrating small lacunar strokes[59,60,62] (Fig. 4–4), the plaques of multiple sclerosis,[85] focal lesions of the temporal lobe,[207] and any lesion in the posterior fossa. Paramagnetic contrast agents that develop a magnetic moment in a magnetic field and alter the radiofrequency signal intensity where they become concentrated are used in MRI, and may be of considerable help in detecting focal lesions.[31] As a rule of thumb, MRI can be considered the most sensitive imaging study to detect chronic lesions, whereas CT excels at visualizing acute lesions. The incompatibility of much medical hardware with the large magnetic fields generated by MRI often precludes its application in the acutely ill patient in emergent circumstances, however. Moreover, long scan times, combined with enclosure in a small space, may limit use in easily agitated dementia patients.

There has not yet been sufficient study of MRI in dementia or AD to assess whether it will prove superior to CT. Which is preferable for a particular patient depends upon availability, cost, and the likelihood of a lesion best imaged by MRI or by CT. It is safe to assume that comparable information about brain atrophy is generated by the two methods, and the same limitations and uses of this parameter in the diagnosis of dementia as described for CT apply equally well to atrophy seen with MRI. MRI may also be useful in recognizing NPH.[20]

Because of the increased sensitivity of

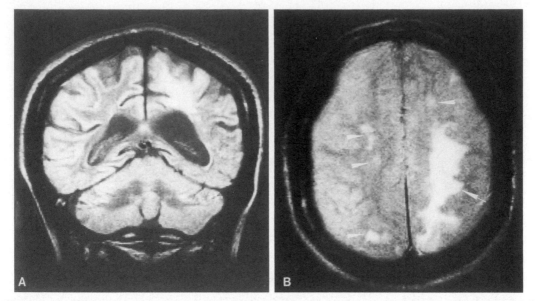

Figure 4–4. MRI in a patient with dementia and a history of hypertension and stroke. The T_2-weighted images (TR 2000, TE 30) demonstrate the power of MRI to provide high-resolution views of the brain in several dimensions. (*A*) A coronal view demonstrates a high-signal lesion that extends through the depth of the superior left parietal cortex, obliterating the gray-white junction. Also note the excellent visualization of the cerebellum, without significant artifact or evidence of stroke. (*B*) A horizontal image in the same patient identifies the same extensive lesion in the left hemisphere, but also shows several smaller areas of increased signal in both hemispheres (*arrowheads*), representing other cerebral infarcts.

MRI for white-matter lesions, many small, so-called "bright spots" can be seen in older individuals with unremarkable CT scans. These "bright spots" are seen in both demented individuals and those with normal cognition, but they are more frequent in patients with cognitive impairment or focal neurologic signs.[209,210] The relation of white-matter changes and cognitive impairment is still controversial. Most studies do find differences between AD and healthy aging.[66,144,165] In a longitudinal study of AD patients, however, Diaz and co-workers[49] found white-matter changes associated with a greater degree of cognitive impairment. Other studies have demonstrated that "bright spots" represent small infarcts. On pathologic examination, some are small lacunar strokes, but others are only widened perivascular spaces or white-matter pallor.[8,188] It has been suggested that the term *leukoariosis* be used to describe the presence of deep white-matter changes in demented elderly patients.[33,94] The relationships

between such lesions seen by CT and those seen by MRI also remain unresolved.[60] Clear criteria have not yet been developed for differentiating pathologic states and normal aging, and further research will be needed before it is clear how these lesions should be interpreted by the clinician. It is safe to say, though, that if no bright spots are seen, the patient does not have MID.

The relative concentrations of various chemical constituents in small brain regions can be measured by magnetic resonance (MR) spectroscopy. The tissue content of metabolically important compounds containing phosphorus, such as adenosine triphosphate and phosphocreatine, or containing carbon, such as lactate, can be examined by MR spectroscopy. In cerebral ischemia, MR spectroscopy has already proven to be an important investigational tool[234] and early investigations with these techniques in dementia are encouraging. A decline in high-energy phosphate metabolism in the parietal cortex in patients with AD and PD with dementia,[89] and alterations in phospholipid metabolism that distinguish degenerative from MID have been observed.[84] Its usefulness in evaluating and understanding diagnosis, however, awaits further work.

RADIONUCLIDE IMAGING

Radionuclide imaging uses a pharmocologic agent as the source of radiation to provide a brain image. Because the distribution of the radioactive agent reflects its biologic properties, this technique has the advantage of being able to examine a variety of physiologic and pharmacologic properties of the brain. Radiopharmaceuticals in use today can be classified on the basis of their isotopic label as either (1) single photon gamma emitters, or (2) positron emitters. Gamma-emitting isotopes have a relatively long half-life and can be used to construct rectilinear (two-dimensional) views of the brain or three-dimensional images using a technique called single photon emission computed tomography (SPECT). Positron-emitting isotopes used in positron emission tomography (PET) have the disadvantage of requiring a cyclotron for their synthesis, but generally provide better resolution. Furthermore, positron-emitting isotopes are available for biologically relevant elements, such as carbon and oxygen, and for other small elements, such as fluorine, which can be easily incorporated into biologically important compounds without substantially changing their chemistry.

Cerebrospinal Fluid Dynamics. Cisternography, originally performed with radioactive iodinated serum albumin (RISA) and now being done using diethylenetriamine pentacetic acid (DTPA) labeled with ytterbium 169 or indium 111, provides an image that reflects CSF dynamics.[160] This method can demonstrate hydrocephalus and aid in the identification of NPH. Unfortunately, it is insufficiently predictive of the success of shunting to recommend its routine use.[106] Consequently, abnormal cisternography should be only one of several indicators used to decide whether surgical treatment should be attempted when ventricular enlargement and dementia coexist. In the presence of the triad of dementia, incontinence, and gait disorder, which suggests NPH, abnormal cisternography provides further evidence that shunt placement should be attempted; it also can be used to monitor shunt function. Cisternography can assess whether periventricular changes noted on CT or MRI are due to altered fluid dynamics. CT cisternography, using a radiopaque dye, or MRI also may be used to assess abnormal spinal fluid dynamics.[20,215]

Regional Cerebral Metabolism. 2-deoxy-2[^{18}F]fluoro-D-glucose (FDG) imaging is the PET counterpart to the 2-[^{11}C]-deoxy-D-glucose technique used to estimate glucose utilization in animals. FDG is taken up by the brain in proportion to the uptake of glucose. Because glucose utilization reflects the brain's energy demands, FDG serves as a measure of neuronal function. Likewise, the utilization of $^{15}O-O_2$ reflects the utilization of oxygen by the brain primarily for oxidative metabolism. AD typically causes predominantly posterior temporoparietal hypometabolism[52,73,157] (Fig. 4-5). The hypometabolism may be bilaterally symmetric or predominantly involve one hemisphere. The region of greatest metabolic impairment corresponds to the patient's behavioral abnormalities,[43,72,91,97] and the severity of symptoms correlates with the degree of hypometabolism.[73]

As seen in Fig. 4-5, the pattern of regional cerebral metabolism differs in various disorders leading to dementia. In progressive supranuclear palsy (PSP), hypometabolism is most prominent in the basal ganglia, brainstem, and frontal cortex.[44,74] In Pick's disease, the frontal cortex is typically hypometabolic.[79,114] PD, when complicated by the presence of dementia, causes a predominantly temporoparietal hypometabolism,[131] and the characteristic feature of MID is the presence of multiple hypometabolic zones throughout the brain.[163] In patients with progressive aphasia without dementia, hypometabolism is limited to the left perisylvian region, whereas in AD with predominant aphasia, accentuated left hemisphere hypometabolism is accompanied by subnormal metabolism in the right hemisphere.[32,72,162] In HD (Fig. 4–6), metabolism of the cerebral cortex is often normal, and hypometabolism primarily occurs in the caudate nucleus and putamen.[132,246] The role of cerebral metabolic imaging in the differential diagnosis of dementia is not yet defined, but the dissimilarity in the pattern of regional cerebral metabolism between disorders that are at times difficult to distinguish clinically suggests that imaging of local glucose and oxygen metabolism may have utility in specific clinical settings.

There has been considerable interest in the use of pharmacologic or behavioral activation during functional brain imaging. In animals, it has now become routine to examine the effects of drugs upon local glucose metabolism using the ^{11}C-deoxyglucose technique. In humans, such methods have not yet been widely used, but both increases (due to neuroleptics) and decreases (due to diazepam) in glucose metabolism can be induced.[47,75] These effects must be considered in interpreting imaging results. Because diazepam in moderate doses causes global but not regional alterations in glucose metabolism in patients with AD, it may be used for sedation to study patients with this diagnosis when only regional comparisons are to be made. It has been hoped that behavioral stimulation would lead to improvement in diagnosis by accentuating differences in how the brain processes information. Although test-retest variability may be reduced by stimulation,[53] and some paradigms cause notable differences in response between demented and normal subjects,[164] individual differences in response and lack of a well-documented and widely used technique have thus

far prevented stimulation studies from achieving diagnostic utility.

Regional Cerebral Blood Flow. Regional cerebral blood flow (rCBF) can also be imaged by radionuclide techniques. Both positron-emitting and single-photon methods are available. Gamma-emitting radiopharmaceuticals such as ^{123}I-IMP,[130] ^{123}I-HIPDM,[58,103] xenon 133,[48,189] and ^{99m}Tc-HM-PAO[57] provide an index of cerebral perfusion and have the additional advantage of being less expensive and more widely available than PET agents that measure cerebral blood flow, such as ^{15}O-H_2O[110] or methane labeled with carbon 11.[102]

In general, rCBF parallels regional cerebral metabolism in dementing disorders. The brain regions most hypometabolic in AD, PSP, and HD are also most hypoperfused[77,139,232] (see Figs. 4–5 and 4–6). Such parallel changes do not occur in cerebrovascular disease, however, when metabolic demands outstrip supply. In the future it may be possible to exploit these differences in helping to identify vasculitis and MID. There is also some evidence that neurogenic cerebrovascular regulation may be altered in PSP, modifying the usual coupling of metabolism and blood flow.[139] Some have also observed an uncoupling during various types of motor or sensory activation.[76] Various drugs and ventilatory status also may alter blood flow but not metabolism.

Single photon imaging of rCBF can discriminate between AD and stroke-related dementia, depression, and normal aging[26,45,86,112,204] (Fig. 4–7). As with metabolism, there are both global and focal temporoparietal reductions in perfusion, which correlate with symptoms, in patients with AD.[46] Imaging of rCBF may be useful in the early diagnosis of AD because flow deficits appear early in the course of the illness. The sensitivity and reliability of rCBF changes in differentiating various forms of early dementia and distinguishing them from depressive pseudodementia will need to be established. As with measurement of metabolism, the role of provocative studies of rCBF during drug or behavioral stimulation remains undetermined.

Neurotransmitter   Distribution. Radiopharmaceuticals that can indicate the distribution and activity of neurotransmitters are being developed with the hope that it may soon be possible to assay neurochemistry noninvasively. Such methods can exploit what is already known about brain biochemistry from postmortem studies and attempt to make similar measurements in vivo. The evolution of these changes may also be observed. A broad range of agents with pharmacologic activity in the brain, including drugs that interact with neurotransmitter receptors (labeled neurotransmitter precursors), and amino acid analogs, have been synthesized. A few are single photon agents,[55] but most have been synthesized with positron-emitting isotopes.[183] Considerable effort still must be spent in defining and confirming models that describe the behavior of these tracers, but many intriguing observations already have been made. For example, in vivo changes in dopamine receptor density have been demonstrated in PSP and HD, and impaired accumulation of ^{18}F-fluorodopa is seen in PD.[11,140,141] Studies of these new neurotransmitter-related agents in demented patients are only just beginning, but clearly such agents have great potential. In vivo markers of cholinergic function are under development and may be of special interest both in AD and in PD with dementia, in which a cholinergic deficit is known to exist. These techniques may also help unravel the mixed dementias by permitting the identification of simultaneous deficits in several functions, such as cholinergic or dopaminergic deficits in the presence of cerebral infarcts. In the future it is conceivable that a variety of physiologic and biochemical parameters will be available for each patient with dementia, so that appropriate therapy can be selected and adjusted based upon the results of brain imaging.

Brain Biopsy

The clinical indications for brain biopsy in patients with dementia are unclear. Although the study of biopsies has contributed to research on dementia, particularly AD,[108,118] the biopsy rarely helps in the management of individual patients, largely owing to the lack of specific therapies for dementias that may be detected by microscopic examination of tissue. If a brain biopsy will not lead to a change in management of an individual patient, then it is probably not justified. Common biopsy diagnoses include AD, Pick's disease, vasculopathy, chronic meningoencephalitis, CJD, and leukodystrophy. Reversible conditions such as tuberculous meningitis, granulomatous angiitis, sarcoidosis, or acute demyelination have been rarely detected.

SUMMARY

The clinical evaluation of patients with dementia requires a working knowledge of the types of dementia and their diagnostic criteria. Such criteria are available for the more common dementing illnesses, such as AD, and are beginning to be formulated for the vascular dementias. The criteria for rarer dementias are not as well specified. The challenge in the early diagnosis of these disorders is to differentiate age-associated memory impairment from early dementia. Clinical evaluation itself includes a neuropsychiatric history, which should include an assessment of the impact of the disease on the individual and family. A family history, looking for evidence of heritable conditions, is essential. A neurologic examination should focus on observing signs of reversible forms of dementia and include an appropriately extensive mental status examination. Selected instruments that may be valuable to assess the cognitive abilities of the patient were described in this chapter and include the Wechsler Adult Intelligence Scale, visuospatial tests, The Wechsler Memory Scale, Selective Reminding Test, Boston Diagnostic Aphasia Evaluation and Boston Naming Test, controlled word association testing, and praxis testing. Standard laboratory tests, including screening blood tests and neuroimaging, were discussed. Lumbar puncture and EEG may be helpful in making a differential diagnosis in some circumstances. CT can be used in routine screening of most patients with dementia, but MRI offers high resolution and a better view of posterior fossa. Cisternography may be useful if NPH is suspected. SPECT and PET are techniques whose roles in clinical practice are currently being evaluated.

REFERENCES

1. Albert ML: Clinical Neurology of Aging. Oxford University Press, New York, 1984.
2. Alexopoulos GS, Abrams RC, Young RC, and Shamoian CA: Cornell Scale for Depression. Biol Psychiatry 23: 271–284, 1988.
3. Amaducci LA, Fratiglioni L, Rocca WA, et al: Risk factors for clinically diagnosed Alzheimer's disease: A case-control study of Italian population. Neurology 16:922–931, 1986.
4. American Academy of Neurology, Therapeutics and Technology Assessment Subcommittee: Assessment: EEG brain mapping. Neurology 39: 1100–1101, 1989.
5. American Psychiatric Association: Diagnostic and Statistical Manual of Mental Disorders, Ed 3, Rev. American Psychiatric Association, Washington, DC, 1987.
6. Applegate WB, Blass JP, and Williams TF: Instruments for the functional assessment of older patients. Current Concepts in Geriatrics 322:1207–1213, 1990.
7. Appleyard ME, Smith AD, Berman P, et al: Cholinesterase activities in cerebrospinal fluid of patients with senile dementia of Alzheimer type. Brain 110:1309–1322, 1987.
8. Awad IA, Johnson PC, Spetzler RF, and Hodak JA: Incidental subcortical lesions identified on magnetic resonance imaging in the elderly. II. Postmortem pathological correlations. Stroke 17:1090–1097, 1986.
9. Awad IA, Spetzler RF, Hodak JA, Awad CA, and Carey R: Incidental subcortical lesions identified on magnetic resonance imaging in the elderly. I. Correlation with age and cerebrovascular risk factors. Stroke 17:1084–1089, 1986.
10. Baloh RW: Neurotology of aging: Vestibular system. In Albert ML (ed): Clinical Neurology of Aging. Oxford University Press, New York, 1984, pp 345–361.
11. Baron JC, Maziere B, Loch C, et al: Loss of striatal [^{76}Br]bromospiperone binding sites demonstrated by positron tomography in progressive supranuclear palsy. J Cereb Blood Flow Metab 6:131–136, 1986.
12. Barry PP and Moskowitz MA: The diagnosis of reversible dementia in the elderly: A critical review. Arch Intern Med 148:1914–1918, 1988.
13. Bartus RT, Dean RL III, Beer B, and Lippa AS: The cholinergic hypothesis of geriatric memory dysfunction. Science 217:408–417, 1982.
14. Benton A: FAS test. In Spreen O and Benton A (eds): Neurosensory Center Comprehensive Examination for Aphasia. University of Victoria, Victoria, BC, 1967.
15. Bentson J, Reza M, Winter J, and Wilson G: Steroids and apparent cerebral atrophy on computed tomography scans. J Comput Assist Tomogr 2: 16–23, 1978.
16. Berg L: Clinical Dementia Rating (CDR). Psychopharmacol Bull 24: 637–639, 1988.
17. Bird TD, Lampe TH, Nemens EJ, Miner GW, Sumi SM, and Schellen-

berg GD: Familial Alzheimer's disease in American descendants of the Volga Germans: Probable genetic founder effect. Ann Neurol 23:25–31, 1988.

18. Bird TD, Sumi SM, Nemens EJ, et al: Phenotypic heterogeneity in familial Alzheimer's disease: A study of 24 kindreds. Ann Neurol 25:12–25, 1989.

19. Blessed G, Tomlinson BE, and Roth M: The association between quantitative measures of dementia and of senile change in the cerebral grey matter of elderly subjects. Br J Psychiatry 114:797–811, 1968.

20. Bradley WG, Kortman KE, and Burgoyne B: Flowing cerebrospinal fluid in normal and hydrocephalic states: Appearance on MR images. Radiology 159:611–616, 1986.

21. Brayne C and Calloway P: Normal aging, impaired cognitive function and senile dementia of the Alzheimer type: A continuum. Lancet 1:1265–1267, 1988.

22. Breen AR, Larson B, Reiffer BU, Vitaliano PP, and Lawrence GL: Cognitive performance and functional competence in co-existing dementia and depression. J Am Geriatr Soc 32:132–137, 1984.

23. Breitner JCS, Silverman JM, Mohs RC, and Davis KL: Familial aggregation in Alzheimer's disease: Comparison of risk among relatives of early- and late-onset cases, and among male and female relatives in successive generations. Neurology 38:207–212, 1988.

24. Brenner RP, Reynold CF, and Ulrich RF: Diagnostic efficacy of computerized spectral versus visual EEG analysis in elderly normal, demented and depressed subjects. Electroencephalogr Clin Neurophysiol 62:110–117, 1988.

25. Breslau J, Starr A, Sicotte N, Higa J, and Bushsbaum MS: Topographic EEG changes with normal aging and SDAT. Electroencephalogr Clin Neurophysiol 72:281–289, 1989.

26. Brinkman SD, Sarwar M, Levin HS, and Morris HH: Quantitative indexes of computed tomography in dementia and normal aging. Radiology 138:89–92, 1981.

27. Brooks RA and DiChiro G: Beam hardening x-ray reconstructive tomography. Phys Med Biol 21:390–398, 1976.

28. Buschke H and Fuld PA: Evaluating storage, retention, and retrieval in disordered memory and learning. Neurology 24:1019–1025, 1974.

29. Carlen PL, Wilkinson DA, Wortzman G, and Holgate R: Partial reversible cerebral atrophy and functional improvement in recently abstinent alcoholics. Can J Neurol Sci 11:441–446, 1984.

30. Carlen PL, Wortzman G, Holgate RC, Wilkinson DA, and Rankin JG: Reversible cerebral atrophy in recently abstinent chronic alcoholics measured by computed tomography scans. Science 200:1076–1078, 1978.

31. Charness ME, Simon RP, and Greenberg DA: Ethanol and the nervous system. N Engl J Med 321:442–454, 1989.

32. Chawluk JB, Mesulam MM, Hurtig H, et al: Slowly progressive aphasia without generalized dementia: Studies with positron emission tomography. Ann Neurol 19:68–74, 1986.

33. Chimowitz MI, Awad IA, and Furhan AJ: Periventricular lesions on MRI. Facts and theories. Stroke 20:963–967, 1989.

34. Claussen C, Laniado M, and Kazner E: Application of contrast agents in CT and MRI (NMR): Their potential in imaging of brain tumors. Neuroradiology 27:164, 1985.

35. Coben LA, Danzigler WL, and Storandt M: A longitudinal EEG study of mild senile dementia of Alzheimer type: Changes at 1 year and 2.5 years. Electroencephalogr Clin Neurophysiol 61:101–112, 1985.

36. Cohen MB, Graham S, Lake R, et al: Diagnosis of Alzheimer's disease and multiple infarct dementia by tomographic imaging of iodine 123-IMP. J Nucl Med 27:769–774, 1986.

37. Cohen MM and Lessell S: Neuro-ophthalmology of aging. In Albert ML (ed): Clinical Neurology of Aging, Oxford

University Press, New York, 1984, pp 313–344.

38. Cook RH, Schneck SA, and Clark DB: Twins with Alzheimer's disease. Arch Neurol 38:300–301, 1981.

39. Cummings JL: Treatable Dementias. In Mayeux R and Rosen W (eds): The Dementias. Raven Press, New York, 1983, pp 165–185.

40. Cummings JL and Benson DF: Dementia: A Clinical Approach. Butterworth & Co, Boston, 1983, pp 1–15.

41. Cummings JL and Duchen LW: Klüver-Bucy syndrome in Pick's disease: Clinical and pathologic correlations. Neurology 31:1415–1422, 1981.

42. Curran JW, Jaffe HW, Hardy AM, Morgan WM, Selik RM, and Dondero TJ: Epidemiology of HIV infection and AIDS in United States. Science 239:533–696, 1988.

43. Cutler NR, Haxby JV, Duara R, et al: Clinical history, brain metabolism and neuropsychological function in Alzheimer's disease. Ann Neurol 18:298–309, 1985.

44. D'Antona R, Baron JC, Samson Y, et al: Subcortical dementia: Frontal cortex hypometabolism detected by positron tomography in patients with progressive supranuclear palsy. Brain 108:785–799, 1985.

45. DeKosky ST, Shih WJ, Coupal J, and Kirkpatrick C: Role of single photon emission computerized tomography (SPECT) in the diagnosis of Alzheimer's disease. Neurology 37:159, 1987.

46. DeKosky ST, Shih WJ, Schmitt FA, Coupal J, and Kirkpatrick C: Assessing utility of single photon emission computed tomography (SPECT) scan in Alzheimer disease: Correlation with cognitive severity. Alzheimer Dis Assoc Disord 4:14–23, 1990.

47. DeLisi LE, Holcomb HH, Cohen RM, et al: Positron emission tomography in schizophrenic patients with and without neuroleptic medication. J Cereb Blood Flow Metab 5:201–206, 1985.

48. Devous MD, Stokely EM, Chehabi HH, and Bonte FJ: Normal distribution of regional cerebral blood flow measured by dynamic single-photon emission tomography. J Cereb Blood Flow Metab 6:95–104, 1986.

49. Diaz JF, Merskey H, Hachinski VC, et al: Improved recognition of leukoaraiosis and cognitive impairment in Alzheimer's disease. Arch Neurol 48:1022–1025, 1991.

50. Doty RL, Deem DA, and Stellar S: Olfactory dysfunction in parkinsonism: A general deficit unrelated to neurologic signs, disease stage, or disease duration. Neurology 38:1237–1244, 1988.

51. Doty RL, Shannon P, Applebaum SL, Giverson R, and Sitsorski L: Smell identification ability: Changes with age. Science 226:1441–1443, 1984.

52. Duara R, Grady C, Haxby J, et al: Positron emission tomography in Alzheimer's disease. Neurology 36:879–887, 1986.

53. Duara R, Gross-Glenn K, Barker WW, et al: Behavioral activation and the variability of cerebral glucose metabolic measurements. J Cereb Blood Flow Metab 7:266–271, 1987.

54. Duffy FH, Albert MS, and McAnulty G: Brain electric activity in patients with senile and presenile dementia of Alzheimer type. Ann Neurol 16:439–448, 1984.

55. Eckelman WC, Reba RC, Rzeszotarski WJ, et al: External imaging of cerebral muscarinic acetylcholine receptors. Science 223:291–293, 1984.

56. Eisendorfer C and Cohen D: Diagnostic criteria for primary neuronal degeneration of Alzheimer's type. J Fam Pract 11:553–557, 1980.

57. Ell PJ, Jaritt PH, Cullum I, et al: Regular cerebral blood flow mapping with 99mTc-labelled compound. Lancet 2:50–51, 1985.

58. Ell PJ, Lui D, Cullum I, Jarritt PH, Donaghy M, and Harrison MJG: Cerebral blood flow studies with 123-iodine-labelled amines. Lancet 1:1348–1352, 1983.

59. Erkinjuntti T: Differential diagnosis between Alzheimer's disease and vascular dementia: Evaluation of common clinical methods. Acta Neurol Scand 76:433–442, 1987.

60. Erkinjuntti T, Ketonen L, Sulkava R, Sipponen J, Vuorialho M, and Iivanainen M: Do white matter changes on MRI and CT differentiate vascular dementia from Alzheimer's disease? J Neurol Neurosurg Psychiatry 50:37–42, 1987.

61. Erkinjuntti T, Laaksonen R, Sulkava R, Syrjalainen R, and Palo J: Neuropsychological differentiation between normal aging, Alzheimer's disease and vascular dementia. Acta Neurol Scand 74:393–403, 1986.

62. Erkinjuntti T, Sipponen JT, Iivanainen M, Ketonen L, Sulkava R, and Sepponen RE: Cerebral NMR and CT imaging in dementia. J Comput Assist Tomogr 8:614–618, 1984.

63. Erkinjuntti T, Wikstrom J, Palo J, and Autio L: Dementia among medical inpatients: Evaluation of 2000 consecutive admissions. Arch Intern Med 146:1923–1926, 1986

64. Eslinger PJ, Damasio H, Graff-Radford N, and Damasio AR: Examining the relationship between computed tomography and neuropsychological measures in normal and demented elderly. J Neurol Neurosurg Psychiatry 47:1319–1325, 1984.

65. Evans DA, Funkenstein HH, Albert MS, et al: Prevalence of Alzheimer's disease in a community population of older persons. Higher than previously reported. JAMA 262:2551–2556, 1989.

66. Fein G, Van Dyke C, Davenport L, et al: Preservation of normal cognitive functioning in elderly subjects with extensive white matter lesion of long duration. Arch Gen Psychiatry 47:220–223, 1990.

67. Ferris E and Levine H: Cerebral arteritis: Classification. Neuroradiology 41:327–341, 1973.

68. Fletcher WA and Sharpe JA: Saccadic eye movement dysfunction in Alzheimer's disease. Ann Neurol 20:464–471, 1986.

69. Flicker C, Ferris SH, and Reisberg B: Mild cognitive impairment in the elderly. Predictors of dementia. Neurology 41:1006–1009, 1991.

70. Folstein MF, Folstein SE, and McHugh PR: "Mini-Mental State," a practical method for grading the cognitive state of patients for the clinician. J Psychiatr Res 12:189–198, 1975.

71. Foncin JF, Salmon D, Supino-Viterbo V, et al: Demence presenile D'Alzheimer transmise dans une familie étendue. Rev Neurol (Paris) 141(3):194–202, 1985.

72. Foster NL, Chase TN, Fedio P, Patronas NJ, Brooks RA, and DiChiro G: Focal cortical changes in Alzheimer's disease demonstrated by positron emission tomography with 18-F-fluorodeoxyglucose. Neurology 33:961–965, 1983.

73. Foster NL, Chase TN, Mansi L, et al: Cortical abnormalities in Alzheimer's disease. Ann Neurol 16:649–654, 1984.

74. Foster NL, Gilman S, Berent S, Morin EM, Brown MB, and Koeppe RA: Cerebral hypometabolism in progressive supranuclear palsy studied with positron emission tomography. Ann Neurol 24:399–406, 1988.

75. Foster NL, VanDerSpek AFL, Aldrich MS, et al: The effect of diazepam sedation on cerebral glucose metabolism in Alzheimer's disease as measured using positron emission tomography. J Cereb Blood Flow Metabol 7:415–420, 1987.

76. Fox PT, Raichle ME, Mintun MA, and Dence C: Nonoxidative glucose consumption during focal physiologic neural activity. Science 241:462–464, 1988.

77. Frackowiak RSJ, Pozzilli C, Legg NJ, et al: Regional cerebral oxygen supply and utilization in dementia. Brain 104:753–778, 1981.

78. Friedland RP, Budinger TF, Ganz E, et al: Regional cerebral metabolic alterations in dementia of the Alzheimer type: Positron emission tomography with [18F]-fluorodeoxyglucose. J Comput Assist Tomogr 7:590–598, 1983.

79. Friedland RP, Jagust WJ, Ober BA, et al: The pathophysiology of Pick's disease: A comprehensive case study. Neurology (Suppl 1)36:268–269, 1986.

80. Gado MH, Coleman RE, Lee KS, Mik-

hael MA, Alderson PO, and Archer CR: Correlation between computerized transaxial tomography and radionuclide cisternography in dementia. Neurology 26:555–560, 1976.

81. Gado MH, Hughes CP, Danziger W, Chi D, Jost G, and Berg L: Volumetric measurements of the cerebrospinal fluid spaces in demented subjects and controls. Radiology 144:535–538, 1982.

82. Gado MH, Hughes CP, Danziger W, and Chi D: Aging, dementia and brain atrophy: A longitudinal computed tomographic study. AJNR 4:699–702, 1983.

83. Gado MH, Patel J, Hughes CP, Danziger W, and Berg L: Brain atrophy in dementia judged by CT scan ranking, AJNR 4:499–500, 1983.

84. Gdowski JW, Brown GG, Levine SR, et al: Patterns of phospholipid metabolism differ between Alzheimer and multi-infarct dementia. Neurology 38(1):268, 1988.

85. Gebarski SS, Gabrielsen TO, Gilman S, Knake JE, Latack JT, and Aisen AM: The initial diagnosis of multiple sclerosis: Clinical impact of magnetic resonance imaging. Ann Neurol 17:469–474, 1985.

86. Gemmell H, Sharp P, Evans N, Besson JAO, Lyall D, and Smith FW: Single photon emission tomography with ^{123}I-isopropylamphetamine in Alzheimer's disease and multi-infarct dementia. Lancet 2:1348, 1984.

87. Goodglass H and Kaplan D: The assessment of aphasia and related disorders, Ed 2. Lea and Febiger, Philadelphia, 1983.

88. vanGool WA and Bolhuis PA: Cerebrospinal fluid markers of Alzheimer's disease. J Am Geriatr Soc 39:1025–1039, 1991.

89. Gorell JM, Bueri JA, Brown GG, et al: Parietal and frontal high-energy cerebral phosphate metabolism in Alzheimer and Parkinson dementia. Neurology 38(1):227, 1988.

90. Goudsmit J, White BJ, Weitkamp LR, et al: Familial Alzheimer's disease in two kindreds of the same geographic and ethnic origin. J Neurol Sci 49:79–89, 1981.

91. Grady CL, Haxby JV, Schlageter NL, Berg G, and Rapoport SI: Stability of metabolic and neuropsychological asymmetries in dementia of the Alzheimer type. Neurology 36:1390–1392, 1986.

92. Gurland BJ, Copeland JRM, Sharpe L, and Kellerner MJ: The geriatric mental status interview (GMS). Int J Aging Hum Dev 7:303–311, 1976.

93. Hachinski VC, Lassen NA, and Marshall J: Multi-infarct dementia. Lancet 2:207–210, 1974.

94. Hachinski VC, Potter P, and Merskey H: Leuko-araiosis. Arch Neurol 44:21–23, 1987.

95. Hammerstrom DC and Zimmer B: The role of lumbar puncture in the evaluation of dementia: The University of Pittsburgh study. J Am Geriatr Soc 33:397–400, 1985.

96. Hayes D and Jerger J: Neurotology of aging: Auditory system. In Albert ML (ed), Clinical Neurology of Aging. Oxford University Press, New York, 1984, pp 362–378.

97. Haxby JV, Duara R, Grady C, Cutler N, and Rapoport SI: Relations between neuropsychological and cerebral metabolic asymmetries in early Alzheimer's disease. J Cereb Blood Flow Metab 5:193–200, 1985.

98. Helkala EL, Laulumaa V, Soininen H, Partenen J, and Riekkinen PJ: Different patterns of cognitive decline related to normal or deteriorating EEG in 3-year follow-up study of patients with Alzheimer's disease. Neurology 41:528–532, 1991.

99. Heston LL, Mastri AR, Anderson VE, et al: Dementia of the Alzheimer's type: Clinical genetics, natural history and associated conditions. Arch Gen Psychiatry 38:1085–1090, 1981.

100. Heyman A, Wilkinson WE, Hurwitz BJ, et al: Alzheimer's disease: Genetic aspects and associated clinical disorders. Ann Neurol 14:507–515, 1983.

101. Heyman A, Wilkinson WE, Hurwitz BJ, et al: Early-onset Alzheimer disease: Clinical predictors of institutionalization and death. Neurology 37:980–984, 1987.

102. Holden JE, Gatley SJ, Hichwa RD, et al: Regional cerebral blood flow using positron emission tomographic measurements of fluoromethane kinetics. J Nucl Med 22:1084–1088, 1981.

103. Holman BL, Lee RGL, Hill TC, Lovett RD, and Lister-James J: A comparison of two cerebral perfusion tracers, N-isopropyl-I-123-p-iodoamphetamine and I-123 HIPDM, in the human. J Nucl Med 25:25–30, 1984.

104. Hubbard BM and Anderson JM: A quantitative study of cerebral atrophy in old age and senile dementia. J Neurol Sci 50, 1981.

105. Hubbard BM and Anderson JM: Age, senile dementia and ventricular enlargement. J Neurol Neurosurg Psychiatry 44:631–635, 1981.

106. Huckman MS: Normal pressure hydrocephalus: Evaluation of diagnostic and prognostic tests. AJNR 2:385–395, 1981.

107. Huff FJ, Auerback BA, Charkravarti A, and Boller F: Risk of dementia in relative of patients with Alzheimer's disease. Neurology 38:786–790, 1988.

108. Hughes CP, Berg L, Danziger W, Coben LA, and Martin RL: A new clinical scale for the staging of dementia. Br J Psychiatry 140:566–572, 1982.

109. Hughes CP and Gado M: Computed tomography and aging of the brain. Radiology 139:391–396, 1981.

110. Hulette CM, Earl NM, and Crain BJ: Evaluation of cerebral biopsies for diagnosis of dementia. Arch Neurol 49:28–31, 1992.

111. Hutchins GD, Hichwa RD, and Koeppe RA: A continuous flow input function detector for $H_2^{15}O$ blood flow studies in positron emission tomography. IEEE Trans Nucl Sci 33:546–549, 1986.

112. Johnson KA, Mueller ST, Walshe TM, English RJ, and Holman BL: Cerebral perfusion imaging in Alzheimer's disease: Use of single photon emission computed tomography and lofetamine hydrochloride I123. Arch Neurol 44:165–169, 1987.

113. Kahn R, Goldfarb A, and Pollack M: Brief objective measures of mental status in the aged. Am J Psychiatry 117:326–328, 1960.

114. Kamo H, McGeer PL, Harrop R, et al: Positron emission tomography and histopathology in Pick's disease. Neurology 37:439–445, 1987.

115. Kaplan E, Goodglass H, and Weintraub S: Boston Naming Test. Lea and Febiger, Philadelphia, 1983.

116. Katz S, Ford AB, Moskowitz RW, Jackson BA, and Jaffee MW: Studies of illness in the aged: The index of ADL. A standardized measure of biological function. JAMA 185:914–919, 1963.

117. Katzman R, Brown T, Fuld P, Peck A, Schechter R, and Schimmel H: Validation of the short Orientation-Memory Concentration test of cognitive impairment. Am J Psychiatry 140:734–738, 1983.

118. Katzman R, Lasker B, Bernstein N, et al: Advances in the diagnosis of dementia: Accuracy of diagnosis and consequences of misdiagnosis of disorders causing dementias. In Terry RD (ed): Aging and the Brain. Raven Press, New York, 1988, pp 17–56.

119. Katzman R and Terry R: The Neurology of Aging. FA Davis, Philadelphia, 1983.

120. Kaye JA, May C, Daly E, et al: Cerebrospinal fluid monoamine markers are decreased in dementia of Alzheimer type with extrapyramidal features. Neurology 38:554–557, 1988.

121. Kirshner HS, Webb WG, Kelly MP, and Wells CE: Language disturbance: An initial symptom of cortical degenerations and dementia. Arch Neurol 41:491–496, 1984.

122. Kitagawa Y, Meyer JS, Tanashashi N, et al: Cerebral blood flow and brain atrophy correlated by xenon contrast CT scanning. Comput Radiol 9:331–340, 1985.

123. Kohlmeyer K, Lehmkuhl G, and Poutska F: Computed tomography of anorexia nervosa. AJNR 4:437–438, 1983.

124. Kokmen E, Beard CM, Offord KP, and Kurland LT: Prevalence of medically diagnosed dementia in a defined United States population: Rochester,

Minnesota. Neurology 39:773–776, 1989.

125. Kokmen E, Chandra V, and Schoenberg BS: Trends in the incidence of dementing illness in Rochester, Minnesota in three quinquennial periods, 1960–1974. Neurology 38:975–980, 1988.

126. Koss E, Haxby JV, deCarli C, Schapiro MB, Friedland RP, and Rapoport SI: Patterns of performance preservation and loss in healthy aging. Developmental Neuropsychology 7(1):99–113, 1991.

127. Kral VA: Senescent forgetfulness: Benign and malignant. Can Med Assoc J 86:257–260, 1962.

128. Kretzschmar K, Nix W, Zschiedrich H, and Philipp T: Morphologic cerebral changes in patients undergoing dialysis for renal failure. AJNR 4:439–441, 1983.

129. Krishnan KRR, Heyman A, Ritchie JC, Utley CM, Dawson DV, and Rogers H: Depression in early-onset Alzheimer's disease: Clinical and neuroendocrine correlates. Biol Psychiatry 24:937–940, 1988.

130. Kuhl DE, Barrio JR, Huang SC, et al: Quantifying local cerebral blood flow by N-isopropyl-p-[^{123}I]-iodoamphetamine (IMP) tomography. J Nucl Med 23:196–203, 1982.

131. Kuhl DE, Metter EJ, and Riege WH: Patterns of local cerebral glucose utilization determined in Parkinson's disease by the (18F) fluorodeoxyglucose method. Ann Neurol 15:419–424, 1984.

132. Kuhl DE, Phelps ME, Markham CH, Metter EJ, Riege WH, and Winter J: Cerebral metabolism and atrophy in Huntington's disease determined by 18 FDG and computed tomographic scan. Ann Neurol 12:425–434, 1982.

133. Kurtzke JF: The current neurologic burden of illness and injury in the United States. Neurology 32:1207–1214, 1982.

134. Kuskowski MA, Malone SM, Mortimer JA, and Dysken MW: Smooth pursuit eye movements in dementia of the Alzheimer type. Alzheimer Dis Assoc Disord 3:157–171, 1989.

135. Lai F and Williams RS: A prospective study of Alzheimer disease in Down syndrome. Arch Neurol 46:849–853, 1989.

136. Larson EB, Reifler BV, Sumi AM, Canfield CG, and Chinn NM: Diagnostic evaluation of 200 outpatients with suspected dementia. Gerontology 40:536–543, 1985.

137. Larson EB, Reifler BV, Sumi AM, Canfield CG, and Chinn NM: Diagnostic tests in the evaluation of dementia: A prospective study of 200 elderly outpatients. Arch Intern Med 146:1917–1922, 1986.

138. Lawton MP and Brody EM: Assessment of older people: Self-maintaining and instrumental activities of daily living. Gerontologist 9:179–186, 1969.

139. Leenders KL, Frackowiak RSJ, and Lees AJ: Steele-Richardson-Olszewski syndrome: Brain energy metabolism, blood flow and fluorodopa uptake measured by positron emission tomography. Brain 11:615–630, 1988.

140. Leenders KL, Frackowiak R, Quinn N, et al: Brain dopamine metabolism in patients with Parkinson's disease measured with positron emission tomography. J Neurol Neurosurg Psychiatry 49:853–860, 1986.

141. Leenders KL, Frackowiak R, Quinn N, and Marsden CD: Brain energy metabolism and dopaminergic function in Huntington's disease measured in vivo using positron emission tomography. Mov Disord 1:69–77, 1986.

142. LeMay M, Stafford JL, Sandor T, Albert M, Haykal H, and Zamani A: Statistical assessment of perceptual CT scan ratings of inpatients with Alzheimer type dementia. J Comput Assist Tomogr 10:802–809, 1986.

143. Leuchter AF, Spar JE, Walter DO, and Weiner H: Electroencephalographic spectra and coherence in the diagnosis of Alzheimer's-type and multi-infarct dementia. Arch Gen Psychiatry 44:993–998, 1987.

144. Leys D, Soetaert G, Petit H, Fauquette A, Pruvo J-P, and Steiling M: Periventricular and white-matter magnetic resonance imaging hyperintensities

do not differ between Alzheimer's disease and normal aging. Arch Neurol 47:524–527, 1990.

145. Lindenbaum J, Healton EB, Savage DG, et al: Neuropsychiatric disorders caused by cobalamin deficiency in the absence of anemia of malrocytosis. N Engl J Med 318:1720–1728, 1988.

146. Lipowski ZJ: Delirium in the elderly patient. N Engl J Med 320:578–582, 1989.

147. Loeb C: Clinical criteria for the diagnosis of vascular dementia. Eur Neurol 28:87–92, 1988.

148. Lopez OL, Swihart AA, Becker JT, et al: Reliability of NINCDS-ADRDA clinical criteria for the diagnosis of Alzheimer's disease. Neurology 40: 1517–1522, 1990.

149. Luxenberg JS, Haxby JV, Creasey H, Sundaram M, and Rapoport SI: Rate of ventricular enlargement in dementia of the Alzheimer type correlates with rate of neuropsychological deterioration. Neurology 37:1135–1140, 1987.

150. Marsden CD and Harrison MJG: Outcome of investigation of patients with presenile dementia. BMJ 2:249–252, 1972.

151. Mayeux R, Stern Y, Hermann A, Greenbaum L, and Fahn S: Correlates of early disability in Huntington's disease. Ann Neurol 20:727–731, 1986.

152. Mayeux R, Stern Y, Rosen J, and Benson DF: Is "subcortical dementia" a recognizable clinical entity? Ann Neurol 14:278–283, 1983.

153. Mayeux R, Stern Y, Rosen J, and Leventhal J: Depression, intellectual impairment and Parkinson's disease. Neurology 31:645–650, 1981.

154. Mayeux R, Denaio J, Hemenegildo N, et al: A population-based investigation of Parkinson's disease with and without dementia: Relationship to age and gender. Arch Neurol 49:492–497, 1992.

155. Mayeux R, Stern Y, and Spanton S: Heterogeneity in dementia of the Alzheimer type: Evidence of subgroups. Neurology 35:453–461, 1985.

156. McGeachie RE, Fleming JO, Sharer LR, and Hyman RA: Diagnosis of Pick's disease by computed tomography. J Comput Assist Tomogr 3:113–115, 1979.

157. McGeer PL, Kamo H, Harrop R, et al: Positron emission tomography in patients with clinically diagnosed Alzheimer's disease. Can Med Assoc J 134:594–607, 1986.

158. McIntyre L and Frank J: Evaluation of the demented patient. J Fam Pract 24:399–404, 1987.

159. McKhann G, Drachman D, Folstein M, et al: Clinical diagnosis of Alzheimer's disease: Report of the NINCDS-ADRDA work group under the auspices of the Department of Health and Human Services Task Force on Alzheimer's disease. Neurology 34:939–944, 1984.

160. Merrick MV: Essentials of Nuclear Medicine. Churchill Livingstone, Edinburgh, 1984.

161. Mesulam M-M: Slowly progressive aphasia without generalized dementia. Ann Neurol 11:592–598, 1982.

162. Mesulam M-M: Primary progressive aphasia: Differentiation from Alzheimer's disease. Ann Neurol 22: 533–534, 1987.

163. Metter E, Mazziotta JC, Itabashi HH, Mankovich, NJ, Phelps ME, and Kuhl DE: Comparison of glucose metabolism, x-ray CT, and postmortem data in a patient with multiple cerebral infarcts. Neurology 35:1695–1701, 1985.

164. Miller JD, DeLeon MJ, Ferris SH, et al: Abnormal temporal lobe response in Alzheimer's disease during cognitive processing as measured by ^{11}C-2-deoxy-D-glucose and PET. J Cereb Blood Flow Metab 7:248–251, 1987.

165. Mirsen TR, Lee DH, Wong CJ, Diaz JF, Fox AJ, and Hackinski VC: Clinical correlates of white matter changes on magnetic resonance imaging scans of the brain. Arch Neurol 48:1015–1021, 1991.

166. Montamat SC, Cusak BJ, and Vestal RE: Management of drug therapy in the elderly. N Engl J Med 321:303–309, 1989.

167. Morris JC, Banker BQ, and Wright D: Hereditary dysphasic dementia and

the Pick-Alzheimer spectrum. Ann Neurol 16:455–466, 1984.

168. Morris JC, Heyman A, Mohs RC, et al: The Consortium to Establish a Registry for Alzheimer's Disease (CERAD). Part I. Clinical and neuropsychological assessment of Alzheimer's disease. Neurology 39:1159–1165, 1989.

169. Morris JC, McKeel DW, Fulling K, Torak RM, and Berg L: Validation of clinical diagnostic criteria for Alzheimer's disease. Ann Neurol 24:17–22, 1988.

170. Morris JC, McKeel DW, Storandt M, et al: Very mild Alzheimer's disease: Informant based clinical, psychometric, and pathologic distinction from normal aging. Neurology 41:469–478, 1991.

171. Naguib M and Levy R: CT scanning in senile dementia. Br J Psychiatry 141:618–620, 1982.

172. Nee LE, Eldridge R, Sunderland T, et al: Dementia of the Alzheimer's type: Clinical and family study of 22 twin pairs. Neurology 37:359–363, 1987.

173. Nee LE, Polinsky RJ, Eldridge R, et al: A family with histologically confirmed Alzheimer's disease. Arch Neurol 40:203–208, 1983.

174. Office of Medical Applications of Research, Consensus Conference on Dementia, National Institutes of Health: Differential diagnosis of dementing diseases. JAMA 258:3411–3416, 1987.

175. Palmert MR, Usiah M, Mayeux R, Raskind M, Tourtellotte WW, and Younkin SG. Soluble derivatives of the β-amyloid protein precursor in cerebrospinal fluid: Alterations in normal aging and in Alzheimer's disease. Neurology 40:1028–1034, 1990.

176. Patterson JV, Michalewski HJ, and Starr A: Latency variability of the components of auditory event-related potentials to infrequent stimuli in aging, Alzheimer-type dementia, and depression. Electroencephalogr Clin Neurophysiol 71:450–460, 1988.

177. Patterson MB, Schnell A, Martin RJ, Mendez MF, Smyth K, and Whitehouse PJ: Assessment of behavioral and affective symptoms in Alz-

heimer's disease. J Geriatr Psychiatry Neurol 3:21–30, 1990.

178. Pearlson GD, Ross CA, Lohr WD, Rovner BW, Chase GA, and Folstein MF: Association between family history of affective disorders and the depressive syndrome of Alzheimer's disease. Am J Psychiatry 147:452–456, 1990.

179. Pedley TA and Miller JA: Clinical neurophysiology of aging and dementia. In Mayeux R and Rosen W (eds): The Dementias. Raven Press, New York, 1983, pp 31–50.

180. Penttila M, Partanen JV, Soininen H, and Reikkinen PJ: Quantitative analysis of occipital EEG in different stages of Alzheimer's disease. Electroencephalogr Clin Neurophysiol 60:1–6, 1985.

181. Perry EK: The cholinergic system in old age and Alzheimer's disease. Age Ageing 9:1–8, 1980.

182. Pfeiffer E: A short portable mental status questionnaire for the assessment of organic brain deficit in elderly patients. J Am Geriatr Soc 22:433–444, 1975.

183. Phelps ME, Mazziotta JC, and Schelbert HR: Positron Emission Tomography and Autoradiography: Principles and Application for the Brain and Heart. Raven Press, New York, 1986.

184. Pizzarello CD: The dimensions of the problem of eye disease among the elderly. Ophthalmology 94:1191–1195, 1987.

185. Rapoport SI, Pettigrew KD, and Schapiro MB: Disconcordance and concordance of dementia of the Alzheimer type (DAT) in monozygotic twins indicate heritable and sporadic forms of Alzheimer disease. Neurology 41:1549–1553, 1991.

186. Rea-Grant A, Blume W, Lag C, Hachinski VC, Fisman M, and Merskey H: The electroencephalogram in Alzheimer type dementia: A sequential quantitative pathological study. Arch Neurol 44:50–54, 1987.

187. Reisberg B, Borenstein J, Salob SP, Ferris SH, Fransen E, and Georgotas A: Behavioral symptoms in Alzheimer's disease: Phenomenology and

treatment. J Clin Psychiatry (Suppl) 48:9–15, 1987.

188. Rezek DL, Morris JC, Fulling KH, and Gado MH: Periventricular white matter lucencies in senile dementia of the Alzheimer type and in normal aging. Neurology 37:1365–1368, 1987.

189. Risberg J: Regional cerebral blood flow measurements by ^{133}Xe inhalation: Methodology and applications in neuropsychology and psychiatry. Brain Lang 9:9–34, 1980.

190. Robins LN, Helzer JE, Crougham J, and Ratcliff KS: National Institute of Mental Health Diagnostic Interview schedule: Its history, characteristics and validity. Arch Gen Psychiatry 38:381–389, 1981.

191. Rocca WA, Luigi AA, and Schoenberg BS: Epidemiology of clinically diagnosed Alzheimer's disease. Ann Neurol 19:415–424, 1986.

192. Ron MA, Toone BK, Garralda ME, and Lishman WA: Diagnostic accuracy in presenile dementia. Br J Psychiatry 134:161–168, 1979.

193. Roos A, Carlton G, and Gibb C: The clinical characteristics of transmissible Creutzfeldt-Jakob disease. Brain 96:1–20, 1973.

194. Rosen WG: Verbal fluency in aging and dementia. Journal of Clinical Neuropsychology 2:135–146, 1980.

195. Rosen WG: The Rosen Drawing Test. Veterans Administration Medical Center, Bronx, NY, 1981.

196. Rosen WG, Mohs RC, and Davis KL: A new rating scale for Alzheimer's disease. Am J Psychiatry 142:1356–1363, 1984.

197. Rosen WG, Terry RD, Fuld PA, Katzman R, and Peck A: Pathological verification of ischemic score in differentiation of dementias. Ann Neurol 7:486–488, 1980.

198. Rowe JW and Khan R: Human aging: Usual versus successful. Science 237:143–149, 1987.

199. Roy-Byrne PP, Weingartner H, Bierer LM, Thompson K, and Post RM: Effortful and automatic cognitive processing in depression. Arch Gen Psychiatry 43:265–267, 1986.

200. Rubin EH, Morris JC, Grant AE, and Vendegna T: Very mild senile dementia of the Alzheimer type: I. Clinical assessment. Arch Neurol 46:379–382, 1989.

201. St George-Hyslop PH, Tanzi RE, Polinsky RJ, et al: The genetic defect causing familial Alzheimer's disease maps on chromosome 21. Science 235:885–890, 1987.

202. Schaumburg HH, Spencer PS, and Ochoa J: The aging human peripheral nervous system. In Katzman R and Terry RD (eds): The Neurology of Aging, FA Davis, Philadelphia, 1983, pp 111–122.

203. Scotti G, Terbrugge K, Malancon D, and Belanger G: Evaluation of the age of subdural hematomas by computerized tomography. J Neurosurg 47:311–315, 1977.

204. Sharp P, Gemmell H, Cherryman G, Besson J, Crawford J, and Smith F: Application of iodine-123-labeled isopropylamphetamine imaging to the study of dementia. J Nucl Med 27:761–768, 1986.

205. Smith JS and Kilch LG: The investigation of dementia: Results in 200 consecutive admissions. Lancet 2:824–827, 1981.

206. Soininen H, Partanen J, Laulumaa V, Helkala E-L, Laakso M, and Riekkinen PJ: Longitudinal EEG spectral analysis in early stage of Alzheimer's disease. Electroencephalogr Clin Neurophysiol 72:290–297, 1989.

207. Sperling MR, Wilson G, Engel J, Babb TL, Phelps M, and Bradley W: Magnetic resonance imaging in intractable partial epilepsy: Correlative studies. Ann Neurol 20:57–62, 1986.

208. Squires KC, Goodin DS, and Starr A: Event related potentials in normal aging and dementia. In Lehmann D and Callaway E (eds): Human Evoked Potentials: Applications and Problems. Plenum Press, New York, 1979, pp 383–396.

209. Steingart A, Hachinski VC, Lau C, and Fox AJ: Cognitive and neurologic findings in subject with diffuse white matter lucencies on computed tomographic scan (Leuko-araiosis). Arch Neurol 44:32–35, 1987.

210. Steingart A, Hachinski VC, Lau C, et al: Cognitive and neurologic findings in demented patients with diffuse white matter lucencies on computed tomographic scan (Leuko-araiosis). Arch Neurol 44:36–41, 1987.

211. Storandt M, Botwinick J, Danziger WL, et al: Psychometric differentiation of mild senile dementia of the Alzheimer type. Arch Neurol 41:497–499, 1984.

212. Sunderland T, Hill JL, Mellow AM, et al: Clock drawing in Alzheimer's disease: A novel measure of dementia severity. J Am Geriatr Soc 37:725–729, 1989.

213. Sunderland T, Rubinow DR, Tariot PN, et al: CSF somatostatin in patients with Alzheimer's disease, older depressed patients and age-matched control subjects. Am J Psychiatry 144:1313–1316, 1987.

214. Syndulko K, Hansch EC, Cohen SN, et al: Long-latency event related potentials in normal aging and dementia. In Courjon J, Maugierer F, and Revol M (eds): Clinical Application of Evoked Potentials in Neurology. Raven Press, New York, 1982, pp 279–285.

215. Takahashi M, Aril H, and Tamakawa Y: Comparison of metrizamide CT cisternography with radionuclide cisternography in abnormal cerebrospinal fluid dynamics. Neuroradiology 16:199–202, 1978.

216. Tariska I: Circumscribed cerebral atrophy in Alzheimer's disease: A pathological study. In Wolstenholme GEW and O'Connor M (eds): Alzheimer's Disease and Related Conditions. J & A Churchill, 1970, pp 51–69.

217. Tatemichi TK: How acute brain failure becomes chronic. A view of the mechanisms of dementia related to stroke. Neurology 40:1652–1659, 1990.

218. Teravainen H and Calne DB: Motor system in normal aging and Parkinson's disease. In Katzman R and Terry RD (eds): The Neurology of Aging, FA Davis, Philadelphia, 1983, pp 85–109.

219. Terry RD, Peck A, DeTeresa R, Schechter R, and Horoupian DS: Some morphometric aspects of the brain in senile dementia of the Alzheimer type. Ann Neurol 10:184–192, 1981.

220. Therapeutics and Technology Assessment Subcommittee, American Academy of Neurology: Assessment: EEG brain mapping. Special Report. Neurology 39:1100–1101, 1989.

221. Tierney MC, Fisher RH, Lewis AJ, et al: The NINCDS-ADRDA Work Group criteria for the clinical diagnosis of probable Alzheimer's disease: A clinicopathologic study of 57 cases. Neurology 38:359–364, 1988.

222. Tierney MC, Snow WG, Reid DW, Zorzitto ML, and Fisher RH: Psychometric differentiation of dementia: Replication and extension of the findings of Storandt and coworkers. Arch Neurol 44:720–722, 1987.

223. Tomlinson BE, Blessed G, and Roth M: Observations on the brains of nondemented old people. J Neurol Sci 7:331–356, 1968.

224. Tsai, FY, Huprich JE, Segall HD, and Teal JS: The contrast-enhanced CT scan in the diagnosis of isodense subdural hematoma. J Neurosurg 50:64–69, 1979.

225. Tweedy J, Reding M, Garcia C, Schulman P, Deutsch G, and Antin S: Significance of cortical disinhibition signs. Neurology 32:169–173, 1982.

226. Uhlman RD and Larson EB: Effect of education on the Mini-Mental State Examination as a screening test for dementia. J Am Geriatr Soc 39:876–880, 1991.

227. Victor M, Adams RD, and Collins G: The Wernicke-Korsakoff Syndrome and Related Neurologic Disorders due to Alcoholism and Malnutrition. FA Davis, Philadelphia, 1989, pp 185–191.

228. Visser SL, Hooijer C, Jonker C, Vantilburg W, and DeRijke W: Anterior temporal focal abnormalities in EEG in normal aged subjects. Correlations with psychopathological and CT main scan findings. Electroencephalogr Clin Neurophysiol 66:1–12, 1987.

229. Wade JPH, Mirsen TR, Hachinski VC, Fisman M, Lau C, and Merskey H: The clinical diagnosis of Alzheimer's disease. Arch Neurol 44:24–29, 1987.

230. Wechsler D: A standardized memory scale for clinical use. J Psychol 19: 87–95, 1945.
231. Wechsler D: Wechsler Adult Intelligence Scale — Revised. Psychological Corporation, San Antonio, TX, 1981.
232. Weinberger DR, Berman KF, Iadorola M, Driesen N, and Sez RF: Prefrontal cortical blood flow and cognitive function in Huntington's disease. J Neurol Neurosurg Psychiatry 51:94–103, 1988.
233. Weisberg LA: Computerized tomographic enhancement patterns in cerebral infarction. Arch Neurol 37:21–24, 1980.
234. Welch KMA, Helpern JA, Robertson WM, and Ewing JR: ^{31}P topical magnetic resonance measurement of high energy phosphates in normal and infarcted brain. Stroke 16:151, 1985.
235. Whitehouse PJ: The concept of subcortical and cortical dementia: Another look. Ann Neurol 19:1–6, 1986.
236. Wilson RS, Fox HJ, Huckman MC, Bacon LD, and Lobick JJ: Computed tomography in dementia. Neurology 32:1054–1057, 1982.
237. Wilson RS, Rosenbaum G, Brown G, Rourke D, Whiteman D, and Griselle J: An index of premorbid intelligence. J Consult Clin Psychol 46:1554–1555, 1978.
238. Wing SD, Norman D, Pollock JA, and Newton TH: Contrast enhancement of cerebral infarcts in computed tomography. Radiology 121:89–92, 1976.
239. Wisniewski KE, Wisniewski HM, and Wen Y: Occurrence of neuropathological changes and dementia of Alzheimer's disease in Down's syndrome. Ann Neurol 17:278–282, 1985.
240. Wolf-Klein GP, Silverstone FA, Levy AP, Brod MS, and Breur J: Screening for Alzheimer's disease by clock drawing. J Am Geriatr Soc 37:730–740, 1989.
241. Wolfson LI and Katzman R: The neurologic consultation at age 80. In Katzman R and Terry RD (eds): The Neurology of Aging. FA Davis, Philadelphia, 1983, pp 221–244.
242. Wolozin BL and Davies P: Alzheimer related protein A68: Alzheimer specific accumulation and detection in cerebrospinal fluid. Ann Neurol 22: 521–526, 1987.
243. Wu S, Schenkenberg T, Wing SD, and Osborn AG: Cognitive correlates of diffuse cerebral atrophy determined by computed tomography. Neurology 31: 1180–1184, 1981.
244. Yamada F, Fukuda S, Samejima H, Yoshii N, and Kudo T: Significance of pathognomonic features of normal pressure hydrocephalus. Neuroradiology 16:212–213, 1978.
245. Yonas H, Wolfson SK, Gur D, et al: Clinical experience with the use of xenon-enhanced CT blood flow mapping in cerebral vascular disease. Stroke 15:443–450, 1984.
246. Young AB, Penney JB, Starosta-Rubinstein S, et al: PET scan investigations of Huntington's disease: Cerebral metabolic correlates of neurological features and functional decline. Ann Neurol 20:296–303, 1986.

Chapter 5

NEURO-PSYCHOLOGICAL ASSESSMENT OF DEMENTIA

Alice Cronin-Golomb, Ph.D.,
Suzanne Corkin, Ph.D., and
T. John Rosen, Ph.D.

THE GOALS OF NEUROPSYCHOLOGICAL ASSESSMENT

The discipline of neuropsychology has its roots in experimental psychology and neurology. Traditionally, neuropsychology was concerned with the assessment of the behavioral consequences of focal brain injury. During the last decade the discipline has grown in scope, partly as a result of investigators' seeking the organic bases of more diffuse disorders of the mind. The study of dementia alone has provided fertile ground for the development of new neuropsychological techniques and for the deployment in new contexts of tests known to be sensitive to focal injury. Equipped with innovative test instru-

ments, neuropsychologists provide a quantitative picture of the mental state of the demented patient that in its breadth, detail, and precision is well beyond that obtainable by neurologists and psychiatrists during a standard clinical interview.

Deterioration of cognitive function is the only positive evidence that leads to a diagnosis of dementia in the living patient. There are no obvious physical manifestations of dementia above the microscopic level, and even the most sophisticated imaging techniques are less sensitive than cognitive testing in distinguishing between demented and healthy elderly individuals. Because dementia is defined behaviorally[8,139] detailed neuropsychological assessment of individuals under evaluation for possible dementing illness clearly is indicated.

Diagnosis

One of the primary goals of neuropsychological examination is to assist clinicians in the differential diagnosis of dementia. A patient who complains of memory loss may be afflicted with one of the various dementing illnesses, with global amnesia of several possible etiol-

130

ogies, or with numerous other conditions.[236] Alternatively, the patient may be exhibiting a relatively benign forgetfulness that often occurs with normal aging.[128] According to one report,[71] older individuals who complain of memory loss and perform poorly relative to the general population meet the "diagnostic criteria" for a nondementing condition called age-associated memory impairment (AAMI). (See Table 4–4; see also Rosen[184] for a critical evaluation of the AAMI construct.) Neuropsychological assessment of a range of cognitive functions indicates whether the patient's deficits are confined to memory, suggesting a diagnosis of global amnesia, or extend to other domains, suggesting a diagnosis of dementia. Amnesias (or circumscribed deficits in other cognitive domains, such as language or visuospatial function) and dementias of different etiologies may be further differentiated, based on specific patterns of sparing and loss of cognitive functions. These patterns indicate the integrity of particular brain areas and thereby permit inferences to be made concerning the localization of pathology.

Clinical Monitoring

After an initial diagnosis has been made, the neuropsychological assessment provides quantitative data for the periodic monitoring of the patient's condition. Specific neurologic disorders are characterized not only by particular patterns of cognitive performance, but also by changes in patterns over time. Hence, like neurologic and psychiatric assessment, neuropsychological evaluation is most useful when performed longitudinally. Mild memory impairment that does not worsen dramatically over time may reflect normal aging. In contrast, an insidious decline of multiple cognitive capacities reflects dementia. In trying to distinguish normal aging from early dementia, it is useful to assess the integrity of several cognitive domains on the patient's initial visit to the clinic and to use these values as a baseline against which performance during subsequent visits can be compared. Baseline and subsequent measures also permit assessment of patients' cognitive responses to internal states and external environmental changes. The cognitive abilities of old people in general and of demented individuals in particular are affected by changes in medication, whether the medication has been prescribed to alleviate symptoms associated with the primary neurologic disorder or to regulate a coexisting medical condition (e.g., high blood pressure). Changes in patients' external environment, such as the introduction of new living arrangements, may also significantly affect cognition.

Research

Besides its uses in diagnosing dementia and monitoring the patient's condition over time, quantitative neuropsychological assessment supports research on the etiology of dementing illnesses such as Alzheimer's disease (AD or SDAT: senile dementia of the Alzheimer type). For example, recent studies have used neuropsychological assessments to characterize subgroups of patients with predominant involvement of a particular cognitive function, or who differ in rate of cognitive deterioration, or who have concomitant parkinsonian neuropathology.[81,130,148] Some behaviorally defined subgroups may reflect genetically based variations of AD, and they may differ in response to treatment with experimental drugs. In the absence of information about possible subgroup classifications, data analyses must treat patient samples as homogeneous, thereby weakening correlations that hold within pathogenetically distinct groups.

Another purpose of neuropsychological assessment in AD is to explore dissociations among cognitive, sensory, and motor functions and then to associate specific functions with particular brain areas or systems. For example, administering memory tasks that assess different kinds of memory (fact learning versus skill learning versus priming) to patients with global amnesia (medial temporal–diencephalic lesions), AD (medial temporal–diencephalic plus cortical lesions), early Huntington's disease (HD) (caudate lesions), and early Parkinson's disease (PD) (putamenal lesions) can provide information about dissociable human memory systems and their neural substrates.[94]

All research is conducted only with the consent of the patient and, if the patient is legally incompetent, with the consent of the primary caregiver.

Treatment

Neuropsychological assessment may help identify whom to treat by what means. Treatment studies based on neurotransmitter replacement[104] usually assume, in the absence of justification, that all patients assigned to a given diagnostic category (e.g., AD) have similar neurotransmitter deficits and similar patterns of neural degeneration. If replacement therapies turn out to be a useful approach to treatment,[104] detailed neuropsychological assessment may help researchers to classify patients into groups that are more homogeneous neurochemically and neuroanatomically, so that specific pharmacotherapies may be matched to patients' particular needs. (See Chapter 13.)

Further, neuropsychological assessment may guide the clinical management of demented patients. Even with diseases that are currently untreatable (e.g., HD and AD), clinicians still have a host of pharmacologic options for treating symptoms. Evaluation of these treatments requires judgments based on subtle behavioral effects. For example, demented patients may suffer from concomitant anxiety, agitation, or depression, states that are generally amenable to treatment, and that may prompt inadvertent overmedication.

The consequent reduction in intellectual function may go unnoticed in view of the obvious expectations that patients will function poorly. The use of neuropsychological assessment procedures to evaluate the effects of different medications and doses should help the clinician to achieve optimal symptomatic relief.

Understanding

The demented patient embodies our worst fear as members of *homo sapiens* — that of "losing our minds," the feature after which we have named our species. Caring for demented people, either professionally as clinicians or personally as friends and family, requires a phenomenological appreciation of their lives and experiences in addition to knowledge gained from disciplines such as epidemiology and neuropathology. Only if we in some sense understand what the world is like to demented patients can we maintain the personal concern and tolerance that these very demanding people require. Because neuropsychological assessment can document the limitations in patients' capacities to perceive, remember, comprehend, and manipulate the world around them, assessment enhances our appreciation of the difficulties patients face. Periodic identification of the spared and impaired abilities during the disease course may be of considerable importance to patients and their caregivers in planning the patients' daily routines. (See Chapter 14.)

The pattern of impairments may be subtler than can be revealed by clinical examination. For example, neuropsychological and neuro-ophthalmologic studies suggest that visual acuity remains intact for much of the course of AD; further, visual field defects are rare.[47,68] Several basic visual capacities (e.g., contrast sensitivity, masking, stereoacuity) and numerous high-order visual capacities, however, seem to show early impairment in some patients. (See Visuospatial Function,

p. 148.) The result may be that, although AD patients ostensibly "see" the world normally, they are insensitive to many forms of visual stimulation and cannot make sense of much of the visual input that they receive: a complex scene may be meaningless and confusing. The neuropsychological literature contains a series of similarly subtle distinctions that help explain the demented patient's world. Regarding memory, certain skills (piano playing) may be retained after associated factual knowledge (the composer's name) has vanished; and regarding language, speech patterns (syntax) may be retained after word meanings (semantic memory) have been lost. By documenting such subtle patterns in demented patients' capacities, neuropsychological assessment contributes to our understanding of the patients as people.

The following sections further describe the usefulness of neuropsychological assessment as a counterpart of the neurologic or psychiatric evaluation. We consider the domains of memory, language, abstract thought, visuospatial function, and attention; point to specific patterns of cognitive impairment and their implications for diagnosis; and indicate when further testing by specialists outside of neuropsychology may be appropriate. The reader who is interested in more comprehensive reviews of the literature pertaining to specific cognitive domains is directed to references 53, 94, 116, 150, and 191 for memory; 107 and 112 for language; 63 for abstract thought; 163 for visuospatial function; and 209 for attention.

NEUROPSYCHOLOGICAL ASSESSMENT: GENERAL CONSIDERATIONS

This section discusses the conditions under which neuropsychological testing is valid and produces interpretable results. The specific issues addressed include subject characteristics, sensory capacities, psychiatric status, and overall mental status.

Subject Characteristics

Clinical populations differ in age, education, socioeconomic status, health history, and native language. Patients in clinics within the same hospital, much less the same city or country, cannot be assumed to be similar with respect to such factors. Premorbid and demographic differences between diagnostic groups may lead to ambiguities in the interpretation of clinical and research data. Because many neuropsychological tests are developed and validated using restricted patient samples and matched samples of control subjects, their validity for populations that differ significantly in demographic factors is suspect. It is imperative that neuropsychologists establish quantitative norms of cognitive performance for local subpopulations, that is, for patients attending a particular hospital, clinic, or private practice. Spouses and siblings of patients are ideal control subjects because they are usually similar in age, socioeconomic status, quality of nutrition and health care, and exposure to regional toxins and other environmental factors.

Sensory Capacities

Sensory deficits can masquerade as deficits in cognition. Thus systematic testing of sensory function, especially in the visual and auditory modalities, is necessary to identify deficits that may contribute to functional difficulties. For example, patients with AD, many of whom display normal visual acuity, nevertheless show impairments in such visual functions as color and depth perception and contrast sensitivity.[58,68,140,190,196] It is unclear whether these impairments in AD are related to pathologic changes sometimes found at autopsy in the optic nerve and retina.[111] Comparing the status of basic and high-order functions in each sensory modality could lead to a better understanding of the relation among deficits in AD. Other dementing illnesses that have been associated with visual changes include progressive supranuclear palsy (PSP),[215] PD,[35,179] and multiple sclerosis.[180] For all patients, the neurologic examination or neuropsychological assessment should include brief measures of visual and auditory acuity. For vision, Snellen-type wall charts are practical, and for audition, the examiner can whisper short phrases at each ear and ask the patient to repeat them. Also, a tuning fork can be used to distinguish bone-conduction from nerve-conduction loss. Referral to a specialist (neuro-ophthalmologist or otolaryngologist) is justified only for patients suspected of having severe sensory disorders, or for research.

Psychiatric Status

A third factor that may affect neuropsychological assessment is the patient's psychiatric status. Conditions such as depression, anxiety, apathy, and psychosis occur in the several dementing disorders and in normal aging. Psychiatric symptoms that could handicap performance on cognitive tests include slow motor behavior, poor attentional focusing, poor concentration, and bizarre associations. The presence of such disturbances can make interpretation of any cognitive impairments problematic. Patients suspected of having dementia should therefore receive rigorous psychiatric screening so that the contribution of psychiatric symptoms to cognition can be explored. The importance of a psychiatric evaluation is underscored by the fact that depression shares many clinical features with dementia; the pattern of cognitive deficits of some depressed individuals has been called "pseudodementia."[91] (See Chapter 12).

Standardized scales often are used to assess the psychiatric status of demented patients. The recently developed Dementia Mood Assessment Scale (DMAS)[220] may prove to be superior to the widely used Hamilton Rating Scale for Depression,[106] upon which the DMAS was based. The Hamilton solicits information about past behavior from the patient, whereas the DMAS solicits information from the caregiver. The latter source is clearly superior when the patient is suspected of having a memory impairment. The Cornell Scale for Depression in Dementia[6] uses information from the patient and from a nursing staff member; it has not yet been validated for noninstitutionalized demented subjects whose caregivers are family members or homeaides. Scales that assess affective behavior and other areas as well include the Schedule for Affective Disorders and Schizophrenia,[211] the Structured Clinical Interview for DSM-III,[213] the Psychiatric Status Schedule,[212] the Symptom Checklist-90R,[79] and the Sandoz Clinical Assessment—Geriatric.[202] These five scales were not specifically designed for use with demented patients. The Behavioral Pathology in Alzheimer's Disease Rating Scale (BEHAVE-AD) uses information drawn from the patient's medical chart to document the presence and severity of paranoid and delusional ideation, hallucinations, activity disturbances, aggressiveness, diurnal rhythm disturbances, affective disturbances, anxieties, and phobias in patients with AD.[181]

Mental Status

A final major factor that bears upon neuropsychological evaluation is the patient's overall mental status. In deciding whether or not a particular patient is sufficiently testable to receive a detailed neuropsychological assessment, it is useful to have a standardized measure of mental status. Although a continuing goal of neuropsychology is to develop tests that are sensitive to changes over time in the patient's pattern of cognitive abilities, there comes a time in the progression of dementia when patients are no longer testable. In the early stages of a dementing process, many cognitive capacities may be normal or at least less affected than others, and patients may have a spotty pattern of test completion.

Mental status examinations are useful in the clinic insofar as they give an overall picture of cognitive functioning in the educationally and socially advantaged individual and grossly document change over time. Clinicians should assess several factors in choosing a mental status examination, including validity and reliability, breadth of coverage (verbal and nonverbal capacities), administration time, and correlation with neuropathologic and cognitive features of dementia. A useful way to measure test-retest reliability in demented patients is to correlate scores on initial test administration with the same patients' scores on retest by the same examiner after an interval of approximately 1 day to 1 month. Interrater reliability is measured by the correlation between the patients' scores on the test administered by two different examiners within a short time. A test is valid if it in fact measures what it claims to measure. Ideally, the mental status examination for dementia should have three characteristics: It should be *sensitive* to the presence of dementia, identifying all individuals who are in fact demented; it should be *specific*, identifying only those who are demented and not miscategorizing healthy people as demented; and it should have high *predictive* value, identifying individuals whose dementia is presently subclinical, meaning that the signs of dementia have not yet appeared. Clinicians want to know not only whether or not the patient is demented, but also whether the patient has a condition that may be treatable, such as the pseudodementia of depressive illness.

Most of the mental status examinations now available are useful in some respects. They provide quantitative information about the overall level of cognitive status; they may be administered quickly at bedside, and after minimal training of the examiner. The methods of data collection, scoring, and interpretation have been standardized. The examinations generally are reliable in terms of test-retest and interrater scoring; they usually correlate highly with scores on tests of specific cognitive capacities and with some anatomic and physiologic measures; and they are sensitive to the progression of dementia over time.

It is important to be aware of the shortcomings of mental status examinations. They have high false-negative rates when used with very mildly demented or highly intelligent subjects (poor sensitivity), and they have high false-positive rates when used with disadvantaged populations (poor specificity). Most mental status examinations are invalid for cross-cultural comparisons, unless they are adapted and standardized for the foreign population of interest. The problems with validity may stem from demographic differences between the patient under examination and patient samples upon which the examinations were standardized. In addition, the brevity of mental status tests limits the depth and breadth of the cognitive assessment. In particular, they commonly neglect nonverbal functions relative to verbal ones. They do not provide information distinguishing among alternative patterns of deficit; that is, individual differences are blurred. Unlike neuropsychological tests such as the Wechsler Adult Intelligence Scale – Revised (WAIS-R),[232] scores on mental status examinations are not interpreted according to the patient's age. It is likely, however, that a particular mental status score attained by a 50-year-old has a different meaning from the same score attained by an 80-year-old. In sum, given the numerous weaknesses of mental status examinations, it is probably advisable to use them as informal screening devices only.

Three mental status tests currently are in wide clinical use: The Blessed Dementia Scale,[23] the Mattis Dementia Rating Scale,[137] and the Mini-Mental State Examination[90] (Table 5–1).

Table 5–1 MENTAL STATUS EXAMINATIONS

Test Instrument	Description	Administration	Relation to Brain Anatomy and Physiology
Blessed Dementia Scale[23]	Two sections: one administered to patient (information, memory, concentration), one to informant (everyday activities, habits, personality, interests, and drives).	15–30 min. Verbal.	Performance correlated with number of cortical amyloid plaques.[23]
Mattis Dementia Rating Scale[137]	Administered to patient. Attention, initiation and perseveration, construction, conceptualization, memory.	20–45 min. Verbal and nonverbal components.	Performance correlated with extent of gray-matter cerebral blood flow.[137]
Mini-Mental State Examination[90]	Administered to patient. Orientation, registration (learning), concentration, recall, language, praxis.	5–10 min. Verbal and nonverbal components.	Performance correlated with findings on computed tomography of the brain.[167,228]

These mental status tests are useful, but they do not substitute for a sensitive and detailed neuropsychological evaluation. That sort of evaluation involves assessing specific cognitive capacities in each of the cognitive domains that are affected in AD and related dementias: memory, language, abstract thought, visuospatial function, and attention. The following sections describe tests that have been used to assess those capacities in patients with age-related neurologic disease. We also present some findings from neuropsychological research on dementia that are relevant to such clinical issues as differential diagnosis and disease progression.

MEMORY

Learning and memory are the processes that permit individuals to modify their behavior through experience by encoding, storing, and retrieving information. These processes probably occur in stages that proceed serially and in parallel, and involve multiple brain regions and systems. Memory processes can be distinguished temporally, that is, in terms of how long material is stored. Iconic or echoic memory lasts milliseconds; short-term, immediate, or primary memory lasts seconds; and long-term or secondary memory survives delay intervals of minutes to years. The terms *immediate memory, short-term memory,* and *primary memory* are used interchangeably to refer to knowledge of the "just past"[117]: events that occurred or facts that were learned a few seconds ago that are recalled immediately (immediate memory)[162] or after the performance of a short distractor task (short-term memory). By contrast, *secondary* or *long-term memory* refers to information from the past minutes, hours, days, or years. Long-term memory is assessed by asking patients to recall or recognize stimulus material (e.g., a story, word list, or drawing) after a delay interval (minutes or longer). *Recent memory* is a nontechnical term, widely used clinically, that refers to information acquired in the recent past, and *remote memory* to knowledge about personal and public events that occurred in past decades.

Memory functions also can be distinguished in terms of material specificity and system specificity. *Material specificity* refers to a memory disorder that is limited to a particular kind of stimulus material.[144] The left hemisphere in most people is relatively specialized for the acquisition of "verbal" material and the right hemisphere for the acquisition of "nonverbal" material. (The verbal-nonverbal dichotomy does not characterize the functions of the two hemispheres adequately,[29] but it does accommodate a large body of empirical findings.) *System specificity* refers to the organization of long-term memory according to components that are dissociable in neurologic disease. It has been proposed that different neural systems mediate memory for events and facts (recall and recognition of personal and public events and of facts); memory for motor and perceptual skills (riding a bi-

cycle, reading words printed backward); and priming (the facilitatory or biasing effect that exposure to a stimulus has on subsequent processing of the same stimulus). It is likely that further dissociations exist within these three categories.[121] Memory capacities in AD and other age-related diseases have been explored using material-specific and system-specific memory tasks. Some of the more appropriate and sensitive tests of explicit memory (when the patient is aware that learning is occurring and/or being measured) assess immediate or short-term verbal memory,[11,169,232,233] recent verbal memory,[183,233] remote verbal memory,[49] immediate nonverbal memory,[57] recent nonverbal memory,[17,166,182,224,225,233] or remote nonverbal memory.[4,192] Tests of implicit memory (when learning occurs without conscious effort) assess perceptual-skill learning,[48,93] motor-skill learning,[51,141] verbal-repetition priming,[101,229] or nonverbal-repetition priming.[230] Summaries of these tests are readily available.[56,107,131] (Table 5–2).

Table 5–2 ASSESSMENT OF MEMORY

Task	Test Name	Task Description
Explicit memory Immediate	Digit Span	Repeat a series of numbers of increasing span immediately after presentation. (A subtest of the Wechsler Memory Scale-R[233] and the WAIS-R[232])
	Block Span (e.g., Corsi Blocks)[57]	Point to a series of blocks of increasing span, in the same order as the examiner, immediately after presentation.
Short-term	Brown-Peterson Distractor Task[11,169]	Hear three letters; count backwards from a given number during delay of 30 seconds or less; recall the three letters.
Long-term (recent)	Word-List Learning	Recall a list of 10 words after a short delay. Words may be related semantically or unrelated. (Rey Auditory-Verbal Learning Test)[183]
	Paired-Associate Learning	Hear a list of word pairs, then recall the second member of each pair upon hearing the first. (Associate Learning subtest of the Wechsler Memory Scale-R)[233]

(continued)

Table 5–2—*Continued*

Task	Test Name	Task Description
	Story Recall	Recall as much of a paragraph-long story as possible after delay. (Logical Memory subtest of the Wechsler Memory Scale-R)[233]
	Benton Visual Retention Test[17]	Briefly view a complex design and reproduce it after a delay.
	Visual Reproduction (Wechsler Memory Scale-R)[233]	(As above)
	Complex Figure Test[166,182,224,225]	(As above)
Remote	Public Events Tests[49]	Recognize or recall past public events of several decades that are described in a written or spoken format.
	Facial Recognition Test of Famous People[4]	Identify faces of famous people categorized by decade.
	Famous Scenes Test[192]	Identify news photographs of famous scenes categorized by decade.
Implicit memory Skill learning	Backward Reading[48]	In multiple sessions, read a series of words that are presented in backwards orientation.
	Pursuit Rotor[51]	In multiple sessions, maintain contact between stylus and disk on a rotating turntable.
	Mirror Tracing[141]	In multiple sessions, trace a figure while looking only at a mirror display of tracing.
Repetition priming	Gollin Incomplete-Pictures Test[53,230]	In two sessions, identify objects or animals represented by fragmented drawings.
	Word-Stem Completion[101,229]	(See text for example)
	Identification of Words Emerging from Noise[96]	Identify words that are initially masked by white noise on a computer screen. Masking lessens over time. Priming refers to the ability to identify words when more heavily masked by noise on subsequent exposures, relative to the original presentation.

Material Specificity

In the early stages of AD, lateralization of deficits is not uncommon: One patient may present with a disproportionate impairment of language and another patient with visuospatial symptoms, suggesting the presence of asymmetric left and right cerebral disease, respectively. Within the domain of memory, the patient with predominantly left-sided initial pathology may have difficulty remembering verbal material but may show relative sparing of nonverbal memory capacities. Conversely, right-sided involvement may cause a predominant loss of nonverbal memory with retention of verbal memory functions. It should be emphasized that lateralization of deficits seems to occur in only a proportion of demented patients, and then only in the early stages of the condition. As the disease progresses, equally devastating loss of verbal and nonverbal functions occurs. Persistence of lateralized dysfunction over time suggests focal rather than widespread involvement of brain tissue and a corresponding diagnosis of a disorder other than one of the dementias, such as unilateral stroke or tumor.

System Specificity

Deficits in explicit memory are the hallmark of global amnesia; they are attributed to lesions of the medial temporal–diencephalic system. That kind of memory may be distinguished from implicit memory, in which recollection is manifested without conscious or deliberate effort.[195] Implicit learning is often preserved in individuals with global amnesia, such as H.M., a well-studied patient with bilateral medial temporal lobectomy for epilepsy,[54] suggesting that skill learning and priming are mediated by brain systems other than the medial temporal–diencephalic system. The hypothesized neural substrates for skill learning and priming include the basal ganglia[146] and cerebellum[226] (skill learning), and posterior neocortex (priming).[121]

Rare instances of preserved memory in demented patients may in some cases be attributable to implicit learning. Such occurrences do not deny the existence of a disorder of explicit memory as required by the diagnosis of dementia.

Immediate and Short-term (Explicit) Memory

Immediate memory span refers to the number of stimulus items a patient can recall (orally for digits, by pointing for blocks) in the original order after minimal delay and no distraction. Patients with AD show deficits in immediate memory as documented by short digit spans (verbal)[232,233] and block spans (nonverbal).[57] Performance on tests of immediate memory appears to worsen in AD as the severity of dementia increases.[53] In contrast to patients with AD, individuals with circum-

scribed global amnesia[53,109,126,210] or PD[149,216] do not show impaired immediate memory. Patients with AD also have a deficit in *short-term memory* relative to normal subjects and to individuals with global amnesia,[53,126,150] as indicated by performance on the Brown-Peterson distractor task.[11,169]

Recent Long-term Memory

AD patients perform poorly on many tests of *explicit memory*, but they may perform normally on some tests of *implicit memory*. Explicit memory tests use a variety of techniques to measure retention after a delay, including free recall, cued recall, delayed matching-to-sample, forced-choice comparison, delayed paired comparison, and continuous recognition.[214] The memory loss is generalized with respect to the kind of stimulus material and the modality of stimulus presentation; story recall is among the more sensitive measures.[210,217,218] In contrast to their performance on tests of explicit memory, patients with AD show normal performance on some tests of implicit learning.[53,83,109,121] in which "previous experiences facilitate performance on a task that does not require conscious or intentional recollection of those experiences."[195] Dissociations among long-term, implicit memory processes distinguish among different types of dementia.

Examples of implicit memory include performing motor or perceptual skills with increasing speed and accuracy,[195] and repetition priming.[195,206] Tests of skill learning include motor tasks such as the pursuit rotor or the tracing of complex figures in a mirror (Fig. 5–1), and perceptual tasks such as the backward reading of words. The measure of learning in each case is the improvement across test sessions. In one repetition priming task, the subject must complete a fragment of a word. If the completion is identical to a previously studied word, thereby indicating a preference for a particular response, prim-

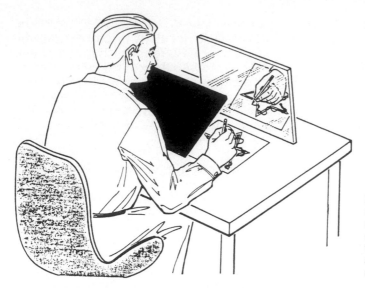

Figure 5–1. Mirror tracing apparatus.[188] Subjects trace the printed star with a stylus as quickly and accurately as possible, trying to stay within the boundaries. The star and hand holding the stylus are seen in mirror-reversed view.

ing has occurred. In a stem-completion priming task, subjects are first exposed to words in a study list (e.g., STANZA). When subsequently presented with three-letter stems (e.g., STA—) and asked to complete them with the first word that comes to mind, normal subjects are influenced by previous exposure to the study list, and often complete the stem to a word in the study list (STANZA) rather than to other, more common words (STAND or STAMP). The response STANZA is evidence of response biasing or priming by processes activated during the study task.

Comparisons of results for different disease groups provide evidence of dissociations among different kinds of implicit memory (e.g., skill learning versus priming) and information about their neural substrates. Subjects with HD (who have severe degeneration of the caudate nucleus) appear to be impaired in learning motor and perceptual skills,[40,109,136] whereas subjects with AD (whose caudate nucleus is relatively normal but who have severe degeneration of medial temporal-lobe structures and of association cortex) may learn some of the same skills normally.[55,83,109] Conversely, deficits in some types of repetition priming have been documented in AD,[55,93,122,207] but

normal priming on some of the same tasks has been observed in HD.[207] This double dissociation of function has prompted the hypothesis that skill learning is dependent upon the caudate nucleus and priming upon association cortex.

Remote Long-term Memory

Remote-memory tests assess recall and recognition of personal and public events from recent decades back through the subject's youth. To date, all tests of remote memory have focused on explicit learning. Performance differs among the several types of dementia and other neurodegenerative disorders, such as PD and Korsakoff's syndrome (KS). Although remote memory is preserved in AD relative to memory for recent events,[192] patients with AD do have poor memory for famous people and events from past decades. As dementia progresses from mild to profound, memories further back in time are lost. The performance of mildly impaired AD patients and patients with PD shows a temporal gradient, with older memories better preserved than more recent ones.[14,192] A similar temporal gradient is seen for patients with

KS,[2,3] whereas patients with HD perform poorly at all decades.[2,3,14] Investigators disagree as to whether the temporal gradient in remote memory has a biologic basis or whether the gradient is caused by items from certain decades having relatively greater salience or greater exposure in the media.[192] The dissociations within the dementias argue in favor of a biologic basis.

Neuropsychological studies of memory in dementia have advanced the clinical characterization of patients and theories about the organization of memory. Assessment of demented patients' recall and recognition of events and facts has documented the severe recent-memory and remote-memory impairment that is the most salient characteristic of the disorder. More comprehensive evaluations of memory, including skill learning and priming tasks in addition to recall and recognition, have clarified the existence of multiple memory systems that are differentially affected in different diagnostic groups. In short, patients with dementia do contribute to our knowledge of brain-behavior relations.

LANGUAGE

Neuropsychological examinations for aphasia have traditionally dissected language in terms of the subject's task (speaking, comprehending, spelling, reading, writing), rather than in terms of psycholinguistic variables (syntax or grammar, semantics or word meanings, phonology or sound patterns). One consequence of the traditional approach has been that language tasks often challenge multiple language capacities simultaneously. Such impure assays hamper precise brain-behavior correlations. Current views about language localization vary considerably. For example, Naeser and Hayward[153] advocate a strong association between Broca's area lesions and speech that is telegraphic and agrammatic, and between Wernicke's area lesions and paraphasic speech and poor comprehension. In contrast, Ojemann and colleagues[165] have evidence of marked intersubject variability in localization of specific language functions within the perisylvian region and beyond. For the future, a promising approach to understanding the neural substrate of language would be to assess specific, psycholinguistically defined components of language as independently as possible[43] and to map each of them onto discrete brain areas. The most common aphasia tests are not based on psycholinguistic principles, but assess a variety of language abilities, including naming[119]; symbolic, semantic, or ideational fluency[18,159,221]; vocabulary[157,158,232]; comprehension[76]; and expressive ability[77,97] (Table 5-3).

Table 5-3 ASSESSMENT OF LANGUAGE

Task	Test Name	Task Description
Naming	Boston Naming Test[119]	Identify line drawings of objects.
	Naming to Definition	Identify a word upon hearing its definition.
Fluency	Symbolic	Name within a designated time interval as many words as possible that begin with, for example, the letter *F*; the letter *A*; the letter *S*. (Controlled Oral Word Association Test)[18]
	Semantic	Name members of categories such as "animals," "colors," "vehicles," "tools," or "birds."[159]

(continued)

Table 5–3—*Continued*

Task	Test Name	Task Description
	Ideational	Name as many different things as you can that you could see when walking down the street; name as many different uses as you can for a brick.[221]
Vocabulary	WAIS-R Vocabulary subtest[232] National Adult Reading Test[157,158]	Hear words and define them. Pronounce phonetically irregular words. (As a measure of premorbid intellectual ability, this test appears to have validity for subjects with AD and MID, among other conditions, but not for HD and KS.)[59]
Comprehension	Simple commands	Respond to spoken or written simple commands such as "Touch your nose with your right index finger."
	Token Test[76]	Manipulate plastic tokens of various sizes and colors according to the examiner's spoken commands.
Expressive Ability	Story Telling	Look at a picture and describe what is going on in it. The subject's oral or written description provides a sample of propositional speech as well as revealing perceptual abilities and integration of picture elements. (Cookie Jar Theft from the Boston Diagnostic Aphasia Examination)[97]
	Reporter's Test[77]	Describe the actions of the examiner who manipulates plastic tokens of various sizes and colors (materials used are the same as for the Token Test, above).
	Reading aloud	Read aloud a passage from a text or newspaper.

Progression of Language Changes

Language stands second only to memory as the cognitive domain most frequently impaired in AD.[112,113,138] Language deficits in the early stages of AD may be noted in word-finding ability (Figure 5–2), discourse analysis, vocabulary, descriptive power, and reading comprehension. Speech may become somewhat slowed. Patients may also perseverate, repeating words or phrases in an inappropriate context. The most sensitive measures of language function early in AD are tests of verbal fluency.[115] Fluency tasks require that patients, within a specified time interval, produce as many words as possible that begin with a given letter (symbolic fluency)[18,227] or that designate members of a given semantic category (semantic or category fluency).[159] In mild AD, symbolic fluency seems to be more impaired than semantic fluency, although the two types are equally impaired in the moderate and severe stages.[186] Storandt and her colleagues[217] used performance on symbolic fluency in combination with three other cognitive tests to distinguish patients with mild AD from healthy older persons. They correctly classified 98% of the subjects. Neither fluency alone

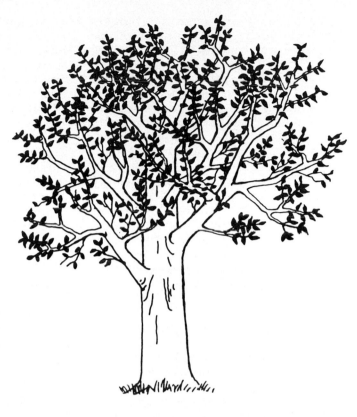

Figure 5–2. Stimulus from the Boston Naming Test.[114,119] Subjects name the depicted object (uncued condition). If they are unable to name the object after a prescribed period of time, the examiner may provide a semantic cue; if failure persists, a phonetic cue may be provided. (From Kaplan et al,[119] with permission.)

nor fluency combined with other tests was useful in differentiating very mild AD patients from healthy subjects or from mild AD patients, however[218]; scores for the very mild group overlapped those for the other groups.

As one would expect, the language deficits seen in the later stages of AD are more extensive than those seen in the early stages.[110] AD patients of moderate severity show extensive perseveration and decreased precision in speech content (e.g., increased circumlocutions). Impairments occur in auditory and reading comprehension as well as in writing ability.[197] At this stage, syntax (grammar) is well preserved relative to semantic knowledge (the understanding of meaning), as is the ability to read aloud.[123,152] Some language errors (e.g., an inability to analyze discourse) result in part from processing deficits consequent to impairments of memory or attention.[82,132]

Severely demented AD patients show profound disruption in language production and comprehension. Some of them become mute or echolalic; others display relatively good production with meaningless content.

In contrast to AD, dementing illnesses that involve the basal ganglia and subcortical nuclei, such as HD, PD, PSP and multi-infarct dementia (MID), deleteriously affect the motor aspects of speech production.[73,173] MID patients show impairment of syntax and the motor components of speech, but sparing of semantic knowledge.[110] Fluency and naming ability do not distinguish AD from MID when the groups are matched for dementia severity.[88] HD patients, like those with MID, commonly make syntactic errors.[98] Further, HD patients were equally impaired on semantic and symbolic fluency, whereas AD patients matched to the HD group for dementia severity were much more deficient on semantic than on symbolic fluency.[38] A number of the language impairments in HD appear to be secondary to other cognitive deficits. For example, impaired confrontation naming may reflect misperception of the stimulus pictures.[173] In Pick's disease, a neurodegenerative disorder of frontal-lobe and temporal-lobe structures, language impairments are prominent, with word-finding difficulty and anomia in the early stages giving way later in the disease to echolalia and mutism.[74] A significant impairment in language abilities typically occurs as an early sign of Pick's disease.[208,231] Word-finding difficulty also occurs in KS,[37,45] as does a mild-to-moderate deficit in semantic and symbolic fluency.[38]

Relation to Demographics

Several studies have linked language dysfunction in AD to specific demographic variables, including age at onset and rate of progression of the disease, and the presence of a family history of AD. Whether language impairment occurs more often in patients who develop AD before the age of 65 than in later-onset cases is a matter of controversy, with multiple reports of negative[198,219] and positive[46,199] findings. The specific language function under study may be important: naming and fluency seem to be impaired regardless of age of onset.[16,72] One study found that auditory comprehension and writing may be especially vulnerable to disruption in early-onset cases.[87] There is no direct evidence, however, of more extensive pathologic change in the left posterior cortex in early-onset AD patients. In regard to rate of progression, language impairment in the early stages has been associated with a more rapid course of disease. This relation was found to hold even when dementia severity was assessed with a behavioral rating scale thought to be independent of language function.[86,125] Finally, it has been suggested that the familial form of AD is more strongly associated with language dysfunction than is the

sporadic form,[31] but Chui and associates found no relation between age at onset and familiality.[46] The question is further complicated by the inherent difficulty of deciding whether or not a case is familial or sporadic: a negative family history may mean merely that too few family members survived to the age when AD is likely to appear or that the original family was too small to permit this question to be addressed.

The predominant language disorders in AD (fluency, naming, and comprehension deficits) all can be attributed to the profound impoverishment of many aspects of semantic memory.[154] Because premorbid semantic knowledge is not affected in pure global amnesia due to lesions of the medial temporal–diencephalic system,[95] the semantic deficit in AD must result from pathology in areas outside the medial temporal–diencephalic system.

ABSTRACT THOUGHT

Abstract thought draws upon two broadly defined capacities. First, "abstraction" is the process of extracting particular features from objects or events. *Concept formation* occurs by identifying features that are common to different objects or events and then generalizing from them. *Problem-solving* tasks demand that subjects abstract relevant information from situations. Second, abstract thought refers to concepts that are "abstract" (containing symbolic and representational features) as distinct from those that are "concrete" (containing features that reflect direct sensory experience). In *set-shifting* tasks, subjects initiate a new concept while suppressing a previously attained concept that is no longer appropriate to the task. Subjects make a series of responses (which may be abstract or concrete) based upon particular features that they have extracted from the test situation. Set shifting occurs when a different set of features are extracted, causing a change in response. Performance on

Table 5–4 ASSESSMENT OF ABSTRACT THOUGHT

Task	Test Name	Task Description
Concept formation	Wisconsin Card Sorting Test[21,102,142]	Sort cards according to unspecified concepts, such as color, shape, or number; the concept changes periodically without warning.
	WAIS-R Picture Arrangement[232]	Arrange several cartoon pictures serially to create a logical storyline.
	Concept Comprehension Test[61,62]	Match a picture of an object or scene to one of a three-choice picture array on the basis of an underlying shared concrete or abstract concept.
	Verbal Fluency	(Tests described under Language)
	WAIS-R Similarities[232]	Hear the names of two objects or concepts and tell how they are similar to each other.
	Proverb Interpretation[99]	Hear proverbs and explain them orally or indicate explanation by pointing to the answer in a multiple-choice array.
Set shifting	Wisconsin Card Sorting Test	(As above)
	Odd Man Out[89]	Choose which of three or four items does not fit the concept being exercised; a second concept periodically alternates with the first one.
	Finger pushing[50]	Learn an initial finger-pushing sequence, then learn a new sequence after the initial one is changed.
	Tactile reversal learning[92]	Choose between two patterned wells to obtain a reward. The rewarded well changes periodically without warning.
	Letter cancellation[222]	Cross out letters on a page according to changing criteria for cancellation.
Problem solving	Word problems[133]	Mentally calculate simple arithmetic and word problems.
	Poisoned Food Problems[9]	Deduce which food is poisoned after presentation of several three-food "meals" and their health outcomes.
	Cognitive Estimate Questions[204]	Apply general knowledge to novel situations (e.g., determine the length of the spine of an average man).
	Hukok Logical Thinking Matrices Test[75]	Choose the member of the nine- to twelve-item array that best completes the 3×3 matrix. Items vary in shape, color, and size, and the same items appear on increasingly difficult trials.

tasks of set shifting depends to a considerable extent on the integrity of the frontal lobes, whereas concept formation and problem solving probably draw on the capacities of multiple brain areas, including the frontal, temporal, and parietal lobes.[63] Tests of abstract thought that are appropriate for demented patients assess concept formation,[21,61,62,99,102,142,232] fluency,[18,159,221] set shifting,[21,50,89,92,102,142,222] and problem solving[9,75,133,204] (Table 5–4).

Concept Use and Set Shifting

Conceptual skills often are impaired in dementia. Verbal fluency is a measure of concept formation; deficits in fluency have already been described above under Language. Studies of semantic (category) fluency have shown that patients with AD can distinguish among major categories of objects, but that the specific semantic information required to distinguish among members within a category either has been lost or cannot be accessed.[115,135] Patients may have difficulty in assessing the relative importance of member attributes to understanding a concept,[103] a finding that is consistent with reports that AD patients produce excessively concrete responses on tests as varied as the WAIS-R Similarities subtest[135,170] and proverb interpretation,[124] which are verbal tests; and the Concept Comprehension Test,[70] which is nonverbal (Fig. 5–3). The tendency to produce concrete responses and to misjudge the relative importance of conceptual attributes implies that at least some semantic information is organized abnormally. This deficit does not seem to hold for category knowledge in particular, however. AD patients showed normal category typicality effects (low-typical exemplars were responded to less quickly than high-typical exemplars),[69,155] and they were normal at ranking triads of category exemplars on the basis of typicality.[69] Interestingly, the deficits seen in concept use may be slight compared with disorders of other cognitive functions in the same patients. On the Concept Comprehension Test, for example, most AD patients, representing a wide range of dementia severity, performed well above chance level, although they performed poorly on certain tests of memory, language, and visuospatial function.

Demented patients with PD showed deficits on conceptual tasks, including Similarities/Differences and proverb interpretation.[24,44] Nondemented PD patients were impaired on the abstract subtest of the Concept Comprehension

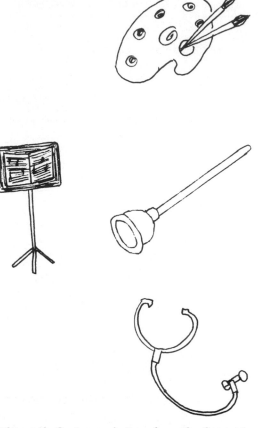

Figure 5–3. A sample item from the Concept Comprehension Test.[61,62] Subjects point to the member of the response array (*right*) that goes best with the target (*left*). Here the music stand is related to the palette because both objects are used in the arts.

Test[65] and on the WAIS-R Picture Arrangement subtest.[164] As in PD, patients with PSP performed subnormally on sorting tasks and Similarities,[134,170] proverb interpretation,[1,67] Picture Arrangement,[134] and the Concept Comprehension Test.[67] Patients with MID outperformed those with AD on Similarities and Picture Arrangement.[168]

Patients with AD and PD differ in performance on tests of set shifting. A widely used test of set shifting, the Wisconsin Card Sorting Test (WCST),[21,102,142] assesses the patient's ability to learn when to switch categories. Four initial cards, containing geometric forms of different shape, color, and number, are used as the basis on which the patient sorts a stack of 128 cards. The examiner does not specify the rule for sorting (for example, sort by color), but tells the patient "right" or "wrong" based on where the patient places each card in relationship to the four initial cards. Without warning to the patient, the criterion is changed after 10 consecutive cards are sorted correctly. A perseverative error occurs when the subject categorizes a card according to a previously but no longer correct sorting criterion. For example, if the patient is sorting according to color and the criterion changes to shape, perseverative responses would occur if the patient continues to sort by color. Although patients with PD, with or without dementia, are consistently impaired on this test in terms of the number of different correct sorts they attain, the deficit may have more than one source. Some workers have attributed poor performance in PD to a predominance of perseverative errors,[89,129] whereas others[28] have found that perseveration did not account for a significant number of errors. In a study comparing AD and PD groups with comparable Blessed Dementia Scale scores, patients with PD performed more poorly on the WCST than did patients with AD (Corkin and associates, unpublished data). Other set-shifting tests on which PD patients show impaired performance include finger pushing (a performance of changing sequences),[50] letter cancellation,[222] and tactile reversal learning.[92]

Problem Solving

Problem solving makes demands on attention and memory. Word problems further call upon verbal comprehension and production, and nonverbal problems may engage visuospatial skills. Attention, memory, language, and visuospatial functions are all impaired in dementia, precluding meaningful interpretation of results on many standard tests of problem-solving ability. Verbal problem solving has not been evaluated successfully in AD, presumably because of the confounding effects of language impairments on the interpretation of test results. Nondemented PD patients have demonstrated normal capacity for deductive reasoning on verbal problem-solving tasks such as Cognitive Estimates,[129] Poisoned Food Problems,[66] (Figure 5–4) and word problems.[67] By contrast, patients with PSP showed poor performance on word problems.[41,67]

It is advantageous to assess nonverbal logical reasoning skills with tests that make minimal visuospatial demands. For example, the Hukok Logical Thinking Matrices Test requires subjects to identify which one of several perceptually simple, colored forms appropriately completes an ordered series.[75] Even mildly demented patients with AD were impaired on this test,[64,70] and individuals with PSP also performed poorly.[67] Nondemented patients with PD appear to have normal deductive reasoning capacities as assessed with the Hukok test[70] and with the Tower of Toronto test,[193] in which subjects follow simple rules in moving a set of discs from one stick to another. Unlike the Hukok test, the Raven's Progressive Matrices (RPM)[177] and Raven's Coloured Progressive Matrices (RCPM)[178] rely on visuospatial function, which is known to be impaired in all dementing illnesses. It is unclear, therefore, whether deficits on the Raven's tests in demented patients reflect impairment of problem solving or of visuospatial function.

One must disregard research findings based on tests of abstract thought that make heavy demands on memory, language, attention, and visuospatial function. Studies that do not impose such demands indicate that demented patients show impairments on particular tests of abstract thought, and that some abstract capacities (e.g., deductive reasoning in AD, set shifting in PD) are more affected than others (e.g., organization of category knowledge, and non-

Meal	Outcome	Possibly Poisoned
tea lamb corn	died	tea lamb corn
tea veal rice	lived	tea* lamb corn
milk beef rice	lived	tea* lamb corn
milk lamb corn	died	tea* lamb corn
coffee veal corn	lived	tea* lamb

*error

Figure 5–4. Poisoned Food Problem.[9,66] Subjects are presented with three-food "meals" and their health outcomes for hypothetical diners ("lived" or "died"). The goal is to deduce the poisoned food. The number of meal/outcome presentations needed to solve the problems ranges from two to five. Shown: Performance by a subject with Parkinson's disease. "Tea" was the answer to the problem that immediately preceded this one. Note that the subject does not eliminate "tea" where appropriate in the current problem, which is otherwise correctly solved.

verbal concept comprehension in AD; problem solving in PD).

VISUOSPATIAL FUNCTION

Two main cortical systems support high-order visual processing, one in the temporal lobe that is concerned with object vision, and one in the parietal lobe that is concerned with spatial vision.[80] The inferior parietal lobule is specialized for spatial perception and visuomotor integration.[7,60] Accordingly, focal lesions in this area may produce visual neglect, constructional apraxia, visual mislocalization, visual disorientation, and topographic and spatial-memory deficits. Like memory, language, and abstract thought, various visuospatial capacities may be affected differentially in the several dementing illnesses. Visuospatial function is unlike the other cognitive domains, however, in that many standard tests depend on motor control and timing. Only tests that do not emphasize these factors are suitable for demented subjects, especially those with motor abnormalities, as in PD, HD, and PSP. Even in AD, some patients have extrapyramidal signs, which could interfere with their test performance.[185] Components of visuospatial function include constructional abilities, which are required in copying,[17,166,182,224,225,233] in drawing (e.g., a Necker cube, a clock, a bicycle), and in assembly[36,232]; personal orientation[147,201,234]; extrapersonal orientation[143,161,200,201,235]; and spatial cognition[19,20,52,227,230] (Table 5–5).

Constructional Abilities

Of the several visuospatial dysfunctions, constructional apraxia may be most familiar to clinicians because it is readily assessed at bedside and is a con-

Table 5–5 ASSESSMENT OF VISUOSPATIAL FUNCTION

Task	Test Name	Task Description
Constructional abilities Copying	Complex Figures Test[166,182,224,225] Benton Visual Retention Test[17] Wechsler Memory Scale-R-Visual Reproduction[233]	Copy exactly the presented figures. (As above) (As above)
Drawing	Necker cube; clock; bicycle	Draw the named objects.
Assembly	WAIS-R Block Design[232]	Replicate the examiner's block construction using individual blocks.
	Stick Test[36]	Copy the examiner's stick pattern (a) exactly as seen; (b) rotated 180 degrees.
Personal (egocentric) orientation	Standardized Road-Map Test of Direction Sense[147]	Trace a dotted pathway on a map and indicate the direction taken at each turn.
	Personal Orientation Test (Body Schema)[201,234]	Indicate parts of the body that are named or numbered on schematic diagrams.
Extrapersonal (allocentric) orientation	Extrapersonal Orientation Test (Locomotor Mazes)[200,201,237]	Translate the lines on a visual map into locomotion by walking the corresponding pattern on a floor map.
	Visually guided stylus mazes[143,161]	Find or retrace a specified route through a matrix of raised blocks using a stylus.
Spatial cognition	Judgment of Line Orientation[19]	Match angled lines to lines of the same orientations that appear in a choice array.
	Test of Facial Recognition[20]	Match pictures of front views of faces with identical front views, side views, or front views taken under different lighting conditions.
	Gollin Incomplete-Pictures Test[53,230]	(Described in Table 5–2: Memory)

sistent manifestation of damage to parietal cortex.[60] Patients with constructional apraxia are unable to assemble forms from given elements, and they often have difficulty in copying or drawing two- or three-dimensional designs. Constructional impairment often appears in the early stages of AD.[163] Patients with PD also have difficulty copying complex figures; analysis of their errors suggests a tendency to form a piecemeal representation of design elements rather than a whole construct.[164]

Personal and Extrapersonal Orientation

Less well known than constructional impairment are several other visuospatial deficits that relate to the disorganization of personal (egocentric) or extrapersonal (allocentric) space. Personal orientation concerns the judgment of the spatial relationship between one's own body and objects external to it. Deficits in personal orientation are associated with lesions to the frontal lobes.

Extrapersonal orientation concerns the ability to assess the spatial relationship that exists between two or more external objects. Impairments in extrapersonal orientation result from parietal lesions, especially in the right hemisphere (see references 39 and 151 for reviews).

Dissociations occur between personal and extrapersonal orientation. For example, Brouwers and colleagues[32] found that construction and manipulation of objects in extrapersonal space (copying the Rey-Osterrieth Complex Figure and use of a stylus maze) were impaired in AD but not in HD, whereas HD but not AD was associated with poor use of a road map that required the subject to negotiate directions in relation to personal orientation (Fig. 5–5). Patients with PD may be impaired relative to normal individuals on road map tests,[105] egocentric spatial localization,[175] and other tests of personal

orientation.[26] PD patients with left-sided motor symptoms, however, also performed poorly on a route-finding test that involved extrapersonal orientation.[26] It would appear, therefore, that the distinction between AD and HD is sharp on tests of personal and extrapersonal orientation, and that both types of test may elicit impaired performance in PD.

The personal orientation deficits of PD and HD patients are reminiscent of the performance of patients with frontal-lobe lesions. It is known that PD and HD patients demonstrate a variety of deficits associated with frontal-lobe lesions.[30,129,223] One may speculate, therefore, that HD and PD patients' deficits in personal orientation are part of a more general frontal-lobe syndrome. The posterior lesions of AD,[34] by contrast, would account for the disorganization of extrapersonal space observed in patients with this disease.

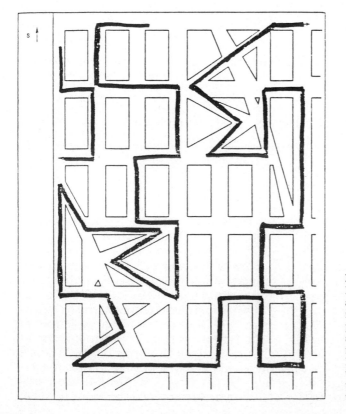

Figure 5–5. Money Road-Map Test of Direction Sense. Subjects watch the examiner trace a route on a map with a marking pen. Then the examiner uses a pencil to retrace the same route, and subjects report at each corner along the route whether to turn to their right or left. Subjects are *not* permitted to turn the map. (From Money.[147] Reprinted with permission of the United Educational Services, Inc., Buffalo, NY.)

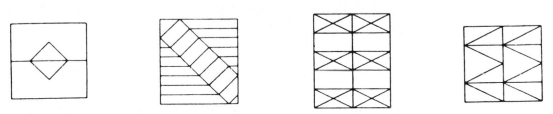

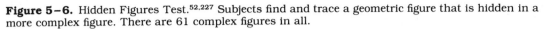

PART IV

Look at the two adjacent figures.
One of them is contained in each of
the drawings below.

In each of the following drawings, mark
that part which is the same as one of the
adjacent figures. Mark only one figure
in each drawing.

Figure 5–6. Hidden Figures Test.[52,227] Subjects find and trace a geometric figure that is hidden in a more complex figure. There are 61 complex figures in all.

Spatial Cognition

Spatial cognition may be described as the mental manipulation of spatial information. It encompasses a wide variety of capacities, including form matching, mental rotation of objects, identification of figures that are embedded in a larger pattern (Fig. 5–6), identification of incomplete figures, and judgment of line orientation. Many of these capacities are subserved by right posterior cortex (see references 160, 163, and 238 for reviews).

Midstage AD is associated with impairments in visuospatial memory and form matching,[187] identification of incomplete pictures on initial presentation,[53] and facial recognition.[237] These deficits may be related to pathology of the right parietal and right temporal lobes,[145] areas that sustain damage in AD.[34]

PD patients show deficits on several aspects of visuospatial function. Impaired capacities include the integration of visual and postural information,[176] spatial orientation,[27] gestural representation,[205] and copying complex figures.[164] However, there is some controversy regarding the extent of visuo-spatial dysfunction in PD. Some[78] claim that impairments appear consistently only on tests with significant motor demands. The fact that tests of some visuospatial capacities require minimal motor involvement[25] suggests that the deficits in visuospatial function go beyond motor impairments. Except for tasks of personal orientation, which are sensitive to frontal-lobe dysfunction (see the preceding section), the neural substrate of visuospatial deficits in PD is yet to be elucidated.

The conclusion that there are widespread deficits in high-order visuospatial function in dementia must be tempered by the lack of information about the contribution of disorders in basic visual capacities (e.g., vernier acuity, contrast sensitivity, stereoacuity) to the high-order deficits. Future research should determine whether basic deficits may in some cases explain the high-order deficits.

ATTENTION

The components of attention include alertness, selectivity, processing capacity, and duration.[174] These components can be evaluated independently and may be impaired selectively in dementing disease. Disorders of one or more of the components of attention can affect a variety of perceptual and cognitive functions by disrupting the control and execution of performance. Demented individuals generally are alert and do not suffer from impairments of consciousness, such as delirium or loss of conscious awareness, but they often do exhibit deficits in selective and sustained attention. Selective attention may be focused (simple reaction time and other tests, including digit span,[232,233] letter cancellation,[222] and identification of hidden figures[100,227]) or divided (Brown-Peterson distractor task,[11,169] Trail Making Test[10]). Several tests also assess sustained attention (Continuous Performance Test,[189] Reporter's Test,[77] or reading aloud) (Table 5–6).

Selective Attention

Selective attention may be described as focused (directed exclusively to a subset of the incoming information) or divided (distributed between two or more subsets of information). Focusing and dividing attention implies the existence of a central executive or control mechanism for attention. The frontal lobes appear to be important to the integrity of the control mechanism.[133,203] Tasks that place high demands on selective attention, especially those that elicit effortful, as opposed to automatic, processing, are performed poorly early in the course of dementia.[118]

The relation between cognition and attention is complex. Performance on many tests of memory, language, and abstract thought is also sensitive to attention. Although primary memory and attention are conceptually distinct, they seem to be difficult to distinguish

Table 5–6 ASSESSMENT OF ATTENTION

Task	Test Name	Task Description
Selective attention Focused	Simple reaction time	Respond vocally or manually as quickly as possible to the appearance of a designated stimulus on a screen.
	Digit Span	Recall a series of numbers of increasing span. (A subtest of the Wechsler Memory Scale-R[233] and the WAIS-R[232])
	Letter Cancellation Test[222]	Cross out letters on a page according to changing criteria for cancellation.
	Hidden Figures Test[100]	Trace the outline of a geometric figure embedded in a more complex one.
Divided	Brown-Peterson distractor task[11,169]	Hear three letters, count backwards from a given number for a specified amount of time, recall the three letters.
	Trail Making Test (B)[10]	Connect consecutively numbered and lettered circles on a page, alternating between the two sequences. (A subtest of the Halstead-Reitan neuropsychological battery[131])
Sustained attention	Continuous Performance Test[189]	Respond vocally or manually to the designated letter whenever it appears on the screen.

from each other in practice.[194] For example, in order to repeat a long string of digits, subjects must attend continuously to the task at hand while placing the digits in a short-term memory store. One can identify patients with AD whose memory impairment seems related specifically to deficits in attentional control (the central executive function)[12] and presumably involves disorders of the frontal lobes. These patients may be contrasted with others for whom memory loss is more likely to have resulted from pathologic changes in the hippocampus.[15] Further, tests of immediate memory (digit span) and short-term memory with distraction (Brown-Peterson distractor task) that are performed poorly by patients with mild AD (as described under Memory) can also be considered to be measures of focused and divided attention, respectively.

Reaction time (RT) tasks are often used to assess selective attention. Patients with AD showed abnormal slowing on tests of simple RT.[13,171] Slowing is even more pronounced on simple RT combined with pursuit tracking[13]; on choice RT[16,171]; and on RT associated with complex tasks such as lexical decision (deciding whether a letter string is a real word) and sentence completion,[156] and word reading.[172] Patients with PD resemble those with AD in showing slowed responses for simple RT[85,108,216] and choice RT.[85,216] Tasks of selective attention that did not use RT and that elicited impaired performance by AD patients include detection of hidden figures,[42] a variety of tasks requiring divided attention,[13] and the cancellation of specific digits or letters on a page.[210] Letter cancellation also is impaired in PD. It is possible that in PD the deficit represents a difficulty in shifting between alternating sets of letters[222] rather than a deficit in selective attention.

Sustained Attention

Sustained attention refers to acts of vigilance that require focused or divided attention over long, uninterrupted sessions, often of more than 30 minutes. During such tasks, subjects must constantly monitor stimulus information and detect small, occasional changes or infrequently occurring specific elements. Deficits in sustained attention on a complex continuous performance task (CPT) have been documented in unspecified senile dementia (i.e., respond to the letter X when it is preceded by an A).[5] On simple CPT (i.e., respond to the letter X whenever it occurs), patients with unspecified senile dementia[5] or PD[216] appear to perform relatively normally. Selective and sustained attention may be assessed in a single test, as in letter cancellation or complex CPT.

SUMMARY

A neuropsychological approach to the study of dementia draws upon, modifies, and extends techniques that have proven valuable in the assessment of focal brain injury and provides new methods of examination that are especially tailored to the characteristics of demented patients. Neuropsychological assessments further a variety of aims, including the diagnosis, treatment, and clinical management of patients, as well as research linking brain systems to behavior. In view of the obvious complexities of human cognition, assessment must be comprehensive. In the clinic, the neuropsychologist evaluates patients' functioning on each of the manifold cognitive and perceptual capacities that support human behavior, including memory, language, abstract thought, visuospatial function, and attention. As evidence of the usefulness of assessments based on this approach, neuropsychological studies have identified numerous dissociations among the cognitive capacities of patients whose dementias differ etiologically. As Brown and Marsden concluded in their recent review,[33] AD, PD, and HD patients manifest many parallel impairments, but each dementing illness appears to be characterized by its own distinct pattern of isolated cognitive deficits.

Proper test administration requires considerable training and practice. Interpreting test results is more difficult still because, for example, patients' age, psychiatric conditions, and education may influence test results, as may any extant sensory impairments. As a more complex example, a given test may measure different capacities in different patients. Even though demented patients may be able to complete a particular task in both the severe and the mild stage of the disease, it is unlikely that they perform the task in the same way in each of the disease stages. Thus proper interpretation of test results requires sensitivity to who the patients are and how the patients are performing tasks, in addition to their success in performing them.

Further complicating test interpretation, a patient's score on a single test may not translate directly into a deficit in a specific cognitive capacity. An observed score may reflect a disorder in a single capacity or it may reflect deficits in a combination of capacities. For example, Corkin[53] concluded that in AD there is an interaction between memory capacities and other cognitive processes such that the observed deficits in both domains are more severe than they would have been in isolation. Good tests are designed to minimize this problem by relying on simple tasks that do not demand contributions from cognitive capacities that the test is not intended to measure. In developing a test, one can exclude irrelevant capacities only if one has an explicit model of what those other capacities are. Thus test designers must start from a specific model of cognition that identifies or segregates individual capacities. In clinical practice, identification of a patient's individual deficits requires careful and comprehensive assessment based on theoretical distinctions between such capacities as implicit versus explicit memory, or syntax versus semantic functions. The complex relations among multiple cognitive capacities,

test design, and test performance bear witness to the difficulties of interpreting the results of assessment procedures.

Because test construction is guided by neuropsychological theories, the rapid pace of theoretical advances in neuropsychology has stimulated parallel advances in clinical assessment procedures. Many of the specific tests and theoretical distinctions discussed here are relatively new, and have emerged from the general "information-processing" paradigm current among psychologists.[84,120,127] In short, the information-processing approach focuses not on observable behavior but rather on what information is passed from one processing stage to the next, and how each stage modifies that information. Thus we neither perceive nor remember the world as it is; we perceive and remember what we have coded. Inevitably, as this dominant paradigm in psychology undergoes change, neuropsychologists will revise their understanding of which capacities and behaviors merit careful assessment, and will modify accordingly the specific tests that support neuropsychological assessment of dementia.

ACKNOWLEDGMENTS

The writing of this chapter was supported by NIH grants 5F32 AG05391 (to A. C.-G.) and AG06605 and AG08117 (to S.C.). We thank Margaret M. Keane, John H. Growdon, Janet Sherman, and Richard Owings for their helpful comments.

REFERENCES

1. Albert ML, Feldman RG, and Willis AL: The 'subcortical dementia' of progressive supranuclear palsy. J Neurol Neurosurg Psychiatry 37:121–130, 1974.
2. Albert MS, Butters N, and Brandt J: Development of remote memory loss

in patients with Huntington's disease. J Clin Exp Neuropsychol 3:1–12, 1981.

3. Albert MS, Butters N, and Brandt J: Patterns of remote memory in amnesic and demented patients. Arch Neurol 38:495–500, 1981.

4. Albert MS, Butters N, and Levin J: Temporal gradients in the retrograde amnesia of patients with alcoholic Korsakoff's disease. Arch Neurol 36:211–216, 1979.

5. Alexander DA: Attention dysfunction in senile dementia. Psychol Rep 32:229–230, 1973.

6. Alexopoulos GS, Abrams RC, Young RC, and Shamoian CA: Cornell scale for depression in dementia. Biol Psychiatry 23:271–283, 1988.

7. Andersen RA: Inferior parietal lobule function in spatial perception and visuomotor integration. In Mountcastle VB, Plum F, and Geiger R (eds): Handbook of Physiology: The Nervous System. American Physiological Society, Bethesda, MD, 1987, pp 483–517.

8. American Psychiatric Association: Diagnostic and Statistical Manual of Mental Disorders, Ed 3, Rev (DSM-III-R). American Psychiatric Association, Washington, DC: 1987.

9. Arenberg D: Concept problem solving in young and old adults. J Gerontol 23:279–282, 1968.

10. Army US: Army Individual Test Battery: Manual of directions and scoring. War Department, Adjutant General's Office, Washington, DC, 1944.

11. Baddeley AD: The Psychology of Memory. Basic Books, New York, 1976.

12. Baddeley AD: Working Memory. Oxford University Press, London, 1986.

13. Baddeley AD, Logie R, Bressi S, Della Sala S, and Spinnler H: Dementia and working memory. Q J Exp Psychol 38A:603–618, 1986.

14. Beatty WW, Salmon DP, Butters N, Heindel WC, and Granholm EL: Retrograde amnesia in patients with Alzheimer's disease and Huntington's disease. Neurobiol Aging 9:181–186, 1988.

15. Becker JT: Working memory and secondary memory deficits in Alz-

heimer's disease. J Clin Exp Neuropsychol 10:739–753, 1988.

16. Becker JT, Huff FJ, Nebes RD, Holland A, and Boller F: Neuropsychological function in Alzheimer's disease: Patterns of impairment and rates of progression. Arch Neurol 45:263–268, 1988.

17. Benton AL: The Revised Visual Retention Test. Psychological Corporation, New York, 1974.

18. Benton AL and Hamsher K: Multilingual aphasia examination. University of Iowa, Iowa City, 1976.

19. Benton AL, Hannay HJ, and Varney NR: Visual perception of line direction in patients with unilateral brain disease. Neurology 25:907–910, 1975.

20. Benton AL and Van Allen MW: Impairment in facial recognition in patients with cerebral disease. Cortex 4:344–358, 1968.

21. Berg EA: A simple objective technique for measuring flexibility in thinking. J Gen Psychol 39:15–22, 1948.

22. Berg L: Mild senile dementia of the Alzheimer type: Diagnostic criteria and natural history. Mt Sinai J Med 55:87–96, 1988.

23. Blessed G, Tomlinson BE, and Roth M: The association between quantitative measures of dementia and of senile change in the grey matter of elderly subjects. Br J Psychiatry 114:797–811, 1968.

24. Boller F: Mental status of patients with Parkinson disease. J Clin Neuropsychol 2:157–172, 1980.

25. Boller F, Passafiume D, Keefe NC, et al: Visuospatial impairment in Parkinson's disease: Role of perceptual and motor factors. Arch Neurol 41:485–490, 1984.

26. Bowen FP: Behavioral alterations in patients with basal ganglia lesions. In Yahr MD (ed): The Basal Ganglia. Raven Press, New York, 1976.

27. Bowen FP, Hoehn MM, and Yahr MD: Alterations in spatial orientation as determined by a route-walking test. Neuropsychologia 10:355–361, 1972.

28. Bowen FP, Kamienny RS, Burns MM, and Yahr MD: Parkinsonism: Effects of levodopa treatment on concept for-

mation. Neurology 25:701–704, 1975.

29. Bradshaw JL and Nettleton NC: The nature of hemispheric specialization in man. Behavioral and Brain Sciences 4:51–91, 1981.

30. Brandt J and Butters N: The neuropsychology of Huntington's disease. Trends Neurosci 118–120, 1986.

31. Breitner JCS and Folstein MF: Familial Alzheimer dementia: A prevalent disorder with specific clinical features. Psychol Med 14:63–80, 1984.

32. Brouwers P, Cox C, Martin A, et al: Differential perceptual-spatial impairment in Huntington's and Alzheimer's dementias. Arch Neurol 41:1073–1076, 1984.

33. Brown RG and Marsden CD: Commentary: "Subcortical dementia": The neuropsychological evidence. Neuroscience 25:363–387, 1988.

34. Brun A and Englund E: Regional pattern of degeneration in Alzheimer's disease: Neuronal loss and histopathological grading. Histopathology 5:549–564, 1981.

35. Bulens C, Meerwaldt JD, Van der Wildt GJ, and Keemink CJ: Contrast sensitivity in Parkinson's disease. Neurology 36:1121–1125, 1986.

36. Butters N and Barton M: Effect of parietal lobe damage on the performance of reversible operations in space. Neuropsychologia 8:205–214, 1970.

37. Butters N, Granholm E, Salmon DP, and Grant I: Episodic and semantic memory: A comparison of amnesic and demented patients. J Clin Exp Neuropsychol 9:479–497, 1987.

38. Butters N, Salmon DP, Heindel W, and Granholm E: Episodic, semantic and procedural memory: Some comparisons of Alzheimer and Huntington disease patients. In Terry RD (ed): Aging and the Brain. Raven Press, New York, 1988, pp 63–87.

39. Butters N, Soeldner C, and Fedio P: Comparison of parietal and frontal lobe spatial deficits in man: Extrapersonal vs personal (egocentric) space. Percept Mot Skills 34:27–34, 1972.

40. Butters N, Wolfe J, Martone M, Granholm E, and Cermak L: Memory dis-

orders associated with Huntington's disease: Verbal recall, verbal recognition and procedural memory. Neuropsychologia 23:729–743, 1985.

41. Cambier J, Masson M, Viader F, Limodin J, and Strube A: Le syndrome frontal de la paralysie supranucleaire progressive. Rev Neurol (Paris) 141:528–536, 1985.

42. Capitani E, Della Sala S, Lucchelli F, Soave P, and Spinnler H: Perceptual attention in aging and dementia measured by Gottschaldt's Hidden Figure Test. J Gerontol 43:157–163, 1988.

43. Caplan D: The biological bases for language. In Newmeyer FJ (ed): Linguistics: The Cambridge Survey. Cambridge University Press, Cambridge (UK), 1988, pp 237–255.

44. Celesia GG and Wanamaker WM: Psychiatric disturbances in Parkinson's disease. Diseases of the Nervous System, 33:577–583, 1972.

45. Cermak, LS, Reale L, and Baker, E: Alcoholic Korsakoff patient's retrieval from semantic memory. Brain Lang 5:215–226, 1978.

46. Chui HC, Teng EL, Henderson VW, and Moy AC: Clinical subtypes of dementia of the Alzheimer type. Neurology 35:1544–1550, 1985.

47. Cogan DG: Visual disturbances with focal progressive dementing disease. Am J Ophthalmol 100:68–72, 1985.

48. Cohen NJ and Squire LR: Preserved learning and retention of pattern-analyzing skill in amnesia: Dissociation of knowing how and knowing that. Science 210:207–209, 1980.

49. Cohen NJ and Squire LR: Retrograde amnesia and remote memory impairment. Neuropsychologia 19:337–356, 1981.

50. Cools AR, Van der Berken JHL, Horstink MWI, Van Spaendonck KPM, and Berger HJC: Cognitive and motor shifting aptitude disorder in Parkinson's disease. J Neurol Neurosurg Psychiatry 47:443–453, 1984.

51. Corkin S: Acquisition of motor skills after bilateral medial temporal lobe excision. Neuropsychologia 6:255–265, 1968.

52. Corkin S: Hidden figures test perform-

ance: Lasting effects of unilateral penetrating head injury and transient effects of bilateral cingulotomy. Neuropsychologia 17:585–605, 1979.

53. Corkin S: Some relationships between global amnesias and the memory impairments in Alzheimer's disease. In Corkin S, Davis KL, Growdon JH, and Usdin E (eds): Alzheimer's Disease: A Report of Progress in Research. Raven Press, New York, 149–164, 1982.

54. Corkin, S: Lasting consequences of bilateral medial temporal lobectomy: Clinical course and experimental findings in H.M. Seminars in Neurology 4:252–262, 1984.

55. Corkin S, Gabrieli JDE, Stanger BZ, et al: Skill learning and priming in Alzheimer's disease. Neurology (Suppl) 36:296, 1986.

56. Corkin S, Growdon JH, Sullivan EV, Nissen MJ, and Huff FJ: Assessing treatment effects: A neuropsychological battery. In Poon LW (ed): Handbook for Clinical Memory Assessment of Older Adults. American Psychological Association, Washington, DC, 1986, pp 156–167.

57. Corsi P: Human memory and the medial temporal region of the brain. McGill University, Montreal. Unpublished doctoral dissertation, 1972.

58. Coyne AC, Liss L, and Geckler C: The relationship between cognitive status and visual information processing. J Gerontol 39:711–717, 1984.

59. Crawford JR, Parker DM, and Besson JAO: Estimation of premorbid intelligence in organic conditions. Br J Psychiatr 153:178–181, 1988.

60. Critchley M: The Parietal Lobes. Arnold, London, 1953.

61. Cronin-Golomb A: Comprehension of abstract concepts in right and left hemispheres of complete commissurotomy subjects. Neuropsychologia 24:881–887, 1986.

62. Cronin-Golomb A: Subcortical transfer of cognitive information in subjects with complete forebrain commissurotomy. Cortex 22:499–519, 1986.

63. Cronin-Golomb A: Abstract thought in aging and age-related neurological disease. In Boller F and Grafman J (eds):

Handbook of Neuropsychology, Vol 4. Elsevier, Amsterdam, 1990, pp 279–309.

64. Cronin-Golomb A, Corkin S, and Growdon JH: Early decline of logical reasoning skills in Alzheimer's disease. Abstracts, Society for Neuroscience 12:1163, 1986.

65. Cronin-Golomb A, Corkin S, and Growdon JH: Relational abilities in Alzheimer's disease and Parkinson's disease. Clinical Neuropsychologist 1:298, 1987.

66. Cronin-Golomb A, Corkin S, and Growdon JH: Impaired problem solving in Parkinson's disease: Influence of set-shifting deficit. Abstracts, Society for Neuroscience 14:218, 1988.

67. Cronin-Golomb A, Corkin S, and Growdon J: Impaired problem solving in progressive supranuclear palsy. Proceedings and Abstracts, Eastern Psychological Association 60:60, 1989.

68. Cronin-Golomb A, Corkin S, Rizzo JF, et al: Visual dysfunction in Alzheimer's disease: Relation to normal aging. Ann Neurol 29(1):41–52, 1991.

69. Cronin-Golomb A, Keane MM, Kokodis A, Corkin S, and Growdon JH: Category knowledge in Alzheimer's disease: Normal organization and a general retrieval deficit. Psychol Aging, in press.

70. Cronin-Golomb A, Rho WA, Corkin S, and Growdon JH: Abstract reasoning in age-related neurological disease. J Neural Transm Suppl 24:79–83, 1987.

71. Crook, T Bartus RT, Ferris SH, et al: Age-associated memory impairment: Proposed diagnostic criteria and measures of clinical change—Report of a National Institute of Mental Health Work Group. Developmental Neuropsychology, 2:261–276, 1986.

72. Cummings JL, Benson DF, Hill MA, and Read S: Aphasia in dementia of the Alzheimer type. Neurology 35:394–397, 1985.

73. Cummings JL, Darkins A, Mendez M, et al: Alzheimer's disease and Parkinson's disease: Comparison of speech

and language alterations. Neurology 38:680–684, 1988.

74. Cummings JL and Duche LW: Klüver-Bucy syndrome in Pick's disease: Clinical and pathologic correlations. Neurology 31:1415–1422, 1981.

75. Daryn E: The Hukok logical thinking matrices test. Eked, Tel Aviv, 1977.

76. De Renzi E and Ferrari C: The Token Test: A sensitive test to detect disturbances in aphasics. Brain 85:665–678, 1962.

77. De Renzi E and Ferrari C: The reporter's test: A sensitive test to detect expressive disturbances in aphasics. Cortex 14:279–293, 1978.

78. Della Sala S, Di Lorenzo G, Giordano A, and Spinnler H: Is there a specific visuospatial impairment in parkinsonians? J Neurol Neurosurg Psychiatry 49:1258–1265, 1986.

79. Derogatis LR: SCL-90: Administration Scoring and Procedures Manual, Revised. Baltimore, MD, 1977.

80. Desimone R and Ungerleider L: Neural mechanisms of visual processing in monkeys. In Boller F and Grafman J (eds): Handbook of Neuropsychology, Vol 3. Elsevier, Amsterdam, 1989, pp 267–299.

81. Ditter SM and Mirra SS: Neuropathologic and clinical features of Parkinson's disease in Alzheimer's disease patients. Neurology 37:754–760, 1987.

82. Emery OB: Language and memory processing in senile dementia Alzheimer's type. In Light LL and Burke DM (eds): Language, Memory, and Aging. Cambridge University Press, New York, 1988, pp 221–243.

83. Eslinger PJ and Damasio AR: Preserved motor learning in Alzheimer's disease: Implications for anatomy and behavior. J Neurosci 6:3006–3009, 1986.

84. Estes WK: The information-processing approach to cognition: A confluence of metaphors and methods. In Estes WK (ed): Handbook of Learning and Cognitive Processes: Human Information Processing, Vol 5. John Wiley & Sons, New York, 1978, pp 1–18.

85. Evarts EV, Teravainen H, and Calne DB: Reaction time in Parkinson's disease. Brain 104:167–186, 1981.

86. Faber-Langendoen K, Morris JC, Knesevich JW, et al: Aphasia in senile dementia of the Alzheimer type. Ann Neurol 23:365–370, 1988.

87. Filley CM, Kelly JM, and Heaton RK: Neuropsychologic features of early- and late-onset Alzheimer's disease. Arch Neurol 43:574–576, 1986.

88. Fischer P, Gatterer G, Marterer A, and Danielczyk W: Nonspecificity of semantic impairment in dementia of Alzheimer's type. Arch Neurol 45:1341–1343, 1988.

89. Flowers KA and Robertson C: The effect of Parkinson's disease on the ability to maintain a mental set. J Neurol Neurosurg Psychiatry 48:517–529, 1985.

90. Folstein MF, Folstein SE, and McHugh PR: "Mini-mental state": A practical method for grading the cognitive state of patients for the clinician. J Psychiatr Res 12:189–198, 1975.

91. Folstein MF and McHugh PR: Dementia syndrome of depression. In Katzman R, Terry RD, and Bick KL (eds): Alzheimer's Disease: Senile Dementia and Related Disorders. Raven Press, New York, 1978, pp 87–93.

92. Freedman M and Oscar-Berman M: Tactile discrimination learning deficits in Alzheimer's and Parkinson's diseases. Arch Neurol 44:394–398, 1987.

93. Gabrieli JDE: Memory systems of the human brain: Dissociations among learning capacities in amnesia. Unpublished doctoral dissertation, Massachusetts Institute of Technology, Cambridge, 1986.

94. Gabrieli JDE: Differential effects of aging and age-related neurological diseases on memory subsystems of the brain. In Boller F and Grafman J (eds): Handbook of Neuropsychology, Vol 5. Elsevier, Amsterdam, 1991, pp 149–166.

95. Gabrieli JDE, Cohen NJ, and Corkin S: The impaired learning of semantic knowledge following bilateral medial temporal-lobe resection. Brain Cogn 7:157–177, 1988.

96. Gabrieli JDE, Merrill FD, and Corkin S: Acquisition of perceptual skills in amnesia due to bilateral medial temporal-lobe (H.M.) or diencephalic lesions. Abstracts, Society for Neuroscience 12:20, 1986.

97. Goodglass H and Kaplan E: Assessment of Aphasia and Related Disorders. Lea & Febiger, Philadelphia, 1972.

98. Gordon WP and Illes J: Neurolinguistic characteristics of language production in Huntington's disease: A preliminary report. Brain Lang 31:1–10, 1987.

99. Gorham DR: A proverbs test for clinical and experiental use. Psychol Rep 1:1–12, 1956.

100. Gottschaldt K: Ueber den Einfluss der Erfahrung auf die Wahrnehmung von Figuren. Psychologische Forschung 8:18–317, 1928.

101. Graf P, Squire LR, and Mandler G: The information that amnesic patients do not forget. J Exp Psychol [Learn Mem Cogn] 10:164–178, 1984.

102. Grant DA and Berg EA: A behavioral analysis of degree of reinforcement and ease of shifting to new responses in a Weigl-type card-sorting problem. J Exp Psychol 38:404–411, 1948.

103. Grober E, Buschke H, Kawas C, and Fuld P: Impaired ranking of semantic attributes in dementia. Brain Lang 26:276–286, 1985.

104. Growdon JH: Biological therapies for Alzheimer's disease. In Whitehouse P (ed): Dementia. FA Davis, Philadelphia, 1992.

105. Growdon JH, Corkin S, Desclos G, and Rosen TJ: Hoehn and Yahr stage predicts the extent of cognitive deficit in Parkinson's disease. Paper presented at the 1987 meeting of the American Academy of Neurology, New York, 1987.

106. Hamilton M: Development of a rating scale for primary depressive illness. Br J Soc Clin Psychol 6:278–296, 1967.

107. Hart S: Language and dementia: A review. Psychol Med 18:99–112, 1988.

108. Heilman KM, Bowers D, Watson RT, and Greer M: Reaction times in Parkinson's disease. Arch Neurol 33:139–140, 1976.

109. Heindel WC, Butters N, and Salmon DP: Impaired learning of a motor skill in patients with Huntington's disease. Behav Neurosci 102:141–147, 1988.

110. Hier B, Hagenlocker K, and Shindler AG: Language disintegration in dementia: Effects of etiology and severity. Brain Lang 25:117–133, 1985.

111. Hinton DR, Sadun AA, Blanks JC, and Miller CA: Optic nerve degeneration in Alzheimer's disease. N Eng J Med 315:485–487, 1986.

112. Huff FJ: Language in normal aging and age-related neurological diseases. In Boller F and Grafman J (eds): Handbook of Neuropsychology, Vol 4. Elsevier, Amsterdam, 1990, pp 251–264.

113. Huff FJ, Becker JT, Belle SH, et al: Cognitive deficits and clinical diagnosis of Alzheimer's disease. Neurology 37:1119–1124, 1987.

114. Huff FJ, Collins C, Corkin S, and Rosen TJ: Equivalent forms of the Boston Naming Test. J Clin Exp Neuropsychol 8:556–562, 1986.

115. Huff FJ, Corkin S, and Growdon JH: Semantic impairment and anomia in Alzheimer's disease. Brain Lang 28:235–249, 1986.

116. Huppert FA: Age-related changes in memory: Learning and remembering new information. In Boller F and Grafman J (eds): Handbook of Neuropsychology, Vol 5. Elsevier, Amsterdam, 1991, pp 123–147.

117. James W: The Principles of Psychology. Henry Holt & Co, New York, 1890.

118. Jorm AF: Controlled and automatic information processing in senile dementia: A review. Psychol Med 16:77–88, 1986.

119. Kaplan E, Goodglass H, and Weintraub S: The Boston Naming Test. Kaplan E and Goodglass H, Boston, 1978.

120. Kazniak AW, Poon LW, and Riege W: Assessing memory deficits: An information-processing approach. In Poon LW (ed): Handbook for Clinical Memory Assessment. American Psychological Association, Washington, DC, 1986, pp 168–188.

121. Keane MM, Gabrieli JDE, Fennema AC, Growdon JH, and Corkin S: Evidence for a dissociation between per-

ceptual and conceptual priming in Alzheimer's disease. Behav Neurosci 5:104–120, 1990.

122. Keane, MM, Gabrieli JDE, Kjelgaard MM, Growdon JH, and Corkin S: Dissociation between two kinds of priming in global amnesia and Alzheimer's disease. Abstracts, Society for Neuroscience 14:1290, 1988.

123. Kempler D, Curtiss S, and Jackson C: Syntactic preservation in Alzheimer's disease. J Speech Hear Res 30:343–350, 1987.

124. Kempler D, Van Lancker D, and Read S: Proverb and idiom comprehension in Alzheimer's disease. Alzheimer Dis Assoc Disord 2:38–49, 1988.

125. Knesevich JW, LaBarge E, and Edwards D: Predictive value of the Boston Naming Test in mild senile dementia of the Alzheimer type. Psychiatry Res 19:155–161, 1986.

126. Kopelman MD: Rates of forgetting in Alzheimer-type dementia and Korsakoff's syndrome. Neuropsychologia 23:623–638, 1985.

127. Kosslyn SM, Flynn RA, Amsterdam JB, and Wang G: Components of high-level vision: A cognitive neuroscience analysis and accounts of neurologial syndromes. Cognition 34:203–277, 1990.

128. Kral VA: Benign senescent forgetfulness. In Katzman R, Terry R, and Bick K (eds): Alzheimer's Disease: Senile Dementia and Related Disorders. Aging, Vol 7. Raven Press, New York, 1978, pp 47–51.

129. Lees AJ and Smith E: Cognitive deficits in the early stages of Parkinson's disease. Brain 106:257–270, 1983.

130. Leverenz J and Sumi M: Parkinson's disease in patients with Alzheimer's disease. Arch Neurol 43:662–664, 1986.

131. Lezak MD: Neuropsychological Assessment. Oxford University Press, New York, 1983.

132. Light LL and Burke DM: Patterns of language and memory in old age. In Light LL and Burke DM (eds): Language, Memory, and Aging. Cambridge University Press, New York, 1988, pp 244–271.

133. Luria AR: Higher Cortical Functions in Man. Basic Books, New York, 1980.

134. Maher ER, Smith EM, and Lees AJ: Cognitive deficits in the Steele-Richardson-Olszewski syndrome (progressive supranuclear palsy). J Neurol Neurosurg Psychiatry 48:1234–1239, 1985.

135. Martin A and Fedio P: Word production and comprehension in Alzheimer's disease: The breakdown of semantic knowledge. Brain Lang 9:124–141, 1983.

136. Martone M, Butters N, Payne M, Becker J, and Sax DS: Dissociations between skill learning and verbal recognition in amnesia and dementia. Arch Neurol 41:965–970, 1984.

137. Mattis S: Mental status examination for organic mental syndromes in the elderly patient. In Bellak L and Karasu TE (eds): Geriatric Psychiatry. Grune & Stratton, New York, 1976, pp 77–121.

138. Mayeux R, Stern Y, and Spanton, S: Heterogeneity in dementia of the Alzheimer type: Evidence of subgroups. Neurology 35:453–461, 1985.

139. McKhann G, Drachman D, Folstein M, et al: Clinical diagnosis of Alzheimer's disease: Report of the NINCDS-ADRDA work group under the auspices of Department of Health and Human Services task force on Alzheimer's disease. Neurology 34:939–944, 1984.

140. Miller E: A note on visual information processing in presenile dementia: A preliminary report. Br J Soc Clin Psychol 16:99–100, 1977.

141. Milner B: Les troubles de la memoire accompagnant des lésions hippocampiques bilaterales. In Physiologie de l'Hippocampe. Centre National de la Recherche Scientifique, Paris, 1962, pp 257–272.

142. Milner B: Effects of different brain lesions on card sorting: The role of the frontal lobes. Arch Neurol 9:90–100, 1963.

143. Milner B: Visually-guided maze learning in man: Effects of bilateral hippocampal, bilateral frontal, and uni-

lateral cerebral lesions. Neuropsychologia 3:317–338, 1965.

144. Milner B: Preface: Material-specific and generalized memory loss. Neuropsychologia 6:175–179, 1968.

145. Milner B: Visual recognition and recall after right temporal-lobe excision in man. Neuropsychologia 6:191–209, 1968.

146. Mishkin M, Malamut B, and Bachevalier, J: Memories and habits: Two neural systems. In Lynch G, McGaugh JL, and Weinberger NM (eds): Neurobiology of Learning and Memory. Guilford Press, New York, 1984, pp 65–77.

147. Money J: A Standard Road Map Test of Direction Sense. Academic Therapy Publications, San Rafael, CA, 1976.

148. Morris JC, Drazner M, Fulling K, et al: Clinical and pathological aspects of parkinsonism in Alzheimer's disease. Arch Neurol 46:651–657, 1989.

149. Morris RG, Downe JJ, Sahakian BJ, et al: Planning and spatial working memory in Parkinson's disease. J Neurol Neurosurg Psychiatry 51:757–766, 1988.

150. Morris RG and Kopelman MD: The memory deficits in Alzheimer-type dementia. Q J Exp Psychol 38:575–602, 1986.

151. Morrow L and Ratcliff G: Neuropsychology of spatial cognition: Evidence from cerebral lesions. In Stiles-Davis J, Kritchevsky M, and Bellugi U (eds): Spatial Cognition: Brain Bases and Development. Lawrence Erlbaum, Hillsdale, NJ, 1988, pp 5–32.

152. Murdoch BE and Chenery HJ: Language disorders in dementia of the Alzheimer type. Brain Lang 31:122–137, 1987.

153. Naeser MA and Hayward RW: Lesion localization in aphasia with cranial computed tomography and the Boston Diagnostic Aphasia Exam. Neurology 28:545–551, 1978.

154. Nebes RD: Semantic memory in Alzheimer's disease. Psychol Bull 106:377–394, 1989.

155. Nebes RD, F Boller, and Holland A: Use of semantic context by patients with Alzheimer's disease. Psychol Aging 1:261–269, 1986.

156. Nebes RD and Madden DJ: Different patterns of cognitive slowing produced by Alzheimer's disease and normal aging. Psychol Aging 3:102–104, 1988.

157. Nelson HE: National adult reading test. Test manual. NFER-Nelson Publishing Co, Windsor (UK).

158. Nelson HE and O'Connell A: Dementia: The estimation of premorbid intelligence levels using the new adult reading test. Cortex 14:232–244, 1978.

159. Newcombe F: Missile Wounds of the Brain. Oxford University Press, London, 1969.

160. Newcombe F and Ratcliff G: Disorders of visuospatial analysis. In Boller F and Grafman J (eds): Handbook of Neuropsychology. Elsevier, Amsterdam, 1989, pp 333–356.

161. Newcombe F and Russell WR: Dissociated visual perceptual and spatial deficits in focal lesions of the right hemisphere. J Neurol Neurosurg Psychiatry 38:73–81, 1969.

162. Norman DA: Memory & Attention: An Introduction to Human Information Processing. John Wiley & Sons, New York, 1976.

163. Ogden JA: Spatial abilities and deficits in aging and age-related disorders. In Boller F and Grafman J (eds): Handbook of Neuropsychology, Vol 4. Elsevier, Amsterdam, 1990, pp 265–278.

164. Ogden JA, Growdon JH, and Corkin S: Impaired ability of patients with Parkinson's disease to shift conceptual set in visuospatial tasks. Int J Neurosci 35:132, 1987.

165. Ojemann G, Ojemann J, Lettich E, and Berger M: Cortical language localization in left, dominant hemisphere. J Neurosurg 71:316–326, 1989.

166. Osterrieth PA: Le test de copie d'une figure complex. Archives de Psychologie 30:206–356, 1944.

167. Pearlson GD and Tune LE: Cerebral ventricular size and cerebrospinal fluid acetylcholine levels in senile dementia of the Alzheimer type. Psychiatry Res 17:23–29, 1986.

168. Perez FI, Rivera VM, Meyer JS, et al: Analysis of intellectual and cognitive performance in patients with multi-infarct dementia, vertebrobasilar insufficiency with dementia, and Alzheimer's disease. J Neurol Neurosurg Psychiatry 38:533–540, 1955.

169. Peterson LR and Peterson MJ: Short-term memory retention of individual verbal items. J Exp Psychol 58:193–198, 1959.

170. Pillon B, Dubois B, Lhermitte F, and Agid Y: Heterogeneity of cognitive impairment in progressive supranuclear palsy, Parkinson's disease, and Alzheimer's disease. Neurology 36:1179–1185, 1986.

171. Pirozzolo FJ, Christensen KJ, Ogle KM, Hansch EC, and Thompson WG: Simple and choice reaction time in dementia: Clinical implications. Neurobiol Aging 2:113–117, 1981.

172. Pirozzolo FJ, Nolan BH, Kuskowski M, et al. Latency and accuracy of word recognition in dementia of the Alzheimer type. Alzheimer Dis Assoc Disord 2:337–341, 1988.

173. Podoll K, Lange HW, and Noth J: Language functions in Huntington's disease. Brain 111:1475–1503, 1988.

174. Posner MI and Boies SJ: Components of attention. Psychol Rev 78:391–408, 1971.

175. Potegal M: A note on spatial-motor deficits in patients with Huntington's disease: A test of a hypothesis. Neuropsychologia 9:233–235, 1971.

176. Proctor F, Riklan M, Cooper IS, and Teuber H-L: Judgement of visual vertical and postural vertical by parkinsonian patients. Neurology 14:287–293, 1964.

177. Raven JC: Guide to the Standard Progressive Matrices. HK Lewis, London, 1960.

178. Raven JC: Guide to Using the Coloured Progressive Matrices. HK Lewis, London, 1965.

179. Regan D and Maxner C: Orientation-selective visual loss in patients with Parkinson's disease. Brain 10:415–432, 1987.

180. Regan D, Silver R, and Murray TJ: Visual acuity and contrast sensitivity in multiple sclerosis: Hidden visual loss. Brain 100:563–579, 1977.

181. Reisberg B, Borenstein J, Salob SP, et al: Behavioral symptoms in Alzheimer's disease: Phenomenology and treatment. J Clin Psychiatry (Suppl)48:9–15, 1987.

182. Rey A: L'examen psychologique dans les cas d'encéphalopathie traumatique. Arch de Psychologie 28:286–340, 1941.

183. Rey A: L'Examen Clinique en Psychologie. Presses Universitaires de France, Paris, 1964.

184. Rosen TJ: Age-associated memory impairment: A critique. European Journal of Cognitive Psychology 2(3):275–287, 1990.

185. Rosen TJ, Growdon JH, and Corkin S: Extrapyramidal signs and dementia progress independently in Alzheimer's disease. Abstracts, Society for Neuroscience 14:103, 1988.

186. Rosen WG: Verbal fluency in aging and dementia. J Clin Neuropsychol 2:135–146, 1980.

187. Rosen WG and Mohs RC: Evolution of cognitive decline in dementia. In Corkin S, Davis KL, and Growdon JH (eds): Alzheimer's Disease: A Report of Progress in Research. Raven Press, New York, 1982, pp 133–139.

188. Rosenzweig MR and Leiman AL: Physiological Psychology. DC Heath, Lexington, MA, 1982.

189. Rosvold HE, Mirsky AF, Sarason I, Bransome ED, and Beck LH: A continuous performance test of brain damage. J Consult Clin Psychol 20:343–350, 1956.

190. Sadun AA, Borchert M, DeVita E, Hinton DR, and Bassi CJ: Assessment of visual impairment in patients with Alzheimer's disease. Am J Ophthalmol, 104:113–120, 1987.

191. Sagar, HJ: Aging and age-related neurological disease: Remote memory. In Boller F and Grafman J (eds): Handbook of Neuropsychology, Vol 4. Elsevier, Amsterdam, 1990, pp 311–324.

192. Sagar HJ, Cohen NJ, Sullivan EV, Corkin S, and Growdon JH: Remote memory function in Alzheimer's disease

and Parkinson's disease. Brain 111:185–206, 1988.

193. Saint-Cyr JA, Taylor AE, and Lang AE: Procedural learning and neostriatal dysfunction in man. Brain, 111:941–959, 1988.

194. Salthouse TA and Prill KA: Inferences about age impairments in inferential reasoning. Psychol Aging 2:43–51, 1987.

195. Schacter DL: Implicit memory: History and current status. J Exp Psychol [Learn Mem Cogn] 13:501–518, 1987.

196. Schlotterer G, Moscovitch M, and Crapper-McLachlan D: Visual processing deficits as assessed by spatial frequency contrast sensitivity and backward masking in normal aging and Alzheimer's disease. Brain 107:309–325, 1984.

197. Schwartz MF, Marin OSM, and Saffran EM: Dissociations of language function in dementia: A case study. Brain Lang 7:277–306, 1979.

198. Selnes OA, Carson K, Rovner B, and Gordon MD: Language dysfunction in early- and late-onset possible Alzheimer's disease. Neurology 38:1053–1056, 1988.

199. Seltzer B and Sherwin I: A comparison of clinical features in early- and late-onset primary degenerative dementia. One entity or two? Arch Neurol 40:143–146, 1983.

200. Semmes J, Weinstein S, Ghent L, and Teuber H-L: Spatial orientation in man after cerebral injury: I. Analysis by locus of lesion. J Psychol 39:227–244, 1955.

201. Semmes J, Weinstein S, Ghent L, and Teuber H-L: Correlates of impaired orientation in personal and extrapersonal space. Brain 86:747–772, 1963.

202. Shader RI, Harmatz JS, and Salzman C: A new scale for clinical assessment in geriatric populations: Sandoz clinical assessment-geriatric (SCAG). J Am Geriatr Soc 22:107–113, 1974.

203. Shallice T: Specific impairments of planning. Philos Trans R Soc Lond [Biol] 298:199–209, 1982.

204. Shallice T and Evans ME: The involvement of the frontal lobes in cognitive estimation. Cortex 14:294–303, 1978.

205. Sharpe MH, Cermak SA, and Sax DS: Motor planning in Parkinson patients. Neuropsychologia 21:455–462, 1983.

206. Shimamura AP: Priming effects in amnesia: Evidence for a dissociable memory function. Q J Exp Psychol 38A:619–644, 1986.

207. Shimamura AP, Salmon DP, Squire LR, and Butters N: Memory dysfunction and word priming in dementia and amnesia. Behav Neurosci 101:347–351, 1987.

208. Sjögren H: Clinical analysis of morbus Alzheimer and morbus Pick. Acta Psychiatr Neurol Scand (Suppl)82:67–115, 1952.

209. Spinnler H: The role of attention disorders in the cognitive breakdown of dementia. In Boller F and Grafman J (eds): Handbook of Neuropsychology, Vol 5. Elsevier, Amsterdam, 1991, pp 79–122.

210. Spinnler H and Della Sala S: The role of clinical neuropsychology in the neurological diagnosis of Alzheimer's disease. J Neurol 235:258–271, 1988.

211. Spitzer RL and Endicott J: Schedule for affective disorders and schizophrenia. New York State Department of Mental Hygiene, New York, 1973.

212. Spitzer RL, Endicott J, Fleiss JL, and Cohen J: The psychiatric status schedule. Arch Gen Psychiatry 23:41–55, 1970.

213. Spitzer RL and Williams JBW: Instruction manual for the structured clinical interview for DSM-III (SCID). New York State Psychiatric Institute, New York, 1985.

214. Squire L: Memory and its disorders. In Boller F and Grafman J (eds): Handbook of Neuropsychology, Vol 3. Elsevier, Amsterdam; 1989, pp 3–267.

215. Steele JC, Richardson JC, and Olszewski J: Progressive supranuclear palsy. Arch Neurol 10:333–359, 1964.

216. Stern Y, Mayeux R, and Cote L: Reaction time and vigilance in Parkinson's disease: Possible role of altered norepinephrine metabolism. Arch Neurol 41:1086–1089, 1984.

217. Storandt M, Botwinick J, Danziger WL, Berg L, and Hughes CP: Psychometric differentiation of mild senile dementia of the Alzheimer type. Arch Neurol 41:497–499, 1984.

218. Storandt M and Hill RD: Very mild senile dementia of the Alzheimer type. II. Psychometric test performance. Arch Neurol 46:383–386, 1989.

219. Sulkava R: Alzheimer's disease and senile dementia of Alzheimer type: A comparative study. Acta Neurol Scand 65:636–650, 1982.

220. Sunderland T, Alterman IS, Yount D, et al: A new scale for the assessment of depressed mood in demented patients. Am J Psychiatry 145:955–959, 1988.

221. Talland GA: Deranged Memory. Academic Press, New York, 1965.

222. Talland GA and Schwab RS: Performance with multiple sets in Parkinson's disease. Neuropsychologia 2:45–53, 1964.

223. Taylor AE, Saint-Cyr JA, and Lang AE: Frontal lobe dysfunction in Parkinson's disease. The cortical focus of neostriatal outflow. Brain 109:845–883, 1986.

224. Taylor LB: Localization of cerebral lesions by psychological testing. Clin Neurosurg 16:269–287, 1969.

225. Taylor LB: Psychological assessment of neurosurgical patients. In Rasmussen T and Marino R (eds): Functional Neurosurgery. Raven Press, New York, 1979.

226. Thompson RF: The neurobiology of learning and memory. Science 223:941–947, 1986.

227. Thurstone LL: A Factorial Study of Perception. University of Chicago Press, Chicago, 1944.

228. Tsai L and Tsuang MT: The mini-mental state test and computerized tomography. Am J Psychiatry 136:436–438, 1979.

229. Warrington EK and Weiskrantz L: Amnesic syndrome: Consolidation or retrieval? Nature 228:628–630, 1970.

230. Warrington EK and Weiskrantz L: New method of testing long-term retention with special reference to amnesic patients. Nature 217:972–974, 1968.

231. Wechsler AF, Verity MA, Rosenschein S, Fried I, and Scheibel AB: Pick's disease: A clinical, computed tomographic, and histologic study with Golgi impregnation observations. Arch Neurol 39:287–290, 1982.

232. Wechsler D: WAIS-R: Wechsler adult intelligence scale–Revised. Psychological Corporation, New York, 1981.

233. Wechsler D: Wechsler memory scale —Revised. Psychological Corporation, New York, 1987.

234. Weinstein S: Deficits concomitant with aphasia or lesions of either cerebral hemisphere. Cortex 1:154–169, 1964.

235. Weinstein S, Semmes J, Ghent L, and Teuber H-L: Spatial orientation in man after cerebral injury: II. Analysis according to concomitant defects. J Psychol 42:249–262, 1956.

236. Whitty CWM and Zangwill OL: Amnesia. Butterworth & Co, London, 1966.

237. Wilson RS, Kaszniak AW, Bacon LD, Fox JH, and Kelly MP: Facial recognition memory in dementia. Cortex 18:329–336, 1982.

238. Young AW and Ratcliff G: Visuospatial abilities of the right hemisphere. In Young AW (ed): Functions of the Right Cerebral Hemisphere. Academic Press, London, 1983, pp 1–32.

Part II

**THE MAJOR
CATEGORIES OF
DEMENTIA**

Chapter 6

DEGENERATIVE DEMENTIAS

Richard H. Civil, M.D.,
Peter J. Whitehouse, M.D.,

Douglas J. Lanska, M.D., M.S.,
and Richard Mayeux, M.D.

DEMENTIA WITHOUT OTHER
  MAJOR NEUROLOGIC SIGNS
DEMENTIA WITH
  EXTRAPYRAMIDAL SIGNS
DEMENTIA ASSOCIATED WITH
  DEGENERATIVE DISORDERS OF
  THE CEREBELLUM
DEMENTIAS ASSOCIATED WITH
  MOTOR NEURON DISEASE
ADULT-ONSET BIOCHEMICAL
  DISORDERS

In the original dementia monograph in this series, diseases causing dementia were categorized into two broad groups: those with potentially reversible or treatable etiologies, and the "diffuse parenchymatous diseases of the central nervous system" (CNS).[133] The latter included the presenile dementias, senile dementias, and other so-called degenerative diseases that were felt to affect "primarily the cells of the nervous system" in the absence of any defined etiology or treatment.[133] The lack of defined cause or known specific therapy is still important in classifying dementing diseases, highlighting the nosologic difficulties encountered in considering the degenerative diseases.[14]

In the broadest of interpretations, the term "degenerative diseases" has in-cluded all disorders in which there is loss of neurologic function due to structural abnormalities of the CNS. Using this definition, a compilation of over 600 neurodegenerative disorders of infancy and childhood has been made — many with well-defined toxic, metabolic, infectious, or immunologic etiologies.[88] In a somewhat more restricted usage, the term *degenerative diseases* encompasses a miscellaneous category of diseases of unknown etiology characterized by gradually progressive disintegration of the nervous system.[3] Inherent in this and many such definitions is the recognition that selective neuronal dysfunction and death is a cardinal feature, and that the pathologic features of diseases of known cause (e.g., cellular inflammatory response, viral inclusion bodies, and so forth) are not prominent features.

Any attempt to define the degenerative diseases must recognize the close historical association that has existed between theories of aging and the degenerative diseases. Early theories invoked the processes of cellular decay, degeneration, and disintegration to explain gradually progressive dysfunction of the nervous system occurring in the senium. These notions were crystallized in the abiotrophy concept of Gowers,[125] in which premature death of cells in the CNS could occur owing to a lack of vital nutrition. A recent extension of this concept proposed that an abiotrophic interaction between aging and the environment might cause the degenerative diseases.[50] Additional proposals including a unifying hypothesis based on trophic factor deficiency[16] and interference of axonal neurofilament transport[109] have attempted to define a biologic basis for selected degenerative CNS diseases. As we learn more about genetic regulation of cell development, neural plasticity, growth factors, exogenous and endogenous neurotoxins, and the biologic basis of normal aging, our understanding of degenerative dementias will improve.

In the absence of a uniformly acceptable definition of the degenerative disease, we will use the clinical and pathologic features commonly encountered in the neurologic literature. Clinical characteristics include insidious onset after a period of normal nervous system function (or static dysfunction in the case of Down's syndrome), gradual progression, increasing incidence with advancing age, and lack of clearly identifiable cause, although a genetic component is often present. In most instances, symptoms attributable to specific regional neuronal systems are present. Common pathologic features include atrophy (often fairly symmetric), regionally selective neuronal loss, and the presence of relatively specific neurohistologic stigmata such as senile plaques, neurofibrillary tangles (NFTs), granulovacuolar degeneration, Lewy bodies, and Hirano bodies.

Unfortunately, we must recognize that these characteristics are not inviolable rules. Clinically similar or even identical degenerative disorders may be familial (inherited cerebello-olivary degeneration of Holmes) or sporadic (sporadic cerebello-olivary degeneration of Marie, Foix, and Alajouanine). Some degenerative diseases may be transmitted as a fully penetrant autosomal dominant trait (Huntington's disease [HD]) whereas others may have no clear hereditary basis (Parkinson's disease [PD]). Lesions may be typically asymmetric in some (Pick's disease) and occasionally glaringly focal in others (primary progressive aphasia). Some conditions due to toxins or vitamin deficiency may selectively involve regional neuronal systems (Wernicke-Korsakoff disease, subacute combined degeneration, 1-methyl-4-phenyl-1,2,3,6-tetra-hydropyridine [MPTP] toxicity) and mimic the idiopathic degenerative disorders.

We must additionally appreciate that our understanding of the term *dementia* is by no means uniform. Almost all would agree that dementia is present when a patient has a global impairment of cognitive function of sufficient severity to interfere with normal social and occupational functioning[68] (see also Chapter 1). Terminologic difficulties emerge in considering individuals with mild impairment who may not be occupationally or socially disabled, or those who have relatively isolated deficits disclosed on detailed neuropsychological assessment.[75,219,220] Many clinicians are rightfully reluctant to label such patients as "demented," presumably reflecting the premise that dementia is present only when an arbitrary threshold of impairment is crossed. This position is not universally accepted, however. A recent monograph emphasized the primacy of deficit multiplicity over symptom severity in defining dementia.[74] It is our intention not to redefine the boundaries of dementia but rather to point out that these boundaries are indistinct. Attempts to characterize the complex matrix of an individual's cognitive, behavioral, and functional capabilities simply as being either "demented" or "not demented" are overly simplistic. Advances in our understanding of the biologic underpinnings and psychological structure of cognition, the effect of "normal aging" on intellectual processes, and the relationship between such normal aging processes and the degenerative diseases will likely alter our future understanding and use of the term *dementia*.

In this chapter we will organize our

discussion of the major degenerative dementias into the following categories: dementia without other major neurologic signs; dementia with extrapyramidal signs; dementia with cerebellar signs; and dementia with motor neuron signs. Finally, we will outline the adult-onset forms of inherited metabolic dementias, which must be kept in mind in any atypical dementing disorder presenting early in adult life. Other parts of the book contain additional discussions of epidemiology (Chapter 1), clinical evaluation (Chapter 4), neuropsychology (Chapter 5), and management (Chapters 13 and 14). The genetics of degenerative disorders (Chapter 2) and the neurobiology of AD, PD, and HD (Chapter 3) are also discussed elsewhere.

DEMENTIA WITHOUT OTHER MAJOR NEUROLOGIC SIGNS

Alzheimer's Disease

In 1907, Alois Alzheimer described what he called a "peculiar disease of the cerebral cortex" in a 51-year-old woman suffering from an inexorably progressive dementing disorder.[11] Although senile dementia and senile plaques (SPs) were well known at the time of his case report, Alzheimer's patient was felt to be clinically and pathologically novel, based on the relatively young age at onset and the presence of the then newly described intracellular inclusions presently known as neurofibrillary tangles (NFTs). In recognition of this apparently unique combination of clinical and pathologic features, the term Alzheimer's disease (AD) was ultimately coined.[14]

Several factors operating in concert have resulted in the recent recognition of AD as "the coming plague of the 21st century."[259] The demographic phenomenon known as the "graying of America," in concert with epidemiologic data indicating a marked increase in the incidence of dementia with ad-

vancing age, have led to projections in which AD will simply overwhelm the resources of limited and often fragmented health care delivery systems in many countries. In the United States alone, as many as 4 million individuals may be afflicted with AD.[96] The cost of caring for these individuals is now over 50 billion dollars annually.[243] These costs are increasing rapidly and are poorly covered by public and private insurance programs (see Chapter 15). Until satisfactory solutions to the multiple biologic and socioeconomic imperatives of AD are found, this disease will continue to be a "looming crisis."[66]

EPIDEMIOLOGY

Descriptive epidemiologic studies measuring the current prevalence of dementing disorders have suggested that severe dementia occurs in 5% to 7% of individuals over age 65. Clinical and autopsy series indicate that more than 90% of such individuals will be diagnosed as suffering from either AD alone, multi-infarct dementia (MID), or mixed AD and MID. The prevalence for AD has been reported to range between 1.9 and 5.8 cases per 100 population aged 65 and over.[278] AD prevalence is slightly higher in women than in men. It is uncertain whether this difference is due solely to the longer life expectancy of women or to some other factors. A recent survey of community residents in East Boston has confirmed that prevalence of AD is strongly associated with age, affecting 3% of individuals aged 65 to 74, 18.7% of individuals aged 75 to 84, and fully 47% of individuals over age 85.[96] Based on unexpectedly high prevalence of dementia in individuals over age 85 demonstrated in this study, possibly due to the inclusion of milder cases than in earlier studies, higher United States prevalence figures for AD have been proposed, with obvious implications for health care policy makers. As always, care must be taken when extrapolating data from studies of single communities to larger populations. Annual incidence figures are harder to obtain but show increases from a rate of 2.4 cases per 100,000 population aged 40 to 60, to 127 cases per 100,000 aged 60 and above. Although many have considered presenile dementia (AD) and senile dementia of the Alzheimer type (SDAT) to represent a single disease entity,[162,197] evidence suggests age-related genetic,[40] clinical,[212,289] and histopathologic[30] heterogeneity in AD

ETIOLOGY

In addition to advancing age, analytic epidemiologic studies have consistently identified genetic factors that contribute to the development of AD[102,141,143] (see Chapter 2). First identified within two decades of Alzheimer's original description, an apparent autosomal dominant form of familial AD (FAD) has been recognized, which probably accounts for less than 1% of AD cases.[216] The relevance of genetic factors and the degree of increased risk for family members in the majority of apparently sporadic AD cases remain less clear. One study has reported that the cumulative incidence of AD in first-degree relatives of AD victims may be as high as 50% in probands surviving to age 87.[40] Based on this observation, it has been suggested that "sporadic" AD may, in fact, be inherited as an autosomal dominant trait with age-dependent penetrance. The Eurodem EC Concerted Action on Epidemiology of Dementia[146] has analyzed family pedigrees of 198 Dutch patients with AD. Individuals who have one or more first-degree relatives with dementia have a fourfold increase in their risk of developing AD; for those with two or more first-degree relatives with dementia, the risk is 40 times normal. Twin studies have demonstrated incomplete concordance in monozygotes, suggesting an additional role for environmental factors that modify gene expression.[65,159,179a,239]

An association between Down's syndrome (DS, trisomy 21) and AD has been recognized since the 1940s.[157] Virtually all individuals with DS surviving to the fourth and fifth decades of life develop the histopathologic stigmata of AD.[92,94,330] In a considerable number of these individuals a dementia syndrome develops, superimposed on the preexisting mental retardation.[244] A recent clinical and pathologic study of such AD/Down's syndrome patients has reported an unusually high frequency of gait disorder and speech deterioration, as well as seizures and myoclonus.[97,331] The genetic implications of this relationship between AD and DS have not gone unexplored. In some FAD families, linkage analysis showed the Alzheimer gene is localized to chromosome 21,[287] which is also the locus of the gene encoding the amyloid precursor protein (APP).[119,122,306,307] These observations led to speculation that in some instances, AD (particularly FAD) might simply result from having more copies of the APP gene. Increased gene dosage, however, has not been demonstrated in FAD.[260,306]

Recently, evidence for genetic heterogeneity in AD has emerged. In some late-onset FAD cases, linkage analysis showed that an additional AD-related gene may be located on chromosome 19.[251] In several FAD families, but not others, specific amino acid substitutions in the APP gene were associated with the presence of AD.[118,235] This relationship between point mutations in the APP gene and the phenotype of AD suggests but does not prove that AD in these families is caused by the amino acid substitution. Moreover, a transgenic mouse that overexpresses the carboxyl end of APP including the β/A4 amyloid protein found in plaques has been found to develop such plaques associated with neurofibrillary tangles and neuronal cell loss.[163a] If transgenic animals with the APP mutations found in AD develop even more severe AD-type changes, the view that these single-codon changes can cause AD in rare families will be even further strengthened (see also Chapters 2 and 3).

Factors variably reported to be associated with increased risk for the development of AD include increasing mother's age at subject's birth, later position in birth order, family history of DS, history of head injury, history of thyroid disease, and female gender. (For review, see references 13, 278.) None of these are strong risk factors, and many of the associations might simply be explained by biases in patient selection. Additionally, smoking history has been negatively associated with AD in case-control studies, suggesting to some that smoking may protect against developing AD.[127] The loss of nicotinic cholinergic receptors in cerebral cortex in AD is also a potential link to this epidemiologic data.[325] Some have claimed that the potential role of head trauma in the development of AD is additionally supported by the "dementia pugilistica" syndrome, which occurs in individuals exposed to repeated blows to the head[277] (see Chapter 11). This progressive syndrome is similar to AD, but it is characterized clinically by dementia with cerebellar, pyramidal, and extrapyramidal features and pathologically by NFTs and senile plaques.[67,277a] Recent reanalysis of several case-control studies detected a significant association between retrospective reports of head injury and the development of AD.[231b]

Considerable and controversial attention has been directed toward the elucidation of an infectious agent in AD. Despite a single report demonstrating spongiform brain changes in hamsters following intracerebral inoculation of buffy coat preparations from patients with AD,[198] the majority of evidence does not suggest an infectious or transmissible etiology for AD. The biologic homologies between the transmissible spongiform encephalopathies and AD may, however, provide clues to understanding the pathophysiology of AD.[43,264,265]

Early studies[69,70] demonstrated increased aluminum content in the brains of patients with AD. High aluminum concentrations have also been detected by some, using microprobe techniques in neurofibrillary-tangle–bearing neurons.[252] Under some experimental circumstances, aluminum can induce intracellular tangles in animals, but their ultrastructure is different from the cytoskeletal pathology in AD.[329] Other groups have not been able to confirm increased whole brain levels of aluminum.[200] A claim[51] that aluminum is the primary constituent of the amyloid core of senile plaques has not been confirmed. Most epidemiologic studies have failed to demonstrate a convincing relationship between aluminum exposure and the development of AD. Studies claiming such an association[204] have been criticized on methodologic grounds. Even if aluminum or other metals accumulate in brains of AD victims, this may represent an epiphenomenon unrelated to the primary (and as yet unknown) etiologic event(s). (See Chapter 13 for discussion of chelation therapy.)

CLINICAL AND
PATHOLOGIC DIAGNOSIS

Criteria for the clinical diagnosis of *probable* AD have been described (see Chapter 1, Table 1–7), and include (1) the presence of a dementia syndrome with deficits in two or more areas of cognition, (2) progressive worsening of memory and other cognitive function over time, (3) a relatively intact level of consciousness, (4) age at onset between 40 and 90 years, and (5) the specific absence of any other systemic or CNS process that could account for the progressive cognitive deterioration.[215] Criteria for the diagnosis of *definite* AD are met when histologic evidence of AD is present in biopsy or autopsy material from patients meeting the criteria for the clinical diagnosis of *probable* AD. Use of these clinical criteria in research centers results in diagnostic accuracy as high as 88% in autopsy series.[312] The importance of factors related to interrater reliability and training issues in research diagnostic settings has been emphasized.[178] Uniform pathologic inclusion criteria for AD have yet to be established and consistently applied.[312] A national study of these issues is under way in the United States as a part of the Consortium to Establish a Registry for

AD (CERAD).[230,231a] Clinical assessment methodologies and standardized pathologic techniques have been incorporated into this multicenter longitudinal study in an effort to identify reliable clinical and pathologic criteria for AD. A recent clinical and pathologic description of "very mild AD" in CERAD patients[100a,231] has reported that truly normal aging may be unaccompanied by neocortical SP and NFT, suggesting that the "presence of these lesions should suggest the possibility of clinically undetected AD."[231]

In the absence of a specific, noninvasive, antemortem diagnostic marker, the clinical diagnosis of AD remains one of exclusion. The evaluation of any patient with suspected cognitive impairment should specifically include a detailed medical history, clinical examination, bedside mental status screening and/or neuropsychological testing, and specific laboratory studies. (See Chapter 4.) The recommended evaluation components have been the subject of several reviews.[62,68,215] For clinical purposes, the presence of AD is likely when evidence of progressive cognitive, behavioral, and functional decline is present, and the medical examination and laboratory tests fail to show evidence of other dementing illnesses. In an effort to emphasize the existence of potentially reversible or "secondary dementias," accounting for as many as 30% of cases in selected series,[153] the term dementia syndrome has been coined.[293,339] In a recent retrospective review of 288 reported cases of dementia from 32 studies, Clarfield[57] found a potentially reversible etiology in 13.2%. Biases of ascertainment in different referral populations likely account for this wide range in reported incidence of reversible dementia. Meta-analysis of treatment efficacy in a subset of patients with potentially reversible disease (151 patients from 10 studies) found that 32 (21%) completely reversed, 81 (54%) partially reversed, and 38 (25%) showed no improvement.[57] Although more than 70 causes of dementia have been tabulated,[243] Clarfield[57] has identified for clinicians six specific conditions that accounted for more than 90% of the partially or completely reversed dementias (Table 6–1). These conditions should be carefully excluded from consideration in all suspected cases of AD. Rarely, brain biopsy may be considered in younger patients with atypical presentation.[151a]

Clinical Heterogeneity. Despite the fact that AD is typically viewed as having few noncognitive manifestations, selected neurologic abnormalities have been found more frequently in patients with AD. In one report, the ex-

Table 6–1 THE MOST COMMON PARTIALLY OR COMPLETELY REVERSIBLE DEMENTIAS

Etiology	Treatment Results		Number of Patients	% of Reversible Dementias
	Partly Reversed	Completely Reversed		
Drug intoxication	17	12	29	28.2
Depression	18	9	27	26.2
Metabolic*	10	6	16	15.5
Normal pressure hydrocephalus	8	3	11	10.7
Subdural hematoma	5	1	6	5.8
Neoplasm	4	0	4	4.0
Other	9	1	10	9.7

*Includes 7 cases due to thyroid disease, 2 calcium abnormalities, and 2 hepatic abnormalities.
Source: Adapted from Clarfield,[57] p. 480.

amination features found more commonly in AD than in control subjects included frontal release signs, olfactory deficits, impaired stereognosis or graphesthesia, gait disorder, tremor, or abnormalities on cerebellar testing.[150] As many as 5% to 10% of Alzheimer patients may have multifocal myoclonus or seizures, particularly late in the course of the illness.[137] The striking heterogeneity of clinical and pathologic features in AD has long since been recognized, and attempts have been made to identify various AD subgroups. One study[212] identified four clinical subgroups: benign, myoclonic, extrapyramidal, and typical AD. Others have reported atypical clinical variants with predominantly focal symptoms including progressive aphasia[128] or right parietal lobe syndrome.[71]

As discussed previously, there is reason to consider age as an important variable in the clinical and pathologic heterogeneity of this disease. In contrast to AD of late onset, early-onset AD has been reported to be characterized by a more common familial pattern of expression,[40] a more rapidly deteriorating course with prominent aphasia,[289] increased pathologic severity,[30] greater loss of choline acetyltransferase activity in the cerebral cortex,[282] and greater loss of neurons in subcortical nuclear structures including the locus ceruleus[30] (see Chapter 3). The additional identification of a subgroup of patients with presumed AD in whom the pathologic changes were characterized by severe hippocampal neuronal loss and astrogliosis in the relative absence of neocortical degenerative change has led some to conclude that AD may be a "hippocampal dementia."[22]

Longitudinal studies and clinicopathologic correlations may ultimately redefine the boundaries of the AD symptom complex. In one recent case report, a single patient with presenile-onset dementia and slowly progressive hemiparesis was found to have pathologically confirmed AD with severe asymmetric involvement of the somatosensory cortex,[155] an area of brain not commonly affected in AD.

Cognition. Efforts to develop and standardize screening mental status exams (Chapter 4) and develop neuropsychological batteries capable of detecting the presence of a primary degenerative dementia are based on the concept that with proper testing, individual dementing diseases may be found to have unique patterns of cognitive impairment (see Chapter 5). In the clinical assessment of any cognitively impaired individual, it is important to recognize several key points. First, given the clinical heterogeneity of AD, it is probably unreasonable to assume that a single or brief "screening" instrument can be developed that will be sensitive enough to detect early cases of AD and broad enough in its testing to capture the range of cognitive deficits and islands of preservation of function that may be present. Nevertheless, the majority of patients with AD will demonstrate memory and language deficits, with additional evidence of impairment frequently found in neuropsychological measures of temporal orientation, visual discrimination, attention, and constructional praxis.[151] Using discriminant function analysis to search for the patterns of deficits on neuropsychological testing that are most powerful in distinguishing AD or dementia cases from healthy subjects, three groups have emphasized the strong discriminative ability of tests of recent memory and verbal fluency.[95,171a,297] It has recently been demonstrated that the simple addition of a measure of verbal fluency (FAS Test) to the Mini-Mental State Examination results in a significant increase in test sensitivity, particularly in those individuals whose test scores fall in the borderline or questionably impaired range.[110]

Behavioral or Psychiatric Symptoms. Although the index case of AD[11] originally presented with changes in personality and paranoia, the behavioral aspects of AD have been relatively neglected despite being a major cause of caregiver stress. (It has subsequently been recognized, however, that functional psychiatric illness can cause cog-

Table 6–2 FREQUENCY AND SEVERITY OF BEHAV-AD SYMPTOMS IN ALZHEIMER'S DISEASE SUBJECTS

	N*	F†	Percent	Severity
Paranoid and Delusional Ideation	34	13	38	
1. Stealing things	34	7	21	2.2
2. Residence is not home	34	5	15	1.2
3. Suspiciousness (other)	32	6	19	1.4
Hallucinations	34	6	18	
4. Visual	30	5	17	2.4
5. Auditory	32	2	6	2.0
Activity Disturbances	34	15	44	
6. Wandering	34	3	9	1.2
7. Purposeless Activity	34	13	38	1.1
8. Inappropriate Activity	34	6	18	1.4
Aggressiveness	34	8	24	
9. Verbal aggressiveness	34	6	18	2.1
10. Physical threats, violence	34	2	6	2
11. Agitation	33	3	9	2.5
Day/Night Disturbance	27	4	15	1.3
Affective Disturbances	34	11	32	
12. Tearfulness	34	11	32	1.9
13. Depressed mood (other)	34	2	6	2
Anxieties and Phobias	34	17	50	
14. Anxiety Re: upcoming events	33	14	42	1.5
15. Other anxieties	34	9	26	1.7
16. Fear of being left alone	32	5	16	1.6
17. Other phobias	34	4	12	2.1

*N = number of subjects rated
†F = frequency symptom was rated present by both raters; severity is averaged over raters and ranges from 0 (least severe) to 3 (most severe).
Source: Adapted from Patterson et al,[249] p. 24.)

nitive impairment or "pseudodementia" [Chapter 12].) In addition, the concomitant occurrence of AD and psychiatric symptoms is commonly encountered in clinical practice.* Behavioral symptoms frequently include anxiety, depression, hallucinations, delusions, agitation, and sleep disturbance.

In a retrospective chart review of 217 outpatients with clinically probable AD, mild depressive symptoms were present in 41%, suspiciousness and paranoia in 36%, anxiety and fearfulness in 31%, and delusions in 30%.[217a] A prospective assessment of noncognitive behavioral and affective symptoms confirmed the extensive behavioral and affective burden in AD patients.[249] In this study, fully 31 of 34 AD subjects had experienced psychiatric symptoms during the week prior to the clinical interview, reflecting significant ongoing psychiatric symptomatology in the great majority of AD subjects (Table 6–2). This study used two newly developed rating scales (BEHAV-AD and the Cornell Scale of Depression in Dementia) specifically designed to assess psychopathology in demented patients.[10,272] Other scales for assessment of noncognitive or behavioral symptoms are under development.

Even if little or no cognitive impairment is present initially, the elderly individual with new-onset psychiatric symptoms is at considerable risk to develop a dementia syndrome. In one reported study of 225 patients evaluated at a dementia clinic, fully 57% of initially nondemented depressed elderly

*References 4, 60, 61, 86a, 179, 269–272, 285, 286, 289.

patients went on to develop a frank dementia syndrome during 3 years of follow-up.[269] The clinical phenomenology,[176a,185,189] neurochemistry,[338] and neuropathology[53,337,340] of major depression in primary dementia are being actively investigated. As a group, patients with primary dementia and major depression have been reported to have reduced cortical norepinephrine levels[338] and increased neuronal loss in the brainstem locus ceruleus and raphe nuclei.[340] The clinical phenomenology, treatment, and neurobiology of nonaffective behavioral disturbances in AD are being similarly investigated.[86,272]

CLINICAL NEUROBIOLOGY

Many attempts have been made to define a specific and relatively noninvasive diagnostic test for AD. Based on the multiplicity of neurochemical brain changes detected at both biopsy and brain autopsy, much effort has focused on an analysis of cerebrospinal fluid (CSF) neurochemical markers in AD. Although reduced lumbar CSF concentrations of acetylcholinesterase (AChE), homovanillic acid (HVA), somatostatin, corticotropin-releasing factor (CRF), adrenocorticotropic hormone (ACTH), and alpha-melanocyte stimulating hormone (α-MSH) have been demonstrated in AD,[19,164,206,266] it has recently been concluded that the relatively modest changes, as well as the significant overlap between AD and control groups, have not allowed for the development of a single neurochemical assay of clinically relevant sensitivity or specificity.[18,314a] Neurochemically distinct subgroups of AD patients may be identifiable related to age of onset (AChE and HVA concentrations reduced in younger AD patients) or the presence of extrapyramidal features (HVA and 5-hydroxyindoleacetic acid [HIAA] concentrations reduced in AD with extrapyramidal features or myoclonus), but their diagnostic utility is uncertain.[18] Another possible marker from CSF for antemortem diagnosis is AChE, the abnormal molecular form of which was found in AD.[236a]

Based on our increased understanding of the neurobiology of SPs and NFTs, attempts have been made to identify soluble protein derivatives of these structures in CSF. Two such proteins, tau and ubiquitin, colocalize with neurofibrillary-tangle–enriched preparations[84] and share antigenic epitopes with paired helical filaments.[232,253] Unfortunately, both of these proteins are normal intraneuronal components of brain tissue, and the search for tau- or ubiquitin-related immunoreactive components in CSF has not yet yielded a specific diagnostic test for AD. A monoclonal antibody, ALZ-50,[333] has been raised against a neuronal antigen, A68, that appears to be greatly enriched in the CSF and brain of patients with AD.[332] It has subsequently been demonstrated that the A68 protein might be a modified form of tau.[232] Despite early encouraging results in CSF, the clinical applicability of such a test is uncertain.[82]

The detection of soluble derivatives of the APP in CSF has led to speculation concerning developing a diagnostic test.[245] The major constituent of amyloid deposits in SP is a 42-43 amino acid protein, molecular weight 4.2 kd, known variably as β-amyloid, β/A4 protein, amyloid β-protein, AβP, or A4 (see Chapters 1 and 3). This protein is derived from a much larger APP, coded for by the gene on chromosome 21 of the human genome. Normal posttranslational processing and proteolytic degradation yield nonamyloidogenic proteins,[292] suggesting that an early event in amyloid formation may involve altered APP processing, which results in the release and subsequent deposition of β-amyloid. Research is currently focusing on the detection of proteolytic degradation products of APPs in the CSF. Such a test may be potentially diagnostic.[245] The potential therapeutic role of altering APP proteolysis is also being explored (see Chapter 13).

The applicability of CNS neuroimaging tests in the diagnosis of AD remains uncertain (see Chapter 4). It is clear that structural imaging studies (computed tomography [CT] and magnetic resonance imaging [MRI]) are useful in the measurement of parenchymal brain volume reduction, and in ruling out non-AD structural brain pathology including subdural hematoma, tumor, stroke, and NPH. Unfortunately, because of the overlap between the normal aged and demented populations, the anatomic appearance of the brain cannot be used to determine the presence or absence of dementia, or to establish the diagnosis of AD.[107] More specific measurements of brain changes, such as progressive reduction in parenchymal volume on CT or MRI, or abnormalities in specific regions of the brain (e.g., hippocampus), might increase diagnostic information, however.[165a]

Physiologic imaging of brain function using positron emission tomography (PET) may prove valuable in the differential diagnosis of dementing disorders.[62] In clinically probable AD, studies of regional cerebral glucose utilization rates[108] and regional cerebral blood flow[263] have indicated the presence of a relatively distinct pattern of bilateral temporal and parietal hypometabolism, with sparing of primary sensory and motor cortices. Even if these findings prove to be relatively specific for AD, financial and logistic considerations may limit the clinical applicability of PET scanning in the routine assessment of dementia.[310]

Based on the assumption that AD may have extra-CNS manifestations, many attempts have also been made to find a specific peripheral diagnostic marker. An extensive literature on such systemic abnormalities in AD exists,[27] and a thorough review is outside the scope of this chapter. Despite reports of various hematologic, fibroblast, endocrine, and blood chemical abnormalities, no specific diagnostic test has yet emerged. Investigations demonstrating abnormal calcium transport,[253a] increased membrane fluidity in platelets,[89,255a,339a] and the presence of amyloid in skin and intestinal biopsy samples[288] have fueled speculation that a systemic marker for AD may be iden-

tified. The demonstration of tau-reactive neurites in olfactory mucosa biopsy specimens in a limited sample of AD subjects has led to the suggestion that such an approach may yet yield a diagnostic test in AD.[301,304] Some have suggested that abnormal serum antibodies to neural antigens may be a marker for the disease.[26,55,90,176,222,236]

Pick's Disease

The recognition of a dementing disorder with predominantly focal neurobehavioral symptoms and circumscribed or lobar cortical atrophy is attributed to Arnold Pick.[254] Shortly after the publication of Pick's description, the histopathology of the disease was described in detail, including accounts of "ballooned cells" as well as rounded, argentophilic, intracytoplasmic inclusion bodies.[12] Subsequently, varying emphasis has been given to clinical aspects, gross atrophic changes, and the presence of argyrophilic intraneuronal inclusions (Pick bodies) in the diagnosis of Pick's disease. In light of this, clinicopathologic characterization of Pick's disease remains controversial.[233]

EPIDEMIOLOGY

The epidemiology of Pick's disease is incompletely characterized, in large part because of clinical difficulties in distinguishing AD and Pick's disease in life.[163] Pick's disease has been estimated to occur with a frequency of 2%[321] to 10%[158] of that of AD. In the Minnesota autopsy series, neuropathologically confirmed Pick's disease accounted for approximately 5% of all progressive dementias.[140] This relatively high reported incidence may primarily reflect immigration of northern Europeans to the Minnesota area. Although familial cases with an apparent autosomal dominant pattern of transmission have been reported,[129] most cases of Pick's disease occur sporadically. Pick's disease usually has its onset between the ages of 40 and 60 years,[75] but extreme cases have been reported with onset as early as age 21 and as late as age 80. In an analysis of 18 cases of Pick's disease with pathologically confirmed Pick bodies, average survival was reported to be 6.3 years for men and 8.4 years for women.[142] In contrast to most large series, which suggest a slight predominance of affected women,[191] a more recent report suggests not only a male predominance of affected individuals, but also an apparent male predominance in the development of progressive degenerative dementia in first- and second-degree relatives of probands with neuropathologically confirmed Pick's disease.[142]

Clinical and pathologic subtypes of Pick's disease have been proposed.[64,233] In one series, which identified a pathologically "generalized" variant of Pick's disease, those cases with extensive atrophy of caudate, substantia nigra, and neocortex had an onset of clinical symptoms in the third and fourth decades of life.[233]

CLINICAL FEATURES

Although early clinical descriptions of Pick's disease emphasized asphasic and apraxic qualities, such an emphasis represented a deliberate attempt to demonstrate that focal signs and symptoms of cerebral dysfunction could be attributed to "senile brain decay."[328] Modern clinical descriptions, however, emphasize the early and predominant changes in personality, insight, and judgment.[75] An apparently distinctive but evanescent pattern of neuropsychological findings has been described in Pick's disease.[170] Others, however, have emphasized that the neuropsychological profile of Pick's disease may be indistinguishable from the frontal dementia seen in amyotrophy-dementia complex (ADC).[227] Elements of the Klüver-Bucy syndrome (hyperorality, hypersexuality, visual agnosia, excessive tactile exploratory behavior) have been reported in the early stages of Pick's disease.[77] As the illness progresses, cognitive processes (including memory and language function) deteriorate. Specific language abnormalities, including semantic anomia,[8] the use of "all-purpose" or generic words, and the emergence of the so-called "gramophone syndrome" (repetitious retelling of stories), are commonly observed but certainly not pathognomonic. Mutism is frequently observed late in the course of this illness. Such alterations in behavior and cognition likely reflect the basal frontotemporal involvement in Pick's disease.

Like AD, Pick's disease essentially remains a diagnosis of exclusion. Features that are suggestive of the diagnosis of Pick's disease include (1) the presence of basal frontotemporal behavioral abnormalities in the relative absence of generalized intellectual decline, (2) asymmetric lobar atrophy on cranial imaging (CT or MRI), and (3) a normal electroencephalogram (EEG). PET scanning has revealed decreased glucose metabolic rate in frontal and/or anterior temporal cortices, a pattern that may be useful in the antemortem distinction of Pick's disease from AD.[160]

NEUROBIOLOGY

The characteristic gross pathology of Pick's disease is marked, circumscribed, often asymmetric, atrophic change of the cerebral cortex in a lobar distribution predominantly affecting either frontal and/or temporal lobes, with sparing of posterior superior temporal gyri. Although occasional cases with selective parieto-ocipital involvement have been reported, such cases are rare, and would need to be distinguished from corticobasal degeneration.[114] At the microscopic level, the major finding in the cerebral cortex is severe neuronal loss and gliosis. Although controversial, the presence of Pick bodies is not necessarily considered to be a sine qua non of the disease.[188,321] Pick bodies were absent in fully two thirds of the cases of Constantinidis.[64] Structures similar to Pick bodies have been reported in Down's syndrome, tuberous sclerosis, and kuru. Swollen chromato-lytic neurons are considered by some to be the most characteristic finding in Pick's disease; but they have been reported not only in Pick's disease with Pick bodies, but also in AD, Lewy body disease, Creutzfeldt-Jakob disease (CJD), and corticodentatonigral degeneration.[58] In Pick's disease, despite its designation as a "cortical" dementia, neuronal loss and astrocytic gliosis frequently are present in parahippocampal and hippocampal regions, the amygdaloid complex, and the caudate nucleus.

At the immunochemical and ultrastructural level, variable findings have been reported. In cases of "classic" Pick's disease, as defined by Munoz-Garcia and Ludwin,[233] Pick bodies reacted with antisera against neurofilament and tubulin components and were ultrastructurally composed of straight fibrils of variable diameter and long-period constricted fibrils. These fibrils share immunocytochemical features with normal and abnormal cytoskeletal structures.[246] In contrast, cytoplasmic inclusion bodies in "generalized" Pick's disease reacted poorly with antineurofilament and antimicrotubule antibodies; contained RNA; and were ultrastructurally composed of straight fibrils coated with a granular material felt to be derived from ribosomes.[267]

The neurochemistry of Pick's disease is less well characterized than that of AD. In contrast to AD, cortical ChAT levels are normal in Pick's disease.[135] Neocortical muscarinic cholinergic receptor binding has been reported to be either normal[334] or significantly reduced.[135] Whether significant cell loss occurs in cholinergic basal forebrain is not clear.[315] Additional analysis of neurotransmitter markers in various subcortical regions, including substantia nigra and globus pallidus, has revealed markedly reduced striatal dopamine concentrations, as well as decreased levels of substance P and GABA 50.[161] Monoamine oxidase (MAO) activity was reported increased in hypothalamus in both forms, MAO-A and MAO-B.

Both forms were decreased in nucleus basalis.[294a]

Slowly Progressive Aphasia Syndromes

In 1982, Mesulam[218] described the clinical and language characteristics of six patients with a slowly progressive disturbance of language apparently without the additional intellectual and behavioral disturbances of dementia. Although cases of presenile dementia presenting as aphasia had been described previously,[320] Mesulam's cases were apparently unique in that the majority did not experience any impairment in functional capability, behavior, or comportment even after 5 to 11 years of follow-up. In all six patients, EEG and CT scans were felt to be focally abnormal; a left temporal lobe biopsy in a single patient was not diagnostic for either Pick's disease or AD.

CLINICAL FEATURES AND DIAGNOSIS

As originally defined, the syndrome of slowly progressive aphasia without generalized dementia represented a behavioral diagnosis, made in the setting of a moderate-to-severe idiopathic, progressive language disorder and minimal to no additional evidence of dementia.[151] A wide range of aphasia profiles, including severe anomic aphasia and progressive dysfluency, have been described. The diagnosis is supported by the presence of focal perisylvian atrophy on CT or MRI imaging and focal perisylvian EEG slowing. PET scanning may show focal hemispheric glucose hypometabolism.

Both the natural history and clinical characteristics of this condition remain controversial. According to Mesulam,[220] some patients with progressive aphasia may remain nondemented for many years, suffering from dementia only in the terminal stages, after 8 to 12 years of disease progression. Mesulam and colleagues have coined the term *primary progressive aphasia* in describing patients with progressive language disturbance and no evidence of dementia on long-term follow-up.[138,220,322] A recent prospective study of eight patients with progressive aphasia, however, has shown that fully seven of eight developed at least mild dementia (CDR grade 1) after only 5 years of disease progression.[138,322] Additional confusion exists regarding the extent of any more generalized intellectual disturbance present in the progressive aphasia syndromes. Poeck and Luzzatti[261] concluded that despite the absence of any functional decline, neuropsychological testing may demonstrate a trend toward generalized impairment.

NEUROBIOLOGY

Although focal perisylvian atrophy is the common anatomic denominator in the progressive aphasia syndromes, diverse etiologies including AD, Pick's disease, and CJD have been identified.[168,196] In some instances, the pathology has been quite nonspecific. Weintraub and associates[322] have speculated that patients with this condition are most likely to have neuronal loss, spongiform degeneration, and gliosis, with the pathologic changes of Pick's disease and AD found less commonly.[138] The relationship between these progressive aphasic syndromes and mixed syndromes of progressive dysphasia and dementia remains to be elucidated.[138]

Progressive Subcortical Gliosis

Progressive subcortical gliosis is a rare, frequently familial, neurodegenerative disorder with onset in the fourth through sixth decades.[183,240,241] The course is progressive over 5 to 30 years. Initially, this disorder is characterized by prominent emotional, personality, and psychiatric changes, with delusions, paranoia, auditory hallucina-

tions, depression, suicidal ideation, and deterioration of judgment, insight, and social behavior. Later, cognitive changes are more pronounced, particularly affecting memory, reasoning, and visual perception. Except for mild naming difficulties, language function is generally spared until late in the course. Muteness may occur in the terminal stages, but affected individuals remain ambulatory. Focal neurologic findings are not part of the syndrome. CT scans show generalized atrophy, and EEGs are normal except for mild slowing late in the illness. Cases of progressive subcortical gliosis cannot be reliably distinguished from Pick's disease clinically.[241]

Neuropathologic examination shows generalized cerebral atrophy with secondary dilation of the lateral ventricles. Microscopic examination shows extensive, severe astrogliosis of the subcortical white matter, particularly at the cortical–white-matter junction. Mild astrogliosis with neuronal loss occurs in the deeper layers of the cerebral cortex, basal, ganglia, brainstem, and spinal cord. No NFTs, SPs, or Pick bodies are detected in the cerebral cortex.[172,315]

Other Dementias without Major Neurologic Signs

Many uncommon dementias are usually reported either as parts of large autopsy series (in which clinical features are often not described) or as individual case reports. Most often, these disorders cannot be clinically differentiated from AD in life. Their classification is confusing due in part to their rarity, to the different pathologic analyses to which they have been submitted, and to the different nosologic schemes used by clinicians and neuropathologists.

VARIANTS OF
COMMON DEMENTIAS

The first category of atypical dementias might best be characterized as variants of the better known, more common dementias such as AD, Pick's disease, and PD. For example, the relative amounts of plaques and tangles can vary in AD. Some have found it acceptable to make the diagnosis of AD with abundant plaques but with no more NFTs than would be found in normal aging.[63,335] As discussed above, a presumed Pick's disease variant with swollen achromatic neurons but no Pick bodies has been described.[58,64]

Any discussion of such "Pick's disease variants" must also acknowledge that certain pathologic similarities exist between Pick's disease and a unique neurologic disorder variously referred to as corticodentatonigral degeneration with neuronal achromasia,[268] corticobasal degeneration,[114] and cortical–basal ganglionic degeneration.[275] While displaying some of the microscopic pathologic hallmarks of Pick's disease,[114] the clinical syndrome of parietal sensory loss, alien limb phenomenon, apraxia, and extrapyramidal features seen in cortical–basal ganglionic degeneration is quite distinct.[275]

Variants of PD with dementia and atypical lesion topology have long since been recognized.[113,175] It is likely that a spectrum of such Lewy-body diseases exists, with lesions confined to the brainstem (typical idiopathic PD), a transitional form with Lewy bodies in both brainstem and neocortex, and a diffuse Lewy-body disease characterized by an early and prominent dementia with widely distributed Lewy and "Lewylike" bodies in brainstem, basal forebrain, and neocortex.[47] Thirteen patients with pathologic changes of AD as well as cortical and subcortical Lewy bodies were felt to constitute a distinct neuropathologic and clinical subset of AD termed the "Lewy-body variant of AD."[136]

Any discussion of variants of the more common dementias must acknowledge that a syndrome may be due to the concurrence of more than one common degenerative disorder.[186] PD can occur with AD and vice versa (see Chapter 3). Although rare, an overlap between HD and AD has also been reported.[274]

DEMENTIAS WITH CHARACTERISTIC PATHOLOGIC FEATURES

A second class of atypical dementias includes those conditions in which the diagnostic neuronal pathology of either AD, Pick's disease, or PD is conspicuously absent. Many of these cases are characterized simply by neuronal loss and subcortical gliosis and are variously referred to as simple atrophy, hippocampal and temporal lobe sclerosis, or frontotemporal atrophy.* Clinical and pathologic heterogeneity characterizes this category. Clark and colleagues[59] have described 22 cases with a clinical history consistent with that of a primary degenerative dementia in whom the anatomic criteria for AD were not met. Of these, 5 had few or nonspecific abnormalities on pathologic examination, 3 had hippocampal and temporal lobe sclerosis, and 2 had cortical degeneration associated with motor neuron disease.

Brun and colleagues have extensively defined the clinical features, regional cerebral blood flow, and pathology of an apparently novel dementing disease which they termed frontal lobe degeneration (FLD) of the non-Alzheimer type.[46,93,132,276] These investigators noted this condition in 10% of 158 autopsied brains. The neuropathologic changes consisted of gray-matter degeneration involving the frontal and anterior temporal lobes, which could be distinguished from Pick's disease, progressive subcortical gliosis, AD, and CJD.[46] The pathologic similarity between FLD and the cortical changes seen in the ALS-dementia complex (see page 193) was noted. The precise relationship between FLD and Pick's disease, however, remains uncertain.[238] Knopman and colleagues[171] have identified an additional, apparently unique

---

*References 33, 59, 167, 281, 291, 294, 299, 328.

non-Alzheimer degenerative disease, which they refer to as "dementia lacking distinctive histology" (DLDH). Minimum pathologic criteria for the diagnosis of DLDH included (1) frontal and temporal or parietal neocortical cell loss and astrocytosis, (2) subcortical cell loss and astrocytosis involving *at least the substantia nigra*, and (3) absent or rare SPs and NFTs, and no Pick or Lewy bodies. Using these criteria, DLDH comprised 3% of their brain bank specimens and was the third most common pathologic cause of dementia, behind only AD and Lewy-body dementia. In contrast to FLD, severe pathologic involvement of the hippocampal formation, substantia nigra, and hypoglossal nuclei was common. The topographic distribution of lesions in frontal and temporal cortex, hippocampus, caudate nucleus, medial thalamus, substantia nigra, and hypoglossal nuclei was felt to suggest the hereditary multiple-system atrophies.

Finally, large autopsy series and pathologic studies using newer immunostaining techniques have disclosed dementia variants with novel pathologic features. For example, Braak and colleagues[35,36] reported eight cases in their series of 56 autopsies that failed to reveal high densities of SPs and NFTs but did show abnormal silver-staining grains distributed throughout the brain substance. These small spindle-shaped grains were found particularly in hippocampus and entorhinal cortex. These authors also identified eight brains that showed these grains in addition to NFTs. An unusual degenerative disorder with intranuclear hyaline inclusions, neuronal intranuclear hyaline inclusion disease, has also been described.[234,300]

DEMENTIA WITH EXTRAPYRAMIDAL SIGNS

Huntington's Disease

HD is an autosomal dominant neurodegenerative disease characterized by abnormal movements, dementia, and psychiatric disturbances.[103,152]

EPIDEMIOLOGY

The prevalence of HD generally ranges from 3 to 7 per 100,000 population in whites of northern European ancestry. The rates are lower in Asian and African populations and are markedly higher in certain isolated populations such as those in Venezuela.[103,131] The incidence rate is approximately 3 to 5 per million population per year. The age-specific incidence rates rise steeply during adolescence and young adulthood, to a maximum of over 7 per million population per year in the 30s. The rates then decline and approach zero by age 70. The duration of the disease generally ranges from 12 to 20 years. Duration does not change appreciably with age of onset in choreic cases, although those with the rigid childhood form of the disease may have a more fulminant course. Reported average annual mortality rates generally vary between 2 and 3 per million population in whites of northern European ancestry.[181] Reported rates for nonwhites are considerably lower. Pneumonia, choking, nutritional deficiencies, mental disorders (leading to self-destructive behavior), and chronic skin ulcers are important factors contributing to death in these individuals.[181,182]

GENETICS

HD is an autosomal dominant genetic disorder with complete penetrance[203] (see Chapter 2). In 1983, Gusella and colleagues[131] identified a DNA marker, D4S10, genetically linked to HD. D4S10 has been localized to the terminal short arm of chromosome 4 within several million base pairs of the HD gene. All HD families tested have shown linkage of the disease to D4S10 irrespective of age of onset, severity of symptoms, or ethnic origin, suggesting a single genetic locus for the disease. The mutation rate is very low.

These genetic advances led to the

availability of a presymptomatic diagnostic test for HD.[184,217] This test requires obtaining DNA samples, usually from lymphocytes, from affected and unaffected individuals in the family. The test is limited in its accuracy by the recombination frequency of the gene and by the availability of specimens from multiple family members. Testing may indicate a high (95% to 99%) chance of having the gene, or not having the gene, or may be inconclusive. Although initial studies indicated that large numbers of individuals at risk for HD might seek such a test, recent surveys suggest that the numbers are smaller.[103,115] The ethical issues of such a test procedure are complex (see also Epilogue).

CLINICAL FEATURES

Initial symptoms of HD are quite varied and include restlessness, clumsiness, altered speech and handwriting, forgetfulness, personality change, depression, and even psychotic behavior. The most characteristic manifestations are the motor abnormalities, which include chorea, ocular motor dysfunction, and disturbances of voluntary movement, particularly initiation of action.[103,184] Chorea usually begins with intermittent movements of the fingers or toes. As the disease progresses, chorea becomes prominent in the head, face, arms, and upper trunk. Ocular motor abnormalities include problems with initiation of voluntary saccades, suppression of reflexive saccades, fixation instability, and slowing of saccade velocities. HD patients are also significantly impaired in their ability to perform rapid voluntary limb movements, a finding not directly related to the chorea or the dementia associated with HD.

COGNITION

The neuropsychological features of HD include problems with concentration (easy distractibility), visuospatial abilities, memory, and executive abilities[37,38,48,156,318] (see Chapter 5). The memory disorder is prominent and characterized by inefficient information storage and faulty retrieval strategies. Although dysarthria may be so severe as to make the patient unintelligible, language function is generally preserved. Praxis and gnosis are also spared until relatively late in the course.

BEHAVIORAL SYMPTOMS

Several types of psychiatric problems are common in HD, including personality change and affective disorders.[49,103a,104] These problems alone or in combination can lead to withdrawal from former activities and friends, and deterioration of work performance, personal appearance, and interpersonal relationships. Personality changes such as apathy, irritability, anxiety, impulsivity, disinhibition, and impaired judgment are particularly frequent, occur early in the illness, and are often severe.

In certain families with HD, major psychiatric illness (including psychotic depression, manic depressive illness,[214] and perhaps schizophrenia[111]) can precede, occur with, or follow the onset of motor and cognitive abnormalities. Affective disorders are the most common, affecting at least half of the patients at some point in their illness.[49,103] So-called intermittent explosive disorder is also found frequently (31%).[103] Schizophrenia occurs less frequently early in the disease but may be found in institutionalized individuals. Although some cases may represent reactive depression, many are endogenous, as evidenced by the episodic nature of the symptoms, the occurrence of mania, the response to pharmacologic treatments, and the occurrence of depression up to 10 years prior to any other evidence of the disease.[104]

DIAGNOSIS

HD is not often confused with other illnesses when a positive family history and typical clinical features are present. Early in the disease, psychiatric difficulties or dementia may precede the characteristic motor abnormalities. False paternity may confuse the clinical picture. Wilson's disease, acanthocytosis, and (in older patients) "senile chorea" may need to be differentiated from true HD. Structural imaging typically shows primarily caudate atrophy, although this need not be well developed even at autopsy.[317] Functional imaging (e.g., PET scanning) to measure glucose utilization or dopamine receptors may show abnormalities early in the disease, even in asymptomatic carriers.[25]

Parkinson's Disease

PD is the most common degenerative disorder involving extrapyramidal systems. In his original 1817 essay, James Parkinson provided an accurate description of the movement disorder ("involuntary tremulous motion") as well as the associated disorder of posture, stance, and gait ("a propensity to bend the trunk forward, and pass from a walking to a running pace").[248] Parkinson also claimed that the senses and intellect were unaffected; ample evidence now exists, however, documenting the frequent occurrence of both cognitive impairment and mood disorder in PD.

EPIDEMIOLOGY

PD is a relatively common disorder, affecting approximately 1 million individuals in North America. The incidence and prevalence of idiopathic PD show dramatic age-related increases. The prevalence of PD is approximately 150 to 200 per 100,000, increasing, after age 65, to nearly 1100 per 100,000.[166] Although familial cases of PD have been reported,[226,262] the finding of a low concordance rate among identical twins suggests that genetic factors play a minimal role in this condition.[120,319]

Given the relatively weak genetic risk for PD, increasing attention is being paid to the possible role of an environmental or toxic agent. The discovery of MPTP (see below, p. 184) and the increasing evidence of an environmental cause for the parkinsonian dementia complex in the Western Pacific highlight nongenetic mechanisms. Moreover, some epidemiologic studies[202] have reported a "protective effect of smoking," although whether this represents either a sampling artifact or else true biologic effect of nicotine or some other component of smoking is not clear.

Although Parkinson did not consider intellectual impairment to be a major portion of the syndrome, in the mid-1800s, Charcot[56] felt that psychic faculties were definitely impaired. Many early authors concluded that the coexistence of dementia and PD represented the chance occurrence of PD and dementing illness such as AD or multi-infarct dementia. Some authors also raised the possibility that drug treatment for parkinsonism could contribute to cognitive impairment (see section on Treatment, p. 185).

A significant literature, however, has accumulated concerning the issue of mental impairment in patients with PD.[28] Pirozzolo and colleagues[258] demonstrated that more than 90% of PD patients given a comprehensive neuropsychological test battery were shown to have some cognitive impairment. Modern epidemiologic surveys have suggested that approximately 10% to 40% of PD patients have dementia.[210] In a comprehensive review of more than 2500 patients described in the studies published over the past 60 years, 15% of PD patients were thought to have dementia.[44] Other groups[117,207,210] also came to overall estimates in the 10% to 15% range. Overall, Mayeux et al[207a] estimate the prevalence of PD-dementia to be 76 per 100,000. In a review of 249 patients followed for almost 5 years, Mayeux and colleagues[207] estimated the incidence rate of dementia in PD to be 69 cases per 1000 person-years of observation. By 85 years of age, more than 65% of the surviving members of this cohort were demented. Advanced age and a family history of dementia may be risk factors for dementia in PD.[146,199] The variable reports of dementia in different studies undoubtedly reflect differences in patient selection, sensitivity of test measures used to detect cognitive impairment, and terminologic issues.

ETIOLOGY

The etiology of idiopathic PD is unclear. A condition resembling idiopathic PD clinically and pathologically can be induced in humans and primates by MPTP administration.[180] This finding has led not only to the development of primate models of PD, but also to speculation that idiopathic PD may result from subclinical exposure to an as-yet-unknown toxic agent.[50] In support of this are epidemiologic data suggesting a higher prevalence of PD in areas of high pesticide use.[120]

Parkinsonism can be associated with arteriosclerosis, although this has been somewhat controversial. Several researchers[52,201,261] have provided evidence that dementia was more likely to occur in PD in the presence of vascular lesions.

Postencephalitic PD[105] and the parkinsonism-dementia complex of Guam[144,145] can also be associated with dementia. The clinical characteristics and frequency of the association with dementia are not well known, however.

COGNITION

The reported range of cognitive impairments in PD is large. Clearly, intellectual problems can be present without impairment severe enough to meet *DSM-III* criteria for dementia.[258]

Bradyphrenia, the slowing of cognitive processing associated with impairment of concentration and apathy,[279] is common in PD. Introduced as a clinical term by Naville in 1922,[237] bradyphrenia has subsequently evolved into a cognitive and behavioral constellation sharing many common features with the so-called frontal lobe syndromes and with depression.[20] Wilson and colleagues[327] were able to demonstrate that the scanning of elements held in short-term memory was slowed in PD. In further distinguishing the cognitive and motoric slowing in PD, the authors failed to demonstrate a relationship between bradyphrenia and bradykinesia. In a more recent study, bradyphrenia was associated with impairment of attention and vigilance and linked to alterations in norepinephrine metabolism.[211]

Some have labeled the pattern of dementia in PD as a "subcortical dementia" characterized by slowed mentation, apathy, depression, and the relative preservation of instrumental cognitive functions like language and praxis.[73,74] Although the behavioral-cognitive syndrome was identified as early as 1922 by Naville,[237] the notion of subcortical dementia enjoyed a rejuvenation that began in the mid-1970s following a description of the dementia syndromes present in progressive supranuclear palsy (PSP)[7] and in HD.[214] Subcortical dementias were contrasted with "cortical dementias" such as AD, in which language, praxis, and gnosis are more impaired. Subsequently, however, the concept of subcortical dementia as a useful nosologic entity has come into question[45,208,325] (see also Chapter 5).

The term "cortical" and "subcortical" dementia are anatomically vague and suggest a relative independence of cortical and subcortical functions that does not exist. In addition, pathology can be found in both cortical and subcortical regions in many of these diseases. The claim for the importance of the distinction rests on whether the clinical features of the two types are separate. Even if we replace the terms "cortical" and "subcortical" with, say, "type A" and "type B," to avoid the pseudoanatomic nature of the terms, it is not yet clear that all dementias can be categorized into two large, superordinate categories. Moreover, because it is difficult to match patients with different dementias on features such as severity of dementia or functional impairment, one must be careful about comparing an early dementia in one condition with a later dementia in another. There are probably as many differences between two "subcortical" dementias such as HD and PD as there are between these disorders and a "cortical" dementia such as AD.[45,257] In addition, not all PD patients show the same pattern of cognitive impairment, because the biologic basis of the dementia may vary in different cases.

Teuber and Proctor[309] may have been the first to identify visuospatial abnormalities in PD. Several early investigators found that patients with PD were not able to perform as well as controls on selected subsets of the Wechsler Adult Intelligence Scale, including block design, picture arrangement, and object assembly.[17,190] Other more specific neuropsychological tests for visuospatial function have also been found to be impaired in PD, including Benton Visual Retention,[316] Hooper Visual Organization Test,[6] and Raven Standard Progressive Matrices.[148]

Most recent papers,[209,256] but not all,[29,34] have confirmed the visuospatial abnormalities. Eye movement abnormalities have been detected in PD[34,305] and may explain some of the visuospatial deficits.[101,290] Defective tracing, delayed recognition of complex visual forms, and impaired judgment of specific spatial relationships have also recently been reported in PD.

Speech difficulties, including hypophonia, dysarthria, stuttering, echolalia, and palilalia, occur frequently.[205,226a] Language problems are said to be relatively rare, but reduced verbal fluency and mild disturbance of confrontation naming can occur. Abnormalities in syntax, semantics, and comprehension have also been reported.[23,76]

BEHAVIORAL OR PSYCHIATRIC SYMPTOMS

The most frequently encountered psychiatric disturbance in idiopathic PD is depression.[209,213] A small number of patients experience depression before any overt motor manifestations appear, and nearly half experience significant depression at some point during their illness. Depression does not appear to be related to disease severity or duration and is not affected by dopamine therapy. Some evidence suggests that depression may be more common in early-onset cases and in those with coexisting dementia.[209] In PD, reduced levels of brain serotonin have been suggested to correlate with the development of depression.[213] Two apparent forms of depression in PD have been described: major depression and dysthymic disorder. The relatively milder affective disorder syndrome, dysthymic disorder, is observed more frequently in PD. It is difficult to detect mild depression in PD, given that bradyphrenia, bradykinesia, and apathy may be attributable to the neurologic condition.

Psychosis (especially delusions and hallucinations) is frequently related to medications in PD patients[52] but can occur as part of the disease process itself[223] (see next section).

RELATIONSHIP BETWEEN TREATMENT AND COGNITIVE IMPAIRMENT

Pharmacologic management of parkinsonian symptoms in the demented patient with PD is difficult. All therapeutic agents for PD, including amantadine, L-dopa, dopamine agonists such as bromocriptine and pergolide, and anticholinergic agents, can increase confusion and produce hallucinations. Confusional episodes in the PD patient are more likely attributable to anticholinergic agents, whereas hallucinations are more likely due to dopamine therapy. Late complications of long-term L-dopa treatment appear in approximately 80% of cases. Most commonly observed are a variety of drug-related movement disorders including end-of-dose akinesia, a variety of dystonic and dyskinetic movements, and the "on-off" phenomenon. Confusion, nightmares, hallucinatory experiences, and frank psychosis may occur in the setting of L-dopa or dopamine-agonist therapy. The emergence of these psychiatric or behavioral symptoms in the cognitively impaired patient requiring symptomatic management of PD is a common therapeutic problem. Useful strategies include a reduction of L-dopa dose with adjunctive therapy with dopamine agonists, initiation of low-dose neuroleptic therapy in an effort to control severe hallucinatory or psychotic episodes, or possibly a therapeutic drug holiday (although these are not without risk). Newer antipsychotic agents such as clozapine may be helpful in such instances. Clozapine apparently produces fewer extrapyramidal side effects than currently available neuroleptics, although it can cause hematologic problems that in rare cases can be fatal.[21]

Selegiline (Eldepryl) recently was approved as an adjunctive therapy in PD to manage the patient who has become unresponsive to dopaminergic drugs or is suffering side effects from those drugs, such as the on-off phenomenon. Two studies[248a,308] have provided some evidence that the use of the drug slows the progression of the disease. The proposed mechanism is the action of Deprenyl as a monoamine oxidase B inhibitor. In animals, this agent prevents the pathologic damage and clinical symptoms produced by MPTP. Further studies are needed to establish whether a drug-induced slowing of the progression of the disease has actually occurred, rather than just symptomatic improvement.

Striatonigral Degeneration

Striatonigral degeneration (SND) is an uncommon neurodegenerative disorder producing dementia and parkinsonism. In the initial description of this condition, several patients clinically diagnosed with PD were found on autopsy to have striking atrophy, neuronal loss, and gliosis in the globus pallidus, putamen and subthalamic region, in addition to depigmentation of the substantia nigra. Based on the

striking striatal degeneration, a distinction from PD was made and the term SND was coined.[2] In the initial description of four patients, mental function was felt to be intact.

CLINICAL FEATURES AND DIAGNOSIS

No clinical features have been found to unequivocally distinguish SND from PD. In a recent retrospective analysis, of 10 cases of autopsy-proven SND, 50% were misdiagnosed in life as PD.[98] Further analysis of these patients suggested that helpful pointers to the diagnosis of SND included unexplained falls, failure to respond to L-dopa, autonomic dysfunction, and absence of rest tremor.[98] Of these 10 cases, one became confused and paranoid after 8 years of illness, and a second developed pseudobulbar emotional lability. Although dementia has been reported to be common in SND,[75] a recently published text suggests that dementia is present only when the SND is part of a larger syndrome in the multiple-system-atrophy spectrum of diseases.[274a] Cranial imaging studies may show selective atrophy of either caudate or putamen.[242] T_2-weighted MRI imaging may reveal low signal intensity in the caudate or putamen, possibly because of iron deposition in these regions. PET scans in "probable" SND patients (no autopsy diagnosis) revealed a 20% reduction in [^{18}F]fluorodeoxyglucose metabolism in the caudate and putamen as well as in the motor and premotor frontal cortex.

NEUROBIOLOGY

As indicated previously, pathologic changes including neuronal loss and gliosis are present in caudate and putamen in SND. Patients with SND who benefit from L-dopa therapy may have a relative preservation of the putamen.[98] Loss of tyrosine hydroxylase immunoreactivity in the medulla may correlate with impairment of autonomic vasomotor control. Immunochemical abnormalities reported in SND include a reduction in tyrosine hydroxylase–immunoreactive neurons in the medulla,[194] reduced expression of met-enkephalin in putamen and ventrolateral globus pallidus,[124] and reduced calcineurin immunoreactivity in the putamen.[123] One recent report on glial cytoplasmic inclusions in SND, olivopontocerebellar atrophy, and Shy-Drager syndrome has suggested that these pathologic factors may be a characteristic cellular change in the multiple-system-atrophy spectrum of diseases.[247]

Progressive Supranuclear Palsy

Long identified as an atypical or "funny" kind of parkinsonism,[80] PSP was first recognized as a distant clinicopathologic entity in 1964 by Steele, Richardson, and Olszewski.[296] PSP is a chronic, progressive disorder characterized clinically by extrapyramidal rigidity, axial dystonia, pseudobulbar lability of affect, swallowing difficulties, severe gait disorder, supranuclear ophthalmoplegia, and dementia.[87,177]

EPIDEMIOLOGY

Little information regarding the epidemiology of PSP is available. Using records of practicing neurologists, the prevalence ratio of PSP in two New Jersey counties with a combined population of slightly over 3/4 million individuals was 1.39/100,000.[121] Given diagnostic difficulties, this figure should be taken as a minimal estimate. In a follow-up study of 41 patients from this study, Davis and colleagues[83] identified no risk factors associated with PSP other than an increased incidence of index cases residing in areas of low population density as adults. Although initial reports suggested a male predominance of disease,[177,296] more recent data reveal no significant sex difference.[121,192] The median age at onset of symptoms is approximately 63 years, with a median survival by life-table analysis of 9.7 years.[121]

CLINICAL FEATURES OF THE DEMENTIA OF PROGRESSIVE SUPRANUCLEAR PALSY

Although dementia was present in seven of the nine patients initially reported,[296] dementia is not a necessary criterion for the diagnosis of PSP.[45,121] In some instances, dementia has been reported to occur in 60% to 80% of PSP patients[192,193] whereas others have reported that IQ in PSP patients may be only slightly below normal.[154] In a discussion of 5 personal cases and review of 42 cases in the literature, Albert and co-workers characterized the neurobehavioral changes of PSP as forgetfulness, slowing of thought processes, emotional or personality changes, and impaired ability to manipulate acquired knowledge in the relative absence of aphasia, apraxia, or agnosia.[7] This behavioral constellation was felt to be unique, and the term "subcortical dementia" was coined. An apparent similarity between the subcortical dementia of PSP and the neuropsychological syndromes seen in bifrontal disease was additionally recognized,[7] and has led to a variety of alternative descriptions, including subcortical or frontosubcortical dementia.[6] PSP patients are impaired on tasks requiring sequential movements and shifting of concepts,[126] as well as on other tests of frontal lobe function,[192] a finding consistent with [^{18}F]fluorodeoxyglucose PET studies showing marked frontal and temporal hypometabolism.[79,106] In addition, PSP patients have been reported to have deficits in visual scanning and search,[100] and in verbal fluency, digit span, verbal memory, and logical memory.[256,257] Disturbances in sleep, depression, obsessive compulsive behavior, and psychosis can also occur.[9,85]

NEUROBIOLOGY

The neurobiology of PSP remains poorly characterized. CT and MRI studies show early involvement of midbrain structures with later atrophy of the pons and frontotemporal regions. As previously mentioned, PET scanning has demonstrated marked frontal cerebral glucose hypometabolism,[79] as well as reduced ^{3}H-spiperone binding in basal ganglia.[284]

Typical neuropathologic findings include neuronal loss associated with gliosis and NFTs most marked in substantia nigra, substantia innominata, the subthalamic nuclear region, pallidum, and superior colliculus. Additional areas involved to a lesser extent include the locus ceruleus, striatum, and a variety of upper brainstem and midbrain structures.[5] The tangles in PSP are most often straight, not twisted as in AD.[303]

The neurochemistry of PSP is characterized by dopamine depletion in the striatum; reduced density of dopamine D-2 receptors in caudate and putamen[255]; reduction in choline acetyltransferase (ChAT) levels in frontal cortex, substantia innominata and basal ganglia; and a variable reduction in GABA-ergic neurotransmitter systems in certain subcortical regions.[284] Alterations in cortical nicotinic[325] and serotonin receptors[195] have also been reported.

The loss of striatal dopamine receptors may explain the poor therapeutic efficacy of dopamine agonist therapy in PSP. The available evidence detailing cortical and subcortical as well as multiple neurotransmitter system abnormalities suggests that it is unwise to think of PSP as being either a purely "subcortical"[72] or "dopaminergic"[20] dementia.

DEMENTIA ASSOCIATED WITH DEGENERATIVE DISORDERS OF THE CEREBELLUM

The role of the cerebellum in supporting normal cognition is as uncertain as the relationship between cerebellar pathology and cognitive impairment in disease.[287a] Acute lesions of the cerebellar hemispheres may result in alterations of arousal, disturbances of memory function, and delirium.[165] Whether these changes actually are due to the cerebellar damage itself or to associated structures such as the brainstem is unclear. Certain acute cerebellar disorders (e.g., hemorrhage) can lead to acute or chronic hydrocephalus with cognitive impairment.[187] The nature and extent of any disturbances in cognition, behavior, or emotional response are variable in different degenerative disorders of the cerebellum. In an earlier volume in this series,[116] minor deficits in memory and attention were felt to be common features of cerebellar disease, but frank dementia was believed to be more likely attributable to pathology in noncerebellar structures.

Several factors may account for these difficulties in understanding the relationship between dementia and cerebellar disease. First, codification of degenerative diseases of the cerebellum has proven difficult. Indeed, a recently proposed classification scheme was presented with apologies to individuals who had previously attempted the classification of chaos.[78] A second difficulty results from our lack of understanding of the role of the cerebellum in human cognition and behavior. In 1985, Botez and colleagues concluded that no convincing evidence existed about the neuropsychological effects of chronic cerebellar disease.[32] Only 4 years later, these authors proposed anatomic correlates for the role of the cerebellum in visuospatial organization of concrete tasks, planning and programming of daily activities, and the speed of information processing.[31] Thompson and colleagues have supported the view that memory traces for classical conditioning of discrete behavioral responses such as eye blink are stored in the cerebellum.[310] Further insights into the functional-anatomic role of the cerebellum in speech and language function have been gleaned from stereotaxic ablation studies,[130] surgical cerebellar hemisphere resection,[273] and functional neuroimaging in aphasic patients.[221] A small body of literature also suggests a possible association between a variety of psychiatric syndromes (including schizophrenia, other psychosis, and depression) and gross or radiographic cerebellar pathology.[134,139] A final problem with understanding the relationship between cerebellar dysfunction and cognition is that assessment of the degree of cognitive impairment is difficult in patients in later stages of cerebellar degeneration syndromes, insofar as dysarthria, ataxia, parkinsonism, and other disabilities may limit testing.

This section will focus on selected degenerative disorders of the cerebellum in which cognitive impairment is a fairly frequently observed attribute (Table 6–3). Those with known metabolic abnormalities and those that occur principally in children will not be considered here (see reference 116 for a review).

Cerebellar Degeneration

In 1907, Gordon Holmes described a hereditary cerebello-olivary degeneration syndrome characterized by gait ataxia and dysarthria with onset in late adulthood.[147] Owing to the rarity of this and related conditions, the incidence, magnitude, and pattern of neuropsychological impairment is unknown, although some cases show dementia in the later stages.[116] Current classification considers the Holmes type of ataxia as a member of autosomal dominant cerebellar ataxias, type I.[298a] Sporadic nonfamilial cases have also been reported, especially in association with cancers such as lymphoma. Cognitive impairment also can occur in paraneoplastic cerebellar degeneration.[15]

Olivopontocerebellar Atrophies

The olivopontocerebellar atrophies (OPCAs) constitute a heterogeneous group of disorders characterized clinically by progressive ataxia, and anatomically by the neuronal degeneration of the cerebellum and brainstem. A sporadic form of OPCA (Dejerine-Thomas) shares similar features with sporadic cerebellar ataxias, and some authors consider this form to be a subgroup of idiopathic late-onset cerebellar ataxia, together with the Ramsay-Hunt type and the Marie-Foix-Alajouanine type.[136a] The cognitive impairment seen in the cerebellar and olivopontocerebellar degenerations has been labeled a dementia of the subcortical type.[75]. In contrast, in the five major OPCA subtypes as defined by Konigsmark,[174] dementia was recognized only in autosomal dominant types III and V, and even then not as a consistent feature.[116] In their review, Cummings and Benson[75] emphasized that dementia appeared to be more common in the autosomal recessive forms of OPCA, and more prominent in those hereditary ataxias associated with the multisystem atrophies.

A recent neuropsychological and autopsy analysis of patients with dominantly inherited OPCA of the Schut type highlights the complexities of understanding the cognitive impairment in OPCA and its biologic basis, as well as the difficulties of comparative studies of the dementias.[169] A unique pattern of memory impairment in tasks of delayed alternation (DA) and delayed response (DR) was reported. In contrast to patients with AD, who have impaired DA and DR, patients with OPCA of the Schut pedigree were impaired only in DA, suggesting impairment of orbitofrontal or temporal lobe systems. A study of the neurochemistry of these cases[169] showed reductions in ChAT in cortex similar to those reported in AD and PD. Thus, in OPCA, the neuropsychological pattern is different even though AD and OPCA share the loss of ChAT, supporting the view that multiple other neurotransmitter systems probably play a role in supporting normal cognition. Perry[253a] suggested four different types of dominantly inherited OPCA based on alteration in neurotransmitter systems, but further analysis is necessary to characterize the relationship between cognitive impair-

Table 6-3 DEGENERATIVE DISEASES ASSOCIATED WITH PROGRESSIVE ATAXIA AND COGNITIVE IMPAIRMENT PRESENTING IN ADULTHOOD

	Inheritance	Age at Onset	Clinical Characteristics[186a,296a]	Dementia; Neuropsychiatric Profile
CEREBELLAR ATAXIAS[186a,296a]				
Autosomal dominant cerebellar ataxia type I	AD	4th–5th decade	Ataxia, ophthalmoplegia, optic atrophy, extrapyramidal signs, amyotrophy	Variable severity, emotional lability, memory complaints
Autosomal dominant cerebellar ataxia type II	AD	2nd–4th decade	Ataxia, pigmentary retinopathy, ophthalmoplegia, extrapyramidal signs	Not reported
Autosomal dominant cerebellar ataxia type III	AD	Over 5th decade	Ataxia, extrapyramidal signs, nystagmus	Not reported
Autosomal dominant cerebellar ataxia type IV	AD	1st–3rd decade	Ataxia, deafness, myoclonus, peripheral neuropathy, generalized tonic-clonic seizures	Not reported
Other autosomal dominant cerebellar ataxias	AD	Variable	Ataxia, extrapyramidal signs, essential tremor, polyneuropathy	Variable
Hereditary periodic ataxia	AD	Variable	Attacks of dysarthria, ataxia, vertigo	Not known
Cerebello-olivary degeneration of Marie-Foix-Alajouanine	Sporadic	5th–6th decade	Ataxia, gait disorder, dysarthria	Variable
Dyssynergia cerebellaris progressiva (Ramsay-Hunt)	Sporadic	5th–6th decade	Ataxia, resting and gross intentional tremor	Not known

OPCA (OLIVOPONTOCEREBELLAR ATROPHY)[253a]

Sporadic OPCA (Dejerine-Thomas)	Sporadic	3rd–5th decade	Ataxia, supranuclear ophthalmoplegia, polyneuropathy, postural hypotension	Variable; usually in late stages, emotionality and euphoria
Type I OPCA (Menzel)	AD	3rd–5th decade	Ataxia, gait disorder, dysarthria, tremor, chorea, optic atrophy	Variable dementia; in one kindred reported progressive dementia and vegetative state
Type II OPCA (Fickler-Winkler)	AR	3rd–5th decade	Ataxia, gait disorder, dysarthria, eye movement disorder	Not reported
Type III OPCA	AD	1st–4th decade	Visual loss, gait ataxia, tremor, supranuclear palsy	Variable incidence, "severe cognitive impairment" reported
Type IV OPCA (Schut)	AD	1st–4th decade	Gait ataxia, impaired position and vibration sense, bulbar palsy, tremor, dysarthria	Frontal symptom dysfunction, impaired delayed alternation
Type V OPCA	AD	Variable	Ataxia, extrapyramidal signs, ophthalmoplegia	Variable severity, described as "subcortical"

AD = autosomal dominant; AR = autosomal recessive
Source: Adapted from Gilman et al,[116] p. 247; and Asbury AK, McKhann GM, and McDonald WI: Diseases of the Nervous System: Clinical Neurobiology. WB Saunders, Philadelphia, 1986.

ment and the pattern of biochemical changes.

Friedreich's Ataxia

Friedreich's ataxia (FA) is a neurodegenerative disease primarily affecting the posterior columns of the spinal cord, the pyramidal tracts, the spinocerebellar tracts, and the cerebellum. Cortical atrophy involving the frontal and parietal lobes has also been described.[42] The clinical symptomatology primarily includes progressive dysarthria with gait, posture, and stance abnormalities owing to sensory and cerebellar system involvement.

The characteristics of the cognitive alterations in FA are poorly defined. Higher cortical functions have been described as being "unaltered" with the exception of emotional lability.[1] Mental status abnormalities ranging from "mental handicaps" to progressive dementia have been reported in 8.5% to 58% of FA patients.[24,81] Other reports have questioned whether intellectual deterioration occurs only in a subpopulation of FA patients (see reference 99 for discussion), or whether FA patients are intellectually normal except for the motor and psychiatric symptoms of this disorder.[81] The syndrome is dominated by personality change, slowing of cognition, and memory disturbances similar to other "subcortical disorders."[75] Tests of nonverbal function,[112] IQ, perception, visual constructive abilities, and three-dimensional mental folding[99] show impairment.

DEMENTIAS ASSOCIATED WITH MOTOR NEURON DISEASE

Motor neuron pathology and dementia occur in several degenerative conditions[282] including the amyotrophic lateral sclerosis (ALS)-parkinsonism dementia complex of Guam,[91,145] the amyotrophy dementia complex (ADC),[228] familial ALS/dementia, and several less common conditions. We will consider only the first two in any detail. Classification schemes have emphasized hereditary factors, age at onset, associated neurologic conditions, and neuropathologic aspects. In one recent review of amyotrophy occurring in multisystem genetic neurologic diseases, motor neuron disease was associated with many other neurodegenerative conditions including HD, Pick's disease, PD, and spinocerebellar degeneration.[280] The co-occurrence of sporadic motor neuron disease and neuropathologically confirmed AD or Pick's disease has generally been attributed to chance.[41,313] Although many definitions of ALS specifically exclude the presence of dementia or extrapyramidal symptoms, approximately 5% to 10% of ALS patients may demonstrate severe dementia or parkinsonism.[313] Whether nondemented patients with sporadic ALS demonstrate a specific pattern of neuropsychological abnormalities[110a,227] remains to be elucidated.

Amyotrophic Lateral Sclerosis—Parkinsonism-Dementia Complex of Guam

Perhaps the most well known of the motor neuron disease-associated dementias is the ALS-parkinsonism-dementia complex of Guam. Epidemiologic evidence suggests that among the native Chamorro population of Guam, ALS and a parkinsonism-dementia syndrome may represent the extremes of phenotypic expression of a single disease process.[144] A pathologically identical mixed syndrome of ALS and parkinsonism with dementia occurs on the Kii Peninsula of Japan, as well as in non-Chamorro residents of the Mariana Islands and in Chamorros residing in the United States. On the island of Guam, 10% of adult deaths in the native Chamorro population result from ALS, and 7% are attributed to the parkinsonism-dementia complex. The prevalence of Guamanian ALS-parkinsonism-dementia complex was reported to be 118 per 100,000, with an average age of onset of 50 years, although the disease may be less frequent now. Men are affected more commonly than women.

The dementia syndrome of the parkinsonism-dementia complex is associated with striking bradykinesia and rigidity. Mental slowing, apathy, and elements of depression occur in the relative absence of aphasia, apraxia, and agnosia — leading to the classification of this syndrome as a "subcortical dementia." Pathologically, gross atrophy is found in a frontotemporal cortical distribution. NFTs in the relative absence of neuritic plaques are present in affected cortical regions as well as in hippocampus, amygdala, and substantia nigra. Such tangles are also found in great abundance in control subjects, however. Severe neuronal loss and depigmentation of the substantia nigra occurs without Lewy body formation. Pathologic changes in the spinal cord include loss of anterior horn cells and the presence of neurofibrillary changes.[75] Environmental factors have been implicated in the pathogenesis of this condition; high aluminum and low calcium in the water supply have been associated with the disease, and the ingestion of betel nut, which contains a neurotoxin, may play a role. Neither of these environmental theories has been proven, however, and any theory needs to explain why the incidence of disease is decreasing.

Amyotrophy-Dementia Complex

Although the pathologic features have been defined only recently,[224,225] sufficient sporadic cases of mixed ALS and progressive dementia without pathologic changes of AD, Pick's disease, or PD have been described both in Japan and in western countries to justify its designation as a distinct clinicopathologic entity. This syndrome has variously been called "classic ALS with dementia,"[326] "dementia of motor neuron disease,"[149] progressive dementia with motor disease,"[224] and "amyotrophy-dementia complex (ADC)."[228]

The clinical features include mild to moderate dementia associated with amyotrophy. In a review of 34 Japanese cases, 68% began with personality changes, 17% with signs and symptoms of motor neuron disease, and 15% with simultaneous occurrence of cognitive-behavioral changes and motor neuron disease.[228] The average age at onset was 53.9 years in these cases, and 15 of 20 other Japanese patients had an onset of illness prior to age 60.[224] Men are more frequently affected than women (sex ratio 1.6 : 1), and the average duration of illness prior to death is approximately 33 months. There have been no reported cases of familial ADC.

The dementia of ADC is described as the frontotemporal or "anterior" type. From the neuropsychological perspective, it may be virtually impossible to distinguish the cognitive syndrome of ADC from Pick's disease.[227] Indeed, the presence of early personality changes in association with predominant frontotemporal atrophy on CT and a normal EEG may lead to an initial incorrect diagnosis of Pick's disease in ADC. Pathologically, slight to moderate atrophy in a predominantly frontotemporal distribution is present. Light microscopic findings include simple atrophy, depigmentation of substantia nigra, and excessive lipofuscin in nerve cells. Spongy changes occur in 90% of cases, and gliosis is frequently present in subcortical white matter of the affected frontal and temporal lobes. No NFTs, Lewy bodies, or Pick bodies have been observed. Extensive neuronal loss and gliosis in substantia nigra may occur in as many as 50% of autopsy cases.[149] Despite the frequent severe involvement of the substantia nigra, no clinical symptoms of extrapyramidal disease have been described.

Table 6–4 CLINICAL MANIFESTATIONS OF ADULT-ONSET FORMS OF INHERITED METABOLIC DEMENTIAS

| | Onset | | | Clinical Features | | | | | | | | | | |
| | Before 50 | After 50 | Course | Dementia | Psychiatric | CST | EPS | Ataxia | Peripheral Neuropathy | Myoclonus/ Seizures | Optic Atrophy | Macular & Retinal Pigmentary Degeneration | Skin | Other Systemic |
Disease														
LEUKOENCEPHALOPATHIES														
Adrenoleukodystrophy	**	—	CP	+	++	+++	+	+	+	++	+	—	++	++
Sulfatide lipidosis (metachromatic leukodystrophy)	**	*	CP	+++	+++	+	+	++	++	++	+	—	—	—
Membranous lipodystrophy (lipomembranous polycystic osteodysplasia)	**	—	CP	+++	++	++	+	+	—	++	—	—	—	+++
Cerebrotendinous xanthomatosis	*	—	CP	+++	+	+++	—	+++	+	+	++	—	+++	++
POLIOENCEPHALOPATHIES														
GM$_2$ gangliosidosis (adult Tay-Sachs disease)	*	—	CP	++	+	++	+	++	—	+	—	—	+	—
Neuronal ceroid lipofuscinosis (Kuf disease)	**	—	CP	+++	+++	+	++	++	—	+++	—	—	+	—
Gaucher disease (type III)	**	—	CP	++	+++	+	+	+	—	+++	—	+	+	++

Disease													
Subacute necrotizing encephalomyelitis (Leigh disease)	*	–	S	++	++	++	+++	++	+++	+++	–	–	–
Hepatolenticular degeneration (Wilson disease)	**	*	CP	++	+++	+	+++	–	+	–	–	–	+++
Hallervorden-Spatz disease	**	*	CP	++	++	++	+++	+	+	–	++	–	–
Choreo-acanthocytosis	**	*	CP	++	++	+++	+	++	++	–	+	–	+++

DIFFUSE ENCEPHALOPATHIES

Disease													
Acute intermittent porphyria	**	*	S	+	+++	+++	+	–	++	–	–	–	++
Fabry disease (angiokeratoma corporis diffusum)	**	*	S	+	+	+	++	–	++	–	+	+++	+++
Adult polyglucosan body disease	**	**	CP	++	++	++	+	+	–	+	–	–	+

CP = chronic progressive; CST = corticospinal tract dysfunction; EPS = extrapyramidal system dysfunction; S = stuttering.
– = does not occur; * = rarely presents at this age; ** = commonly presents at this age; + = present to a variable degree in some cases; ++ = moderate involvement seen in many cases; +++ = prominent involvement seen in the majority of cases.

ADULT-ONSET BIOCHEMICAL DISORDERS

Adult-onset forms of inherited metabolic dementias are rare, particularly in individuals over age 50.[3,173] Although sulfatide lipidosis (metachromatic leukodystrophy), Wilson's disease, Hallervorden-Spatz syndrome, choreoacanthocytosis, adult polyglucosan body disease, and acute intermittent porphyria can present in individuals over 50, onset is much more common under age 50. In all of these conditions, prominent nonneuronal systemic involvement and/or involvement of multiple neural systems occurs. For example, corticospinal tract dysfunction, extrapyramidal system dysfunction, ataxia, peripheral neuropathy, myoclonus, seizures, optic atrophy, and retinal degenerations are common.

Following the classification scheme of Dyken and Krawiecki,[88] adult-onset metabolic dementing disorders have been classified into leukoencephalopathies, polioencephalopathies, corencephalopathies, and diffuse encephalopathies (Table 6–4).

In the leukoencephalopathies, the major pathologic change is in the subcortical white matter, whereas in the polioencephalopathies, the major clinical or anatomic involvement is in the cerebral cortex. *Corencephalopathies* is a term coined by Dyken and Krawiecki[88] to refer to neurodegenerative disorders in which the principal pathology occurs in deep telencephalic, diencephalic, or mesencephalic structures, including both gray and white matter. Diffuse encephalopathies include those with widespread anatomic involvement. As is typical of childhood-onset leukoencephalopathies, there are prominent early motor signs in adult-onset leukoencephalopathies, particularly reflecting corticospinal tract dysfunction. Extrapyramidal system dysfunction, ataxia, and peripheral neuropathy are less common features. Seizures occur late in the course of these conditions. Blindness may occur owing to involvement of geniculo-calcarine pathways or optic nerves, but is generally less common than in childhood-onset forms of these disorders. For the polioencephalopathies, myoclonus or seizures are common and are frequently early presenting signs. Motor signs appear late and peripheral nerves are generally spared. Optic atrophy is not seen. The corencephalopathies are characterized by early and prominent extrapyramidal system involvement.

In some of these conditions the biochemical defect has been identified, and specific laboratory studies are helpful in diagnosing a majority of them.[88,173,250] CNS imaging (CT or MRI) can suggest a class of disorders (e.g., leukoencephalopathies), or may support a clinical diagnosis, but rarely are disease-specific abnormalities identified. Specific disease diagnosis requires tissue biopsy or assay of deficient enzymes or accumulating metabolites (Table 6–5).

A few of these conditions (Wilson's disease, cerebrotendinous xanthomatosis) are treatable. In others (adrenal leukodystrophy, subacute necrotizing encephalomyelitis, and acute intermittent porphyria), promising new therapies are being developed. None of these conditions is likely to be confused with AD when standard criteria are applied.

SUMMARY

In this chapter we have considered degenerative diseases as disorders characterized by selective neuronal dysfunction of progressive and unknown etiology. Many degenerative dementias are not associated with other major neurologic signs, at least early in the illness. AD is the prototypical disorder in this category and the most common cause of dementia. Other, rarer conditions, including Pick's disease and a variety of other syndromes that have recently been described, are characterized by neuronal loss and atrophy without specific pathologic stigmata. HD and PD are progressive degenerative dementias associated with extrapyramidal signs and are important because of the clues they provide about genetic and environmental determinants of degenerative dementias. Although rare, progressive degenerative dementias can also be associated with pathologies in cerebellar and motor neuron systems. In individuals in early adulthood, it is important to consider adult-onset forms of biochemical disorders most often associated with children, particularly if the presentation is atypical.

Table 6–5 GENETICS AND BIOCHEMISTRY OF ADULT-ONSET FORMS OF INHERITED METABOLIC DEMENTIAS

Disease	Transmission	Biochemical Defect	Major Accumulating Metabolites
LEUKOENCEPHALOPATHIES			
Adrenoleukodystrophy	XLR	Defective peroxisomal fatty acid oxidation	Very long chain saturated fatty acids (VLCFA)
Sulfatide lipidosis (metachromatic leukodystrophy)	AR	Arylsulfatase A (sulfatide sulfatase)	Sulfatide
Membranous lipodystrophy (lipomembranous polycystic osteodysplasia)	AR	?	?
Cerebrotendinous xanthomatosis	AR	Defective bile acid synthesis	Cholestanol
POLIOENCEPHALOPATHIES			
GM$_2$ Gangliosidosis (adult Tay-Sachs disease)	AR	Hexosaminidase A	GM$_2$ ganglioside
Neuronal ceroid lipofuscinosis (Kuf disease)	AR(AD)	?	Ceroid lipofuscin; dolichol
Gaucher disease (type III)	AR	Acid β-glucosidase and glucocerebrosidase	Glucocerebroside
CORENCEPHALOPATHIES			
Subacute necrotizing encephalomyelitis (Leigh disease)	AR/S	Defect in activation mechanism of pyruvate dehydrogenase complex	?
Hepatolenticular degeneration (Wilson disease)	AR	Defective copper metabolism	Copper
Hallervorden-Spatz disease	AR/S	? cysteine dioxygenase	Iron in basal ganglia
Choreo-acanthocytosis	AR/S	?	?
DIFFUSE ENCEPHALOPATHIES			
Acute intermittent porphyria	AD	Uroporphyrinogen I synthetase (porphobilinogen deaminase)	Excretion of excess porphyrin precursors (porphobilinogen and delta-aminolevulinic acid)
Fabry disease (angiokeratoma corporis diffusum)	XLR	Alpha-galactosidase A	Ceramide trihexoside
Adult polyglucosan body disease	S(?AR)	?	?

AR = autosomal recessive; AD = autosomal dominant; S = sporadic; XLR = x-linked recessive.

REFERENCES

1. Adams JH, Corsellis JAN, and Duchen LW (eds): Greenfield's Neuropathology. John Wiley & Sons, New York, 1984.
2. Adams RD, VanBogaert L, and Vander Eecken H: Striato-nigral degeneration. J Neuropathol Exp Neurol 23:584, 1964.
3. Adams RD and Victor M: Principles of Neurology, Ed 3. McGraw-Hill, New York, 1985, pp 753–759.
4. Agbayewa MO: Earlier psychiatric morbidity in patients with Alzheimer's disease. J Am Geriatr Soc 34:561–564, 1986.
5. Agid Y, Javoy-Agid F, Ruberg M, et al: Progressive supranuclear palsy: Anatomoclinical and biochemical considerations. In Yahr MD and Bergmann KJ (eds): Advances in Neurology, Vol 45. Raven Press, New York, 1986, pp 191–206.
6. Albert ML: Subcortical dementia. In Katzman R, Terry RD, and Bick KL (eds): Alzheimer's Disease, Senile Dementia and Related Disorders. Raven Press, New York, 1978, pp 173–180.
7. Albert ML, Feldman RG, and Willis AL: The "subcortical dementia" of progressive supranuclear palsy. J Neurol Neurosurg Psychiatry 37: 121–130, 1974.
8. Albert ML, Goodglass H, Helm N, Rubens AB, and Alexander MP: Disorders of human communication 2. In Clinical Aspects of Dysphasia. Springer-Verlag, New York, 1981.
9. Aldrich MS, Foster NL, White RF, et al: Sleep abnormalities in progressive supranuclear palsy. Ann Neurol 25(6):577–581, 1989.
10. Alexopoulos GS, Abrams RC, Young RC, et al: Cornell scale for depression in dementia. Biol Psychiatry 23:271–284, 1988.
11. Alzheimer A: Uber eine eigenartige Erkrankung der Hirnrinde. Allgemeine Zeitschrift für Psychiatrie und Psychisch-Gerichtliche Medizin 64: 146–148, 1907.
12. Alzheimer A: Uber eigenartige krankheitsfalle des spateren alters. Z Neurol 4:356–385, 1911.
13. Amaducci LA, Fratiglioni L, Rocca WA, et al: Risk factors for clinically diagnosed Alzheimer's disease: A case-control study of an Italian population. Neurology 36:922–931, 1986.
14. Amaducci LA, Rocca WA, and Schoenberg BS: Origin of the distinction between Alzheimer's disease and senile dementia: How history can clarify nosology. Neurology 36:1497–1499, 1986.
15. Anderson NE, Posner JB, Sidtis JJ, et al: Paraneoplastic cerebellar degeneration. Ann Neurol 23(6):533–540, 1988.
16. Appel SH: A unifying hypothesis for the cause of amyotrophic lateral sclerosis, parkinsonism, and Alzheimer disease. Ann Neurol 10:499–505, 1981.
17. Asso D: WAIS scores in a group of Parkinson patients. Br J Psychiatry 115:555–556, 1969.
18. Atack JR: Cerebrospinal fluid neurochemical markers in Alzheimer's disease. In Boller F, Katzman R, Rascol A, Signoret J-L, and Christen Y (eds): Biological Markers of Alzheimer's Disease. Springer-Verlag, New York, 1989, pp 1–16.
19. Atack JR, Beal MF, May C, et al: CSF somatostatin and neuropeptide Y: Concentrations in aging and in dementia of the Alzheimer type with and without extrapyramidal signs. Arch Neurol 45:269–274, 1988.
20. Bachman DL and Albert ML: The dopaminergic syndromes of dementia. In Pilleri G and Tagliavini F (eds): Brain Pathology, Vol 1. Brain Anatomy Institute, Bern, Switzerland, 1984, pp 91–119.
21. Baldessarini RJ and Frankenburg FR: Drug therapy: Clozapine—a novel anti-psychotic agent. N Engl J Med 324(11):746–754, 1991.
22. Ball MJ, Hachinski VC, Fox A, et al: A new definition of Alzheimer's disease: A hippocampal dementia. Lancet 1:14–16, 1985.
23. Bayles KA: Language and Parkinson

disease. Alzheimer Dis Assoc Disord 4(3):171–180, 1990.

24. Bell J, Carmichael EA, quoted by Tyrer JH: Friedreich's ataxia. In Vinken PJ, Bruyn GW (eds), Handbook of Clinical Neurology, Vol 21. Elsevier North Holland, New York, 1975, pp 319–364.

25. Berent S, Giordani B, Lehtiner S, et al: Positron emission tomographic scan investigations of Huntington's disease: Cerebral, metabolic correlates of cognitive functions. Ann Neurol 23:541–546, 1988.

26. Blass JP, Baker AC, Li-Wen Ko, Sheu RK-F, and Black RS: Expression of "Alzheimer antigens" in cultured skin fibroblasts. Arch Neurol 48:709–717, 1991.

27. Blass JP and Zemcov A: Alzheimer disease: A metabolic systems degeneration? Neurochem Pathol 2:103–114, 1984.

28. Boller F: Mental status of patients with Parkinson's disease. Journal of Clinical Neuropsychology 2:157–172, 1980.

29. Boller F: Visuospatial impairment in Parkinson's disease: Role of perceptual and motor factors and of disease stage. Unpublished doctoral dissertation, Case Western Reserve University, Cleveland, OH, 1982.

30. Bondareff W, Mountjoy CQ, Roth M, Rossor MN, Iversen LL, and Reynolds GP: Age and histopathologic heterogeneity in Alzheimer's disease. Arch Gen Psychiatry 44:412–417, 1987.

31. Botez MI, Botez T, Elie R, and Attig E: Role of the cerebellum in complex human behavior. Ital J Neurol Sci 10:291–300, 1989.

32. Botez MI, Gravel J, Attig E, and Vezina J-L: Reversible chronic cerebellar ataxia after phenytoin intoxication: Possible role of cerebellum in cognitive thought. Neurology 35:1152–1157, 1985.

33. Bowen DM, Benton JS, Spillane JA, et al: Choline acetyltransferase activity and histopathology of frontal neocortex from biopsies of demented patients. J Neurol Sci 57:191–202, 1982.

34. Bowen FP: Behavioral alterations in patients with basal ganglia lesions. In Yahr MD (ed): The Basal Ganglia. Raven Press, New York, 1976, pp 169–177.

35. Braak H and Braak E: Argyrophilic grains: Characteristic pathology of cerebral cortex in cases of adult onset dementia without Alzheimer changes. Neurosci Lett 76:124–127, 1987.

36. Braak H and Braak E: Cortical and subcortical argyrophilic grains characterize a disease associated with adult onset dementia. Neuropathol Appl Neurobiol 15:13–26, 1989.

37. Brandt J, Folstein SE, Folstein MF, et al: Differential cognitive impairment in Alzheimer's disease and Huntington's disease. Ann Neurol 23:555–561, 1988.

38. Brandt J, Quaid KA, Folstein SE, et al: The neuropsychology of Huntington's disease. International Neuropsychiatry Society 9:118–120, 1986.

39. Brandt J, Quaid KA, Folstein SE, et al: Presymptomatic diagnosis of delayed-onset disease with linked DNA markers: The experience in Huntington's disease. JAMA 261:3108–3114, 1989.

40. Breitner JCS, Silverman JM, Mahs RD, et al: Familial aggregation in Alzheimer's disease: Comparison of risk among relatives of early- and late-onset cases, and among male and female relatives in successive generations. Neurology 38:207–212, 1988.

41. Brion S, Psimaras A, Chevalier JF, et al: Association of Pick's disease and amyotrophic lateral sclerosis. Encephale 6:259–286, 1980.

42. Brown JR: Disease of the cerebellum. In Baker AB (ed): Clinical Neurology, Vol 3. Hoeber Medical Division, Harper Brothers, New York, 1962, pp 1406–1455.

43. Brown P, Goldfarb LG, and Gajdusek DC: The new biology of spongiform encephalopathy: Infectious amyloidoses with a genetic twist. Lancet 337:1019–1022, 1991.

44. Brown RG, Marsden CD: How com-

mon is dementia in Parkinson's disease. Lancet 2:1262–1265, 1984.

45. Brown RG, Marsden CD: 'Subcortical Dementia': The neuropsychological evidence. Neuroscience 25(2):363–387, 1988.

46. Brun A: Frontal lobe degeneration of non-Alzheimer type. I. Neuropathology. Arch Gerontol Geriatr 6:193–208, 1987.

47. Burkhardt CR, Filley CM, Klein-schmidt-DeMasters BK, et al: Diffuse Lewy body disease and progressive dementia. Neurology 38:1520–1528, 1988.

48. Butters N, Sax D, Montgomery K, and Tarlow S: Comparison of the neuropsychological deficits associated with early and advanced Huntington's disease. Arch Neurol 35:585–589, 1978.

49. Caine ED and Shoulson I: Psychiatric syndromes in Huntington's disease. Am J Psychiatry 140:728–733, 1983.

50. Calne DB, Eisen A, McGeer E, and Spence P: Alzheimer's disease, Parkinson's disease, and motoneurone disease: Abiotrophic interaction between aging and environment? Lancet 2:1067–1070, 1986.

51. Candy JM, Oakley EA, and Klenowski J: Aluminosilicates and senile plaque formation in Alzheimer's disease. Lancet 1:354–357, 1986.

52. Celesia GG and Wannamaker WM: Psychiatric disturbances in Parkinson's disease. Dis Nerv Syst 33:577–583, 1972.

53. V.Chan-Pallay and Asan E: Alterations in catecholamine neurons of the locus coeruleus in senile dementia of the Alzheimer type and in Parkinson's disease with and without dementia and depression. J Comp Neurol 287:373–392, 1989.

54. Chandra V, Kokmen E, Schoenberg BS, and Beard CM: Head trauma with loss of consciousness as a risk factor for Alzheimer's disease. Neurology 39:1576–1578, 1989.

55. Chapman J, Bachar O, and Lorezyn AD: Antibodies to cholinergic neurons in Alzheimer's disease. J Neurochem 51:479–485, 1988.

56. Charcot JM: De la paralysie agitante. Gazette hebdomadaire de médecine et de chirurgie 8:765–767, 1861.

57. Clarfield AM: The reversible dementias: Do they reverse? Ann Intern Med 109:476–486, 1988.

58. Clark AW, Manz HJ, White CL III, et al: Cortical degeneration with swollen chromatolytic neurons: Its relationship to Pick's disease. J Neuropathol Exp Neurol 45(3):268–284, 1986.

59. Clark AW, White CL III, Manz HJ, et al: Primary degenerative dementia without Alzheimer pathology. Can J Neurol Sci 13:462–470, 1986.

60. Cohen-Mansfield J: Agitated behaviors in the elderly: II. Preliminary results in the cognitively deteriorated. J Am Geriatr Soc 34:722–727, 1986.

61. Cohen-Mansfield J and Billig N: Agitated behaviors in the elderly: I. A conceptual review. J Am Geriatr Soc 34:711–721, 1986.

62. Consensus Conference, Office of Medical Applications of Research, NIH: Differential diagnosis of dementing diseases. JAMA 258:3411–3416, 1987.

63. Constantinidis J: Is Alzheimer's disease a major form of senile dementia? Clinical, anatomical, and genetic data. In Katzman R, Terry RD, and Bick KL (eds): Alzheimer's Disease, Senile Dementia and Related Disorders. Aging Series, Vol 7. Raven Press, New York, 1978, p 15.

64. Constantinidis J, Richard J, and Tissot R: Pick's disease: Histological and clinical correlations. Eur Neurol 11:208–217, 1974.

65. Cook RH, Schneck SA, Clark DB, et al: Twins with Alzheimer's disease. Arch Neurol 38:300–301, 1981.

66. Cook-Deegan RM and Whitehouse PJ: Alzheimer's disease and dementia: The looming crisis. Issues in Science and Technology 3:52–63, 1987.

67. Corsellis JAN, Bruton CJ, and Freeman-Browne D: The aftermath of boxing. Psychol Med 3:270–303, 1973.

68. Council on Scientific Affairs: Dementia. JAMA 256:2234–2238, 1986.

69. Crapper DR, Krishman SS, and Dalton AJ: Brain aluminum distribution in Alzheimer's disease and experimental neurofibrillary degeneration. Science 180:511–513, 1973.

70. Crapper DR, Krishman SS, and Dalton AJ: Aluminum, neurofibrillary degeneration and Alzheimer's disease. Brain 99:67–80, 1976.

71. Crystal HA, Horoupian DS, Katzman R, and Jotkowitz S: Biopsy-proved Alzheimer disease presenting as a right parietal lobe syndrome. Ann Neurol 12:186–188, 1982.

72. Cummings JL: Subcortical dementia: Neuropsychology, neuropsychiatry, and pathophysiology. Br J Psychiatry 149:682–697, 1986.

73. Cummings JL: Introduction. In Cummings JL (ed): Subcortical Dementia. Oxford University Press, New York, 1990, pp 3–16.

74. Cummings JL: Subcortical mechanisms and human thought. In Cummings JL (ed): Subcortical Dementia. Oxford University Press, New York, 1990, pp 251–259.

75. Cummings JL and Benson DF: Dementia: A clinical approach. Butterworth & Co, Boston, 1983.

76. Cummings JL and Benson DF: Psychological dysfunction accompanying subcortical dementias. Annu Rev Med 39:53–61, 1988.

77. Cummings JL and Duchen LW: The Klüver-Bucy syndrome in Pick's disease. Neurology 31:1415–1422, 1981.

78. Currier RD: A classification for ataxia. In Duvoisin RC and Plaitakis A (eds): The Olivopontocerebellar Atrophies. Raven Press, New York, 1984, pp 1–4.

79. D'Antona R, Baron JC, Samson Y, et al: Subcortical dementia: Frontal cortex hypometabolism detected by positron tomography in patients with progressive supranuclear palsy. Brain 108:785–799, 1985.

80. Daroff RB: Progressive supranuclear palsy: A brief personalized history. Yale J Biol Med 60:119–122, 1987.

81. Davies DL: Psychiatric changes associated with Friedreich's ataxia. J Neurol Neurosurg Psychiatry 12:246–250, 1949.

82. Davies P: Potential diagnostic markers for Alzheimer's disease. In Boller F, Katzman R, Rascol A, Signoret J-L, and Christen Y (eds): Biological Markers of Alzheimer's Disease. Springer-Verlag, New York, 1989, pp 17–22.

83. Davis PH, Golber LI, Duvoisin RC, and Schoenberg BS: Risk factors for progressive supranuclear palsy. Neurology 38:1546–1552, 1988.

84. Delacourte A, Flament S, Défossez A, et al: Tau 64 and Tau 69: Two early biochemical markers of neurofibrillary degeneration. In Boller F, Katzman R, Rascol A, Signoret J-L, and Christen Y (eds): Biological Markers of Alzheimer's Disease. Springer-Verlag, New York, 1989, pp 37–55.

85. Destee A, Gray F, Parent M, et al: Obsessive-compulsive behavior and progressive supranuclear palsy. Rev Neurol (Paris) 146(1):12–18, 1990.

86. Devanand DP, Sackeim HA, and Mayeux R: Psychosis, behavioral disturbance, and the use of neuroleptics in dementia. Compr Psychiatry 29(4):387–401, 1988.

86a. Drevets WC and Rubin EH: Psychotic symptoms and the longitudinal course of senile dementia of the Alzheimer type. Biol Psychiatry 25:35–68, 1988.

87. Duvoisin RC, Golbe LI, and Lepore FE: Progressive supranuclear palsy. Can J Neurol Sci 14:547–554, 1987.

88. Dyken P and Krawiecki N: Neurodegenerative diseases of infancy and childhood. Ann Neurol 13:351–364, 1983.

89. Eagger S, Hajimohammadreza I, Fletcher K, Levy R, and Brammer M: Platelet membrane fluidity, family history, severity and age of onset in Alzheimer's disease. International Journal of Geriatric Psychiatry (United Kingdom) 5/6:395–400, 1990.

90. Eisdorfer C, Cohen D, and Buckley CE III: Serum immunoglobulins and cognition in the impaired elderly. In Katzman R, Terry RD, and Bick KL (eds): Alzheimer's Disease: Senile

Dementia and Related Disorders. Aging, Vol 7. Raven Press, New York, 1978, pp 401–407.

91. Elizan TS, Hirano A, Abrams BM, Need RL, et al: Amyotrophic lateral sclerosis and Parkinsonism-dementia complex on Guam: Neurological reevaluation. Arch Neurol 14:356–368, 1966.

92. Ellis WG, McCulloch JR, and Corley CL: Presenile dementia in Down's syndrome: Ultrastructural identity with Alzheimer's disease. Neurology 24:101–106, 1974.

93. Englund E and Brun A: Frontal lobe degeneration of non-Alzheimer type. IV. White matter changes. Archives of Gerontology and Geriatrics 6:235–243, 1987.

94. Epstein CJ: Down's syndrome and Alzheimer's disease: Implications and approaches. In Katzman R (ed) Biological Aspects of Alzheimer's disease. Banbury Report No. 15, Cold Spring Harbor Laboratory, 1983, pp 169–182.

95. Eslinger PJ, Damasio AR, Benton AL, and Van Allen M: Neuropsychologic detection of abnormal mental decline in older persons. JAMA 253:670–674, 1985.

96. Evans DA, Funkenstein HH, Albert MS, et al: Prevalence of Alzheimer's disease in a community population of older persons: Higher than previously reported. JAMA 262:2551–2556, 1989.

97. Evenhuis HM: The natural history of dementia in Down's syndrome. Arch Neurol 47:263–267, 1990.

98. Fearnley JM and Lees AJ: Striato nigral degeneration. Brain 113:1823–1842, 1990.

99. Fehrenbach RA, Wallesch W, and Claus D: Neuropsychologic findings in Friedreich's Ataxia. Arch Neurol 41:306–308, 1984.

100. Fisk JD, Goodale MZ, Burkhart G, and Barnett HJM: Progressive supranuclear palsy: The relationship between ocular motor dysfunction and psychological test performance. Neurology 32:698–705, 1982.

100a. Flicker C, Ferris SH, and Reisberg B:

Mild cognitive impairment in the elderly: Predictors of dementia. Neurology 41:1006–1009, 1991.

101. Flowers KA and Downing AC: Predictive control eye movements in Parkinson's disease. Ann Neurol 4:63–66, 1978.

102. Folstein MF and Powell D: Is Alzheimer's disease inherited? A methodological review. Integrative Psychiatry 2:163–176, 1984.

103. Folstein SE: Huntington's disease: A disorder of families. Johns Hopkins University Press, Baltimore, MD 1989.

103a. Folstein SE: The psychopathology of Huntington's disease. In McHugh PR and McKusick VA (eds): Brain and Behavior. Raven Press, New York, 1991, pp 181–191.

104. Folstein SE and Folstein MF: Psychiatric features of Huntington's disease: Recent approaches and findings. Psychiatric Developments 2:193–205, 1983.

105. Forno LS and Alvord EC Jr: The pathology of parkinsonism, Part 1. Some new observations. In McDowell F and Markham C (eds): Recent Advances in Parkinson's Disease. FA Davis, Philadelphia, 1971, pp 120–130.

106. Foster NL, Gilman S, Berent S, and Hichwa RD: Distinctive patterns of cerebral glucose metabolism in progressive supranuclear palsy and Alzheimer's disease studied with positron emission tomography (abstr). Neurology (Suppl 1):36:338, 1986.

107. Friedland RP: Brain imaging and cerebral metabolism. In Boller F and Grafman J (eds): Handbook of Neuropsychology. Elsevier, New York, 1990, pp 197–211.

108. Friedland RP, Budinger TF, Ganz E, et al: Regional cerebral metabolic alterations in dementia of the Alzheimer type: Positron emission tomography with [^{18}F]fluorodeoxyglucose. J Comput Assist Tomogr 7:590–598, 1983.

109. Gajdusek DC: Interference with axonal transport of neurofilament. A common pathogenetic mechanism in

slow virus infections, Alzheimer's disease, amyotrophic lateral sclerosis and mental intoxications of the CNS. Discussions in Neurosciences 3:33–35, 1986.

110. Galasko D, Klauber MR, Hofstetter CR, Salmon DP, Lasker B, and Thal LJ: The Mini-Mental State Examination in the early diagnosis of Alzheimer's disease. Arch Neurol 47: 49–52, 1990.

110a. Gallassi R, Montagna P, Morreale A, et al: Neuropsychological, electroencephalogram and brain computed tomography findings in motor neuron disease. Eur Neurol 25:115–120, 1989.

111. Garron DC: Huntington's chorea and schizophrenia. In Barbeau A, Chase TN, and Paulson GW (eds): Huntington's Chorea. Advances in Neurology, Vol 1. Raven Press, New York, 1973.

112. Geoffroy G, Barbeau A, Breton G, et al: Clinical description and roentgenologic evaluation of patients with Friedreich's ataxia. Can J Neurol Sci 3:279–286, 1976.

113. Gibb WRG: Idiopathic Parkinson's disease and the Lewy body disorders. Neuropathol Appl Neurobiol 12: 223–234, 1986.

114. Gibb WRG, Luthent PJ, and Marsden CD: Corticobasal degeneration. Brain 112:1171–1192, 1989.

115. Gilliam TC, Bucan M, MacDonald ME, et al: A DNA segment in coding two genes very tightly linked to Huntington's disease. Science 238:950–952, 1987.

116. Gilman S, Bloedel JR, and Lechtenberg R: Disorders of the Cerebellum. FA Davis, Philadelphia, 1981, p 194.

117. Girotti F, Soliveri P, Carella F, et al: Dementia and cognitive impairment in Parkinson's disease. J Neuro Neurosurg Psychiatry 51:1498–1502, 1988.

118. Goate AM, Chartier-Harlin M-C, Mullan M, et al: Segregation of a missense mutation in the amyloid precursor protein gene with familial Alzheimer's disease. Nature 349: 704, 1991.

119. Goate AM, Haynes AR, Owen MJ, et al: Predisposing locus for Alzheimer's disease on chromosome 21. Lancet 1:352–355, 1989.

120. Golbe LI: The genetics of Parkinson's disease: A reconsideration. Neurology (Suppl 3)40:7–14, 1990.

121. Golbe LI, Davis PH, Schoenberg BS, and Duvoisin RC: Prevalence and natural history of progressive supranuclear palsy. Neurology 38: 1031–1034, 1988.

122. Goldgaber D, Lerman MI, McBride OW, Saffiotti U, and Gajdusek DC: Characterization and chromosomal localization of a cDNA encoding brain amyloid of Alzheimer's disease. Science 235:877–880, 1987.

123. Goto S and Hirano A: Inhomogeneity of the putaminal lesion in striatonigral degeneration. Acta Neuropathol (Berl) 80:204–207, 1990.

124. Goto S, Hirano A, and Mutsumoto, S: Met-enkephalin immunoreactivity in the basal ganglia in Parkinson's disease and striatonigral degeneration. Neurology 40:1051–1056, 1990.

125. Gowers WR: A lecture on abiotrophy. Lancet 1:1002–1007, 1902.

126. Grafman J, Litvan I, Gomez C, et al: Frontal lobe function in progressive supranuclear palsy. Arch Neurol 47(5):553–558, 1990.

127. Graves AB, van Dujin CM, Chandra V, et al: Alcohol and tobacco consumption as risk factors for Alzheimer's disease: A collaborative reanalysis of case-control studies. Int J Epidemiol 20(2):S48–57, 1991.

128. Green J, Morris JC, Sandson J, et al: Progressive aphasia: A precursor of global dementia? Neurology 40:423–429, 1990.

129. Groen JJ: Hereditary Pick's disease. In Becker PE (ed): Humangenetik: Ein kurzes Handbuch, Vol 5. Georg Thieme Verlag, Stuttgart, West Germany, 1967.

130. Guidetti B and Fraioli B: Neurosurgical treatment of spasticity and dyskinesias. Acta Neurochir Suppl 24:27 39, 1977.

131. Gusella JF, Wexler NS, Conneally

PM, et al: A polymorphic DNA marker genetically linked to Huntington's disease. Nature 306:134–238, 1983.

132. Gustafson L: Frontal lobe degeneration of non-Alzheimer type. II. Clinical picture and differential diagnosis. Archives of Gerontology and Geriatrics 6:209–223, 1987.

133. Haase GR: Diseases presenting as dementia. In Wells CE (ed): Dementia. FA Davis, Philadelphia, 1971, pp 164–207.

134. Hamilton NG, Frick RB, Takahashi T, and Hopping MW: Psychiatric symptoms and cerebellar pathology. Am J Psychiatry 140:1322–1326, 1983.

135. Hansen LA, Deteresa R, Tobias H, et al: Neocortical morphometry and cholinergic neurochemistry in Pick's disease. Am J Pathol 131:507–518, 1988.

136. Hansen LA, Salmon D, Galasko D, et al: The Lewy body variant of Alzheimer's disease: A clinical and pathologic entity. Neurology 40:1–8, 1990.

136a. Hardig AE: Cerebellar and spinocerebellar disorders. In Bradley WG, Daroff RB, Fenichel GM, and Marsden CD (eds): Neurology in Clinical Practice, Vol 2: The Neurological Disorders. Butterworth & Co, Boston, pp 1603–1623, 1989.

137. Hauser WA, Morris ML, Heston LL, and Anderson VE: Seizures and myoclonus in patients with Alzheimer's disease. Neurology 36:1226–1230, 1986.

138. Heath PD, Kennedy P, and Kapur N: Slowly progressive aphasia without generalized dementia. Ann Neurol 13:687–688, 1983.

139. Heath RG, Franklin DE, and Shraberg D: Gross pathology of the cerebellum in patients diagnosed and treated as functional psychiatric disorders. J Nerv Ment Dis 167:585–592, 1979.

140. Heston LL and Mastri AR: Age at onset of Pick's and Alzheimer's dementia: Implications for diagnosis and research. J Gerontol 37:422–424, 1982.

141. Heston LL, Mastri AR, Anderson VE, and White J: Dementia of the Alzheimer type: Clinical genetics, natural history, and associated conditions. Arch Gen Psychiatry 38:1085–1090, 1981.

142. Heston LL, White JH, and Mastri AR: Pick's disease—Clinical genetics and natural history. Arch Gen Psychiatry 44:409–411, 1987.

143. Heyman A, Wilkinson WE, Stafford JA, et al: Alzheimer's disease: A study of epidemiological aspects. Ann Neurol 15:335–341, 1984.

144. Hirano A, Kurland LT, Krooth BS, and Lessell J: Parkinsonism-dementia complex, an endemic disease on the island of Guam. I. Clinical features. Brain 84:642–661, 1961.

145. Hirano A, Malamud N, Elizan TS, and Kurland LT: Amyotrophic lateral sclerosis and parkinsonism-dementia complex on Guam. Arch Neurol 15:35–51, 1966.

146. Hofman A, Schulte W, Tanja TA, et al: History of dementia and Parkinson's disease in 1st-degree relatives of patients with Alzheimer's disease. Neurology 39:1589–1592, 1989.

147. Holmes G: A form of familial degeneration of the cerebellum. Brain 30:466, 1907.

148. Horn S: Some psychological factors in parkinsonism. J Neurol Neurosurg Psychiatry 37:27–31, 1974.

149. Horoupian DS, Thal L, Katsman R, et al: Dementia and motor neuron disease: Morphometric, biochemical, and Golgi studies. Ann Neurol 16:305–313, 1984.

150. Huff FJ, Kalaria RN, Boller F, et al: The neurologic examination in patients with probable Alzheimer's disease. Arch Neurol 44:929–932, 1987.

151. Huff FJ, Becker JT, Belle SH, Nebes RD, Holland AL, and Boller F: Cognitive deficits and clinical diagnosis of Alzheimer's disease. Neurology 37:1119–1124, 1987.

151a. Hulette CM, Earl NL, and Crain BJ: Evaluation of cerebral biopsies for the diagnosis of dementia. Arch Neurol 49:28–31, 1992.

152. Huntington G: On chorea. Adv Neurol 1:33–35, 1872.

153. Hutton JT: Results of clinical assessment for the dementia syndrome: Implications for epidemiologic studies. In Schuman LM and Mortimer JA (eds): The Epidemiology of Dementia. Oxford University Press, New York, 1981, pp 62–69.

154. Jackson JA, Jankovic J, and Ford J: Progressive supranuclear palsy: Clinical features and response to treatment in 16 patients. Ann Neurol 13:273–278, 1983.

155. Jagust WJ, Davies P, Tiller-Borcich JK, and Reed BR: Focal Alzheimer's disease. Neurology 40:14–19, 1990.

156. Jason GW, Pajurkova EM, Suchowersky O, et al: Presymptomatic neuropsychological impairment in Huntington's disease. Arch Neurol 45:769–773, 1988.

157. Jervis GA: Early senile dementia in mongoloid idiocy. Am J Psychiatry 105:102–106, 1948.

158. Jervis GA: Alzheimer's disease. In Minkler J (ed): Pathology of the Nervous System, Vol 2. McGraw-Hill, New York, 1971, pp 1385–1395.

159. Kallman FJ and Sander G: Twin studies on senescence. Am J Psychiatry 106:29–36, 1949.

160. Kamo H, McGeer PL, Harrop R, et al: Positron emission tomography and histopathology in Pick's disease. Neurology 37:439–445, 1987.

161. Kanazawa I, Kwak S, Sasaki H, et al: Studies on neurotransmitter markers of the basal ganglia in Pick's disease, with special reference to dopamine reduction. J Neurol Sci 83:63–74, 1988.

162. Katzman R: Senile dementia of the Alzheimer type—defining a disease. In Maddox GL and Auld E (eds): Proceedings of seminars 1976–1980. Duke University Council on Aging, Durham, NC, 1981, pp 19–40.

163. Katzman R: Differential diagnosis of dementing illness. Neurol Clin 4:329–340, 1986.

163a. Kawabata S, Higgins GA, and Gordon JW: Amyloid plaques, neurofibrillary tangles and neuronal loss in brains of transgenic mice overexpressing a coterminal fragment of human amyloid precursor protein. Nature 354:476–478, 1991.

164. Kaye JA, May C, Atack JR, et al: Cerebrospinal fluid neurochemistry in the myoclonic subtype of Alzheimer's disease. Ann Neurol 24:647–650, 1988.

165. Keschner M, Bender MB, and Strauss I: Mental symptoms in cases of subtentorial tumor. Archives of Neurobiology and Psychiatry 37:1–15, 1937.

165a. Kesslak JP, Malciouglu O, and Cotman CW: Quantification of magnetic resonance scans for hippocampal and parahippocampal atrophy in Alzheimer's disease. Neurology 41:51–54, 1991.

166. Kessler H: Epidemiological studies of Parkinson's disease. III: A community based study. Am J Epidemiol 96:242–254, 1972.

167. Kim RC, Collins GH, Parisi JE, et al: Familial dementia of adult onset with pathologic findings of a non-specific nature. Brain 104:61–78, 1981.

168. Kirschner HS, Tanridag O, Thurman L, et al: Progressive asphasia without dementia: Two cases with focal spongiform degeneration. Ann Neurol 22:527–532, 1987.

169. Kish SJ, Robitaille Y, El-Awar M, et al: Non–Alzheimer-type pattern of brain cholineacetyltransferase reduction in dominantly inherited olivopontocerebellar atrophy. Ann Neurol 26(3):362–367, 1989.

170. Knopman DS, Christensen KJ, Schut LJ, et al: The spectrum of imaging and neuropsychological findings in Pick's disease. Neurology 39:362–368, 1989.

171. Knopman DS, Mastri AR, Frey WH, et al: Dementia lacking distinctive histologic features: A common non-Alzheimer degenerative dementia. Neurology 40:251, 1990.

171a. Knopman DS and Rybert S: A verbal memory test with high predictive accuracy for dementia of the Alzheimer type. Arch Neurol 46:141–145, 1985.

172. Kobayashi K, Kurachi M, Gyoubu T, et al: Progressive dysphasic dementia with localized cerebral atrophy:

Report of an autopsy. Clin Neuropathol 9(5):254–261, 1990.

173. Kolodny EH and Cable WJ: Inborn errors of metabolism. Ann Neurol 11:221–232, 1982.

174. Konigsmark BW and Weiner LP: The olivopontocerebellar atrophies: A review. Medicine 49:227–241, 1970.

175. Kosaka K, Yoshimira M, Ikeda K, and Budka H: Diffuse type of Lewy body disease: Progressive dementia with abundant cortical Lewy bodies and senile changes of varying degree — A new disease? Clin Neuropathol 3: 185–192, 1984.

176. Kraus LJ: Decreased natural killer cell activity in Alzheimer's disease. Soc Neurosci Abstr 9:115, 1984.

176a. Krishnan KRR, Heyman A, Ritchie JC, et al: Depression in early-onset Alzheimer's disease: Clinical and neuroendocrine correlates. Biol Psychiatry 24:337–340, 1988.

177. Kristensen MO: Progressive supranuclear palsy: 20 years later. Acta Neurol Scand 71:177–189, 1985.

178. Kukull WA, Larson EB, Reifler BV, Lampe TH, Yerby M, and Hughes J: Interrater reliability of Alzheimer's disease diagnosis. Neurology 40:257–260, 1990.

179. Kumar A, Koss E, Metzler D, and Moore A: Behavioral symptomatology in dementia of the Alzheimer type. Alz Dis Assoc Disord 2:342–355, 1988.

179a. Kumar A, Schapiro MB, Grady CL, et al: Anatomic, metabolic, neuropsychological and molecular genetic studies of three pairs of identical twins discordant for dementia of the Alzheimer type. Arch Neurol 48: 160–168, 1991.

180. Langston JW, Bollard P, Tetrud JW, and Irwin I: Chronic parkinsonism in humans due to a product of meperidine-analog synthesis. Science 219:979–980, 1983.

181. Lanska DJ, Lavine L, Lanska MJ, and Schoenberg BS: Huntington's disease morality in the United States. Neurology 38:769–772, 1988.

182. Lanska DJ, Lanska MJ, Lavine L, and Schoenberg BS: Conditions associated with Huntington's disease at death: A case-control study. Arch Neurol 45:878–880, 1988.

183. Lanska DJ, Lanska MJ, Lavine L, and Schoenberg BS: Familial progressive subcortical gliosis. Neurology (Suppl 1)39:252, 1989.

184. Lanska DJ and Whitehouse PJ: Huntington's disease. Neurology Neurosurgery Update Series 8(11):1–8, 1989.

185. Lazarus LW, Newton N, Cahler B, et al: Frequency and presentation of depressive symptoms in patients with primary degenerative dementia. Am J Psychiatry 144:41–45, 1987.

186. Leverenz J and Sumi SM: Parkinson's disease in patients with Alzheimer's disease. Arch Neurol 43: 662–664, 1986.

187. Levine DN, Grek A, and Calvanio R: Dementia after surgery for cerebellar stroke: An unrecognized complication of acute hydrocephalus? Neurology 35:568–571, 1985.

188. Lindgren AGH: The patho-anatomical classification of morbus Alzheimer and morbus Pick. Acta Neurol Scand 82:119–152, 1952.

189. Liston EH, Jarvik LF, and Gerson S: Depression in Alzheimer's disease: An overview of adrenergic and cholinergic mechanisms. Compr Psychiatry 28(5):444–457, 1987.

190. Loranger AW, Goodell H, McDowell FH, Lee JE, and Sweet RD: Intellectual impairment in Parkinson's syndrome. Brain 95:405–412, 1972.

191. Luers T and Spatz H: Picksche krankheit (progressive umschriebene grosshirnatrophic). In Scholz W (ed): Handbuch der speziellen pathologischen Anatomie und Histologie, BD 13. Springer-Verlag, Berlin, pp 614–715, 1957.

192. Maher ER and Lees AJ: The clinical features and natural history of the Steele-Richardson-Olszewski syndrome (progressive supranuclear palsy). Neurology 36:1005–1008, 1986.

193. Maher ER, Smith EM, and Lees AJ: Cognitive deficits in the Steele-Richardson-Olszewski syndrome (pro-

gressive supranuclear palsy). J Neurol Neurosurg Psychiatry 48:1234–1239, 1985.

194. Malessa S, Hirsch EC, Cervera P, Duyckaerts C, and Agid Y: Catecholaminergic systems in the medulla oblongata in parkinsonian syndromes: A quantitative immunohistochemical studying Parkinson's disease, progressive supranuclear palsy, and striatonigral degeneration. Neurology 40:1739–1743, 1990.

195. Maloteaux JM, Vanisberg MA, Laterre C, et al: [³H]GBR 12935 binding to dopamine uptake sites: Subcellular localization and reduction in Parkinson's disease and progressive supranuclear palsy. Eur J Pharmacol 156(3):331–340, 1988.

196. Mandell AM, Alexander MP, and Carpenter S: Creutzfeldt-Jakob disease presenting as isolated aphasia. Neurology 39:55–58, 1989.

197. Mann DMA: The neuropathology of Alzheimer's disease: A review with pathogenetic, aetiological and therapeutic considerations. Mech Ageing Dev 3:215–255, 1985.

198. Manuelidis EE, deFigueireda JM, Kim JH, et al: Transmission studies from blood of Alzheimer's disease patients and healthy relatives. Proc Natl Acad Sci USA 85:4898, 1988.

199. Marder K, Flood P, Cote L, and Mayeux R: A pilot study of risk factors for dementia in Parkinson's disease. Mov Disord 5:156–161, 1990.

200. Markesbery WR, Ehmann WD, Hossain TIM, et al: Instrumental neutron activation analysis of brain aluminum in Alzheimer's disease and aging. Ann Neurol 10:511–516, 1981.

201. Martilla RJ and Rinne UK: Dementia in Parkinson's disease. Acta Neurol Scand 54:431–441, 1976.

202. Martilla RJ and Rinne UK: Smoking and Parkinson's disease. Acta Neurol Scand 62:322–325, 1980.

203. Martin JB and Gusella JF: Huntington's disease: Pathogenesis and management. N Engl J Med 315:1267–1276, 1986.

204. Martyn CN, Baker DJ, Osmond C, et al: Geographical relationship between Alzheimer's disease and aluminum in drinking water. Lancet 1:59, 1989.

205. Matison R, Mayeux R, Rosen J, and Fahn S: "Tip-of-the-tongue" phenomenon in Parkinson's disease. Neurology 32:567–570, 1982.

206. May C, Rapoport SI, Tomai P, Chrousos GP, and Gold PW: Cerebrospinal fluid concentrations of corticotropin releasing hormone (CRH) and corticotropin (ACTH) are reduced in patients with Alzheimer's disease. Neurology 7:535–538, 1986.

207. Mayeux R, Chen J, Mirabello E, et al: An estimate of the incidence of dementia in idiopathic Parkinson's disease. Neurology 40:1513–1516, 1990.

207a. Mayeux R, Denero J, Hemenigildo N, et al: A population-based investigation of Parkinson's disease with and without dementia: Relationship to age and gender. Arch Neurol 49:492–497, 1992.

208. Mayeux R, Stern Y, Rosen J, and Benson F: Is "subcortical dementia" a recognizable clinical entity? Ann Neurol 14:278–283, 1983.

209. Mayeux R, Stern Y, Rosen J, and Leventhal J: Depression, intellectual impairment, and Parkinson's disease. Neurology 31:645–650, 1981.

210. Mayeux R, Stern Y, Rosenstein R, et al: An estimate of the prevalence of dementia in idiopathic Parkinson's disease. Arch Neurol 45:260–263, 1988.

211. Mayeux R, Stern Y, Sano M, Cote L, and Williams JBW: Clinical and biochemical correlates of bradyphrenia in Parkinson's disease. Neurology 37:1130–1134, 1987.

212. Mayeux R, Stern Y, and Spanton S: Heterogeneity in dementia of the Alzheimer type: Evidence of subgroups. Neurology 35:453–461, 1985.

213. Mayeux R, Stern Y, and Williams JBW: Clinical and biochemical features of depression in Parkinson's disease. Am J Psychiatry 143:756–759, 1986.

214. McHugh PR and Folstein MF: Psychi-

atric syndromes of Huntington's chorea: A clinical and phenomenologic study. In Benson DF and Blumer D (eds): Psychiatric aspects of neurologic disease. Grune & Stratton, New York, 1975.

215. McKhann G, Drachman D, Folstein M, Katzman R, Price D, and Stadian E: Clinical diagnosis of Alzheimer's disease: Report of the NINCDS-ADRDA work group under the auspices of Department of Health and Human Services Task Force on Alzheimer's Disease. Neurology 34: 939–944, 1984.

216. Meggendorfer F: Uber die hereditare disposition zur dementia senilis. Zeitschrift für Neurologic und Psychiatrie 101:387–405, 1926.

217. Meissen GJ, Meyers RH, Mastromauro CA, et al: Predictive testing for Huntington's disease with use of a linked DNA marker. N Engl J Med 318:535–542, 1988.

217a. Mendez MF, Martin RJ, Smyth KA, and Whitehouse PJ: Psychiatric symptoms associated with Alzheimer's disease. J Neuropsychiatry and Clinical Neuroscience 2:28–33, 1990.

218. Mesulam M-M: Slowly progressive aphasia without generalized dementia. Ann Neurol 11:592–598, 1982.

219. Mesulam M-M: Dementia: Its definition, differential diagnosis and subtypes. JAMA 253:2559–2561, 1985.

220. Mesulam M-M: Primary progressive aphasia — differentiation from Alzheimer's disease. Ann Neurol 2: 533–534, 1987.

221. Metter EJ, Kempler D, Jackson CA, et al: Cerebellar glucose metabolism in chronic aphasia. Neurology 37:1599–1606, 1987.

222. Miller AE, Neighbaur PA, Katzman R, et al: Immunological studies in senile dementia of the Alzheimer type: Evidence for enhanced suppressor cell activity. Ann Neurol 10:506–510, 1981.

223. Mindham RHS: Psychiatric symptoms in parkinsonism. J Neurol Neurosurg Psychiatry 33:188–191, 1970.

224. Mitsuyama Y, Lagaoh H, Ata K, et al: Progressive dementia with motor neuron disease: An additional case report and neuropathological review of 20 cases in Japan. Eur Arch Psychiatry Neurol Sci 235:1–8, 1985.

225. Mitsuyama Y, Takamiya S: Presenile dementia with motor neuron disease. Arch Neurol 36:592–593, 1979.

226. Mjones H: Paralysis agitan, a clinical and genetic study. Acta Psychiatr Scand 54:1–195, 1949.

226a. Mlosh AG: Diagnosis and treatment of Parkinsonian dysarthria. In Kuller WC (ed): Handbook of Parkinson's Disease. Marcel Decker, New York, 1992, pp. 227–254.

227. Montgomery GK and Erickson LM: Neuropsychological perspectives in amyotrophic lateral sclerosis. Neurol Clin 5:61–81, 1987.

228. Morita K, Halya H, Ikeda T, Namba M: Presenile dementia combined with amyotrophy: A review of 34 Japanese cases. Archives of Gerontology and Geriatrics 6:263–277, 1987.

229. Morris JC, Cole M, Banker BQ, and Wright D: Hereditary dysphasic dementia and the Pick-Alzheimer spectrum. Ann Neurol 16:455–466, 1984.

230. Morris JC, Heyman A, Mohs RC, et al: The Consortium to Establish a Registry for Alzheimer's Disease (CERAD). Part I. Clinical and neuropsychological assessment of Alzheimer's disease. Neurology 39:1159–1165, 1989.

231. Morris JC, McKeel DW, Storandt M, et al: Very mild Alzheimer's disease: Informant based clinical, psychometric and pathologic distinction from normal aging. Neurology 41:469–478, 1991.

231a. Morris JC, Mohs RC, Rogers H, et al: The Consortium to Establish a Registry for Alzheimer's Disease (CERAD). Clinical and neuropsychological assessment of Alzheimer's disease. Psychopharmacol Bull 4:641–652, 1988.

231b. Mortimer JA, von Duijn CM, Clayton D, et al: Head trauma as a risk factor for Alzheimer's disease: A collaborative re-analysis of case-control studies. Int J Epidemiol 20(supp 2):528–535, 1991.

232. Mulvihill P and Perry G: Immunoaffinity demonstration that paired helical filaments of Alzheimer disease share epitopes with neurofilaments, MAP2 and tau. Brain Res 484:150–156, 1989.

233. Munoz-Garcia D and Ludwin SK: Classic and generalized variants of Pick's disease: A clinicopathological, ultrastructural, and immunocytochemical comparative study. Ann Neurol 16:467–480, 1984.

234. Munoz-Garcia D and Ludwin SK: Adult-onset neuronal intranuclear hyaline inclusion disease. Neurology 36:785–790, 1986.

235. Murrell J, Martin H, Bernardino G, and Benson D: A mutation in the amyloid precursor protein associated with hereditary Alzheimer's disease. Science 254:97–99, 1991.

236. Nandy K: Brain-reactive antibodies in aging and senile dementia. In Katzman R, Terry RD, and Pick KL (eds): Alzheimer's Disease: Senile Dementia and Related Disorders. Aging, Vol 7. Raven Press, New York, 1978, pp 503–512.

236a. Navarathan DS, Priddle JD, McDonald B, et al: Anomalous molecular form of acetylcholinesterase in cerebrospinal fluid in histologically diagnosed Alzheimer's disease. Lancet 337:447–450, 1991.

237. Naville F: Études sur les complications et les scquelles mentales de l'encéphalite épidémique. La Bradyphrénie. Encéphale 17:369–375, 423–436, 1922.

238. Neary D: Non-Alzheimer dementia. Neurology and Neurosurgery 2:457–459, 1989.

239. Nee LE, Eldridge R, Sunderland T, et al: Dementia of the Alzheimer type: Clinical and family study of 22 twin pairs. Neurology 37:359–363, 1987.

240. Neumann MA: Pick's disease. J Neuropath Exp Neurol 8:255–282, 1949.

241. Neumann MA and Cohn R: Progressive subcortical gliosis: A rare form of pre-senile dementia. Brain 90:405–427, 1967.

242. O'Brien C, Sung JH, McGeachie RE, and Lee MC: Striatonigral degeneration: Clinical, MRI, and pathologic correlation. Neurology 40:710–711, 1990.

243. Office of Technology Assessment, US Congress: Losing a Million Minds: Confronting the Tragedy of Alzheimer's Disease and Other Dementias. Publication No. OTA-BA-323. US Government Printing Office, Washington, DC, 1987.

244. Oliver C and Holland AJ: Down's syndrome and Alzheimer's disease: A review. Psychol Med 16:307–322, 1986.

245. Palmert MR, Usiak M, Mayeux R, Raskind M, Tourtellotte WW, and Younkin SG: Soluble derivatives of the β amyloid protein precursor in cerebrospinal fluid: Alterations in normal aging and in Alzheimer's disease. Neurology 40:1028–1034, 1990.

246. Palo J, Haltia M, Carpenter S, Karpati G, and Mushynski W: Neurofilament subunit-related proteins in neuronal intranuclear inclusions. Ann Neurol 15:322–328, 1984.

247. Papp MI, Kahn JE, and Lantos PL: Glial cytoplasmic inclusions in the CNS of patients with multiple system atrophy (striatonigral degeneration, olivopontocerebellar atrophy and Shy-Drager syndrome). J Neurol Sci 94:79–100, 1989.

248. Parkinson J: An Essay on the Shaking Palsy. Sherwood, Neely and Jones, London, 1817.

248a. Parkinson Study Group: Deprenyl forestalls disability in early Parkinson's disease: A controlled clinical trial. N Engl J Med 321:1364–1371, 1989.

249. Patterson MB, Schnell A, Martin RJ, et al: Assessment of psychiatric symptoms in Alzheimer's disease. J Geriatr Psychiatry Neurol 3:21–30, 1990.

250. Percy AK: The inherited neurodegenerative disorders of childhood: Clinical assessment. J Child Neurol 2:82–97, 1987.

251. Pericak-Vance MA, Bebout JL, Gaskell PC, et al: Linkage studies in fa-

milial Alzheimer's disease: Evidence for chromosome 19 linkage. Am J Hum Genet, 48:1034–1050,1991.

252. Perl DP and Brady AR: Alzheimer's disease: X-ray spectrometric evidence of aluminum accumulation in neurofibrillary angle-bearing neurons. Science 208:297–299, 1980.

253. Perry G, Mulvihill P, Fried VA, Smith HT, Grundke-Iqbal I, and Iqbal K: Immunochemical properties of ubiquitin conjugates in the paired helical filaments of Alzheimer disease. J Neurochem 52:1523–1528, 1989.

253a. Perry TL: Four biochemically different types of dominantly inherited olivopontocerebellar atrophy. Adv Neurol 44:205–216, 1984.

253b. Peterson C, Gibson GE, Blass JP, et al: Altered calcium uptake in cultured skin fibroblasts from patients with Alzheimer's disease. N Engl J Med 312:1063–1064, 1985.

254. Pick A: On the relation between aphasia and senile atrophy of the brain (1892). In Rottenberg DA and Hochberg FH (eds); Schoene WC (trans): Neurological Classics in Modern Translation. Hafner Press, New York, 1977, pp 35–40.

255. Pierot L, Desnos C, Blin J, et al: D1- and D2-type dopamine receptors in patients with Parkinson's disease and progressive supranuclear palsy. J Neurol Sci 86(2–3):291–306, 1988.

255a. Piletz JE, Sarasua P, Whitehouse P, and Chotani M: Intracellular membranes are more fluid in platelets of Alzheimer's disease patients. Neurobiol Aging 12:401–406, 1991.

256. Pillon B, Dubois B, L'Hermitte F, and Agid Y: Heterogeneity of intellectual impairment in progressive supranuclear palsy: Parkinson's disease and Alzheimer's disease. Neurology 36: 1179–1185, 1986.

257. Pillon B, Dubois B, Ploska A, and Agid Y: Severity and specificity of cognitive impairment in Alzheimer's, Huntington's and Parkinson's diseases and progressive supranuclear palsy. Neurology 41: 634–643, 1991.

258. Pirozzolo FJ, Hansch EC, Mortimer JA, et al: Dementia in Parkinson's disease: A neuropsychological analysis. Brain Cogn 1:71–83, 1982.

259. Plum F: Dementia as an approaching epidemic. Nature 279:269, 1979.

260. Podlisny MB, Lee G, and Selkoe DJ: Dosage of the amyloid β precursor protein in Alzheimer's disease. Science 238:669–671, 1987.

261. Poeck K and Luzzatti C: Slowly progressive aphasia in three patients: The problem of accompanying neuropsychological deficit. Brain 111: 151–168, 1988.

262. Pollock M and Hornabrook RW: The prevalence, natural history and dementia of Parkinson's disease. Brain 89:429–448, 1966.

263. Prohovnik I, Smith G, Sackeim HA, Mayeux R, and Stern Y: Gray-matter degeneration in presenile Alzheimer's disease. Ann Neurol 25: 117–124, 1989.

264. Prusiner SB: Prions and neurodegenerative diseases. N Engl J Med 317:1571, 1987.

265. Prusiner SB: Prions Causing Degenerative Neurological Diseases. Ann Rev Med 38:381–398, 1987.

266. Raniero I, May C, Laye JA, Friedland RP, and Rapoport SI: CSF α-MSH in dementia of the Alzheimer type. Neurology 38:1281–1284, 1988.

266a. Rapoport SI, Pettigrew KD, and Schapiro MB: Disconcordance and concordance of dementia of the Alzheimer type (DAT) in monozygotic twins indicate heritable and sporadic forms of Alzheimer's disease. Neurology 41:1549–1553, 1991.

267. Rasool CG and Selkoe DJ: Sharing of specific antigens by degenerating neurons in Pick's disease and Alzheimer's disease. N Engl J Med 312:700–705, 1985.

268. Rebeiz JJ, Kolodny EH, and Richardson EP Jr: Corticodentatonigral degeneration with neuronal achromasia. Arch Neurol 18:20–33, 1968.

269. Reding M, Haycox J, Blass J, et al: Depression in patients referred to a dementia clinic: A three-year prospective study. Arch Neurol 42:894–896, 1985.

270. Reifler BV, Larson E, and Hanley R: Coexistence of cognitive impairment and depression in geriatric outpatients. Am J Psychiatry 139:623–625, 1982.

271. Reifler BV, Larson E, Teri L, and Paulsen M: Dementia of the Alzheimer's type and depression. J Am Geriatr Soc 34:855–859, 1986.

272. Reisberg B, Borwenstein J, Salah SP, et al: Behavioral symptoms in Alzheimer's disease: Phenomenology and treatment. J Clin Psychiatry 48:9–15, 1987.

273. Rekatc HL, Grubb RL, Aram DM, et al: Muteness of cerebellar origin. Arch Neurol 42:697–698, 1985.

274. Reyes MG, Lang AE, Lewis A, et al: Dementia of the Alzheimer's type and Huntington's disease. Neurology 35:273–277, 1985.

274a. Riley DE and Lang AE: Movement disorders. In Bradley WG, Daroff RB, Fenichel GM, and Marsden CD (eds): Neurology in Clinical Practice. Butterworth & Co, Boston, MA, 1989, pp 1572–1575.

275. Riley DE, Lang AE, Lewis A, et al: Cortical-basal ganglionic degeneration. Neurology 40:1203–1212, 1990.

276. Risberg J: Frontal lobe degeneration of non-Alzheimer type III. Regional cerebral blood flow. Archives of Gerontology and Geriatrics 6:225–233, 1987.

277. Roberts AH: Brain Damage in Boxers. Pittman, London, 1969.

277a. Roberts GW, Allsop D, Bruton C: The occult aftermath of boxing. J Neurol Neurosurg Psychiatry 53:373–378, 1990.

278. Rocca WA, Amaducci LA, Schoenberg BS, et al: Epidemiology of clinically diagnosed Alzheimer's disease. Ann Neurol 19:415–424, 1986.

279. Rogers D, Lees AJ, Trimble M, and Stern GM: Concept of bradyphrenia: A neuropsychiatric approach. In Yahr MD and Bergmann KJ (eds): Advances in Neurology. Raven Press, New York, 1986, pp 447–450.

280. Rosenberg RN: Amyotrophy in multisystem genetic diseases. In Rowland LP (ed): Human Motor Neuron Diseases. Raven Press, New York, 1982, pp 149–157.

281. Rossor M, Garrett NJ, Johnson AL, et al: A postmortem study of the cholinergic and GABA systems in senile dementia. Brain 105:313–330, 1982.

282. Rossor MN, Iversen LL, Reynolds GP, Mountjoy C, and Roth M: Neurochemical characteristics of early and late onset types of Alzheimer's disease. BMJ 288:961–964, 1984.

283. Rowland LP: Diverse forms of motor neuron diseases. In Rowland LP (ed): Human Motor Neuron Diseases. Raven Press, New York, 1982, pp 1–11.

284. Ruberg M, Javoy-Agid F, Hirsch E, and Scatton B: Dopaminergic and cholinergic lesions in progressive supranuclear palsy. Ann Neurol 18:523–529,1985.

285. Rubin EH, Drevetz WC, Burke WJ, et al: The nature of psychotic symptoms in senile dementia of the Alzheimer type. J Geriatr Psychiatry Neurol 1:16–20, 1988.

286. Ryden MB: Aggressive behavior in persons with dementia who live in the community. Alz Dis Assoc and Disord 2:342–355, 1988.

287. St George-Hyslop PH, Tanzi RE, Polinsky RJ, et al: The genetic defect causing familial Alzheimer's disease maps on chromosome 21. Science 235:885–890, 1987.

287a. Schmahmann JD: An emerging concept: The cerebellar contribution to higher function. Arch Neurol 48:1178–1187, 1991.

288. Selkoe DJ: Beta-amyloid precursor protein of Alzheimer's disease occurs as a 110- to 135-kilodalton membrane-associated protein in neural and non-neural tissues. Proc Natl Acad Sci U S A 85:7341, 1988.

289. Seltzer B and Sherwin I: A comparison of clinical features in early and late onset primary degenerative dementia. Arch Neurol 40:143–146, 1983.

290. Shibasaki H, Tsuji S, Kuroiwa Y, et al: Oculomotor abnormalities in Parkinson's disease. Arch Neurol 36:360–364, 1979.

291. Sims NR, Bowen DM, Smith CC, et al:

Glucose metabolism and acetylcholine synthesis in relation to neuronal activity in Alzheimer's disease. Lancet 1:333–335, 1980.

292. Sisodia SS, Koo EH, Beyreuther K, Unterbeck A, and Price L: Evidence that β-amyloid protein in Alzheimer's disease is not derived by normal processing. Science 248: 492–495, 1990.

293. Small GW, Jarvik LF: The dementia syndrome. Lancet 2:1443–1446, 1982.

294. Smith WT, Turner E, Sim M, et al: Cerebral biopsy in the investigation of presenile dementia. II. Pathological aspects. Br J Psychiatry 112:127–133, 1966.

294a. Sparks DL, VanWoeltz M, and Markesbery R: Alteration in brain monoamine oxidase activity in aging, Alzheimer's disease and Pick's disease. Arch Neurol 48:718–721, 1991.

295. Spitzer, RL: DSM-III-R Case Book: A Learning Companion to the Diagnostic and Statistical Manual of Mental Disorders, Ed 3. American Psychiatric Press, Washington, DC, 1989.

296. Steele JC, Richardson JC, and Olszewski J: Progressive supranuclear palsy. Arch Neurol 10:333–359, 1964.

297. Storandt M, Botwinick RJ, Danziger WL, et al: Psychometric differentiation of mild senile dementia of the Alzheimer type. Arch Neurol 41: 497–499, 1984.

298. Stoudemire A, Hill C, Gulley LR, and Morris R: Neuropsychological and biomedical assessment of depression-dementia syndromes. Journal of Neuropsychiatry and Clinical Neurosciences 1:347–361, 1989.

298a. Stumpf DA: Friedreich's ataxia and other ataxias. In Tyler HR and Dawson DM (eds): Current Neurology Vol 1. Houghton Mifflin, Boston, 1978, pp 86–110.

299. Sulkava R, Haltia M, Paetau A, et al: Accuracy of clinical diagnosis in primary degenerative dementia: Correlation with neuropathologic findings. J Neurol Neurosurg Psychiatry 46:9–13, 1983.

300. Sung JH, Ramirez-Lassepas M, Mastri AR, and Larkin SM: An unusual degenerative disorder of neurons associated with a novel intranuclear hyaline inclusion (neuronal intranuclear hyaline inclusion disease). J Neuropathol Exp Neurol 39(2):107–130, 1980.

301. Tabaton M, Cammarata S, Mancardi GL, Cordone G, Perry G, and Loeb C: Abnormal tau-reactive filaments in olfactory mucosa in biopsy specimens of patients with probable Alzheimer's disease. Neurology 41: 391–394, 1991.

302. Tabaton M, Whitehouse PJ, Perry G, et al: ALZ 50 recognizes abnormal filaments in Alzheimer's disease and progressive supranuclear palsy. Ann Neurol 24:407–413, 1988.

303. Takahashi H, Oyanagi K, Takeda S, et al: Occurrence of 15-nm-wide straight tubules in neocortical neurons in progressive supranuclear palsy. Acta Neuropathol (Berl) 79(3): 233–239, 1989.

304. Talamo BR, Rudel RA, Kosik KS, et al: Pathological changes in olfactory neurons in patients with Alzheimer's disease. Nature 337:736–739, 1989.

305. Talland GA: Cognitive function in Parkinson's disease. J Nerv Ment Dis 135:196–205, 1962.

306. Tanzi RE, Bird ED, Latt SA, and Neve RL: The amyloid β protein gene is not duplicated in brains from patients with Alzheimer's disease. Science 238:666–669, 1987.

307. Tanzi RE, St. George-Hyslop PH, Haines JL, et al: The genetic defect in familial Alzheimer's disease is not tightly linked to the amyloid beta protein gene. Nature 329:156, 1987.

308. Tetrud JW, Langston JW: The effect of Deprenyl (selegiline) on the natural history of Parkinson's disease. Science 245:519–522, 1989.

309. Teuber H and Proctor F: Some effects of basal ganglia lesions in subhuman primates and man. Neuropsychologic 2:85–93, 1964.

310. Therapeutics and Technology Assessment Subcommittee of the American Academy of Neurology: As-

sessment: Positron emission tomography. Neurology 1:163–167, 1991.

311. Thompson RF: The neurobiology of learning. Science 233:941, 1986.

312. Tierney MC, Fisher RH, Lewis AJ, et al: The NINCDS-ADRDA work group criteria for the clinical diagnosis of probable Alzheimer's disease: A clinicopathologic study of 57 cases. Neurology 38:359–364, 1988.

313. Tyler HR: Nonfamilial amyotrophy with dementia or multisystem degeneration and other neurological disorders. In Rowland LP (ed): Human Motor Neuron Diseases. Raven Press, New York, 1982, pp 173–179.

314. Uhl GR, Hilt DC, Hedreen JC, Whitehouse PJ, and Price DL: Pick's disease (lobar sclerosis): Depletion of neurons in the nucleus basalis of Meynert. Neurology 3:1470–1473, 1983.

314a. VanGool WA and Bolhuis PA: Cerebrospinal fluid markers of Alzheimer's disease. JAGS, 39:1025–1039, 1991.

315. Verity A and Wechsler AF. Progressive subcortical gliosis of Neumann: A clinicopathologic study of two cases with review. Archives Gerontology and Geriatrics 6:245–261, 1987.

316. Villardita C, Smirni P, lePira F, et al: Mental deterioration, visuoperceptive disabilities and constructional apraxia in Parkinson's disease. Acta Neurol Scand 66:112–120, 1982.

317. Vonsattel JP, Myers RH, Stevens TJ, et al: Neuropathological classification of Huntington's disease. J Neuropathol Exp Neurol 44:559–577, 1985.

318. Wallesch CW and Fehrenbach RA: On the neurolinguistic nature of language abnormalities in Huntington's disease. J Neurol Neurosurg Psychiatry 51:367–373, 1988.

319. Ward CD, Duvoisin RC, Ince SE, et al: Parkinson's disease in 65 pairs of twins and in a set of quadruplets. Neurology 33:815–824, 1983.

320. Wechsler AF: Presenile dementia presenting as aphasia. J Neurol Neurosurg Psychiatry, 40:303–305, 1977.

321. Wechsler AF, Verity MA, Rosenschein S, Fried I, and Scheibel AB: Pick's disease: A clinical, computed tomographic, and histological study with Golgi impregnation observations. Arch Neurol 39:287–290, 1982.

322. Weintraub S, Rubin NP, and Mesulam M-M: Primary progressive aphasia: Longitudinal course, neuropsychological profile, and language features. Arch Neurol 47:1329–1335, 1990.

323. Wells CE: The symptoms and behavioral manifestations of dementia. In Wells CE (ed): Dementia. FA Davis, Philadelphia, 1971, pp 2–11.

324. Whitehouse PJ: Understanding the etiology of Alzheimer's disease. Neurol Clin 4:427–437, 1986.

325. Whitehouse PJ, Martino AM, Antuono PG, et al: Nicotinic acetylcholine binding sites in Alzheimer's disease. Brain Res 371:146–151, 1986.

326. Wikstrom J, Pateau A, Palo J, et al: Classic amyotrophic lateral sclerosis with dementia. Arch Neurol 39:681–683, 1982.

327. Wilson RS, Kazniak AW, Klawans HL, and Garron DC: High speed memory scanning in parkinsonism. Cortex 16:67–72, 1980.

328. Wilson SAK: Neurology, Vol 2. Williams & Wilkins, Baltimore, MD, 1941.

329. Wisniewski HM, Yen GW, and Lidskey AA: Aluminum-induced neurofibrillary changes in rabbit retina: ERG and morphological studies. J Neuropathol Exp Neurol 37:708, 1978.

330. Wisniewski KE and Wisniewski HM: Age associated changes and dementia in Down's syndrome. In Reisberg R (ed): Alzheimer's Disease: The Standard Reference. Free Press, New York, 1983, pp 319–326.

331. Wisniewski KE, Wisniewski HM, and Wen GY: Occurrence of neuropathological changes and dementia of Alzheimer's disease in Down's syndrome. Ann Neurol 17:278–282, 1985.

332. Wolozin BL and Davies P: Alzheimer related protein A68: Alzheimer spe-

cific accumulation and detection in cerebrospinal fluid. Ann Neurol 22:521–526, 1987.

333. Wolozin BL, Pruchnicki A, Dickson DW, and Davies P: A neuronal antigen in the brains of Alzheimer patients. Science 232:648–650, 1986.

334. Yates CM, Simpson J, Maloney AF, and Gordon A: Neurochemical observations in a case of Pick's disease. J Neurol Sci 48(2):257–263, 1980.

335. Yen SH, Dikran S, Houroupian MD, and Terry R: Immunocytochemical comparison of neurofibrillary tangles in senile dementia of Alzheimer type. Progressive supranuclear palsy and postencephalitic parkinsonism. Ann Neurol 13:172–175, 1983.

336. Yoshimura M: Cortical changes in the parkinsonian brain: A contribution to the delineation of "diffuse Lewy body disease." J Neurol 229:17–32, 1983.

337. Zubenko GS and Moossy J: Major depression in primary dementia: Clinical and neuropathological correlates. Arch Neurol 45:1182–1186, 1988.

338. Zubenko GS, Moossy J, and Kopp U: Neurochemical correlates of major depression in primary dementia. Arch Neurol 47:209–214, 1990.

339. Zubenko GS, Moossy J, Martinez AJ, et al: Neuropathologic and neurochemical correlates of psychosis in primary dementia. Arch Neurol 48: 619–624, 1991.

339a. Zubenko GS, Weysylko M, Cohen BM, and Boller F: Family study of platelet membrane fluidity in Alzheimer's disease. Science 238:539, 1987.

340. Zweig RM, Ross CA, and Hedreen JC: The neuropathology of aminergic nuclei in AD. Ann Neurol 24:233–242, 1988.

Chapter 7

VASCULAR DEMENTIAS

John Marshall, M.D.

**MULTI-INFARCT DEMENTIA
BINSWANGER'S DISEASE
DISORDERS OF CEREBRAL BLOOD
    FLOW**

Pathologists of the 19th century laid great emphasis on cerebral arteriosclerosis as a cause of dementia, recognizing various morphologic types, although not always relating the histologic changes to etiology, as would be done today. Among these was arteriocapillary fibrosis, described by Gull[31] in 1872. This was characterized by intimal thickening, reduplication of the elastic lamina, and hypertrophy of the muscular coat, affecting mainly small arteries and arterioles and leading to occlusion of the latter. Its association with left ventricular hypertrophy and renal sclerosis indicates that it was what would now be called hypertensive vascular disease. The studies of Charcot and Bouchard[12] had previously revealed the development of microaneurysms on the striate arteries in this type of vascular disease.

The status of senile, involutional, or decrescent arteriosclerosis of Allbutt[2] as a separate disease entity is less clear. The muscular layer of medium and larger arteries was atrophied and replaced by connective tissue. There was patchy overgrowth of the intima with fatty change, calcification, loss of endothelium, and thrombus formation, a picture that probably mainly represented atheromatous change.

The link between the changes in the vessels and those in the parenchyma was far from clear, particularly because the distinction between vascular disease and Alzheimer's disease (AD) had not yet been made. The état criblé described by Durand-Fardel[18] consisted of numerous minute spaces around small arteries, giving cribriform appearance to the parenchyma. The spaces probably arose from damage to perivascular tissue caused by the effects of pulsation of arteries that had lost their elasticity.

This condition was distinguished from the état lacunaire described by Marie,[49] in which small areas of softening less than 1 cm in diameter were found mainly in the distribution of the striate arteries (Fig. 7–1). Many years later, Miller Fisher[22] showed these to be associated with occlusion of small vessels, the walls of which were affected by hypertensive lipohyalinosis and fibrinoid necrosis. It is this condition that is most relevant to the present consideration of vascular dementia.

In addition to these more gross changes, diffuse cellular changes in response to ischemia came to be recognized. Nerve cells appeared shrunken, with small, dark-staining nuclei and cytoplasm that stained poorly with basic dyes and appeared eosinophilic on hematoxylin-and-eosin staining. Microglia increased, and subsequently there was shrinkage of tissue and gliosis.

Against this background of prolific morphologic observations with rather

215

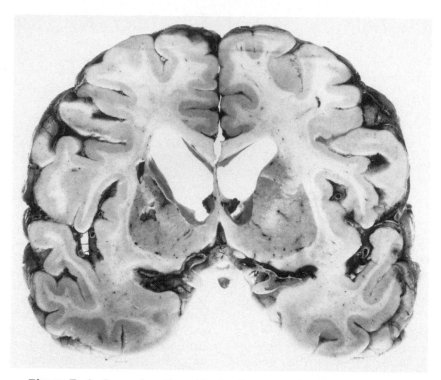

Figure 7–1. Coronal section of brain showing multiple small lacunes.

tenuous links to pathogenesis, clinical practice responded with an ill-founded certainty. Dementia in the older age groups was firmly attributed to "cerebral arteriosclerosis," the term "arteriosclerotic dementia" being freely applied. The diagnosis carried with it the underlying assumption that arteriosclerotic changes in cerebral arteries gradually starved the brain of its blood supply and so caused dementia. The unwarranted nature of this assumption is dealt with later in the chapter, on page 224.

It must of course be remembered that in 1907, when Alzheimer[3] described the condition that bears his name, it was considered to be a disease of the presenium. The fact that it occurs in the older age groups and, indeed, is the major cause of mental deterioration in the later decades, was not appreciated. Moreover, intellectual decline, when present, was often attributed to the arteriopathy and even to one or two small

areas of softening often found in the brains of older people. In 1977, in an earlier book in this series, Tomlinson[80] lamented that "the tendency to ascribe dementia to the ischemic lesion is common among clinicians and pathologists." As late as 1983, the journal *Stroke* published an article entitled "Vascular Dementia — Still Overdiagnosed."[11]

The difficulty of diagnosing vascular dementia was compounded by the problem of distinguishing changes caused by disease, be it Alzheimer's or vascular, from those attributable to normal aging. This problem was encountered in both clinical assessment and morphologic studies. What degree of memory impairment is part of the normal aging process? How many senile plaques or what volume of cerebral softening can be accepted as a normal accompaniment of aging?

Clarification of these issues has gradually been achieved during the last two decades. Recognition of the fact that AD is the major cause of dementia in old age has been a major step forward, enabling study of vascular dementia to be concentrated on cases that truly have vascular dementia and not AD with some concomitant vascular changes. The introduction of techniques for measuring cerebral blood flow and metabolism has contributed to the elucidation of the mechanism by which dementia is produced in patients with cerebral vascular disease. The pathologic studies of Tomlinson and colleagues[81,82] and the emphasis given by Hachinski and his associates[33] to the role of multiple small infarcts in the genesis of dementia have helped to link the clinical, pathologic, and metabolic aspects of vascular dementia.

MULTI-INFARCT DEMENTIA

The most common cause of vascular dementia is loss of cerebral parenchyma through multiple small infarctions in subjects who are usually hypertensive. Other causes of vascular dementia will also be addressed in this chapter, but the main focus will be on multi-infarct dementia (MID), the second most common cause of dementia in the elderly.

Epidemiology and Risk Factors

Despite the increasing importance of dementia as a medical and social problem in developed countries, reliable data about its epidemiology are as yet sparse.[55] This is particularly true in the case of vascular dementia. Several factors have contributed to this lack of data. First is the problem of distinguishing dementia from the decline in mental function that may accompany normal aging. Even when armed with an acceptable definition, there is the operational problem of applying it to individual cases. Furthermore, it is a problem

to ascertain in the community a condition which is not easily recognized in its milder forms, and, when recognized, may be concealed.

These difficulties are compounded when an effort is made to determine the epidemiology of a specific form of dementia such as MID. Even if all the cases of dementia in a defined population could be reliably ascertained, the problem would remain of distinguishing those caused by MID from those attributable to other causes, in particular AD. Differentiation on clinical grounds alone, although improving, is far from perfect. The use of neuroimaging can increase the reliability of the diagnosis but as yet can only be applied to small numbers of cases. Despite these difficulties, anatomico-clinical studies using discriminant function analysis have shown that vascular dementia can be distinguished from other forms, with a high degree of reliability.[79]

For these reasons, the available information on the epidemiology of MID is based largely on hospital series and autopsy studies, with all the epidemiologic limitations these types of data impose. Among the more useful clinical data is a series of 106 cases with an initial diagnosis of dementia, reported by Marsden and Harrison.[50] First to be noted is that 15 were in fact not demented, 8 of whom suffered from depression. In 28, a firm "neurologic" diagnosis was made, such as neoplasm, Creutzfeldt-Jakob disease, and so on. This high proportion likely reflects the fact that the series is from a neurologic hospital. There were 8 cases called "arteriosclerotic dementia" (which would now be called MID), and 48 labeled cerebral atrophy of unknown cause." The majority of these latter cases were undoubtedly examples of AD. Thus approximately 8% of the series had MID.

Contributing to the problem is the fact that cerebral biopsy is thought to be justified only in selected cases. Also, because of the distribution of the lesions, the result is more likely to be positive in AD or viral illness than in MID, in which the lacunes are situated deep in the cerebral hemispheres. Thus biopsy series report a preponderance of cases of AD.[13,71,72]

Perhaps the most satisfactory studies from the epidemiologic standpoint have been those of Roth, Tomlinson, and colleagues.[81,82] Interviews were conducted on a random sample of 309 people over age 65 living at home, to determine whether or not they had a mental disorder and, if so, of what type. Simultaneously, a census of individuals in hospitals or nursing homes within the area was carried out and interviews conducted. Organic brain disease was found to be present in 10%. What the authors referred to as senile and arteriosclerotic syndromes were equally present, although there was an excess of arteriosclerotic syndromes in men.[42] The diagnoses were based on carefully applied clinical criteria.

These clinical observations were followed by pathologic studies of the brain of mentally normal and of demented old people from the same community.[81,82] Among the 50 demented, 50% were judged to have AD; 12% to have certain MID, and 5%, probable; 8% had both AD and MID. Thus the more exacting pathologic criteria indicate that in sound terms alone, 20% of organic dementia in the older age groups is caused by MID.[16]

The risk factors for MID are essentially those for cerebrovascular disease.[41] Among these is age; MID appears mainly in those 60 to 75 years old. Precise figures are not available, but there is an impression that the proportion of MID in the demented population over age 75 falls, presumably because those at risk have died of some form of vascular accident, MID being part of vascular disease as a whole. Vascular dementia is not seen in younger people except in association with specific conditions such as systemic lupus erythematosus, large arteriovenous malformations, and other disorders discussed later in this chapter.

The incidence of MID is slightly higher among men than among women.

Among the preventable risk factors, hypertension is paramount. Indeed, it is uncommon to encounter MID in someone who is not hypertensive. When this does occur, it is usually in relation to a specific condition giving rise to multiple small-vessel occlusions.

The other risk factors for cerebrovascular disease in general, such as abnormal lipid levels, glucose intolerance, obesity, and cigarette smoking, do not appear to carry any specific predisposition to MID. The level of hematocrit may, however, be an exception. There is evidence that a raised hematocrit is associated with impaired psychological function, which improves after venesection.[89] Prolonged exposure to a raised hematocrit level might produce irreversible change.

Finally, clinical observation of mental change in early heart failure and data on cerebral blood flow (CBF) suggest that impaired cerebral perfusion associated with cardiac failure may be a risk factor. The etiologic role of impaired cerebral perfusion will be discussed later.

Genetics

There is no evidence of a specific genetic factor for MID. As explained above, the main risk factors for MID are age and hypertension. Hypertension itself has a multifactorial genetic predisposition, but the reasons some untreated hypertensives succumb to left ventricular failure, others to renal failure, others to cerebral hemorrhage, and still others to MID does not appear to be genetically determined.

Clinical Features

MID may present in a variety of ways, depending on the sites of the earliest infarcts. It is generally uncommon for all the early lesions to develop in neurologically "silent" areas. When this does occur, the cumulative loss of parenchyma reaches the point at which dementia is the sole presentation. More frequently, one or more of the earliest lesions gives rise to a neurologic event or deficit that prompts the patient or family to seek medical attention. At this stage, careful examination may reveal a degree of memory and cognitive impairment that had hitherto escaped notice.

A typical event bringing the patient to attention is an episode of so-called confusion. This term fails to denote the precise nature of the disturbance. Most often, it refers to loss of orientation for place or time. This results in inappropriate behavior such as wandering in the night, which is labeled as confusion. Alternatively, there may be a specific neurologic defect, such as apraxia for dressing, or loss of topographical orientation, so that the patient loses his way in familiar surroundings. These and many other specific neurologic deficits are mistakenly labeled as confusion. Transient dysphasic difficulties, especially receptive, are particularly liable to similar mislabeling. This point is of importance because, without precise diagnosis, there is danger of overlooking other causes of specific neurologic defects, or of general metabolic upsets, such as uremia.

Gait disturbance is another presenting complaint. This is typically the "marche à petits pas" characterized by short, shuffling, and often rapid steps. The feet are slightly apart, though not grossly so, as in an ataxic gait. The posture is usually upright or slightly tilted backwards, in contrast to parkinsonism, in which there is usually a flexed posture.

Yet another presentation may involve pseudobulbar palsy. The patient may previously have experienced a mild stroke that passed almost unnoticed. A second contralateral stroke, which again may have been mild in itself, gives rise to a pseudobulbar picture, with heightened emotional response that the patient finds difficult to control, difficulty swallowing, and altered voice.

The development of extrapyramidal features is yet another way in which MID may present. The patient's physical and mental activities are noted to have become slower, with some loss of facial expression and a shuffling gait. Formal examination reveals general slowness of movement and a degree of extrapyramidal rigidity.

Finally, urinary difficulties may be the reason for the patient's seeking clinical attention.[45] Frequency, urgency, and incontinence may develop. In men, these may be attributed to prostatic hypertrophy and in women, to vaginal prolapse, but frequently the difficulties are neurologic in origin.

The dementia itself, though sharing features with other forms of dementia, has a characteristic overall pattern. Memory impairment is an early and cardinal feature. Typically, recent memory is most affected, the patient forgetting where he has put things, arrangements for the day, and recent instructions. There is no confabulation to cover up the deficit, which is a source of embarrassment and anxiety for the patient. In contrast, long-term memory is preserved, events from early life being retained and accurately recalled.

Cognitive tests are affected in patchy fashion. The patient is unable to cope with money transactions, calculations, forms to be completed, or written instructions. He has difficulty dealing with new and unfamiliar situations and cannot readily learn new material.

Impaired emotional control is a striking feature. The patient is easily moved to tears and is unable to control this manifestation in circumstances in which he formerly would have done so. Even more embarrassing is inappropriate emotional response, such as laughter in serious situations.

Preoccupation with real or imagined somatic symptoms is frequently present and may lead to numerous medical consultations to no avail, particularly if the underlying dementia is not recognized.

Judgment becomes impaired and may lead to imprudent statements, unwise financial decisions, or social gaffes. As the disease progresses, disinhibition may develop and lead to uncharacteristic sexual misdemeanors.

Most of these manifestations also

**Table 7–1 DIAGNOSTIC FEATURES
OF MULTI-INFARCT DEMENTIA**

Hypertension
Age 60–75 years
Abrupt onset, often associated with neurologic incident
Stepwise progression
Frequent impairment of emotional control
Relative preservation of personality
Mild but definite neuropsychological and neurologic abnormalities

occur in other forms of dementia. The feature that distinguishes MID is the relatively abrupt onset, often associated with some neurologic incident such as a transient ischemic attack, and the stepwise progression. Unlike with AD, relatives of MID victims are often able to date the onset of decline, although careful questioning may reveal earlier changes that were unremarked. MID may also show short periods of improvement within the overall picture of general decline.

A further distinguishing feature is the relative preservation of the personality. The patient still gives the impression of being someone with a distinctive personality who communicates and establishes a degree of relationship, whereas in AD the personality becomes dimmed, and one has a feeling of no longer talking to a person. The relative preservation of personality in MID is accompanied by a degree of insight into failing capacity, which is a source of distress to the patient.

At the time the patient comes for evaluation, examination of the physical as well as the mental state is often helpful diagnostically. The patient is almost always hypertensive and may show evidence that this has been longstanding, with changes in the retinal arteries and left ventricular hypertrophy.

On neurologic examination, there may be traces of a mild residual hemiparesis with slight increase of tone, asymmetry of the tendon reflexes, and an equivocal or extensor plantar response. Alternatively, signs suggestive of pseudobulbar palsy may be present,

with dysarthria and brisk jaw jerk and brisk tendon reflexes bilaterally.

The gait may be abnormal with a marche à petits pas, or there may be a suggestion of extrapyramidal rigidity. Resistance to passive movement of the limbs, which seems almost voluntary but is not (gegenhalten), may be present.

Often present, but equally often overlooked, are neuropsychological deficits such as various forms of agnosia (in particular, visual), apraxtic difficulties, elements of dysphasia, and problems with topography and orientation.

In summary, MID, although sharing features with other forms of dementia as well as with other types of cerebrovascular diseases, has a constellation of features that in most instances make it readily recognizable. These features are listed in Table 7–1.

These distinguishing characteristics are so constant that they have been incorporated by Hachinski and colleagues[32] into an "ischemic score." (See Chapter 1, Table 1–9.) The systematic observation of factors such as abrupt onset, stepwise progression, and emotional incontinence is associated with evidence of cerebrovascular disease. A score of 4 or less makes it highly likely that the patient is not suffering from MID. In practical terms, this means that he or she has AD. A score of 6 or more suggests MID. The score has been validated by autopsy[68] and other studies, and its wide use indicates that it has been found to be of practical value. There is some overlap, of course, as some patients have the changes of both

MID and Alzheimer's, but this does not occur with sufficient frequency to deprive the Hachinski score of its value in clinical practice.

The time course of MID is extremely variable, depending on the occurrence of unpredictable cerebrovascular and cardiovascular events. It is these, rather than the dementia itself, that determine the life span. Of 115 cases of MID, 12% were alive after 6 years, as against an expected survival of 45%. This contrasted with 218 cases of AD, in which 21% survived 6 years against 48% expected. On the other hand, the mean duration of survival for MID and Alzheimer's was 5.2 and 5.7 years, respectively.[54] Among the MID patients, 40% were said to have died of "dementia," the effective cause appearing to be bronchopneumonia. Thirty percent died of a cerebrovascular accident; surprisingly, no mention was made of cardiac deaths.

In another series,[8] 50% of cases of MID survived 6.7 years from onset, compared with 8.1 years for AD. The cause of death was not reported.

Neuropsychology

Neuropsychological testing plays an important role in the diagnosis and management of MID. It must be made clear at the outset, however, that there are no neuropsychological deficits specific to vascular disease. Individual deficits are related to the site of lesions, not to their pathology. Nevertheless, since vascular lesions show a predilection for certain sites because of the anatomy of the cerebral circulation and the presence or absence of collateral vessels, a characteristic overall pattern of neuropsychological deficits is often present in vascular dementia.

The lesions underlying MID are usually small lacunar infarcts deep in the white matter in the distribution of the striate arteries. Isolated lacunes cause no demonstrable deficit unless they happen to be in a "neurologically eloquent" area such as the ventrolateral nucleus of the thalamus, giving a hemisensory deficit,[21] or the internal capsule, producing a pure motor hemiplegia.[24] These are examples of the so-called lacunar syndromes described by Fisher.[23]

When lacunes are confined to "silent" areas, they produce no demonstrable effect until their aggregate volume is sufficient to impair memory and cognitive function, which will be reflected in the results of psychological tests such as the Wechsler Adult Intelligence Scale (WAIS). Such general impairment of memory and cognitive function is uncommon in MID because the development of the dementia is usually interspersed with minor vascular events, giving rise to transient or permanent neurologic and neuropsychological deficits. Just as careful neurologic examination of a patient with MID can reveal mild but definite neurologic signs, so skilled neuropsychological testing can uncover dysphasic, apraxic, and agnostic difficulties.

Cortical infarcts are particularly liable to develop in the posterior cerebral territory and in the watershed areas between the middle and posterior cerebral arteries, so that subtle and sometimes bizarre manifestations of visual function are not uncommon.[70] Apart from classical hemianopsia, the patient may present with cortical blindness, loss of ability to recognize faces or colors, and other forms of visual agnosia. Because however, the specific nature of the deficit is often undiagnosed, however, the patient may simply be described as "confused."

Involvement of the parietal lobe of the minor hemisphere can give rise to topographic and constructional deficits. Although many functions may be involved, lesions in the major hemisphere may produce highly discrete deficits, such as dyslexia without dysgraphia, sometimes called "pure word blindness."

The overall picture of MID is therefore general impairment of memory and cognitive function with additional specific neuropsychological deficits of "cortical" type. The other characteristic feature is the tendency of the deficits to wax and wane.

Neuroimaging

Neuroimaging has an important role in the diagnosis of vascular dementia, apart from its general value in excluding unexpected, space-occupying lesions in neurologically silent areas of the brain, subdural hematomas, and normal pressure hydrocephalus, all of which may present with dementia. (See also Chapter 4.)

COMPUTED TOMOGRAPHY

Computed tomography (CT) scanning may show evidence of cerebral atrophy with ventricular enlargement and widening of cortical sulci. This appearance is common to cerebral atrophy from any cause. In MID, however, some infarcts, large or small, probably will also be seen as low-density lesions. These are most commonly lacunar in type and are seen deep in the white matter (Fig. 7–2).

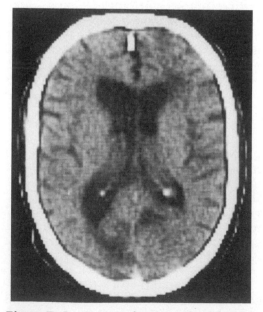

Figure 7–2. CT scan showing enlarged ventricles, widened cortical sulci, and multiple lacunar infarcts.

They may be associated with one or more small cortical infarcts.

A single lacune does not establish the diagnosis of MID. Neuropathologic studies[81] of healthy older people have shown some manifestation of vascular disease in a number of them, both in the arteries themselves and in the brain parenchyma, in the form of small infarcts. Many people with AD will also have a few vascular lesions.

CT scans show similar findings. The difficulty is compounded by the fact that not all lacunes are visible on the scan. Lacunes, when seen, must therefore be related to the clinical picture as a whole, to the presence or absence of hypertension, to the steplike or gradual mode of progression, and to other features contained in the Hachinski score. The CT scan should be regarded as an additional tool that could help to distinguish MID from Alzheimer's.

MAGNETIC RESONANCE IMAGING

The same principles apply to the role of magnetic resonance imaging (MRI). This form of imaging is not able to recognize vascular lesions as such. The appearance of the individual lacunes is indistinguishable, for example, from that of plaques of demyelination. However, besides lacunes deep in the white matter, small cortical infarcts are likely to be present. In addition, the altered signal from the periventricular white matter is likely to be uniform, whereas in demyelination, although diffuse, it is likely to be more patchy (Fig. 7–3). The overall picture of MID is therefore distinguishable from demyelination in most cases, although not in all. The advantage of MRI is its greater sensitivity; it will detect more lacunes when these are present than will CT scanning, and so contribute to the evaluation of the role of the lacunes in causing the dementia.

ANGIOGRAPHY

It might be thought that angiography would be particularly helpful in the

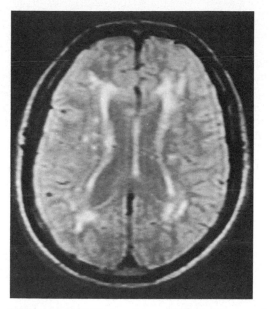

Figure 7–3. MRI showing multiple lacunes and heightened periventricular signal.

diagnosis of vascular dementia, but generally this has not proved to be so. In exceptional cases, when the dementia is due to severe occlusive disease of the extracranial arteries, to multiple small-vessel occlusions, to a large arteriovenous malformation, or to ectasia of the basilar artery, the angiogram will be helpful. In MID, however, the changes are unremarkable. Radiographic magnification techniques can show irregularities in the caliber of arteries, occlusion of vessels, retrograde filling, and other manifestations of vascular disease.[77] Instead, these changes are more likely to be encountered in atheroma than in hypertensive vascular disease, which usually gives rise to MID.

In individuals, it is difficult to determine the significance of changes. The angiographic appearance of the carotid bifurcation differs significantly between patients with strokes and transient ischemic attacks and those with cerebral tumors in the incidence of stenosis and occlusion, but not in the incidence of minor irregularities.[34] There is therefore even less expectation of seeing a significant difference in the cerebral arteries. Because the primary

cause of MID, hypertension, affects mainly small arteries and arterioles, the changes are undetectable by conventional angiography.

Etiology

The importance of CBF for the function of the brain is reflected in the fact that although the brain contributes only 2% to body weight, it takes 20% of cardiac output. It is therefore hardly surprising that reduction in CBF has long been thought to be associated with dementia.

Evidence to support this hypothesis has been scarce. It was not until 1945, when Kety and Schmidt[44] introduced the nitrous oxide clearance method, that it became possible to measure CBF in humans reliably. The introduction of the radioisotope clearance method in the early 1960s, first with krypton 85,[38] brought the methodology to the bedside.

Technologic advances did not solve all problems. There remained the question as to whether CBF declines with normal aging, as do many other physiologic functions. In 1956, Kety himself reviewed all published data on CBF in humans and concluded that CBF does decline with normal aging.[43] Data from the literature were not entirely satisfactory to answer this question, however, because although the subjects reported were free from gross evidence of cerebrovascular disease, they were not normal.

Accordingly, in 1963 Dastur and colleagues[17] measured CBF in a group of old people in whom they had made strenuous efforts to exclude any abnormality. They found a CBF of 58 mL/100 g per minute, compared with 62 mL/100 g per minute in a group of young people; the difference was insignificant. This seemed to contradict the view that CBF declines with normal aging. Later studies,[25,78,88] which included positron emission tomography (PET), however, showed a reduction in CBF with normal aging. This should be considered when assessing CBF in patients with cerebrovascular disease.

Also, CBF is responsive to cerebral metabolism. A reduction in cerebral metabolism from whatever cause will be accompanied by a reduction in CBF, which may be misinterpreted as a cause rather than an effect. CBF data must therefore be interpreted with great circumspection.

There is an abundance of published evidence that CBF is reduced in dementia and that the reduction is roughly proportional to the degree of dementia.* There is also evidence that the reduction in CBF is greater in vascular dementia than in AD,[32,68] although other investigators deny this.[37,59] That reduction in CBF does not cause vascular dementia is shown by the fact that the cerebral arteries are capable of delivering more blood in response to a rise in CO_2. CBF is low because metabolic demand is low. If the latter were to rise, the demand for increased CBF could be met, at least in part. The cerebral arteries are not so "hardened" that they cannot supply more blood.

Although CO_2 responsiveness is not lost in vascular dementia, it is reduced slightly.[32,90] In contrast, it is normal in AD. Thus, although low CBF cannot be the primary cause of vascular dementia, impaired responsiveness to changing metabolic demands may be a contributory factor. What, then, is the primary cause?

There is good evidence from neuropathologic studies and, more recently, from brain imaging during life, that the primary cause of vascular dementia is loss of brain parenchyma through infarction. This occurs in two major forms. Occlusion of major cerebral vessels, whether by embolus or thrombus, may give rise to large infarcts if collateral circulation cannot meet the deficit. These infarcts most commonly result only in neurologic deficit such as hemiplegia or hemianopsia, without evidence of dementia. In some instances, however, there may be associated dementia, particularly if the infarcts are multiple and bilateral.[47]

The more characteristic pathology in MID is a multiplicity of small infarcts of lacunar size (less than 1 cm diameter) and distributed mainly, though not exclusively, in the territory of the striate vessels. These lacunes, when small and numerous, give rise to the état lacunaire of classical neuropathology. They may vary in size and in some cases are associated with larger infarcts.

It was in this context that the term "multi-infarct dementia" was coined.[33] There is thus a gradation from the classic état lacunaire with multiple small infarcts, through larger lacunes (sometimes called "giant" lacunes), to large infarcts with or without lacunes elsewhere (Fig. 7–4).

The underlying vascular pathology for the lacunar state is almost always hypertensive vascular disease. This produces changes in the cerebral arterioles, particularly in the distribution of the striate arteries. The changes have been variously described as fibrinoid necrosis or lipohyalinosis and are asso-

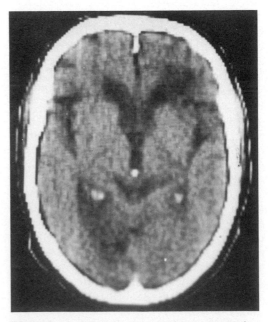

Figure 7–4. CT scan showing large occipital infarct with small lacunar infarcts elsewhere.

*References 26, 27, 32, 37, 48, 57, 58, 73.

ciated with the formation of microan-eurysms of Charcot-Bouchard type.[12]

Through serial sections, Fisher[22] traced the course of an artery supplying the territory in which a lacune occurred and demonstrated occlusion of the vessel. Thus the lacunar state is the result of multiple small-vessel occlusions secondary to changes wrought in the vessel wall by hypertension.

The pathologic studies of Tomlinson and his colleagues[81,82] showed the importance of the volume of infarcted parenchyma in the production of dementia. Cerebral softening can be found in as many as 50% of mentally normal people over 65 years, but the volume of infarcted tissue is less than 50 mL. Above this volume, a history of dementia is increasingly common, and it is unusual to find a subject with more than 100 mL of softening who is not demented.

The volume of infarction is not, however, the only factor to be taken into account; the site of the lesions is also important. Interference with neurotransmitter systems of the brain plays a crucial role in dementia. Small lacunes in critical sites may well produce effects far beyond what might be expected from their volume. The heavy concentration of lacunes deep in the cerebral hemisphere may well be a significant factor in the production of dementia.

Although MID is most commonly associated with hypertension, the condition most likely to give rise to occlusion of many small vessels, the association is not invariable. Conditions producing multiple very small emboli can have a similar effect, and dementia due to this cause is well recognized.

Management

Treatment must be directed at hypertension, almost invariably the primary cause of MID. Particular emphasis is placed on prevention. Detection of hypertension in the community is the first step, followed by careful monitoring of the effectiveness of treatment.

If MID is already present, treatment of hypertension is made more difficult by the patient's limited compliance. Nevertheless, every effort should be made to control the blood pressure by involving relatives in the administration of drugs. Retarding the progress of the changes in the arterial walls by lowering pressure makes it less likely that new lacunes will develop.

The blood pressure must be lowered slowly and cautiously, however. In hypertensive patients the range of blood pressure over which autoregulation of the cerebral circulation is maintained is shifted to the right. Sudden lowering of blood pressure to levels that may be within the normal range for autoregulation may induce hypotensive symptoms in patients who have been hypertensive for a long time. Gradually lowering the blood pressure over a period of a few weeks avoids this difficulty.

There is no evidence that anticoagulants influence the course of MID, and in view of the presence of hypertension, they are contraindicated. There is likewise no evidence that antiplatelet agents are beneficial, but as their use does not pose a particular hazard, they may be given. Evidence[11a] that aspirin may reduce the incidence of stroke in patients with TIAs suggests that it might prevent the development of further lacunes in MID.

BINSWANGER'S DISEASE

History

In 1894, Binswanger[10] reported on eight patients under the title "Encephalitis subcorticalis chronica progressiva." These were patients in whom progressive dementia had developed in midlife. At autopsy, extensive involvement of the white matter of the cerebral hemispheres was observed. Later publications by other authors added histologic observations. These publications included a major review by Olszewski,[63] who added two cases of his own. He also proposed the term "subcortical arteriosclerotic encephalopathy" which is now often used, although the eponymous title is still popular. A more recent review in 1987[6] lists the many subsequent publications.

Clinical Features

The dementia appears in the 50- to 70-year-old age group among those who have almost invariably been hypertensive. Although Biemond[9] pointed to features that might enable the diagnosis to be made in life, the clinical picture is similar to MID; specific neuropsychological deficits, however, are uncommon. Progressive memory failure and cognitive impairment are punctuated by neurologic, strokelike episodes. The onset is abrupt in about one third of cases. About 43% have a gradual progression punctuated by acute neurologic events, whereas in an equal number progress occurs gradually, without acute events. In a minority, the dementia does not appear to progress, but the patient has repeated strokes.

Mental Status Testing

Neurologic examination reveals mild but definite focal signs including gait disorder, pseudobulbar features, and mild pyramidal or extrapyramidal signs. Because the clinical picture is very similar to MID, the diagnosis was only made at autopsy prior to the introduction of CT. Among patients dying with a vascular dementia, a number would be found with the changes of Binswanger's disease. In Tokyo a study[83] of 1000 brains showed 45 with Binswanger's disease; these constituted 6.7% of those with cerebrovascular disease of any kind.

Neuropsychology

The neuropsychological picture of Binswanger's disease is characterized by impairment of memory and cognitive function, often with alteration of mood and poor control. Specific deficits, such as dysphasia, apraxia, or agnosia, are less commonly found than in MID. The neuropsychological profile is similar to that of so-called "subcortical dementia."

Neuroimaging

The advent of CT scanning brought the condition to prominence, when diffuse low density throughout the white matter of the cerebral hemisphere was observed (Fig. 7–5). In some of these cases, subsequent pathologic examination confirmed the presence of Binswanger's disease. The scan appearances must be interpreted in light of the clinical picture, as these changes are not unique to Binswanger's disease.

In 1987, Hachinski and associates[33a] coined the term "leuko-araiosis for the low-density white-matter lesions seen

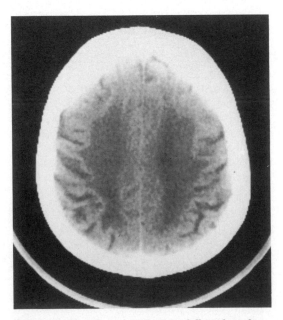

Figure 7–5. CT scan showing diffuse low density in white matter in Binswanger's disease.

on the CT scan. These lesions are seen in normal aging and in association with hypertension, a history of strokes, focal neurologic signs, and dementia of MID, Alzheimer, and Binswanger types. Similar appearances may also be seen on the CT scan after severe head injury and in cerebral edema from a variety of causes. These changes are caused mainly by ischemia leading to thinning and loss of myelin, but nonishcemic causes may also have a role in some cases.

The reported incidence of the CT-scan abnormality depends very much on the origin of the series. When the presence of radiologic evidence of cerebral atrophy was the criterion for selection of 1700 patients, 1.6% showed the changes of Binswanger's disease, whereas among 4742 scans of patients with mental deterioration or cerebrovascular disease, the incidence of Binswanger's disease was 5%.[30]

MRI demonstrates white matter lesions well (Fig. 7–6), although hyperlucencies can be seen in intellectually intact individuals without a history of stroke, especially in periventricular areas.

Neurobiology

Pathologic changes in Binswanger's disease are consistent and characteristic.[63] The lateral ventricles are enlarged and the white matter of the cerebral hemispheres is obviously puckered and discolored. Histologically, the early change is swelling of myelin sheaths, with subsequent loss of myelin and oligodendrocytes. Axis cylinders are relatively spared but undergo fragmentation in advanced lesions. Astrocytes are prominent. The loss of tissue leads to scattered minute cavities in the white matter. The changes are not fluent but distributed patchily throughout the white matter.

The vessels mainly affected are the long penetrating arteries, which are thickened and show the lipohyalinosis and fibrosis of hypertensive vascular disease. Cortical arteries are generally spared.

Although the pathologic changes are concentrated in the white matter in the territory of the long penetrating arteries, systematic examination of the rest of the brain reveals lacunar infarcts in a high proportion of cases and cortical infarcts in a minority.

Etiology and Prognosis

Binswanger's disease is part of the spectrum of hypertensive vascular disease. It is not clear why in some cases this produces mainly multiple infarcts and MID, in others diffuse white matter changes and Binswanger's disease, and in yet others cerebral hemorrhage. Although these conditions overlap to a degree, they differ distinctly in the nature and site of the most prominent lesions. The natural history of Binswanger's disease shares the progressive course of

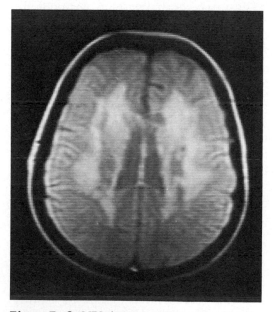

Figure 7–6. MRI showing white matter changes in Binswanger's disease.

MID, with life expectancy of only a few years.

DISORDERS OF CEREBRAL BLOOD FLOW

Extracranial Occlusive Disease

A primary reduction in CBF is the consequence of severe extracranial stenosis by atheroma. Usually the internal carotid arteries are involved bilaterally, with occlusion on one side and high-grade stenosis on the other. In addition, one or more vertebral arteries may be compromised by stenosis or congenital narrowing, and the external carotid arteries—an important collateral system—may also be diseased.

This type of severe disease most often presents as a stroke, but in some instances (presumably because occlusion has developed slowly, allowing time for some collateral circulation to develop) there is no neurologic incident, and the patient presents with dementia.

Digital subtraction angiography provides a relatively noninvasive method of diagnosing occlusive and stenotic disease. It should be carried out in those cases of vascular dementia in which there are such clinical features as bruits or inequality of the blood pressure in both upper limbs.

PET has helped to illuminate this situation. When extracranial occlusive disease is of moderate severity, the cerebral hemodynamic state may be normal. When occlusion reaches a degree at which there is significant reduction of perfusion pressure, the cerebral vessels respond by dilating; in cases of unilateral occlusion of the internal carotid artery, the dilation is detectable by PET as an increased cerebral blood volume (CBV) in the cerebral hemisphere as compared with the opposite side. The dilation can also be detected by unilateral reduction of CO_2 responsiveness measured by the ^{133}Xe clearance technique. When cerebral vasodilation is no longer sufficient to maintain adequate CBF, increased oxygen extraction ratio (OER) develops. This situation has been well documented by Gibbs and associates,[28] a number of whose patients presented with dementia. Increasing the CBF by surgical means may improve the clinical situation, although the number of patients in whom this has been demonstrated is small.

Aortic Arch Syndrome

A similar situation may be created by the lesions of the aortic arch syndrome (Takayasu's disease, pulseless disease). Here, the lesions are more proximal, being situated at the origins of the great vessels from the arch of the aorta. The effect is the same. Angiography confirms the diagnosis.

Ectasia of the Basilar Artery

Rarely, atheromatous disease in the basilar artery causes tortuosity and enlargement of the vessel sufficiently marked to warrant the description of fusiform aneurysmal dilation.[1,53] Most frequently, patients seek medical attention for symptoms of pressure on a cranial nerve, but some patients present with dementia.

The mechanism for the dementia is complex. The tortuosity of the artery distorts the anatomy of its branches, impairing blood flow through them. In addition, the enlargement of the artery may be sufficient for it to act as a space-occupying lesion, producing hydrocephalus.

Prognosis is poor and treatment of no avail.

Arteriovenous Malformations

Ninety percent of patients with cerebral arteriovenous malformations (AVMs) present with hemorrhage, epilepsy, or headache.[65] Of these, a number will also show evidence of dementia.

It is difficult to determine from the literature how frequently dementia is seen. All reports agree that dementia is rarely the presenting symptom, but they differ widely in how often it occurs when a patient presents with other symptoms. Estimates vary from virtual absence[14] to 50%,[62] with several in between.[46,51,65,76] The reason for the scatter is that most reports are not primarily concerned with the presence or absence of dementia, so that the thoroughness with which it was sought is varied.

The only report to address specifically the question of the frequency of dementia in patients with a cerebral AVM[87] found no reduction in full-scale IQ, and no impairment of verbal performance with left-sided AVMs or of visuoconstructive performance with right-sided AVMs. Despite this negative result, there can be no doubt that some patients with cerebral AVMs do become demented, some severely so.[62,76] The dementia seems to be related to the size of the AVM and possibly to its localization on the medial aspect of the cerebral hemisphere.[65]

The cause of the dementia in large cerebral AVMs is commonly steal of blood from the cerebral cortex by shunting through the malformation. Angiographic observation may show a difference in the circulation time between the AVM and the brain of as much as 3 seconds.[84] A ^{133}Xe clearance curve recorded over an AVM shows a huge spike representing rapid transit of isotope through the AVM, with little clearance through the underlying cortex.[60]

Other mechanisms may also play a part and are operative with both small and large malformations. Repeated minor bleeds, some of which may be clinically silent, damage the underlying cerebral cortex. Widespread hemosiderin staining and atrophy of the cortex can frequently be seen in surgery or at autopsy.[65] Subarachnoid hemorrhage may also give rise to communicating hydrocephalus, and AVMs in the posterior fossa may cause obstructive hydrocephalus.[65]

Prevention of dementia in patients with large cerebral AVMs that cannot be excised is difficult. Selective occlusion of feeding vessels produces only a temporary reduction in blood flow through the malformation as new channels develop.

Multiple Small-Vessel Occlusions

EMBOLI

Any condition that gives rise to multiple emboli may cause dementia if cerebral embolizations occur in sufficient number to produce the critical volumetric loss of brain parenchyma. Such conditions include rheumatic endocarditis with atrial fibrillation, infective endocarditis, and atrial myxoma.[36]

An unusual form of generalized occlusion of small arteries and veins has been described in three patients presenting with dementia.[85] The brain was the site of multiple small infarcts, especially in the watershed areas. No source of emboli was found; the vessels themselves were histologically normal but were the site of multiple thromboses. Only one of the three patients had adequate hematologic investigation; platelet survival time was shortened, but this could have been a consequence of the thromboses rather than a primary disturbance.

VASCULITIDES

A wide variety of arteritis and collagen disorders may involve the cranial arteries.[69] The striking feature is the selectivity of the different disease processes. Giant-cell arteritis, for example, affects extracranial and ciliary arteries and rarely involves cerebral vessels. In systemic lupus erythematosus, on the other hand, as many as half the patients have cerebral involvement, many showing organic cerebral impairment.[4,20] The disease can be controlled to some extent by steroids and immunosuppression. Polyarteritis nodosa may also affect cerebral vessels, and about one third of patients show evidence of some form of central nervous system involvement during the course of their illness.[64] In a minority, this takes the form of organic cerebral impairment with focal neurologic disturbance such as hemiplegia.

The rare condition of granulomatous angiitis of the central nervous system, which is distinct from giant-cell arteritis, may also present as a rapidly progressive dementia.[35] Multiple low-density lesions are seen on the CT scan[56] and multiple small ischemic lesions are found at autopsy.

CEREBRAL AMYLOID ANGIOPATHY

Cerebral amyloid angiopathy has attracted considerable attention, particularly because of a possible relationship to AD. The involvement of cortical arteries causes multiple small cortical infarcts and hemorrhages[61] and may present as dementia.[39]

Cerebral Insufficiency

HISTORY

The term "cerebral insufficiency" is unsatisfactory but is deliberately used here to call attention to a problem of clinical classification that remains unresolved. The term originated from the concept that impaired cerebral function may be due to an insufficient blood flow to the brain for its metabolic needs.

CLINICAL FEATURES

Undoubtedly, there is a clinical state in patients with cerebrovascular disease, short of dementia, in which cerebral function is reversibly impaired. The clinical manifestations are often subtle. The patients concentration is impaired, and tasks that could previously be undertaken without trouble cause worry. Because of this the patient is less enthusiastic about new undertakings, and even familiar tasks are felt to be a burden. The patient tires easily and readily becomes irritable with people and things. Formal examination (including memory testing) fails to reveal anything significant. It is difficult to distinguish this symptomatology from that seen in anxiety and mild depression. Indeed, the patient may feel depressed.

That this state may be related to the cerebral circulation is indicated by the fact that it may appear following myocardial infarction, taking weeks or months to resolve. Even more striking are the instances in which the symptoms appear as a patient slips into cardiac failure, resolve as cardiac status is restored, and recur with further manifestations of cardiac failure. In the latter situation, definite signs of impaired cerebral function may appear, such as poor orientation and memory failure. Cardiac arrhythmias, which impair CBF, can also cause this syndrome.

NEUROPSYCHOLOGY

Considerable neuropsychological data indicate mild cognitive impairment in patients with cerebrovascular disease who do not have clinical dementia. Although the data are not beyond challenge, hypertensive patients have been found to perform less well in a variety of neuropsychological tests.[5,66] Similarly, patients with cardiac disease have been found to perform less well,[29,75] and performance may improve after heart surgery for valvular disease.[40]

The whole subject is fraught with difficulties. Expert clinical assessment must be combined with skilled neuropsychological testing, particularly when the effects of therapy are being studied. Not infrequently, however, one arm of the partnership does not match the other in quality. This is unfortunate, as it usually means that intriguing data cannot be fully substantiated. Despite these shortcomings, the overall thrust of the literature confirms the clinical impression of a state short of ischemia in which higher cerebral function is impaired. Whether this is a precursor of vascular dementia is not known, but certainly it deserves attention as a state for which therapeutic intervention might be most rewarding.

ETIOLOGY

When CBF becomes inadequate for metabolic requirements, the first response is an increase in OER. This response has not been found in MID, where, although CBF is low, OER is normal, indicating that the low flow is mainly the result of reduced metabolic demand. The decline of CBF appears to begin before the onset of symptoms of MID, however. In a 7-year prospective study of 181 normal, healthy volunteers with a mean age of 70.6 years, 3.3% developed AD and 5.5%, MID.[67] The reason for the higher incidence of MID was that, although healthy at the start of the study, many of the subjects had significant risk factors for vascular disease. Serial CBF measurements were made, and it was noted that in the subjects who developed AD, CBF remained normal until symptoms appeared, and then it fell rapidly. In the MID group, on the other hand, CBF began to decline as much as 2 years before the onset of symptoms.

It seems unlikely that the volume of "silent" infarcts caused the decline in CBF before symptoms appeared. An alternative explanation is that the normally close coupling between CBF and metabolism became impaired in some way. CO_2 responsiveness, although not abolished, is certainly lessened.[24,32] This impairment may have an effect on the fine-tuning of CBF to metabolism short of producing frank ischemia.

Support for this hypothesis is provided by the observation that cognitive impairment fluctuates during the development of MID, and the fluctuations correlate with the level of CBF.[52] Furthermore, the levels of homovanillic acid (HVΛ) and 5 hydroxyindoleacetic acid (5-HIAA) in the cerebrospinal fluid (which fall after a frank ischemic lesion) are reduced in MID.[74] This fall may be a consequence of global depletion of dopamine and serotonin in the brain as a result of circulatory impairment.

MANAGEMENT

Vigorous management of patients at this stage is necessary if the more definitive state of MID is to be prevented. Vascular risk factors must be treated. In particular, hypertension must be controlled, and the cardiac status must be evaluated and remedied when necessary.

The role of vasodilator drugs in this situation is controversial. The rationale for their use was the hypothesis that low CBF is the cause of the clinical state, but this is not the case. Moreover, cerebral vasodilation does not guarantee an increase of CBF. If cerebral vasodilation is accompanied by a dilation of systemic arteries, a fall in blood pressure will occur; if autoregulation is impaired, CBF may be reduced.

Vasodilators may have some effect, however. Controlled clinical trials have given variable results.[15] Improved performance on psychological testing is frequently claimed, but practical clinical benefit is reported less often. Although problems of trial design and execution make evaluation of the data difficult, vasodilators cannot be entirely dismissed as without value.

SUMMARY

Next to AD, vascular causes are probably the second most common etiology of dementia in the elderly. It is sometimes difficult to distinguish between patients with true vascular dementia and those with AD who have concomitant vascular changes, as some vascular changes are common in normal aging. Advances in neuroimaging and techniques for measuring cerebral blood flow and metabolism, however, are helping to elucidate the mechanisms by which vascular disease leads to dementia, and should aid in the timely diagnosis of vascular dementias.

Multiple small infarctions are the most frequent cause of vascular dementia. They almost always occur in hypertensive individuals, commonly 60 to 75 years of age. Neurologic deficits may precede or accompany the appearance of dementia, and the clinician faced with a "confused" patient should try to determine the precise nature of the "confusion" so that potentially treatable causes can be ruled out. An abrupt onset and stepwise progression are common. Generally, recent memory is most affected, with other patchy cognitive losses. Emotional control is usually lost, yet the personality is relatively preserved, unlike the presentation of AD. Treatment of the underlying hypertension may retard the progress of the dementia.

Binswanger's disease, which also occurs almost exclusively in hypertensive individuals, is characterized by diffuse changes in the white matter, mainly in the territory of the long penetrating arteries. The clinical picture is similar to that of MID, although specific neuropsychological deficits are less common. In most cases the dementia progresses gradually; acute neurologic events also may occur.

The compromise of the cerebral blood flow by the occlusion or severe stenosis of extracranial arteries may result in dementia even without a stroke or other neurologic incident, and should be looked for if bruits or inequality of blood pressure in the upper limbs is detected. Other conditions, such as aortic arch syndrome, ectasia of the basilar artery, or arteriovenous malformations, may have similar effects. Patients with impaired CBF (often cardiogenic) may show mild cognitive impairment that is sometimes confused with depression. Vigorous management of such patients may prevent the development of MID.

REFERENCES

1. Alajouanine T, Le Beau J, and Houdart R: La symptomatologie tumorale des volumineux anévrysmes des artères vertébrales et basilaires. Rev Neurol (Paris) 80:321, 1948.
2. Allbutt TC: Arteriosclerosis. Macmillan, London, 1925.
3. Alzheimer A: Über eine eigenartige Erkrankung der Hernrinde. Allgemeine Zeitschrift für Psychiatrie 64: 146, 1907.
4. Appenzeller O and Williams RC: Cerebral lupus erythematosus. Ann Intern Med 90:430, 1979.
5. Apter NS, Halstead WC, and Heimburger RF: Impaired cerebral functions in essential hypertension. Am J Psychiatry 107:808, 1951.
6. Babikian V and Ropper AH: Binswanger's disease: A review. Stroke 18:2, 1987.
7. Bademosi O, Falase AO, Jaiyesimi F, and Bademosi A: Neuropsychiatric manifestations of infective endocarditis: A study of 95 patients at Ibadan, Nigeria. J Neurol Neurosurg Psychiatry 39:325, 1976.
8. Barclay LL, Zemcov A, Blass JP, and Sansone J: Survival in Alzheimer's disease and vascular dementias. Neurology 35:834, 1985.
9. Biemond A: On Binswanger's subcortical arteriosclerotic encephalopathy and the possibility of its clinical recognition. Psychiatr Neurol Neurochir 73:413, 1970.
10. Binswanger O: Die Abgrenzung der allgemeinen progressiven Paralyse. (Referate erstattet auf der Jahresversammlung des Vereins Deutschr Irrenarzte zu Dresden am 20 September 1894). Berliner Klinische Wochenschrift 31:1103, 1137, and 1180, 1894.
11. Brust JCM: Vascular dementia— still overdiagnosed. Stroke 14:298, 1983.
11a. Canadian Cooperative Study Group: A randomized trial of aspirin and sulfinpyrazone in threatened stroke. N Engl J Med 299:53, 1978.
12. Charcot JM and Bouchard C: Nouvelles recherches sur la pathogenie de l'hemorrhagie cérébral. Arch Physiol Norm Path 1:110, 643 and 725, 1868.
13. Coblenz JM, Mattis S, Zingesser LH, Kasoff SS, Wisniewski HM, and Katz-

man R: Presenile dementia. Arch Neurol 29:299, 1973.

14. Constans JP and Assal G: Evolution de la symptomatologie neuropsychologique d'une série d'anevrismes arterioveineux opérés. Neurochirurgie 14:201, 1971.

15. Cook P and James I: Cerebral vasodilators. N Engl J Med 305:1508, 1981.

16. Corsellis JAN: Mental Illness and the Aging Brain. Oxford University Press, London, 1983.

17. Dastur DK, Lane MH, Hansen DB, et al: Effects of aging on cerebral circulation and metabolism in man. In Birren JE, Greenouse SW, Sokoloff L, and Yarrow MR (eds): Human Aging: A Biological and Behavioral Study. USPHS Publication No 986, US Government Printing Office, Washington, DC, 1963, p 59.

18. Durand-Fardel C-L-M: Les Maladies des Vieillards, Ed 2. Germer-Bailliere, Paris, 1873.

19. Faer MJ, Mead JH, and Lynch RD: Cerebral granulomatous angiitis. American Journal of Roentgenology 129:413, 1977.

20. Feinglass EJ, Arnett FC, Dorsch CA, Zizic TM, and Stevens MB: Neuropsychiatric manifestations of systemic lupus erythematosus. Medicine (Baltimore) 55:323, 1976.

21. Fisher CM: Pure sensory stroke involving face, arm, and leg. Neurology 15:76, 1965.

22. Fisher CM: The arterial lesions underlying lacunes. Acta Neuropathol (Berl) 12:1, 1969.

23. Fisher CM: Lacunar strokes and infarcts: A review. Neurology 32:871, 1982.

24. Fisher CM and Curry HB: Pure motor hemiplegia of vascular origin. Arch Neurol 13:30, 1965.

25. Frackowiak RSJ: Measurement and imaging of cerebral function in aging and dementia. In Swaab DF, Fliers E, Mirmira M, VanGool WA, and Van-Haaren F (eds): Progress in Brain Research, Vol 70. Elsevier, Amsterdam, 1986, p 69.

26. Frackowiak RSJ, Pozzilli C, Legg NJ, et al: Regional cerebral oxygen supply and utilization in dementia. A clinical and physiological study with oxygen 15 and positron tomography. Brain 104:753, 1981.

27. Freyham FA, Woodford RB, and Kety SS: Cerebral blood flow and metabolism in psychosis of senility. J Nerv Ment Dis 113:445, 1951.

28. Gibbs JM, Frackowiak RSJ, and Legg NJ: Regional cerebral blood flow and oxygen metabolism in dementia due to vascular disease. Gerontology (Suppl 1)32:84, 1984.

29. Goldman H, Kleinman KM, Snow MY, Bidus DR, and Korol B: Correlation of diastolic blood pressure and signs of cognitive dysfunction in essential hypertension. Diseases of the Nervous System 35:571, 1974.

30. Goto K, Ishii N, and Fukasawa H: Diffuse white matter disease in the geriatric population. Radiology 141:687, 1981.

31. Gull WW and Sutton HG: On the pathology of the morbid state commonly called chronic Bright's disease with contracted kidney (arterio-capillary fibrosis). Med chir Trans 55:273, 1872.

32. Hachinski VC, Iliff LD, Zilkha E, et al: Cerebral blood flow in dementia. Arch Neurol 32:632, 1975.

33. Hachinski VC, Lassen NA, and Marshall J: Multi-infarct dementia: A case of mental deterioration in the elderly. Lancet 2:207, 1974.

33a. Hachinski VC, Potter P, and Merskey H: Leuko-araiosis. Arch Neurol 44:21, 1987.

34. Harrison MJG and Marshall J: Angiographic appearance of carotid bifurcation in patients with completed stroke, transient ischaemic attacks, and cerebral tumour. BMJ 1:205, 1976.

35. Hughes JT and Brownell B: Granulomatous giant-cell arteritis of the central nervous system. Neurology 16:293, 1966.

36. Hutton JT: Atrial myxoma as a cause of progressive dementia. Arch Neurol 38:533, 1981.

37. Ingvar DH and Gustafson L: Regional cerebral blood flow in organic dementia with early onset. Acta Neurol Scand (Suppl 43)46:42, 1970.

38. Ingvar DH and Lassen NA: Regional blood flow of the cerebral cortex determined by krypton 85. Acta Physiol Scand 54:325, 1962.
39. Jellinger K: Cerebrovascular amyloidosis with cerebral hemorrhage. J Neurol 214:195, 1977.
40. Juolasmaa A, Outakoski J, Hirvenoja R, Tienari P, Sotaniemi K, and Takkunen J: Effect of open heart surgery on intellectual performance. J Clin Neuropsychol 3:181, 1981.
41. Kannel WB and Wolf P: Vascular Disease of the Central Nervous System, Ed 2. Churchill Livingstone, London, 1983.
42. Kay DWK, Beamish P, and Roth M: Old age mental disorders in Newcastle upon Tyne. Part 1: A study of prevalence. Br J Psychiatry 110:146, 1964.
43. Kety SS: Human cerebral blood flow and oxygen consumption as related to aging. Res Publ Assoc Res Nerv Ment Dis 35:31, 1956.
44. Kety SS and Schmidt CF: The determination of cerebral blood flow in man by the use of nitrous oxide in low concentrations. Am J Physiol 143:53, 1945.
45. Kotsoris H, Barclay LL, Kheyfets S, Hulyalkar A, and Dougherty J: Urinary and gait disturbances as markers for early multi-infarct dementia. Stroke 18:138, 1987.
46. Krenchel NJ: Intracranial Racemose Angiomas: A Clinical Study. Universitetsforlaget, Aarhus, Denmark, 1961.
47. Ladurner G, Iliff LD, and Lechner H: Clinical factors associated with dementia in ischaemic stroke. J Neurol Neurosurg Psychiatry 45:97, 1982.
48. Lassen NA, Feinberg I, and Lane MH: Bilateral studies of cerebral oxygen uptake in young and aged normal subjects and in patients with organic dementia. J Clin Invest 39:491, 1960.
49. Marie P: Des foyers lacunaires de désintégration et de différents autres états cavicaires du cerveau. Revue de Médecine (Paris) 21:281, 1901.
50. Marsden CD and Harrison MJG: Outcome of investigation of patients with presenile dementia. BMJ 2:249, 1972.
51. McKenzie I: The clinical presentation of the cerebral angioma. Brain 76:184, 1953.
52. Meyer JS, Judd BW, Rogers RL, and Mortel KF: Cognition fluctuates in multi-infarct dementia. Stroke 18:297, 1987.
53. Michael WF: Posterior fossa aneurysms simulating tumours. J Neurol Neurosurg Psychiatry 37:218, 1974.
54. Molsa PK, Marttila RJ, and Rinne UK: Alzheimer's disease and multi-infarct dementia. Acta Neurol Scand 74:103, 1986.
55. Mortimer JA and Schuman LM (eds): The Epidemiology of Dementia. Oxford University Press, New York, 1981.
56. Nurick S, Blackwood W, and Mair WPG: Giant cell granulomatous angiitis of the central nervous system. Brain 95:133, 1972.
57. O'Brien MD and Mallett BL: Cerebral cortex perfusion rates in dementia. J Neurol Neurosurg Psychiatry 33:497, 1970.
58. Obrist WD, Chivian E, Cronqvist S, and Ingvar DH: Regional cerebral blood flow in senile and presenile dementia. Neurology 20:315, 1970.
59. Obrist WD, Thompson HK, Wang HS, and Wilkinson, WE: Regional cerebral blood flow estimated by [133]Xenon inhalation. Stroke 6:245, 1975.
60. Oeconomos D, Kosmaoglou B, and Prossalentis A: rCBF studies in patients with arteriovenous malformations of the brain. In Brock M (ed): Cerebral Blood Flow. Clinical and Experimental Results. Springer-Verlag, Berlin, 1969, p 146.
61. Okazaki H, Reagan TJ, and Campbell J: Clinicopathologic studies of primary cerebral amyloid angiopathy. Mayo Clin Proc 54:22, 1979.
62. Olivecrona H and Riives J: Arteriovenous aneurysms of the brain. Archives of Neurology and Psychiatry 59:567, 1948.
63. Olszewski J: Subcortical arteriosclerotic encephalopathy: Review of the literature on the so-called Binswanger's disease and presentation of two cases. World Neurology 3:359–375, 1962.

64. Parker HL and Kernohan JW: Central nervous system in periarteritis nodosa. Mayo Clin Proc 24:43, 1949.

65. Paterson JH and McKissock W: A clinical survey of intracranial angiomas with special reference to their mode of progression and surgical treatment: A report of 110 cases. Brain 79:233, 1956.

66. Reitan RM: Intellectual and affective changes in essential hypertension. Am J Psychiatry 110:817, 1954.

67. Rogers RL, Meyer JS, Mortel KF, Mahurin RK, and Judd BW: Decreased cerebral blood flow precedes multi-infarct dementia, but follows senile dementia of Alzheimer type. Neurology 36:1, 1986.

68. Rosen WG, Terry RD, Fuld PA, Katzman R, and Peck A: Pathological verification of ischemic score in differentiation of dementias. Ann Neurol 7:486, 1979.

69. Ross-Russell RW: Less common varieties of cerebral arterial disease. In Ross-Russell RW (ed): Vascular Disease of the Central Nervous System, Ed 2. Churchill Livingstone, New York, 1983, p 368.

70. Ross-Russell RW and Bharucha N: The recognition and prevention of border-zone cerebral ischaemia during cardiac surgery. Q J Med 47:303, 1978.

71. Sim M, Turner E, and Smith WT: Cerebral biopsy in the investigation of presenile dementia. I. Clinical aspects. Br J Psychiatry 112:119, 1966.

72. Sim M, Turner E, and Smith WT: Cerebral biopsy in the investigation of presenile dementia. II. Pathological aspects. Br J Psychiatry 112:127, 1966.

73. Simard D, Olesen J, Paulson OB, Lassen NA, and Skinhoj E: Regional cerebral blood flow and its regulation in dementia. Brain 94:273, 1971.

74. Smirne S, Francheschi M, Truci G, et al: Homovanillic acid and 5-hydroxyindoleacetic acid modifications in CSF of patients with stroke and multi-infarct dementia. Stroke 16:1003, 1985.

75. Spieth W: Cardiovascular health status, age and psychological performance. J Gerontol 19:277, 1964.

76. Svein HJ and McRae JA: Arteriovenous anomalies of the brain. Fate of patients not having definitive surgery. J Neurosurg 23:23, 1965.

77. Taveras JM and Wood EH: Diagnostic Neuroradiology. Williams & Wilkins, Baltimore, MD, 1964.

78. Thomas DJ, Zilkha E, Redmond S, et al: An intravenous ^{133}xenon clearance technique for measuring cerebral blood flow. J Neurol Sci 40:53, 1979.

79. Todorov AB, Go RCP, Constantinidis J, and Elston RC: Specificity of the clinical diagnosis of dementia. J Neurol Sci 26:81, 1975.

80. Tomlinson BE: The pathology of dementia. In Wells CE (ed): Dementia, Ed 2. FA Davis, Philadelphia, 1977, pp 113–153.

81. Tomlinson BE, Blessed G, and Roth M: Observations on the brains of non-demented old people. J Neurol Sci 7:331, 1968.

82. Tomlinson BE, Blessed G, and Roth M: Observations on the brains of demented old people. J Neurol Sci 11:205, 1970.

83. Tomonaga M, Yamanoushi H, Tohgi H, and Kameyama M: Clinicopathologic study of progressive subcortical vascular encephalopathy (Binswanger type) in the elderly. J Am Geriatr Soc 30:524, 1982.

84. Tonnis W, Schiefer W, and Walter W: Signs and symptoms of supratentorial arteriovenous aneurysms. J Neurosurg 15:471, 1958.

85. Torvik A, Endresen KM, Abrahamsen AF, and Godal HC: Progressive dementia caused by an unusual type of generalized small vessel thrombosis. Acta Neurol Scand 47:137, 1971.

86. Valentine AR, Moseley IF, and Kendall BE: White matter abnormality in cerebral atrophy: Clinicoradiological correlations. J Neurol Neurosurg Psychiatry 43:139, 1980.

87. Waltimo O and Putkonen A-R: Intellectual performance of patients with

intracranial arteriovenous malformations. Brain 97:511, 1974.

88. Wang HS and Busse EW: Correlates of regional cerebral blood flow in elderly community residents. In Harper M, Jennett B, Miller D, and Rowan J (eds): Blood Flow and Metabolism in the Brain. Churchill Livingstone, London, 1975, pp 8–17.

89. Willison JR, du Boulay GH, Paul EA, et al: Effect of high haematocrit on alertness. Lancet 1:846, 1980.

90. Yamamoto M, Meyer JS, Sadai F, and Yamaguchi F: Aging and cerebral vasodilator responses to hypercarbia: Responses in normal aging and in persons with risk factors for stroke. Arch Neurol 37:489, 1980.

Chapter 8

VIRAL DEMENTIAS

Justin C. McArthur, M.B., B.S., M.P.H.,
Raymond P. Roos, M.D., and
Richard T. Johnson, M.D.

DEMENTIA AS A SEQUELA OF
  ACUTE INFECTIONS
VIRUS INFECTIONS CAUSING
  PROGRESSIVE DEMENTIA
PROGRESSIVE MULTIFOCAL
  LEUKOENCEPHALOPATHY — A
  DEMYELINATING DISEASE AS A
  CAUSE OF DEMENTIA
CREUTZFELDT-JAKOB DISEASE —
  A NONINFLAMMATORY DISEASE
  AS A CAUSE OF DEMENTIA

Viral infections of the central nervous system (CNS) cause varied signs and symptoms because of the selective vulnerability of different neural cell populations to different viruses. When the cerebral cortex or cortical-cortical connections are a major site of infection, disorders of consciousness and mentation may be salient findings. If this infection is acute and self-limited, a static intellectual deficit may persist; if the infection is slow or chronic, progressive mental deterioration may occur.

Some viruses, such as rubella and cytomegaloviruses, infect primarily the fetal brain, thereby causing congenital mental dysfunction which may be severe or subtle.[109,110] Others, such as herpes simplex virus and some arboviruses, can cause severe, acute encephalitis with ensuing static dementia. Direct damage of neural cells appears to be important in the subsequent neural dysfunction. Several slowly evolving infections of the CNS cause progressive dementia as a major clinical feature and may play a role in these varied pathogenetic mechanisms. Newly recognized mechanisms of neural dysfunction such as noncytopathic neuronal infection that interferes with neurotransmitters or trophic factors (so-called luxury functions[186]) may hold clues to understanding other forms of dementia. Dementia may result from a chronic inflammatory encephalitis, as in subacute sclerosing panencephalitis, progressive rubella panencephalitis, and chronic tick-borne encephalitis; from subcortical demyelination, as in progressive multifocal leukoencephalopathy; or from noninflammatory cortical neuronal degeneration, as in Creutzfeldt-Jakob disease (CJD). The most recently described dementia of viral etiology is human immunodeficiency virus (HIV) encephalopathy, in which pathogenetic mechanisms remain uncertain.

The recognition of the viral etiology of a dementia relies on the analysis of historical and laboratory features. The appearance in summertime of a neurologic illness coincident with a local epidemic of encephalitis must suggest an arboviral infection. In a sporadic case of fulminant encephalitis with frontotemporal localization, herpes simplex encephalitis is the primary consideration. The development of progressive dementia in an individual with a history of intravenous drug use or homosexual activity should suggest the possibility of HIV infection. In postinfectious encephalomyelitis, the onset of neurologic symptoms usually follows a viral exanthema by several weeks. More chronic causes of dementia such as progressive multifocal leukoencephalopathy and CJD must be distinguished from idiopathic degenerative conditions, familial disorders such as olivopontocerebellar atrophy, toxic exposure to heavy metals or chemicals, neoplasms, and paraneoplastic processes.

A serologic analysis is helpful in some of the acute infectious processes, particularly the arboviral encephalitides. Analysis of cerebrospinal fluid (CSF) is rarely diagnostic in itself, but the presence of lymphocytic pleocytosis, elevated protein, and increased immunoglobulin indicates an inflammatory or infective process. The intrathecal synthesis of antibody, as measured by the presence of specifically directed oligoclonal bands or an elevated IgG index, can indicate the presence of viral replication within the CNS. Imaging studies are helpful in documenting localized infections such as herpes simplex encephalitis, or diffuse white-matter changes such as postinfectious encephalomyelitis; and in excluding neoplasms, cerebrovascular disease, or the effects of trauma. Specific diagnostic clues for a variety of acute and chronic viral causes of dementia are discussed in this chapter.

DEMENTIA AS A SEQUELA OF ACUTE INFECTIONS

Many viruses can invade the CNS in the course of acute systemic infection. In viral meningitis presumably only the meninges are involved, causing fever, headache, meningismus, and a CSF pleocytosis. In encephalitis, signs of parenchymal involvement include seizures, focal neurologic deficits, and disorders of consciousness. Postinfectious encephalomyelitis may cause the same signs but usually develops after initial recovery from an exanthema or respiratory or enteric infection.

The same spectrum of viruses causes both acute meningitis and encephalitis. Some viruses, such as the enteroviruses and mumps, tend to cause benign meningitis, whereas others, such as arboviruses and herpes simplex virus, tend to cause severe encephalitis with permanent residua.[170] Even the enteroviruses, however, can cause mild encephalitis; sequelae occasionally are seen in children, particularly in those less than 1 year old. In one series,[221] 3 of 19 cases had sequelae involving speech and language development, and 5 had slight intellectual or behavioral abnormalities. Similarly, sequelae are unusual in mumps encephalitis, although severe residua involving disorders of mentation rarely may be seen.[134]

Arbovirus Encephalitis

Nervous system infections with the arthropod-borne encephalitis viruses can lead to severe sequelae (Table 8–1). In fatal arbovirus encephalitis, infection of neurons, with neuronal death and neuronophagia, is prominent. Perivascular inflammation is widespread but is usually more intense in gray matter. One hundred forty-eight cases of arboviral encephalitis were reported in the United States in 1987.[37] In Eastern, Western, and California (LaCrosse subtype) virus encephalitides, permanent deficits are common in the very young. In general, Eastern encephalitis has a low rate of subclinical infection, a high mortality rate, and a very high frequency of severe sequelae in survivors. In one series, the majority of survivors under 5 years of age had mental retardation, speech problems, and seizures.[69] Western encephalitis has a much higher and more variable rate of inapparent infections and a very low rate of sequelae after clinical disease. Nevertheless, major mental and motor deficits are found in half the patients under 1 month of age who contract the disease. A delay in the clinical appear-

Table 8–1 ARTHROPOD-BORNE ENCEPHALITIS VIRUSES

Type	Ratio of Subclinical Infection : Severe Infection	Approximate Mortality	Frequency of Sequelae
Eastern Equine	2–4 : 1	25–50%	Very high
Western Equine	58–1150 : 1	<1%	Very low
California (LaCrosse)	High	<1%	Low
Venezuelan Equine	High	<5%	High (<15 years)
St. Louis	2–64 : 1	<5%	High (>40 years)

Source: Adapted from Evans,[68] p. 369.

ance of deficits has suggested that Western encephalitis virus might cause chronic infection in infants, but Finley's studies suggest instead that the acute disease affects cerebral ontogenesis and that neurologic deficits that become manifest later are not caused by persistent infection.[71] California (LaCrosse subtype) encephalitis causes inapparent infection in adults but can produce a clinical encephalitis in children, with rare residual deficits.[7,43] LaCrosse is the principal cause of endemic arboviral CNS infections in the United States.[37] Venezuelan equine encephalitis, a recognized cause of encephalitis in this country, can produce severe sequelae or death in individuals under 15, usually causes subclinical disease or a mild influenzal syndrome in individuals 15 to 50, and is associated with a self-limited encephalitis with complete recovery in patients over age 50.[64] St. Louis encephalitis appears to differ from the other North American arbovirus encephalitides because mortality and morbidity are greater among adults over 40 years of age. In one follow-up study of 52 patients, 60% of elderly patients had persistent memory deficits 1 year after infection.[236]

Arboviral encephalitis should be considered if there is a known epidemic involving mosquitos, equines, and humans. Late summer is the most common time for cases of arbovirus encephalitis to appear, and there may be a history of environmental risk factors that support breeding of mosquitos, such as discarded tires or hollow trees. Specific diagnosis is based on virus isolation or serologic evidence of a fourfold or greater rise in antibodies between early and convalescent specimens.

Herpes Simplex Virus Encephalitis

CLINICAL FEATURES

In adults, herpetic encephalitis is usually due to type 1 herpes simplex virus and is usually not associated with visceral or cutaneous herpetic disease. Infection and pathologic changes are predominantly in orbitofrontal and medial temporal lobes, giving more focal neurologic signs and stereotyped residual mental deficits.[8,59,126,171] Encephalitis may develop abruptly or evolve over a number of days. When clinical disease evolves insidiously, bizarre behavior, hallucinations, and other psychiatric manifestations may be evident for several days before seizures (focal or generalized) and focal signs, such as hemiparesis or aphasia, develop. Confusion may progress to stupor or coma.

CSF pleocytosis and elevated protein are usually found, with variable numbers of red cells. A low CSF glucose level within the first 5 days of illness increases the likelihood of an alternative treatable diagnosis and should be an indication for biopsy.[217] Focal electroencephalographic (EEG) abnormalities are found in about 80% of biopsy-proven cases.[175] The EEG often is distinctive, with repetitive, periodic sharp and slow wave complexes, usually localized in the frontal or frontotemporal area, against a diffusely slow background activity.[235] Contrast-enhanced CT scans or magnetic resonance imaging (MRI) may aid in localization, demonstrating frontotemporal lesions and swelling in the majority of cases. EEG abnormalities often precede CT scan changes. The MRI detects changes earlier than CT and has greater sensitivity.[218a]

PATHOLOGY

Although the encephalitis is usually bilateral, focal involvement of one inferior frontal or temporal lobe may suggest an abscess or tumor. The microscopic appearance is that of intense edema and necrosis, perivascular inflammation, intranuclear inclusion bodies, and often necrosis with small hemorrhages. The diagnosis is difficult, because virus is usually not recoverable from CSF and because herpes simplex virus serum antibody can increase nonspecifically in the course of other infections. Definitive diagnosis can be made only by antigen demonstration or virus isolation from brain biopsy or autopsy material.[108,133] In a recent multicenter treatment trial, only 69 of 208 patients who underwent biopsy for clinically suspected herpes simplex encephalitis had this diagnosis confirmed,[261] documenting that other conditions may mimic herpes simplex encephalitis and emphasizing the importance of biopsy in the pre-MRI era. The most commonly confused diagnoses include cerebrovascular disease, tumors, bacterial and fungal infections, and other viral encephalitides.[262] The recent use of the polymerase chain reaction technique in detecting herpes simplex virus in the CSF holds new promise as a diagnostic technique.[216]

TREATMENT

The actual morbidity and mortality of herpes simplex virus encephalitis depend on the promptness with which therapy is instituted. Earlier studies demonstrated that the outcome of herpes simplex encephalitis was affected by age and the level of consciousness prior to starting therapy.[262] Survival from untreated herpes simplex encephalitis is typically followed by severe cognitive impairment, primarily in the areas of new verbal learning, memory, and naming. Bizarre behavior reminiscent of the Klüver-Bucy syndrome has also been described.[97] Young patients who were alert at the start of treatment were four times more likely to survive than elderly patients who were comatose at the outset. Several recent trials have confirmed the heightened efficacy of acyclovir over vidarabine.[233] In the largest study, Whitley and the National Institute of Allergy and Infectious Disease (NIAID) Collaborative Antiviral Study Group[261] demonstrated a mortality of 13% for acyclovir recipients 1 month after therapy, compared with 43% in those randomized to receive vidarabine. Morbidity was reduced from 86% in the vidarabine group to 62% with acyclovir treatment. A trial comparing a combination of vidarabine and acyclovir with acyclovir alone is under way.

It is now recognized that much of the early mortality results from brain swelling and herniation, so that aggressive management of cerebral edema with corticosteroids and hyperventilation may also improve survival in herpes simplex encephalitis.

Despite the improvements in diagnosis and treatment, herpes simplex encephalitis has a 30% to 50% case-fatality rate, and severe deficits may occur in a large percentage of survivors. Even in patients treated with acyclovir who have a "good" clinical outcome and who have normal Mini-Mental State examination scores, significant cognitive impairment can be detected.[93] The localization of necrosis to the inferior frontal and temporal lobes frequently leads to a severe amnestic syndrome (Korsakoff's psychosis), although a more global dementia, in addition to motor abnormalities and seizures, may also be seen.[59] Memory is the most affected cognitive function in mild forms

Table 8-2 POSTINFECTIOUS ENCEPHALOMYELITIS

		Rate per per 100,000	Case Fatality Rate(%)	Major Sequelae
Exanthemata:	Measles	100	20	Frequent
	Varicella	10*	5	10%
	Rubella	20*	20	Very rare
Nonexanthemata:	Mumps	Rare*	Rare	Rare
	Epstein-Barr	Rare	Rare	Rare
	Influenza	Rare	Rare	Rare
Vaccinations:	Vaccinia	0.5-1600†	25	Common
	Rabies-Semple	10-300‡	15	Comon
	Influenza	?§	Uncommon	Rare
	Measles	?§	Rare	Rare
	Rabies-DEV	4¶,§	12	Common
	Rabies-HDCV	None**	0	None

*The exact frequency of acute disseminated encephalitis (ADE) is difficult to estimate because of the frequency of toxic encephalopathy or direct infection and the paucity of autopsy-proven cases.

†Vaccination no longer widely used. The wide variation in incidence is unexplained.

‡Semple neural-tissue vaccine is still widely used outside U.S.

§The incidence of ADE is so low as to be indistinguishable from the background rate.

¶Duck-embryo vaccine (DEV). No longer used in the U.S.

**Human diploid cell vaccine (HDCV): has been used in the U.S. since 1980, and although there are two reported cases of neuroparalytic illness, there are no documented instances of ADE.

Source: Adapted from Johnson et al,[129] p. 73.

of herpes simplex encephalitis, with good recovery.[138]

Postinfectious Encephalomyelitis

Postinfectious encephalomyelitis may also lead to permanent sequelae, such as mental retardation or subtle neuropsychological impairment.[1,128,129,239,249] Most commonly associated with measles, postinfectious encephalomyelitis also occurs with other exanthemous infections such as vaccinia, varicella, and rubella and with a variety of nonexanthematous diseases, including mumps, influenza, Epstein-Barr virus infections, and *M. pneumoniae* infections[129] (Table 8-2). Persistent sequelae occur frequently with measles, and far less commonly with the other exanthemata. Rabies vaccines prepared in neural tissues (Semple vaccine) produces an acute demyelinating encephalomyelitis in as many as 1:400 vaccinations.[112] This post-rabies-vaccine encephalomyelitis appears to be the clinical equiva-

lent of experimental allergic encephalomyelitis.

ETIOLOGY

The clinical and pathologic similarities between experimental allergic encephalomyelitis and postinfectious encephalomyelitis suggest that common pathogenetic mechanisms are involved.[128] Both processes have perivenular inflammation with lymphocytes, macrophages, and plasma cells, accompanied by demyelination. Can viral infections in some way stimulate an autoimmune response within the CNS? There is no evidence of measles virus replication in the brain in measles encephalomyelitis,[86,174] and the lack of intrathecal antibody synthesis in most patients suggests a lack of antigen in brain.[130] On the other hand, a variety of abnormalities of immune regulation are found during measles, and many patients with encephalomyelitis show lymphoproliferative responses to myelin basic protein.[130] The autoimmune disease may occur due to lack of immune regulation or to molecular mimicry (a phenomenon in which sequence similarities between viral polypeptides and encephalitogenic myelin proteins might induce an autoimmune demyelinating disease).

TREATMENT

There is no proven benefit to the use of hyperimmune γ-globulin, corticosteroids, or adrenocorticotrophic hormone (ACTH).[129] Supportive treatment must be aggressive.

VIRUS INFECTIONS CAUSING PROGRESSIVE DEMENTIA

Viruses were classically associated with acute, evanescent infections but now have been recognized also to cause slowly progressive, degenerative neurologic diseases. The term "slow virus infections" originated in veterinary literature in reference to sheep diseases such as visna and scrapie.[230] The term is applied to infections with long incubation periods followed by slowly progressive disease leading to death. Slow viral infections can be caused by conventional viruses such as visna, or by unconventional agents such as the scrapie agent.

Some conventional viruses grow rapidly in cell cultures but are modulated in the intact host to cause slowly progressive disease; lentiviruses causing visna in sheep and the acquired immunodeficiency syndrome in humans are examples. Conventional viruses also can cause slow infections because of defective virus replication, as in subacute sclerosing panencephalitis, or because of defects of the host's immune response, as in progressive multifocal leukoencephalopathy.

The unconventional agents are responsible for the subacute spongiform viral encephalopathies, which include the human diseases kuru, Creutzfeldt-Jakob, and the Gerstmann-Sträussler variant. Although these agents replicate, they are unconventional in that they are resistant to treatments that inactivate viruses, they lack antigenicity, and they cannot be definitively visualized by electron microscopy.

Human Immunodeficiency Virus Type 1 Encephalopathy

CLINICAL FEATURES

Within the first year or two of clinical experience with HIV-1 infection, it became apparent that many patients developed cognitive impairment.[23,154] At first, the psychomotor slowing and mental dulling was mistakenly attributed to "depression," "delirium," or an "adjustment disorder," or confused with opportunistic infections of the nervous system. It is obvious now, however, that a definable dementia develops in association with infection with HIV-1, known as HIV-1 encephalopathy (HIVE).[36a,180] This has also been termed HIV-related dementia, subacute encephalitis, AIDS encephalopathy, and AIDS dementia complex. Surveillance data from the Centers for Disease Control indicate that the incidence of HIVE has a bimodal character (Fig. 8–1), with an incidence of 2.2% in the age range 20 to 29, rising to 6.0% in those aged 60 to 69. Dementia is evident in 20% to 40% of patients with AIDS by the time of death, and 90% of patients dying with AIDS show histologic evidence of a subacute encephalitis, the pathologic correlate of HIVE.[50,179,183] HIVE develops only rarely during the incubation period of HIV infection, before constitutional symptoms, immune deficiency, and opportunistic processes develop.[162,181] Although several groups have described high rates of neuropsychological test abnormalities in healthy HIV-1–infected homosexual men (in CDC groups II or III)[95,125] and in intravenous drug users,[231] the clinical significance of these findings is uncertain because these neuropsychological abnormalities are not necessarily progressive and may reflect the effects of low education, age, and alcohol and drug

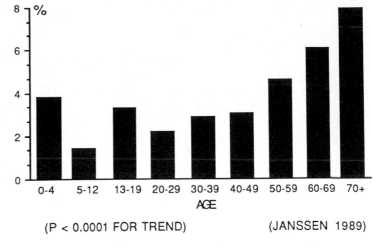

(CDC CASES: USA 9/1/87 - 12/31/88)

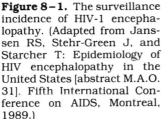

Figure 8–1. The surveillance incidence of HIV-1 encephalopathy. (Adapted from Janssen RS, Stehr-Green J, and Starcher T: Epidemiology of HIV encephalopathy in the United States [abstract M.A.O. 31]. Fifth International Conference on AIDS, Montreal, 1989.)

(P < 0.0001 FOR TREND)   (JANSSEN 1989)

use, rather than HIV-1 infection. Information about the prevalence of HIVE has come from a longitudinal study in nearly 2000 HIV-1–seropositive and –seronegative homosexual men underway in the Multicenter AIDS Cohort Study.[164] In this study the prevalence of HIVE in individuals without AIDS or constitutional symptoms was less than 1% and the frequency of neuropsychological impairment in HIV carriers was not significantly higher than in appropriate controls.[164] These findings have been confirmed by Janssen and colleagues[124] and Goethe and colleagues.[90]

The clinical syndrome occurs in all groups at risk for HIV-1 infection, including children. In fact, in children progressive encephalopathy may occur early, antedating opportunistic infections.[67] Clinical features in children include microcephaly and developmental delay, leading to loss of milestones, with death occurring within the first few years of life. The proportion of infected infants born to seropositive mothers may be as high as 65%, based on frequency data obtained from HIV-1–infected mothers who had already delivered an infected infant.[219] The

diagnosis of HIV-1 infection in infants is complicated by the fact that current serologic techniques may produce a false-positive result because of the presence of maternally derived anti–HIV-1 IgG. Polymerase chain reaction technologies will be helpful in detecting small quantities of viral DNA, thus indicating the presence of true infection.

Typically, HIVE develops and progresses in parallel with the later stages of AIDS and is associated with marked immune deficiency. The clinical manifestations of HIVE suggest predominantly subcortical involvement, at least initially.[180] A typical presentation includes apathy and inertia, depressive symptoms, and withdrawal from usual activities. The early symptoms are often subtle and may be overlooked or confused with psychiatric complaints. Patients complain of slowing of mental processing, a reduction in mental flexibility, poor short-term memory, and difficulties with reading comprehension. Family and friends will notice behavioral changes such as a loss of initiative or "spark," depressive symptoms, social withdrawal, and a decline in spontaneity. Specific neuropsychological

Table 8–3 CLINICAL STAGING OF THE AIDS DEMENTIA COMPLEX*

Stage	Characteristics
Stage 0 (normal)	Normal mental and motor function
Stage 0.5 (equivocal/subclinical)	Absent, minimal, or equivocal symptoms without impairment of work or capacity to perform ADL. Mild signs (snout response, slowed ocular or extremity movements) may be present. Gait and strength are normal.
Stage 1 (mild)	Able to perform all but the more demanding aspects of work or ADL but with unequivocal evidence (signs or symptoms that may include performance on neuropsychological testing) of functional intellectual or motor impairment. Can walk without assistance.
Stage 2 (moderate)	Able to perform basic activities of self-care but cannot work or maintain the more demanding aspects of daily life. Ambulatory, but may require a single prop.
Stage 3 (severe)	Major intellectual incapacity (cannot follow news or personal events, cannot sustain complex conversation, considerable slowing of all outputs) or motor disability (cannot walk unassisted, requiring walker or personal support, usually with slowing and clumsiness of arms as well).
Stage 4 (end stage)	Nearly vegetative. Intellectual and social comprehension and output are at a rudimentary level. Nearly or absolutely mute. Paraparetic or paraplegic with urinary and fecal incontinence.

*Developed at Memorial Sloan Kettering Center.
Source: From Price RW and Brew BJ,[199] p. 1080.

features include (1) bradyphrenia or psychomotor slowing as demonstrated by tests like finger-tapping, Grooved Pegboard, reaction time, and others; (2) memory disturbance, typically somewhat milder than occurs with cortical dementias, including frequent sparing of recognition memory; and (3) visuospatial abnormalities, as demonstrated by tests like the Rey Complex Figure and Block Design (WAIS-R). Deficits of "executive" or frontal-lobe–type functions also occur and can be documented by tests like the World Fluency Test, Wisconsin Card Sorting, and the Category Test. (See Chapter 5.) With advancing dementia, new learning and memory deteriorate, mental processing slows further, and language impairment becomes more obvious. The terminal phases of the syndrome are characterized by a global deterioration with severe psychomotor retardation and mutism. The dementia may progress rapidly over a few weeks or months. In one series of 30 patients with HIVE, the mean interval from first symptoms to death was 5.6 months.[162] Price and colleagues[199] have developed a staging scheme (Table 8–3) that is useful both in clinical practice and in conducting research studies.

Neurologic examination is often normal in the early stages of HIVE, although careful examination may demonstrate impaired rapid eye and limb movements and diffuse hyperreflexia. As HIVE progresses, increased tone develops, particularly in the lower extremities, and is usually associated with tremor, clonus, release signs, and hyperactive reflexes. Some of these signs may reflect the effects of an accompanying AIDS-related myelopathy.[193] Abnormalities of eye movements, including impaired smooth tracking, slowing of saccades, and inaccuracy of antisaccades, are common. Retinal changes may be seen, most commonly the presence of "cotton-wool" spots, but these are not pathognomonic for HIVE and occur frequently in nondemented individuals.[196]

Differential diagnosis is particularly difficult in the early stages of HIVE because the initial symptoms can be confused with depression or anxiety disorders or with the effects of psy-

Table 8–4 CLINICAL FEATURES USEFUL FOR
DIAGNOSIS OF HIV-1–RELATED
ENCEPHALOPATHY/DEMENTIA

HIV-1 seropositivity (Western blot confirmation)
History of *progressive* cognitive/behavioral decline with apathy, memory loss, slowed mental processing
Neurologic exam: diffuse CNS signs including slowed rapid eye/limb movements, hyperreflexia, hypertonia, and release signs
Neuropsychological assessment: progressive deterioration on serial testing in at least two areas including frontal lobe, motor speed, and nonverbal memory
CSF analysis: nonspecific abnormalities of IgG and protein, HIV-1 isolation, and intrathecal synthesis of anti–HIV-1; exclusion of neurosyphilis and cryptococcal meningitis
Imaging studies: diffuse cerebral atrophy with ill-defined white matter rarefaction (on MRI), exclusion of opportunistic processes
Absence of major psychiatric disorder or active substance abuse
Absence of metabolic derangement (e.g., hypoxia, sepsis)

choactive substances. Often, detailed historical information from friends, family, or co-workers is helpful, and psychiatric consultation may be indicated. Differentiation from infections such as cerebral toxoplasmosis, cytomegalovirus encephalitis, neurosyphilis, and cryptococcal or tuberculous meningitis is critical because specific therapies are available for these conditions. HIVE is not an inevitable consequence of HIV infection; altered mental status in any patient should be evaluated thoroughly and not simply ascribed to the effects of HIVE.

Precise criteria do not yet exist for diagnosing HIVE, yet dementia has recently been included by the Centers for Disease Control as one of the conditions to establish a diagnosis of AIDS.[36a] Table 8–4 lists features that may be helpful in establishing this diagnosis in clinical practice.

LABORATORY FINDINGS

CSF abnormalities are frequently found in neurologically *normal* HIV carriers, and also in subjects with minor neuropsychological abnormalities. Thus CSF analysis is not specific for HIVE (Fig. 8–2). CSF analysis is impor-

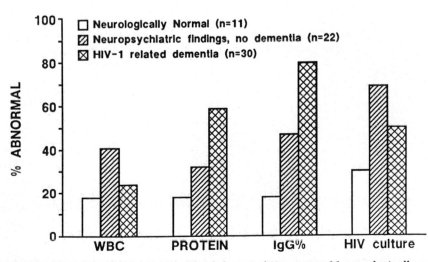

Figure 8–2. The frequency of cerebrospinal fluid abnormalities among 11 neurologically normal HIV-1 seropositive men, 22 HIV-1 seropositives with minor neuropsychological abnormalities, and 30 with HIV-1 encephalopathy.

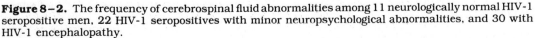

tant, however, to exclude opportunistic infections in the patient with suspected HIVE. Although no single CSF test or combination of tests can reliably diagnose HIVE at present, a completely normal CSF profile, with no abnormalities of protein or IgG, points away from the diagnosis. The most frequent CSF abnormalities in 30 patients with HIVE were an elevated total protein (in 17 of 26 patients [65%]) and immunoglobulin (IgG) fraction (in 4 of 5 individuals [80%]).[162] Oligoclonal bands are less frequent and myelin basic protein levels are not usually elevated. Intrathecal synthesis of anti–HIV-1 IgG appears to correlate with the presence of progressive dementia but is also present in up to 45% of neurologically normal individuals with HIV infection.[253] The CSF is usually acellular but may show a mild lymphocytic pleocytosis. T lymphocytes are distributed in CSF in a similar pattern to their distribution in peripheral blood, with reduced proportions of T helper cells and inverted T-helper: T-suppressor ratios.[166] CSF B2 microglobulin appears to be a marker for the presence of HIV encephalopathy, elevated levels correlating with the clinical severity of the dementia.[18]

Radiologic features include cerebral atrophy and white-matter rarefaction. Imaging studies are important in the evaluation of suspected HIVE to exclude mass lesions. Diffuse cerebral atrophy[155,180] can often be observed to progress in parallel with the clinical deterioration (Fig. 8–3). Both CT and MRI appear to be equally sensitive in demonstrating the atrophy in early HIVE (Fig. 8–4A).[162] MRI, however, more readily demonstrates white-matter abnormalities in HIVE, which appear as ill-defined areas of increased signal intensity on T_2-weighted images.[155,200] These often evolve from small, ill-defined hyperintensities seen in deep white matter in patients with early HIVE (Fig.

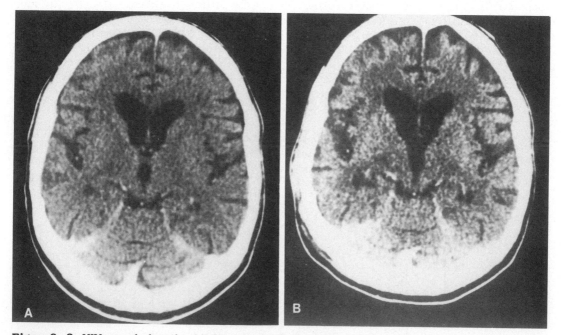

Figure 8–3. HIV encephalopathy: (A) CT scan of a 36-year-old intravenous drug user with AIDS-related complex and early AIDS-related dementia. Mild frontotemporal atrophy and ventricular enlargement are seen. (B) CT scan of same patient 3 months later, with far-advanced HIV-1 encephalopathy. Severe frontotemporal atrophy and ventriculomegaly are noted, with attenuation of the periventricular white matter.

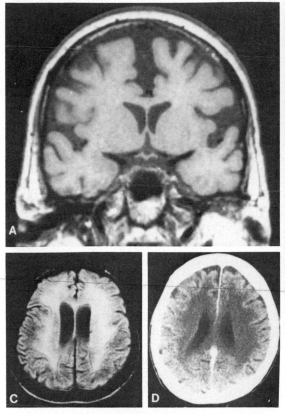

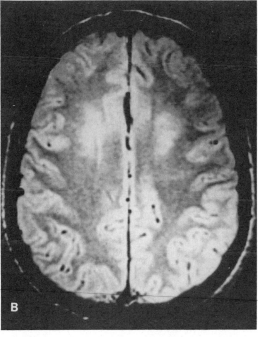

Figure 8–4. HIV encephalopathy: (A) MRI (T₁-weighted image) of 33-year-old homosexual man with early AIDS-related dementia showing moderate diffuse cerebral atrophy and hydrocephalus ex vacuo. (B) MRI (T₂-weighted image) of same patient, showing larger areas of abnormal signal intensity in the white matter (*arrows*). No mass effect is present. (C) MRI (T₂-weighted image) of 38-year-old bisexual man with late-stage HIV-1 encephalopathy demonstrating enlargement of the ventricles, cerebral atrophy, and diffuse abnormalities throughout the white matter. (D) CT scan obtained at the same time from the same patient as (C), showing moderate ventriculomegaly. White-matter attenuation is seen, although the changes are far less striking than those observed on MRI.

8–4B) to more diffuse abnormalities in severely demented individuals (Fig. 8–4C,.D). It is uncertain how often MRI abnormalities can be identified before the development of cognitive symptoms. Discrete white-matter hyperintensities ("unidentified bright objects") are relatively common even in the age group at most risk for HIV infection, and are probably of no pathologic significance.[165]

Both single photon emission computed tomography (SPECT) and positron emission tomography (PET) have been studied in small numbers of individuals with HIVE. Using PET, Rottenberg and colleagues[215] demonstrated subcortical hypermetabolism in the early stages of HIVE, with later progression to cortical and subcortical hypometabolism. Normalization of PET abnormalities has also been shown with azidothymidine (AZT) administration.[267] With SPECT, abnormalities in cerebral blood flow have been identified in most individuals with HIVE and in neurologically normal HIV-1 carriers, raising the possibility that SPECT might be a useful predictive tool.[148] Neither of these techniques is widely available, however, and their interpretation and quantitation is difficult. Their usefulness in detection of HIVE or in assessing treatment effects remains to be determined.

EEG has not been systematically

studied in either the diagnosis or staging of HIVE. In the late stages of HIVE a diffuse slowing is frequently noted,[180] but in less advanced stages of dementia the EEG may be normal in 50% of patients.[162] The specificity of EEG in differentiating psychiatric disorders from early dementia is uncertain, and in general EEG adds little information to the evaluation of suspected HIVE.

PATHOLOGIC FEATURES

Cerebral atrophy is common in patients with HIVE, often occurring in a frontotemporal distribution. Multiple small nodules containing macrophages, lymphocytes, and microglia (termed microglial nodules) are scattered throughout both gray and white matter of the brain, appearing more commonly in white matter and the subcortical gray matter of the thalamus, basal ganglia, and brainstem (Fig. 8–5A).[50] Although these inflammatory nodules are frequently identified in HIVE, they are not specific for this disorder and have been described with other CNS infections, including cytomegalovirus encephalitis occurring after renal transplantation.[58] The number of nodules does not correlate with the severity of the dementia.[179] Multinucleated giant cells are characteristically seen (Fig. 8–5B).[30,207,226] The combination of multinucleated giant cells, microglial nodules, and perivenular inflammation has been termed *subacute encephalitis*[179,183,227,237] and has been identified in 90% of patients dying with AIDS or AIDS-related complex (ARC).[50] The presence of multinucleated giant cells correlates both with the degree of dementia and with the detection of HIV-1 nucleic acid sequences by Southern blot analysis.[142,201] These giant cells have been posited as markers of HIV-1 replication, because HIV-1 forms giant multinucleated cells in culture.[84] Perivascular infiltrations of lymphocytes and monocyte/macrophages are also frequently seen.[50,179,207,264] The inflammatory infiltrates, multinucleated giant cells, and endothelial cells have been demonstrated to contain viral nucleic acid sequences.[264] In general, these pathologic changes affect white matter more than gray. Another striking pathologic feature also involves white matter, and includes both discrete areas of focal demyelination[183] and more widespread and diffuse rarefaction or vacuolation of white matter (Fig. 8–5C).[140,179] This leukoencephalopathy probably gives rise to the abnormal appearance of white matter on MRI.

A vacuolar (spongiform) myelopathy has been described to occur in association with HIVE[50,193]

EVIDENCE FOR HIV-1 AS THE CAUSATIVE AGENT

Initially cytomegalovirus (CMV) was incriminated as the cause of HIVE.[237] Although disseminated systemic CMV infection is very frequent in AIDS, in only a minority of cases of HIVE can CMV be identified within the CNS.[179,183] Using immunocytochemical staining, Wiley and colleagues demonstrated CMV antigens in 31 of 93 (33%) brains at autopsy, with two histopathologic patterns: microscopic infarctions and microglial nodules.[263] HIV-1 now is presumed to cause HIVE,[83,118,153,226] but the actual pathogenetic mechanisms remain unexplained,[131] and it is possible that an in vivo interaction between HIV-1 and other viruses such as CMV may be important.[263] There have been preliminary reports of neurologic disease appearing with HIV-2, a distinct type of retrovirus prevalent in Western Africa.[29] As yet, however, the spectrum of clinical disease with HIV-2 has not been mapped.

The evidence for HIV-1 as the causative agent rests on morphologic identification of the virus,[66,101] intrathecal synthesis of antibody,[65,206,253] virus isolation,[50,118,153,241] immunocytochemical staining for viral antigens,* and in situ

---

*References 50, 75, 101, 201, 204, 254, 264.

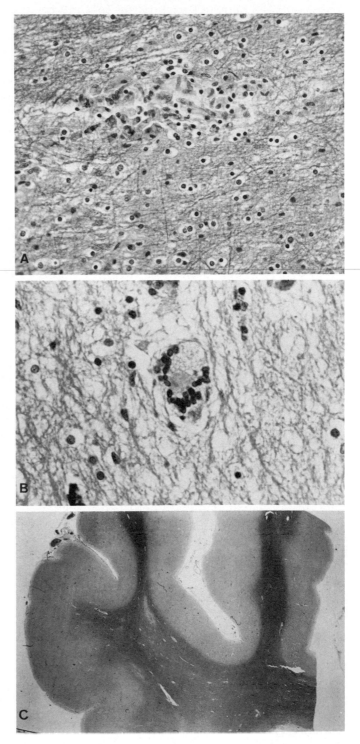

Figure 8–5. HIV-1 encephalopathy: High-power photomicrographs from centrum semiovale of a patient dying with advanced AIDS-related dementia, demonstrating (A) a microglial nodule, and (B) a multinucleated giant cell (hematoxylin-eosin stain, magnification × 800). (C) Low-power photomicrograph of cerebral cortex from same patient. There is marked rarefaction of the subcortical white matter in places (arrows), whereas other areas appear to have normally staining myelin (luxol–fast blue stain, magnification × 10). (Courtesy of Dr. S. Becker.)

hybridization.[142,228,264] In one of the first reports, viral DNA and RNA sequences were detected within the inflammatory nodules in brains from patients with HIVE.[228] The viral DNA, by Southern blot analysis, showed higher concentrations within the brain than in samples of spleen, lymph node, liver, or lung. Other investigators have demonstrated HIV-1–like particles within multinucleated giant cells, and also free within the extracellular space.[66,101]

In patients with HIVE, virus isolation studies have recovered HIV-1 from both brain and CSF.[118] The antemortem isolation of HIV-1 from a brain biopsy of a homosexual man with AIDS-related dementia has also been described.[153] The same investigators also cultured HIV-1 from the CSF of 13 of 14 patients, including 1 without neurologic symptoms. HIV-1 can be isolated from CSF in up to 30% of neurologically normal HIV-1–infected individuals[163] (see Fig. 8–2), suggesting that the brain is an early target for HIV-1 infection. Primary cultures obtained from a brain biopsy specimen of an individual with HIVE revealed that the cells expressing virus in the primary explant cultures were derived from a monocyte-macrophage lineage.[83]

LOCALIZATION AND NEUROTROPISM OF HIV-1

By immunocytochemical identification of viral structural proteins and by in situ hybridization, HIV-1 has been localized within macrophages and multinucleated cells in the microglial nodules and areas of perivascular inflammation.* Two groups of investigators have reported a striking involvement of capillary endothelial cells.[256,264] The virus is found with greater frequency in the white matter and subcortical areas than in the cortex.[241] Some investigators have provided evidence of

viral replication within parenchymal cells, including astrocytes, and possibly within neurons.[75,204,241] In one study, careful ultrastructural examination of brain biopsies from 7 patients with HIVE revealed small numbers of budding HIV-1 virions within cells that were identified as oligodendrocytes and astrocytes by double immuno-staining for myelin basic protein and HIV-1 p24 core protein.[101] It is possible that these cells could, in fact, have been microglial cells. Other investigators using combined immunocytochemistry and in situ hybridization detected involvement of capillary endothelial cells in 7 of 12 patients with HIVE, but in only 1 case was HIV-1 identified within neurons and glial cells.[264] In summary, the majority of studies have consistently shown that HIV-1 infection is more frequent in macrophages and multinucleated giant cells, and that the deep white matter is more commonly involved than the gray matter. Whether parenchymal cells such as oligodendrocytes or neurons ever contain replicating virus remains uncertain.

Several groups of investigators have focused on the cell tropism of HIV-1 and have demonstrated productive infection within different brain-derived cell lines in vitro, including human fetal brain cells and cells of astrocytic origin.[40,53] Distinct strains of HIV-1 isolated from the nervous system of the same individual appear to have different tropisms in vitro.[144] It has been suggested that certain strains of HIV-1 are noncytocidal and replicate with greater efficiency within cells of neural origin than do other strains.[4] Expression of the T_4 antigen has been demonstrated in cell lines of astrocytic origin, raising the possibility that HIV-1 might selectively bind to cell surface receptors on parenchymal cells and thus cause infection.[54] Productive infection can take place in cells that do not express the CD4 antigen, although the level of replication is several orders of magnitude less than in cell lines of CD4 lymphocytes or macrophages. The relevance of these in vitro studies to the situation in

---

*References 50, 75, 101, 142, 179, 201, 204, 254, 264.

vivo is uncertain. It is to be hoped that these avenues of research may eventually help explain the differences among patients in susceptibility to HIVE and the variability often seen in the rate of cognitive decline.

HIV-1 probably gains access to the CNS from the bloodstream, either by direct infection of capillary endothelial cells,[131] or more likely by ingress of infected macrophages, the "Trojan-horse" hypothesis.[102] Despite several in vitro studies demonstrating that both astrocytes[53] and oligodendrocytes[101] can act as targets for HIV-1 infection and that cells of astrocytic origin can express CD_4 antigen,[54] these parenchymal cells are unlikely primary targets for HIV-1 infection.

PATHOGENETIC MECHANISMS

The pathogenetic mechanisms involved in the production of HIVE remain obscure, in that profound dementia sometimes occurs with relatively mild neuropathologic changes.[50,201] For example, in one study of 10 demented patients, moderate or severe subacute encephalitis was observed in 8, yet 2 had only mild pathologic abnormalities.[50] By contrast, up to 90% of patients with AIDS will have pathologic abnormalities, but not all will display manifestations of dementia.[50] Using in situ hybridization techniques, less than 0.01% of circulating total mononuclear cells contain HIV-1 RNA,[111] and in the nervous system only a small fraction of cells within inflammatory nodules or capillary endothelial cells contain viral antigens, even in individuals with advanced dementia.[75]

This discrepancy between the small concentrations of replicating HIV-1 present and the severity of the dementia suggests that other factors besides direct cellular damage by HIV-1 may be of importance in pathogenesis.[132] First, the release of cytokines locally from infected lymphocytes and/or macrophages might impair cellular functioning or modify neurotransmitter function.[131,179] Alternatively, these sol-uble factors might cause the leukoencephalopathy that has been observed both focally and diffusely in subcortical regions, and which probably contributes significantly to the clinical manifestations.[101] The precise mechanisms underlying these changes in white matter have not yet been defined, but the similarities to the lesions of postinfectious encephalomyelitis or visna infection suggests that the changes may result from immune-mediated mechanisms or as a form of "bystander demyelination" mediated by proteases and other products of activated macrophages.[111,176,178] Second, the possibility of direct neuronal infection and cell killing or damage has been raised. The absence of productive infection in neurons and the apparently normal neuronal population densities make this premise unlikely. Other viruses (for example, JC virus see p. 256) can produce demyelination by direct infection of oligodendrocytes,[177] but there is little evidence for this with HIV-1 infection. Third, the role of calcium flux has been suggested as important with the descriptions that gp120 (the envelope glycoprotein of HIV-1) increases the amount of free intracellular calcium and might lead to neuronal damage in the same manner that calcium is thought to be neurotoxic in other neurologic disorders, including stroke.[60] Fourth, based on autoradiographic methods, it has been suggested that CD4-like antigen receptors exist in the hippocampus, amygdala, and cortex.[116] These receptors may be binding sites for an endogenous neurotransmitter, vasoactive intestinal polypeptide.[117] Despite the lack of congruity between the described topographic distribution of the CD4-like antigens and the localization of HIV-1, it has been postulated that by binding to these CD4-like receptors, the envelope glycoprotein of HIV-1 interferes with naturally occurring neurotransmitters, including vasoactive intestinal polypeptide.[192] A pentapeptide, peptide T, has been synthesized that appears to prevent neuronal death in cell cultures.[17] Preliminary phase-1 trials have demonstrated minimal antiviral or immunologic effects but have suggested improvement in cognitive functioning in patients with impaired neuropsychological performance.[19] This novel and intriguing hypothesis needs to be confirmed by expanded studies with more extensive controls. An antiviral effect that was initially described has not been confirmed by other investigators.[238] Finally, the question of the potential for brain dysfunction to result from exposure to toxins has been raised by recent studies demonstrating greatly elevated levels of quinolinic acid (an excitatory neurotoxic metabolite of tryptophan).[115]

In summary, the clinical, radiologic, and pathologic features of HIVE suggest predominantly subcortical involvement with prominent leukoencephalopathy and relative sparing of the cortex. The frequent CSF abnormalities in the early stages of infection and the neuropathologic abnormalities in more than 90% of patients dying with AIDS suggest that viral invasion of the CNS occurs in the majority of HIV-1-infected patients, yet not all develop progressive dementia. The role of differences in neurovirulence among strains of HIV-1 may be of importance in explaining this discrepancy. Whether an indirect effect of HIV-1 on neural cells causes HIVE, whether the cause is the release of soluble factors evoked by infection, or whether other viruses or infectious agents are involved remains unknown. Questions regarding the timing and route of initial CNS invasion also will require clarification through careful prospective studies.

TREATMENT OF HIVE

Despite the unresolved questions in pathogenesis, specific antiviral agents have already been used in the treatment of HIVE. Preliminary studies with AZT in four demented individuals showed promising improvements in clinical functioning, neuropsychological performance, and, in one case, nor-malization of PET scans.[94] Evidence from the multicenter licensing trial[72] of AZT in patients with AIDS or ARC suggests that AZT may improve or stabilize neuropsychological function at least temporarily.[218] Epidemiologic evidence has suggested that the more widespread and earlier use of AZT might reduce the incidence of HIVE. Portegies[197] documented a drop in the incidence of HIVE from 53% before AZT was available to 10% after its widespread use. Peptide T and newer antivirals, including pyrimidine analogues such as dideoxyinosine (ddI), have demonstrated some efficacy for neurologic disorders when used in phase 1 trials.

As with other CNS viral infections, early initiation of antimicrobial therapy is likely to be essential in stabilizing or restoring brain function. This makes it critical to understand better the earliest clinical manifestations of HIVE and develop screening tests that are both sensitive *and* specific. An epidemic of HIVE in young adults both in the United States and in African nations is probable. If 225,000 Americans are alive with AIDS in 1993, and 30% develop HIVE, that translates to 68,000 cases during that year alone,[37a] a figure seven times the annual incidence of multiple sclerosis.

Subacute Sclerosing Panencephalitis

This disorder occurs in a worldwide distribution but is rare, striking fewer than 50 new patients in 1979 in the United States.[242] It has been decreasing in incidence since that year. There is about one case of subacute sclerosing panencephalitis (SSPE) per million cases of primary measles. The onset of SSPE is usually between the ages of 2 and 21, with a mean age of onset of 7.2 years,[127] but cases have been documented in the third decade of life.[31] Males are affected nearly three times as frequently as females, and whites are affected four times more frequently than blacks.[172] The condition does not cluster in families but is more common in rural areas, particularly on farms.[20,52,123] The attack rate is 10 times higher in unvaccinated children with a history of measles than in vaccinated children,[173] and patients frequently have a history of having had clinical measles infection before reaching age 2.[20,52] These epidemiologic observations may no longer be valid for the small group of patients that presently have SSPE.

CLINICAL FEATURES

Typically, a previously normal child has insidious changes in behavior and a subtle decline in intellect, which usually manifests as a deterioration in school performance.[74] Weeks or months later, myoclonic jerks develop. A characteristic EEG is frequently seen, consisting of repetitive discharges of high-amplitude slow waves followed by a flat background, the "suppression burst" pattern.[159] Chorioretinitis, papilledema, and optic atrophy are not infrequent.[73,182,210] As dementia and myoclonus progress, corticospinal tract signs, cerebellar signs, rigidity, and dystonia may develop. Eventually, the patient lapses into a mute, stuporous, rigid state with autonomic instability evidenced by temperature fluctuations and sweating abnormalities.

Most cases have an insidious onset and progress to death in 1 to 3 years. Approximately 10% of patients have a fulminant course causing death within 3 months;[89,122] another 10% survive 4 to 10 years, occasionally with transient remissions.[122]

The CSF is usually normocellular, with a normal glucose and protein content. An increase in γ-globulin is due to oligoclonal IgG that corresponds, in large part, to measles antibody. These elevated levels of measles antibody have been found in the serum and CSF of virtually all cases of SSPE and are crucial in establishing a diagnosis. A reduced serum-to-CSF ratio of measles antibody is found, suggesting intrathecal production of antibodies. CSF contains antibodies reacting with multiple antigens of the measles virion, although the predominant reaction is against the internal nucleocapsid antigen,[2,184] often with an absence of antibody against the matrix (M) protein by Western immunoblot analysis.[107,257]

PATHOLOGY

The histopathologic lesions in SSPE are usually most severe in the posterior cerebral hemispheres, with lesser involvement of brainstem, cerebellum, spinal cord, and retina. A sclerosing panencephalitis is present, with perivascular and leptomeningeal mononuclear cell infiltration, neuronophagia, and microglial proliferation.[245] In addition, neuronal loss, gliosis, and variable degrees of demyelination are observed. Inclusions corresponding to the filamentous nucleocapsids of measles virus are found in the nuclei and cytoplasm of neurons and glia.[113]

ETIOLOGY

In the original descriptions of the inclusions in SSPE, Dawson[48,49] suggested a viral etiology but it was not until Bouteille's description of the ultrastructural similarities between the inclusions and the nucleocapsids of paramyxoviruses that the specific link with measles virus was established.[16] In 1967, Connolly and co-workers[45] demonstrated exceptionally high levels of measles antibody in serum and CSF of three patients with SSPE, as well as evidence of measles virus antigen in brain tissue by immunofluorescent staining. In 1968, measles virus cytopathic effect was seen in two cultures derived from brain of patients with SSPE,[11] and subsequently complete infectious measles virus was isolated using cocultivation techniques.[119,191] Virus cannot be isolated directly from the brain of patients with SSPE, but requires either cocultivation or explantation.[103,136] Patients with SSPE may lack antibody to a viral protein, the M protein, despite high levels of antibody to other viral proteins.[257] Despite these observations, evidence of M protein has been detected within the CNS of some SSPE patients.[188] Absence of serum antibodies to M protein occurs in more than 50% of convalescent uncomplicated measles patients[96] and has been reported in a case complicated by acute encephalitis[106] and in an immunosuppressed child with measles inclusion body encephalitis.[214] Different groups of investigators have put forward diverse explanations for the absence of M protein, including defective protein translation[34] and excessively rapid protein degradation.[229] The glycosylated envelope proteins may also be reduced in concentration, and it seems likely that either defective production or overly rapid turnover of envelope proteins probably accounts for the absence of enveloped extracellular virions.

Recent cloning and sequencing studies have begun to clarify the above observations regarding M protein. These studies have directly demonstrated a remarkable degree of mutation in the M gene, as well as in other measles virus genes.[35] The M gene had an average of 12 expressed and 8 silent nucleotide changes per 1000 bases of the coding region. This extraordinarily high number of mutations alters the antigenicity of M protein and thereby can fail to trigger a detectable anti-M immunoprecipitating antibody response in the SSPE patient.[6] Mutations in viruses from three of four cases studied caused partial deletions in the gene for F, an envelope glycoprotein, perhaps impairing efficient viral budding. Another interesting feature of these studies, not yet completely understood, is the apparent "biased hypermutation" of these genes. In the case of the M gene isolated from one case, about 50% of the uridine residues were mutated to cytosine, whereas in another case more than 20% of the adenine residues of the F gene were changed to guanine. This high frequency and nonrandom nature of the mutations may reflect the presence of a persistent infection (with an absence of the normal selective pressure) and the presence of an unusual enzyme activity in the CNS.[10]

No abnormality of the immune system has been identified to account for the persistent infection,[14] although the ability of measles infections to alter cell-mediated immunity transiently during both natural[251] and experimental infections[167] may be important in the induction of persistent infection. Gene mutations may account for this defective infection, with cell-to-cell spread producing a persistent slow virus infection with failure of host clearance despite normal immune responses.[103] The frequency with which measles develops before the age of 2 years in patients with SSPE may be pertinent; the interactive role of CNS development and measles infection has yet to be fully explored.[41] The residual presence of maternal antibody may modulate infection and increase the likelihood of a defective infection.

TREATMENT

A variety of immunosuppressive and antiviral agents, including isoprinosine,[104] have been tried without any demonstrated benefit in patients with SSPE. Recent reports have suggested that interferon leads to a remission, but these studies have been uncontrolled and have involved relatively few patients.[121,189] The myoclonus occasionally responds to clonazepam (Klonopin).

Progressive Rubella Panencephalitis

CLINICAL FEATURES

Progressive rubella panencephalitis, a slowly progressive illness, is a rare, late manifestation of congenital rubella infection.[246,258] Cerebellar degeneration and deterioration in mental function beginning in the second decade of life are characteristic. Progressive panencephalitis also has been reported in scattered cases with postnatal rubella.[152,256]

PATHOLOGY

Histopathology of three cases showed a subacute-to-chronic panencephalitis with meningeal and perivascular lymphocytic and plasma-cell infiltration, microglial nodules, gliosis, and mild neuronal loss.[258]

ETIOLOGY

Rubella virus is occasionally isolated from the brain,[47,258] but in general neither viral antigens nor virions can be demonstrated in brain tissue. No recent cases have been reported and none appear to have resulted from the last major epidemic of rubella in 1964. Thus strain variation of virus may be a factor in the apparent disappearance of progressive rubella panencephalitis.

Other Chronic Encephalitides

In addition to SSPE and rubella, chronic encephalitis has been described as an opportunistic infection of immunosuppressed individuals and as a persistent sequela of tick-borne encephalitis. In children with agammaglobulinemia, enteroviruses such as poliovirus can persist within the CNS, producing progressive motor and mental deficits.[168] Occasionally, immunosuppressed adults develop encephalitis with adenovirus[212] or cytomegalovirus.[58]

A chronic inflammatory encephalitis has been described in the former Soviet Union[225] and in North America[205] in patients with epilepsia partialis continua and associated progressive mental and motor deterioration. As many as 83% of patients with the Russian form, Kozhevnikov's epilepsy, have an antecedent history of acute tick-borne encephalitis,[143] and virus has been isolated from blood, CSF, and brain tissue.[42,145] Nonspecific febrile illness of some sort precedes the onset of seizures in more than 50% of the North American cases,[205] but no virus has been isolated.

Limbic encephalitis associated with carcinoma,[46] Behçet's disease,[38] uveomeningoencephalitis syndrome,[209] and Vilyuisk's encephalitis of the Commonwealth of Independent States (formerly the Soviet Union)[194] have also been identified as putative chronic viral encephalitides, although the etiology of these conditions has not been firmly established.

PROGRESSIVE MULTIFOCAL LEUKOENCEPHALOPATHY — A DEMYELINATING DISEASE AS A CAUSE OF DEMENTIA

Clinical Features

Progressive multifocal leukoencephalopathy (PML) is an opportunistic infection occurring in immunologically compromised individuals. Until 1982, more than half the cases were associated with lymphoproliferative disease, and many of the remainder with sarcoidosis, tuberculosis, and neoplasms.[208] Cases have also occurred in patients undergoing vigorous immunosuppression in order to maintain renal allografts[158] or to treat systemic lupus erythematosus.[259] Since the recognition of AIDS in 1981, however, the majority of cases occur in the setting of the cellular immune deficiency caused by infection with HIV-1. A few well-documented cases have been reported in individuals with no known history or autopsy evidence of an underlying disease.[28]

PML is a worldwide disease. Prior to the AIDS epidemic, the average age of onset was in the sixth decade; the youngest reported patient was 18 years old.[177] Patients develop progressive multifocal neurologic signs such as hemiparesis, aphasia, seizures, intellectual decline, personality change, gait abnormalities, and visual problems.[208] Cerebellar, brainstem, and spinal cord signs are less common. A terminal stage with prominent dementia, motor deficits, and coma ensues. Occasional

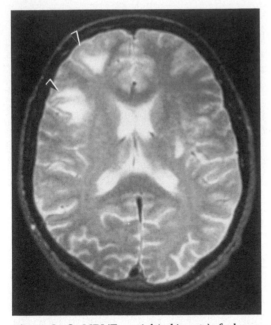

Figure 8–6. MRI (T$_2$-weighted image) of a homosexual male presenting with aphasia and hemiparesis. Two discrete areas of hyperintensity are seen within the white matter of the left hemisphere (*arrows*). Cerebral biopsy confirmed progressive multifocal leukoencephalopathy (PML).

cases have been reported with courses longer than 10 years and with transient remissions.[137,240] In cases associated with AIDS, death usually occurs 3 to 6 months after onset.[12] CT scans typically show nonenhancing hypodensities of cerebral white matter that do not cause mass effect,[147] but MRI scan appears to offer heightened sensitivity in the diagnosis of PML[146] (Fig. 8–6). The EEG is typically abnormal, progressing from focal to diffuse delta activity. The CSF is generally normal except for occasional protein elevation.

Pathology

The primary lesions are subcortical foci of demyelination, with relative sparing of axons. In demyelinated areas astrocytes are large, with bizarre mitotic figures, and abnormal nuclear and chromatin forms. Oligodendrocytes are absent within these areas and surrounding oligodendrocytes are enlarged, with intranuclear inclusions.[5] In 1965, two groups independently reported electron microscopic demonstration of papovaviruslike particles corresponding to the oligodendroglial inclusion bodies (Fig. 8–7); the particles were thought to resemble the polyoma-simian virus 40 (SV40) group of papovaviruses.[232,268]

Etiology

Despite numerous attempts, virus was not isolated from PML until 1971, when Padgett and co-workers,[187] using primary cultures of human fetal brain, isolated a new papovavirus, the JC virus. Weiner and co-workers,[259] subsequently isolated a variant of SV40 virus, another papovavirus, from two cases of PML. In subsequent cases, JC virus has been the virus isolated or identified by immune electron microscopy.[177] Two subgroups of JC virus isolates have been described on the basis of their restriction enzyme patterns.[99,211]

Pathogenesis

Serologic studies have demonstrated that primary infection with JC virus has occurred in 80% of young adults; no overt clinical signs have been associated with this infection.[81,187,224] SV40 virus antibodies, however, occur much less commonly.[222] In 1971, another new papovavirus, BK virus, was found in the urine of a renal transplant patient who had no neurologic disease,[82] but this has not yet been implicated in PML. It is assumed that immunosuppression results in activation of a latent papovavirus causing PML, but an alternative explanation is that a primary infection with a papovavirus in a naive immunosuppressed individual leads to PML.

Inoculation of JC, SV40, or BK viruses in experimental animals pro-

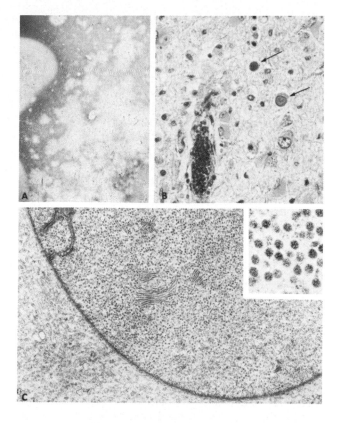

Figure 8–7. Progressive multifocal leukoencephalopathy: (*A*) Patchy demyelination unrelated to vessels, merging into confluent lesions (LFB stain, magnification × 8) (Armed Forces Institute of Pathology [AFIP] Neg. No. 68-9405). (*B*) Oligodendrocytes with enlarged nuclei (*arrows*) occur within early demyelinated lesions. Note absence of perivascular leukocytes (hematoxylin and eosin stain, magnification × 350) (AFIP Neg No. 68-9404). (*C*) Oligodendrocyte with enlarged nucleus filled with spheroidal and filamentous papovirus particles (× 20,000). (*Inset*) Magnification of virus particles in *C* (× 80,000). (From Lampert PW: Autoimmune and virus-induced demyelinating diseases. Am J Pathol 92:176, 1978, with permission.)

duces tumors[63,223,255] but not demyelination. Spontaneous PML due to SV40 has been reported in macaques with underlying systemic diseases, especially lymphoma.[98] The transgenic introduction of the early genes of JC virus into mice gives rise to gene expression selectively in oligodendrocytes and to failure of normal myelin formation.[234,247] These studies may furnish clues to the understanding of the pathogenesis of the myelin damage in PML.

CREUTZFELDT-JAKOB DISEASE — A NONINFLAMMATORY DISEASE AS A CAUSE OF DEMENTIA

Clinical Features

CJD is a worldwide disease occurring with an approximate incidence of 1 per million population per year.[21,23,77] An extensive epidemiologic study identified 230 pathologically verified cases in France over a 15-year period, yielding an annual incidence of 0.29 per million.[22] Geographic variations in incidence of CJD have been noted,[160] including an apparent focus among Libyan Jews,[135] a northern preponderance in 69 North American cases,[15] and two clusters among United Kingdom cases.[161] It seems likely that these apparent "foci", represent flawed case ascertainment or unrecognized familial clusters.[120a]

CJD affects equal numbers of men and women and has a peak incidence in the age group 55 to 65, although patients in their 20s and their 70s have been described.[22,248] As many as 10% of cases may be familial,[248] with a pattern most consistent with autosomal dominant inheritance.[70] Affected relatives within the same pedigree have similar clinical and pathologic findings.[70] Familial cases tend to have earlier onsets than sporadic cases.[213]

In its most characteristic dramatic presentation and course, CJD is fairly stereotyped.[51] The first symptoms of disease are often subtle and may initially be overlooked. Insidious mental deterioration is the most common presentation, occurring initially in 64% of patients, although in up to 20% the initial phase of disease develops rapidly over a few days.[22] Cerebellar and visual complaints accounted for 34% and 17%, respectively, of the early manifestations. All cases eventually become severely demented, usually within 6 months, and as the disease advances a majority of patients will develop stimulus-sensitive myoclonus and pyramidal, cerebellar, and extrapyramidal disturbances. Lower motor neuron signs appeared in only 11%.[22] EEG abnormalities are uncommon in the initial stages of presentation, but during the course of their disease, 80% of patients will develop periodic EEG complexes, either triphasic, 1-cycle/second sharp waves or a burst-suppression pattern. The CSF is typically acellular, although mildly elevated CSF protein values are occasionally found. The disease has an average duration of less than 8 months, and the patient dies in a terminal state of mute, akinetic rigidity with frequent seizures and myoclonic jerking. Some patients have a longer-than-average duration of illness and have prominent speech and language abnormalities resembling the so-called slowly progressive aphasias.[25]

Although the diagnosis of typical CJD cases is relatively straightforward, the rarer, more atypical clinical presentations are frequently misdiagnosed. The slowly progressive forms of CJD cannot easily be differentiated from AD on the basis of neuropsychological testing. The recent description of HIVE mandates exclusion of HIV-1 infection, particularly in younger patients presenting with putative CJD. Patients with the amyotrophic form of CJD may cause diagnostic difficulties because they may

have early lower motor neuron signs, later dementia, a prolonged course (over 2 years) and neither myoclonus nor a characteristic EEG.[3] Similarly, some individuals develop prominent cerebellar signs (Brownell-Oppenheimer variant[27]) and the disease may be mistaken for paraneoplastic cerebellar degeneration or multiple sclerosis. Another atypical presentation involves predominantly visual deterioration (Heidenhain's syndrome[169]).

Pathology

CJD is a member of the group of "subacute spongiform encephalopathies," along with scrapie, kuru, transmissible mink encephalopathy, and spongiform encephalopathy of captive mule deer, cows, and elk. The histopathologic hallmarks of subacute spongiform encephalopathies are neuronal loss, astrocytosis, and cytoplasmic vacuolation of neurons and astrocytes (status spongiosus)[151] (Fig. 8–8).

In CJD the neuronal loss can have a predilection for the anterior horn (the amyotrophic form), the cerebellum (the Brownell-Oppenheimer variant,[27] the "ataxic form" of CJD[92]) or the parietal and occipital lobes (Heidenhain's syndrome).[169] Astrocytosis of the gray matter may be prominent enough to suggest a diagnosis of astrocytoma.[213] The status spongiosus, of varying severity, corresponds under electron microscopy to vacuolated and swollen neuronal processes and perikaryal cytoplasm; spongiform changes occur less frequently in astrocytic processes.[150] Curled membrane fragments are found within the vacuoles.

The histopathologic abnormalities are characteristic but not pathognomonic. The neuronal loss and gliosis are frequent pathologic features of other degenerative diseases, and in some cases of CJD the spongiosus is insignificant, and white matter changes are seen.

Plaques are found in the cerebellum in more than 10% of cases of CJD[76] and

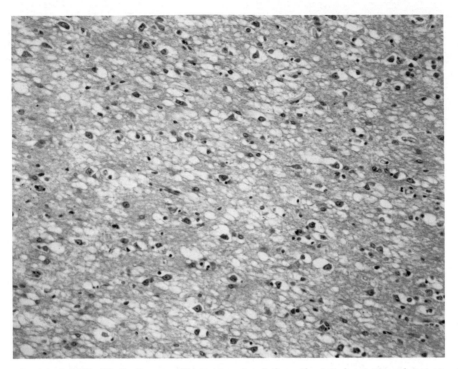

Figure 8–8. Creutzfeldt-Jakob disease: Photomicrograph from the insular cortex showing extensive spongiform changes (hematoxylin and eosin stain, magnification × 150). (Courtesy of Dr. Robert Wollman.)

all cases of Gerstmann-Sträussler syndrome and are similar to the plaques seen in kuru and scrapie. In the latter disease these plaques have been found identical at an ultrastructural level to the senile plaques of Alzheimer's disease (AD).[265]

Etiology

The absence of clinical signs of inflammation in CJD, such as fever or CSF pleocytosis, or of histopathologic findings of inclusion bodies or inflammatory infiltrates, made a viral etiology seem unlikely in the past.[252] The transmissibility of CJD was finally determined, however, through studies of kuru and scrapie.

Kuru, a subacute cerebellar disease occurring in the Fore linguistic group and their immediate neighbors in New Guinea, was described by Gajdusek and Zigas[80] in 1957. The disease was initially considered to be a genetic disorder that primarily affected adult females and young children of both sexes, causing death in less than 1 year. Clues to kuru's etiology were supplied in 1959 by Hadlow,[105] a veterinary neuropathologist, who remarked on the epidemiologic, clinical, and pathologic similarities between kuru and scrapie, a neurodegenerative disease of sheep and goats. Scrapie was known to be experimentally transmissible with an incubation period of several years, and Hadlow postulated that kuru might be a slow virus infection transmissible to subhuman primates.

Gajdusek, Gibbs, and Alpers inoculated suspensions of kuru-affected brain intracerebrally into a variety of animals including chimpanzees. Finally, 20 and 21 months after inoculation, two chimpanzees developed an ataxic disease and died 5 to 9 months later with pathologic evidence of sub-acute spongiform encephalopathy.[79] Numerous human cases of kuru have now been transmitted to chimpanzees, other primates, mink, guinea pigs, and hamsters, with incubation periods varying from 10 to 82 months.[68]

Klatzo and co-workers,[139] in an initial description of kuru pathology, re-marked on the similar histopathology of CJD. Attempts at transmission of CJD were soon initiated and in 1968, a chimpanzee developed subacute spon-giform encephalopathy 13 months after inoculation with filtered CJD-affected brain suspension.[87] CJD has now been transmitted from numerous cases of sporadic CJD and familial CJD cases from separate pedigrees.[248] By contrast, no confirmed transmission from spo-radic and familial AD has been re-ported. An initial report of transmission from two AD patients could not be re-produced after a repeat inoculation of the original material.[94]

The incubation period of CJD varies from 11 to 71 months or longer in the chimpanzee. Transmission of CJD to other monkey species, the domestic cat, mice,[26,244] rats, goats, hamsters, and guinea pigs[156] has also been reported,[68] but not all cases of CJD transmit to these species. Human-to-human trans-mission has been documented after corneal transplantation,[61] in two cases where stereotaxic electrodes were reused,[13] after dura mater grafts,[36] and most recently in young adults who had received human growth hormone injec-tions prepared from pooled cadaveric pituitaries.[24,88,141,198]

Despite the evidence of both acciden-tal and experimental transmission of CJD, the pathogenesis and mode of spread of sporadic CJD remain obscure. Horizontal contact spread appears to be very uncommon in CJD.[15] There are two reports of conjugal cases of CJD, although both involve questionable diagnoses.[85,161] There are rare reports of CJD in medical or paramedical personnel.[79]

The extreme scarcity of cases among health care workers and among spouses of affected patients seems sur-prising considering the successful transmissibility via parenteral and even oral inoculation, the apparent sus-ceptibility of most primates, the hardi-ness and high infectivity of the trans-missible agent, and the agent's presence in nonneural tissue. The rar-ity of obvious horizontal transmission may possibly be explained by low titers of the CJD agent in body fluids, thereby preventing transmission by conven-tional routes. Both blood and urine have been found infectious in human CJD,[157,243] but saliva, stool, and other body fluids have not been determined to be infectious.[44] The kuru agent, simi-larly believed to be absent from body fluids or present in only low concentra-tions, has never spread to visitors to the kuru area.[77] Presumably the subacute spongiform encephalopathies can be laterally transmitted by gross contami-nation by tissue, as exemplified by pre-sumed transmission of CJD by corneal transplantation, spread of kuru during endocannibalism,[78] possible transmis-sion of scrapie by placental inges-tion,[190] and spread of transmissible mink encephalopathy by natural can-nibalism of mink.[77] The genetics of the host may also be important in suscepti-bility, especially with respect to the par-enteral route of transmission.

The successful oral transmission of some subacute spongiform encephalo-pathies has aroused interest in the di-etary history of CJD patients. Suggested sources have included ingestion of in-completely cooked scrapie-infected ma-terial,[78] eating hog brain,[15] and in Li-byan Jews, the consumption of ovine brain and eyes.[114] There is no convinc-ing evidence that dietary factors are im-portant, and the cluster of cases among Libyan Jews is now considered a famil-ial one.[120a]

The physical and chemical properties of the transmissible CJD agent appear to be similar to those of the scrapie agent.[78] The scrapie agent is filterable but is more resistant to heat, ultraviolet inactivation, ultrasonication, and for-malin than known conventional viruses. The lack of a detectable antibody response and the absence of recognizable viral particles in the spongiform encephalopathies initially suggested that these agents might be unusual, naked nucleic-acid–containing structures, such as viroids of plants.[57] Studies failed to identify an agent-specific nucleic acid in infectious preparations, however, leading to speculation that the causative agents of scrapie and other spongiform encephalopathies represented "small *proteinaceous infectious* particles" or "prions."[202] Subsequently, a protein named PrP was found to copurify with infectivity, but PrP proved to be a normal endogenous protein of brain and other tissues.[185] In scrapie a modified form of PrP that is proteinase-K resistant accumulates; this appears to be a posttranslational modification of PrP, called PrP^{sc}.[9] Prusiner and co-workers[203] speculate that PrP^{sc} disrupts normal membrane processing, leading to formation of vacuoles, but the cloned protein has not been shown to transmit disease. Recent data regarding familial spongiform encephalopathies have emphasized the importance of PrP. Studies have suggested that the PrP gene is tightly linked to the gene that governs the length of the incubation period of scrapie in mice.[32,33,260] Following inoculation with hamster prions (PrP^{sc}), transgenic mice that harbor the hamster PrP gene develop scrapie with an incubation period characteristic of hamsters, not mice.[220] These studies demonstrate the importance of the PrP gene in modulating the susceptibility to and the length of the incubation period of transmissible spongiform encephalopathies.

Genetic factors also play a role in CJD, especially in the cases that appear to be dominantly inherited and transmissible. The elucidation of how an apparently hereditary disease is also transmissible has implications in studies of other familial neurologic diseases. Of great interest has been the finding of mutations in the PrP gene among affected individuals belonging to pedigrees with Gerstmann-Sträussler-Scheinker (GSS) syndrome, an autosomal dominantly inherited form of CJD.[91,120] This finding raises the possibility that the altered PrP produced by this mutant gene may become deposited in the brain and thereby result in spongiform encephalopathy. The latter situation would be analogous to that found with familial amyloidotic polyneuropathy, in which mutated transthyretin gene leads to amyloid deposition.[62] Recently, transgenic mice expressing the GSS-syndrome mutant PrP were reported to develop a degenerative brain disease.[120b] It remains unclear whether this disease is identical to scrapie, implicating the mutant PrP as the etiologic agent.

The finding of PrP gene mutations in individuals with the GSS syndrome has implications for our thinking about the pathogenesis of sporadic CJD as well as about the transmissibility of a "genetic" disease.[70] In sporadic CJD, a somatic (GSS-like) mutation of PrP in the CNS might lead to PrP deposition; this deposition may cause modification of PrP in the brain into a protease-resistant form (PrP^{sc}), with its subsequent deposition into the brain and the induction of spongiform encephalopathy. Unfortunately, the role of somatic mutation of PrP in the pathogenesis of the spongiform encephalopathies may be difficult to prove. Experimental transmission of spongiform encephalopathy may occur because PrP^{sc} accumulates in the brain following inoculation and leads to modification of the normal PrP and induction of spongiform encephalopathy.

Fibrils are found in preparations of brains of animals or humans with spongiform encephalopathies. These fibrils or rods contain PrP, but again, whether they represent the infectious agent or a host-derived product secondary to infection remains unknown.

Genetic factors seem to be important in all of the subacute spongiform encephalopathies. Kuru was originally thought to be a genetic disease, and family studies continue to stress the role of genetic factors.[78] Susceptibility of sheep to scrapie appears to be under genetic control,[56] as does the length of the incubation period in different breeds of mice.[55]

SUMMARY

The recognition of viral agents in the causation of dementing diseases has clarified certain confused clinical and pathologic disease entities. Not until the measles virus became implicated was it generally accepted that Dawson's "inclusion encephalitis,"[48,49] Pette and Doring's "panencephalitis,"[195] and van Bogaert's "subacute sclerosing leukoencephalitis"[250] were a single disease, now called SSPE. More than 10 separately named syndromes can be unequivocally considered CJD as a result of transmission studies. It is apparent that greater understanding of etiology can help redefine clinical and pathologic definitions of diseases. The implication of viruses in the etiology of some chronic neurologic diseases has stimulated virologic investigations of other degenerative neurologic processes.

Unfortunately, despite numerous therapeutic attempts with both antiviral agents and immunotherapeutic drugs, no satisfactory treatment now exists for most forms of acute or chronic encephalitis, PML, or CJD. Rational treatment for these diseases must await a better understanding of pathogenetic mechanisms. Acyclovir has convincingly been shown to reduce the mortality of herpes simplex encephalitis and the severity of residual neurologic deficits in survivors. One feature complicating therapeutic considerations in acute and chronic encephalitides, including HIV-related dementia, is that irreversible cerebral damage probably has occurred by the time the first clinical symptoms appear. For this reason, prophylaxis and vaccination are desirable — especially against agents implicated in not-uncommon disease states, such as measles virus in postinfectious encephalomyelitis and SSPE, and against HIV-1. For the next decade the most rapidly rising viral cause of dementia will be HIV-1; physicians must anticipate and plan for an epidemic of HIV-1 – related dementia in young adults.

ACKNOWLEDGMENTS

The writing of this chapter was supported by NIAID contract AI-72634 and NINDS grant 1 PO1 NS 26643.

The authors are appreciative of helpful discussions with Drs. Ola Selnes, Scott Becker, Jonathan Glass and Jack Griffin. We acknowledge the clinical and technical support of Julie McArthur and Carol Schlough and the dedication of the medical and nursing staff of The Johns Hopkins Hospital.

REFERENCES

1. Aarli JA: Nervous complications of measles: Clinical manifestations and prognosis. Eur Neurol 12:79–93, 1974.
2. Ahmed A, Strong DM, Sell KW et al: Demonstration of a blocking factor in the plasma and spinal fluid of patients with subacute sclerosing panencephalitis. J Exp Med 139:902–924, 1974.
3. Allen IV, Dermott E, Connolly JH, and Hurwitz LJ: A study of a patient with the amyotrophic form of Creutzfeldt-Jakob disease. Brain 94:715–724, 1971.
4. Anand R, Siegal F, Reed C, Cheung T, Forlenza S, and Moore J: Non-cytocidal natural variants of human immunodeficiency virus isolated from AIDS patients with neurological disorders. Lancet 2:234–238, 1987.
5. Astrom K-E, Mancall EL, and Richardson EP Jr: Progressive multifocal leukoencephalopathy. Brain 81:93–111, 1958.
6. Ayata M, Hirano A, and Wong TC: Structural defect linked to nonrandom mutations in the matrix gene of Biken strain subacute sclerosing

pancephalitis virus defined by cDNA cloning and expression of chimeric genes. J Virol 63:1162–1173, 1989.

7. Balfour HH, Siem RA, Bauer H, and Quie PG: California arbovirus (La Crosse) infections. I. Clinical and laboratory findings in 66 children with meningoencephalitis. Pediatrics 52: 680–691, 1973.

8. Baringer JR: Human herpes simplex virus infections. In Thompson RA and Green JR (eds): Infectious Diseases of the Central Nervous System. Raven Press, New York, 1974.

9. Basler K, Oesch B, Scott M, et al: Scrapie and cellular PrP isoforms are encoded by the same chromosomal gene. Cell 46:417–428, 1986.

10. Bass BL, Weintraub H, Cattaneo R, and Billeter MA: Biased hypermutation of viral RNA genomes could be due to unwinding/modification of double-stranded RNA. Cell 56:331, 1989.

11. Baublis JV and Payne FE: Measles antigen and syncytium formation in brain cell cultures from subacute sclerosing panencephalitis (SSPE). Proc Soc Exp Biol Med 129:593–597, 1968.

12. Berger JR, Kaszowitz B, Post MJD, and Dickinson G. Progressive multifocal leukoencephalopathy associated with human immunodeficiency virus infection: A review of the literature with a report of sixteen cases. Ann Int Med 107:78–87, 1987.

13. Bernoulli C, Siegfried J, Baumgartner G, et al: Danger of accidental person-to-person transmission of Creutzfeldt-Jakob disease by surgery. Lancet 1:478–479, 1977.

14. Blaese RM and Hofstrand H: Immunocompetence of patients with SSPE. Arch Neurol 32:494–495, 1975.

15. Bobowick AR, Brody JA, Matthews MR, Roos R, and Gadjdusek DC: Creutzfeldt-Jakob Disease: A casecontrol study. Am J Epidemiol 98:381–394, 1973.

16. Bouteille M, Fontaine C, Vedrenne C, and Delarue J: Sur un cas d'encé-phalitie subaique à inclusions. Etude anatomoclinique et ultrastructurale. Rev Neurol (Paris) 113:454–458, 1965.

17. Brenneman D, Buzy J, Ruff M, et al: Peptide T sequences prevent neuronal cell death produced by the protein (gp120) of the human immunodeficiency virus. Drug Development Research 15:361–369, 1988.

18. Brew BJ, Ghalla R, Paul M, Schwartz M, and Price RW: CSF β2 microglobulin as a marker of the presence and severity of AIDS dementia complex (abstract TH.B.P.233). Fifth International Conference on AIDS, Montreal, June 1989.

19. Bridge PT, Goodwin FK, Heseltine NR, Eaton E, and Parker ES: Peptide T phase I study: Neuropsychiatric results (abstract W.B.O.45a). Fifth International Conference on AIDS, Montreal, June 1989.

20. Brody JA and Detels R: SSPE: A zoonosis following aberrant measles. Lancet 2:500–501, 1970.

21. Brown P: An epidemiologic critique of Creutzfeldt-Jakob disease. Epidemiol Rev 2:113–135, 1980.

22. Brown P, Cathala F, Castaigne P, and Gajdusek DC: Creutzfeldt-Jakob disease: Clinical analyses of a consecutive series of 230 neuropathologically verified cases. Ann Neurol 20:597–602, 1986.

23. Brown P, Cathala F, Raubertas RF, Gajdusek DC, and Castainge P: The epidemiology of Creutzfeldt-Jakob disease: Conclusion of a 15-year investigation in France and review of the world literature. Neurology 37:895–904, 1987.

24. Brown P, Gajdusek DC, Gibbs CJ Jr, and Asher DM: Potential epidemic of Creutzfeldt-Jakob disease from human gowth hormone therapy. N Engl J Med 313:728–731, 1985.

25. Brown P, Rodgers-Johnson P, Cathala F, Gibbs CJ Jr, and Gajdusek DC: Creutzfeldt-Jakob disease of long duration: Clinicopathological characteristics, transmissibility, and differential diagnosis. Ann Neurol 16: 295–304, 1984.

26. Brownell B, Campbell MJ, Greenham LW, and Peacock DB: Experimental transmission of Creutzfeldt-Jakob disease. Lancet 2:186–187, 1975.

27. Brownell B and Oppenheimer DR: An ataxic form of subacute presenile polioencephalopathy (Creutzfeldt-Jakob disease). J Neurol Neurosurg Psychiatry 28:350–361, 1965.

28. Brun A, Nordenfeldt E, and Kjellén L: Aspects on the variability of progressive multifocal leukoencephalopathy. Acta Neuropathol (Berl) 24:232–243, 1973.

29. Brun-Vezinet F, Katlama C, Roulot D, et al: Lymphadenopathy-associated virus type 2 in AIDS and AIDS-related complex. Lancet 1:128–132, 1987.

30. Budka H: Multinucleated giant cells in brain: A hallmark of the acquired immune deficiency syndrome (AIDS). Acta Neuropathol (Berl) 69:253–258, 1986.

31. Cape CA, Martinez AJ, Robertson JT, Hamilton R, and Jabbour JT: Adult onset of subacute sclerosing panencephalitis. Arch Neurol 28:124–127, 1973.

32. Carlson GA, Kingsbury DT, Goodman PA, et al: Linkage of prion protein and scrapie incubation time genes. Cell 46:503–511, 1986.

33. Carp RI, Moretz RC, Natelli M, and Dickinson AG: Genetic control of scrapie incubation period and plaque formation in I mice. J Gen Virol 68:401–407, 1987.

34. Carter MJ, Willcocks MM, and ter Meulen V: Defective translation of measles virus matrix protein in a subacute sclerosing panencephalitis cell line. Nature 305:153–155, 1983.

35. Cattaneo R, Schmid A, Spielhofer P, et al: Mutated and hypermutated genes of persistent measles viruses which caused lethal human brain diseases. Virology 173:415–425, 1989.

36. Centers for Disease Control: Rapidly progressive dementia in a patient who received a cadaveric dura mater graft. MMWR 36:49–55, 1987.

36a. Centers for Disease Control: Revision of the CDC surveillance case definition for acquired immunodeficiency syndrome. MMWR (Suppl 1S)36:3S–15S, 1987.

37. Centers for Disease Control: Arboviral infections of the central nervous system. MMWR 37:506, 513, 1988.

37a. Centers for Disease Control: Projected numbers of AIDS cases: United States, January 1989 to December 1993. MMWR 39:110–112, 117–119, 1990.

38. Chajek T and Fainaru M: Behçet's disease: Report of 41 cases and a review of the literature. Medicine (Baltimore)54:179–196, 1975.

39. Chaput M, Claes V, Portetelle D, et al: The neurotrophic factor neuroleukin is 90% homologous with phosphohexose isomerase. Nature 332:454–455, 1988.

40. Cheng-Meyer C, Rutka JT, Rosenbaum ML, McHugh T, Sites DP, and Levy JA: Human immunodeficiency virus can productively infect cultured human glial cells. Proc Natl Acad Sci U S A 84:3526–3530, 1987.

41. Choppin PW, Richardson CD, Merz DC, Hall WW, and Scheid A: The functions and inhibition of the membrane glycoproteins of paramyxoviruses and myxoviruses and the role of the measles virus M protein in subacute sclerosing panencephalitis. J Infect Dis 143:352–363, 1981.

42. Chumakov MP, Vorob'jeva NN, and Bel'Jajeva AL: Study of the ultraviral encephalitides. III. Kozhevnikov's epilepsy and tick-borne encephalitis. Zh Nevropatol Psikhiatr 13:63–68, 1944.

43. Chun RWM, Thompson WH, Grabow JD, and Matthews CG: California arbovirus encepahlitis in children. Neurology 18:369–375, 1968.

44. Committee on Health Care Issues, American Neurological Association: Precautions in handling tissues, fluids, and other contaminated materials from patients with documented or suspected Creutzfeldt-Jakob disease. Ann Neurol 19:75–77, 1986.

45. Connolly JH, Allen IV, Hurwitz LJ, and Millar JH: Measles-virus antibody and antigen in subacute sclerosing panencephalitis. Lancet 1:542–544, 1967.

46. Corsellis JAN, Goldberg CJ, and Norton AR: "Limbic encephalitis" and its association with carcinoma. Brain 91:481–496, 1968.

47. Cremer NE, Oshiro LS, Weil MS, Lennette EH, Itabashai HH, and Carnay J: Isolation of rubella virus from brain in chronic progressive panencephalitis. J Gen Virol 29:143–153, 1975.

48. Dawson JR: Cellular inclusions in cerebral lesions of lethargic encephalitis. Am J Pathol 9:7–15, 1933.

49. Dawson JR: Cellular inclusions in cerebral lesions of epidemic encephalitis: Second report. Arch Neurol 31: 685–700, 1934.

50. de la Monte SM, Ho DD, Schooley RT, Hirsch MS, and Richardson EP: Subacute encephalomyelitis of AIDS and its relation to HTLV-III infection. Neurology 37:562–569, 1987.

51. Denny-Brown D: Discussion. Transactions of the American Neurological Association 85:149–150, 1960.

52. Detels R, McNew J, Brody JA, and Edgar AH: Further epidemiological studies of subacute sclerosing panencephalitis. Lancet 2:11–14, 1973.

53. Dewhurst S, Bresser J, Stevenson M, Sakai K, Evinger-Hodges MJ, and Volsky DJ: Susceptibility of human glial cells to infection with human immunodeficiency virus (HIV). FEBS Lett 213:138–143, 1987.

54. Dewhurst S, Stevenson M, and Volsky DJ: Expression of the T4 molecule (AIDS virus receptor) by human brain-derived cells. FEBS Lett 213: 133–137, 1987.

55. Dickinson AG, Meikle MH, and Fraser H: Identification of a gene which controls the incubation period of some strains of scrapie agent in mice. J Comp Pathol 78:293–299, 1968.

56. Dickinson AG, Stamp JT, Renwick CC, and Rennie JC: Some factors controlling the incidence of scrapie in Cheviot sheep infected with a Che-

57. Diener TO: PrP and the nature of the scrapie agent. Cell 49:719–721, 1987.

58. Dorfman LJ: Cytomegalovirus encephalitis in adults. Neurology 23: 136–144, 1973.

59. Drachman DA and Adams RD: Herpes simplex and acute inclusion-body encephalitis. Arch Neurol 7:61–79, 1962.

60. Dreyer FB, Kaiser PK, Hoffman JT, and Lipton SA: HIV-1 coat protein neurotoxicity prevented by calcium channel antagonists. Science 248: 364–367, 1990.

61. Duffy P, Wolf J, Collins G, DeVoe AG, Steeten B, and Cowen D: Possible person-to-person transmission of Creutzfeldt-Jakob disease. N Engl J Med 290:692–693, 1974.

62. Dwulet FE and Benson MD: Primary structure of an amyloid prealbumin and its plasma precursor in a heredofamilial polyneuropathy of Swedish origin. Proc Natl Acad Sci U S A 81:694–698, 1984.

63. Eddy BE, Borman GS, Grubbs GE, and Young RD: Identification of the oncogenic substance in rhesus monkey kidney cell cultures as simian virus 40. Virology 17:65–75, 1962.

64. Ehrenkranz NJ and Ventura AK: Venezuelan equine encephalitis virus infection in man. Annu Rev Med 25:9–14, 1974.

65. Elovaara I, Iivanainen M, Valle S-L, Suni J, Tervo T, and Lahdevirta J: CSF protein and cellular profiles in various stages of HIV infection related to neurological manifestations. J Neurol Sci 78:331–342, 1987.

66. Epstein LG, Sharer LR, Cho ES, Myenhofer M, Navia B, and Price RW: HTLV-III/LAV-like particles in the brains of patients with AIDS encephalopathy. AIDS Res Hum Retroviruses 1:447, 1985.

67. Epstein LG, Sharer LR, Joshi VV, et al: Progressive encephalopathy in children with acquired immunodeficiency syndrome. Ann Neurol 17: 488–496, 1985.

68. Evans AS: Viral Infections of

Humans, Ed 2. Plenum Publishing, New York, 1984.

69. Feemster RF: Eastern equine encephalitis: Sequelae. Neurology 8: 883, 1958.

70. Ferber RA, Wiesenfeld SL, Roos RPI, Bobowick AR, Gibbs CJ Jr, and Gajdusek DC: Familial Creutzfeldt-Jakob disease: Transmission of the familial disease to primates. In Subirana A, Espadaler JM, and Burrows EH (eds): Proceedings of the 10th International Congress of Neurology. Excerpta Medica International Congress. Series No 296, Amsterdam, 1973.

71. Finley KH, Fitzgerald LH, Richter RW, Riggs N, and Shelton JN: Western encephalitis and cerebral ontogenesis. Arch Neurol 16:140–164, 1967.

72. Fischl MA, Richman DD, Grieco MH, et al: The efficacy of azidothymidine (AZT) in the treatment of patients with AIDS and AIDS-related complex. N Engl J Med 317:185–191, 1987.

73. Font RL, Jenis EH, and Tuck KD: Measles maculopathy associated with subacute sclerosing panencephalitis. Arch Pathol Lab Med 96: 168–174, 1973.

74. Freeman JM: The clinical spectrum and early diagnosis of Dawson's encephalitis. J Pediatr 75:590–603, 1969.

75. Gabuzda DH, Ho DD, de la Monte SM, Hirsch MS, Rota TR, and Sobel RA: Immunohistochemical identification of HTLV-III antigen in brains of patients with AIDS. Ann Neurol 20: 289–295, 1986.

76. Gajdusek DC: Hypothesis: Interference with axonal transport of neurofilament as a common pathogenetic mechanism in certain diseases of the central nervous system. N Engl J Med 312:714–719, 1985.

77. Gajdusek DC and Gibbs CJ Jr: Subacute and chronic diseases caused by atypical infections with unconventional viruses in aberrant hosts. In Pollard M (ed): Perspectives in Virology, Vol 8. Academic Press, New York, 1973.

78. Gajdusek DC and Gibbs CJ Jr: Slow virus infections of the nervous system and the laboratories of slow, latent, and temperate virus infections. In Tower DC (ed): The Nervous System, Vol 2. Raven Press, New York, 1975.

79. Gajdusek DC, Gibbs CJ Jr, and Alpers M: Experimental transmission of a kuru-like syndrome to chimpanzees. Nature 209:794–796, 1966.

80. Gajdusek DC and Zigas V: Degenerative disease of the central nervous system in New Guinea. The endemic occurrence of "kuru" in the native population. N Engl J Med 257:974–978, 1957.

81. Gardner SD: Prevalence in England of antibody to human polyomavirus (BK). BMJ 1:77–78, 1973.

82. Gardner SD, Field AM, Coleman DV, and Hulme B: New human papovavirus (BK) isolated from urine after renal transplantation. Lancet 1: 1253–1257, 1971.

83. Gartner S, Markovits P, Markovitz DM, Betts RF, and Popovic M: Virus isolation from and identification of HTLV-III/LAV-producing cells in brain tissue from a patient with AIDS. JAMA 256:2365–2371, 1986.

84. Gartner S, Markovits P, Markovitz DM, Kaplan MH, Gallo RC, and Popovic M: The role of mononuclear phagocytes in HTLV-III/LAV infection. Science 233:215–219, 1986.

85. Garzuly F, Jellinger K, and Pilz P: Subakute spongiose Encephalopathie (Jakob-Creutzfeldt Syndrom) Klinische-morphologische Analyse von 9 Fallen. Archiv für Psychiatrie und Nervenkrankheiten 214:207–227, 1971.

86. Gendelman HE, Wolinsky JS, Johnson RT, Pressman NJ, Pezeshkpour GH, and Boisset GF: Measles encephalomyelitis: Lack of evidence of viral invasion of the central nervous system and quantitative study of the nature of demyelination. Ann Neurol 15:353–360, 1984.

87. Gibbs CJ Jr, Gajdusek DC, Asher DM, et al: Creutzfeldt-Jakob disease (spongiform encephalopathy):

Transmission to the chimpanzee. Science 161:388–389, 1968.

88. Gibbs CJ Jr, Joy A, Heffner R, et al: Clinical and pathological features and laboratory confirmation of Creutzfeldt-Jakob disease in a recipient of pituitary-derived human growth hormone. N Engl J Med 313:734–738, 1985.

89. Gilden DH, Rorke LB, and Tanaka R: Acute SSPE. Arch Neurol 32:644–646, 1975.

90. Goethe KE, Mitchell JE, Marshall DW, et al: Neuropsychological and neurological function of human immunodeficiency virus seropositive asymptomatic individuals. Arch Neurol 46:129–133, 1989.

91. Goldgaber D, Goldfarb LG, Brown P, et al: Mutations in familial Creutzfeldt-Jakob disease and Gerstmann-Sträussler-Scheinker's syndrome. Exp Neurol 106:204–206, 1989.

92. Gomori AJ, Partnow MH, Horoupian DS, and Hirano A: The ataxic form of Creutzfeldt-Jakob disease. Arch Neurol 29:318–323, 1973.

93. Gordon B, Selnes OA, Hart J Jr, Hanley DF, and Whitley RJ: Long-term cognitive sequelae of acyclovir-treated herpes simplex encephalitis. Arch Neurol 47:646–647, 1990.

94. Goudsmit J, Marrow CH, Asher DM, et al: Evidence for and against the transmissibility of Alzheimer disease. Neurology 30:945–950, 1980.

95. Grant I, Atkinson JH, Hesselink JR, et al: Evidence for early central nervous system involvement in the acquired immunodeficiency syndrome (AIDS) and other human immunodeficiency virus (HIV) infections. Ann Intern Med 107:828–836, 1987.

96. Graves M, Griffin DE, Johnson RT, et al: Development of antibody to measles virus polypeptides during complicated and uncomplicated measles virus infections. J Virol 49:409–412, 1984.

97. Greenwood R, Bhalla A, Gordon A, and Roberts J: Behavior disturbances during recovery from herpes simplex encephalitis. J Neurol Neurosurg Psychiatry 46:809–817, 1983.

98. Gribble DH, Haden CC, Schwartz LW, and Henrickson RV: Spontaneous progressive multifocal leukoencephalopathy (PML) in macaques. Nature 254:602–604, 1975.

99. Grinnel BW, Padgett BL, and Walker DL: Comparison of infectious JC virus DNAs cloned from human brain. J Virol 45:299–308, 1983.

100. Gurney ME, Heinrich SP, Lee MR, and Yin H-S: Molecular cloning and expression of neuroleukin, a neurotrophic factor for spinal and sensory neurons. Science 234:566–574, 1986.

101. Gyorkey F, Melnick JL, and Gyorkey P: Human immunodeficiency virus in brain biopsies of patients with AIDS and progressive encephalopathy. J Infect Dis 155:870–876, 1987.

102. Haase AT: Pathogenesis of lentivirus infection. Nature 322:130–136, 1986.

103. Haase AT, Gantz D, Eble B, et al: Natural history of restricted synthesis and expression of measles virus genes in subacute sclerosing panencephalitis. Proc Natl Acad Sci U S A 82:3020–3024, 1985.

104. Haddad FS and Risk WS: Isoprinosine in 18 patients with subacute sclerosing panencephalitis: A controlled study. Ann Neurol 7:185–188, 1980.

105. Hadlow WJ: Scrapie and kuru. Lancet 2:289–290, 1959.

106. Hall WW and Choppin PW: Evidence for lack of synthesis of the M polypeptide of measles virus in brain cells in subacute sclerosing panencephalitis. Virology 99:443–447, 1979.

107. Hall WW, Lamb RA, and Choppin PW: Measles and SSPE virus proteins: Lack of antibodies to the M protein in patients with subacute sclerosing panencephalitis. Proc Natl Acad Sci U S A 76:2047–2051, 1979.

108. Hanley DF, Johnson RT, and Whitley RT: Yes, brain biopsy should be a prerequisite for herpes simplex encephalitis treatment. Arch Neurol 44:1289–1290, 1987.

109. Hanshaw JB, Morley AW, Gaev L, and Abel V: CNS sequelae of congeni-

tal cytomegalovirus infection. In Krugman S and Gershon AA (eds): Progress in Clinical and Biological Research, Vol 3. Alan R Liss, New York, 1975.

110. Hardy JB, McCracken GH Jr, Gildeson MR, and Sever JL: Adverse fetal outcome following maternal rubella after the first trimester of pregnancy. JAMA 207:2414–2420, 1969.

111. Harper ME, Marselle LM, Gallo RC, and Wong-Staal F: Detection of lymphocytes expressing human T-lymphotropic virus type III in lymph nodes and peripheral blood from infected individuals by in situ hybridization. Proc Natl Acad Sci U S A 83:772–776, 1986.

112. Hemachudha T, Phanuphak P, Johnson RT, Griffin DE, Tatanavongsiri J, and Siriprasomsu P: Neurologic complications of Semple-type rabies vaccine: Clinical and immunologic studies. Neurology 37:550–556, 1987.

113. Herndon RM and Rubinstein LJ: Light and electron microscopic observations of the development of viral particles in the inclusions of Dawson's encephalitis (subacute sclerosing panencephalitis). Neurology 18:8–28, 1968.

114. Herzberg L, Herzberg BN, Gibbs CJ Jr, Sullivan W, Amyx H, and Gajdusek DC: Creutzfeldt-Jakob disease: Hypothesis for high incidence in Libyan Jews in Israel. Science 186:848, 1972.

115. Heyes MP, Brew BJ, Markey SP, Martin A, Price RW, and Ribinow D: Quinolinic acid concentrations are increased in plasma and cerebrospinal fluid in AIDS and correlates with AIDS dementia (abstract Th.B.P.232) 5th International Conference on AIDS, Montreal, June 1989.

116. Hill JM, Farrar WL, and Pert CB: Localization of the T4 antigen/AIDS virus receptor in monkey and rat brain: Prominence in cortical regions. Psychopharmacol Bull 22:689–694, 1986.

117. Hill J, Ruff M, and Pert C: AIDS as a

neuropeptide disorder: Peptide T, VIP, and the HIV receptor. Psychopharmacol Bull 24:315–319, 1988.

118. Ho DD, Rota TR, Schooley RT, et al: Isolation of HTLV-III from cerebrospinal fluid and neural tissues of patient with neurologic syndromes related to the acquired immunodeficiency syndrome. N Engl J Med 313:1493–1497, 1985.

119. Horta-Barbosa L, Fuccillo DA, Sever JL, and Zeman W: Subacute sclerosing panencephalitis: Isolation of measles virus from a brain biopsy. Nature 221:974, 1969.

120. Hsiao K, Baker HF, Crow TJ, et al: Linkage of a prion protein missense variant to Gerstmann-Sträussler syndrome. Nature 338:342–344, 1989.

120a. Hsiao K, Meiner Z, Kahana E, et al: Mutation of the prion protein in Libyan Jews with Creutzfeldt-Jakob disease. N Engl J Med 324:1091–1097, 1991.

120b. Hsiao K, Scott M, Foster D, et al: Spontaneous neurodegeneration in transgenic mice with mutant prion protein. Science 250:1587–1590, 1990.

121. Huttenlocher PR, Picchietti DL, Roos RP, et al: Intrathecal interferon in subacute sclerosing panencephalitis. Ann Neurol 19:303–305, 1986.

122. Jabbour JT, Duenas DA, and Modlin J: SSPE: Clinical staging, course, and frequency. Arch Neurol 32:493–494, 1975.

123. Jabbour JT, Duenas DA, Sever JL, Krebs HM, and Horta-Barbosa L: Epidemiology of subacute sclerosing panencephalitis (SSPE). A report of the SSPE Registry. JAMA 220:959–962, 1972.

124. Janssen RS: Neuropsychological abnormalities in HIV infection. Ann Neurol 26:592–600, 1989.

125. Janssen RS, Saykin AJ, Kaplan JE, et al: Neurological symptoms and neuropsychological abnormalities in lymphadenopathy syndrome. Ann Neurol (Suppl)23:S17–S18, 1988.

126. Johnson KP, Rosenthal MS, and Lerner PI: Herpes simplex encephali-

tis: The course in five virologically proven cases. Arch Neurol 27:103–105, 1972.

127. Johnson RT: Subacute sclerosing panencephalitis. J Infect Dis 121:227–230, 1970.

128. Johnson RT: The pathogenesis of acute viral encephalitis and postinfectious encephalomyelitis. J Infect Dis 155:359–364, 1987.

129. Johnson RT, Griffin DE, and Gendelman HE: Postinfectious encephalomyelitis. Semin Neurol 5:180–190, 1985.

130. Johnson RT, Griffin DE, Hirsch RL, et al: Measles encephalomyelitis—clinical and immunologic studies. N Engl J Med 310:137–141, 1984.

131. Johnson RT and McArthur JC: AIDS and the brain. Trends Neurosci 9:1–4, 1986.

132. Johnson RT, McArthur JC, and Narayan O: The neurobiology of human immunodeficiency virus infections. FASEB J 2:2970–2981, 1988.

133. Johnson RT, Olson LC, and Beuscher EL: Herpes simplex virus infections of the nervous system: Problems in laboratory diagnosis. Arch Neurol 18:260–264, 1968.

134. Johnstone JA, Ross CAC, and Dunn M: Meningitis and encephalitis associated with mumps infection: A 10-year survey. Arch Dis Child 47:647–651, 1972.

135. Kahana E, Alter M, Braham J, and Sofer D: Creutzfeldt-Jakob disease: Focus among Libyan Jews in Israel. Science 183:90–91, 1973.

136. Katz M and Koprowski H: The significance of failure to isolate infectious viruses in cases of subacute sclerosing panencephalitis. Archiv für Gesamte Virusforschung 41:390–393, 1973.

137. Kepes JJ, Chou SM, and Prince LW: Progressive multifocal leukoencephalopathy with 10-year survival in a patient with non-tropical sprue: Report of a case with unusual light and electron microscopic features. Neurology 25:1006–1012, 1975.

138. Klapper PE, Cleator GM, and Longson M: Mild forms of herpes encephalitis. J Neurol Neurosurg Psychiatry 47:1247–1250, 1984.

139. Klatzo I, Gajdusek DC, and Zigas V: Pathology of kuru. Lab Invest 8:799–847, 1959.

140. Kleihues P, Lang W, Burger PC, et al: Progressive diffuse leukoencephalopathy in patients with acquired immune deficiency syndrome (AIDS). Acta Neuropathol (Berl) 68:333–339, 1985.

141. Koch TK, Berg BO, De Armond SJ, and Gravina RF: Creutzfeldt-Jakob disease in a young adult with idiopathic hypopituitarism. Possible relation to the administration of cadaveric human growth hormone. N Engl J Med 313:731–733, 1985.

142. Koenig S, Gendelman HE, DalCanto MC, et al: Detection of AIDS retroviral RNA in nonlymphoid cells in the brain of an AIDS patient with encephalopathy. Clin Res 34:722A, 1986.

143. Komandenko NI, Ilyenko VI, Platonov VG, and Panov AG: The clinical picture and some problems of the pathogenesis of progressive forms of tick-borne encephalitis. Zh Nevropatol Psikhiatr 72:1000–1007, 1972.

144. Koyanagi Y, Miles S, Mitsuyasu RT, Merrill JE, Vinters HV, and Chen ISY: Dual infection of the central nervous system by AIDS viruses with distinct cellular tropisms. Science 236:819–822, 1987.

145. Kraminskaja NN, Meierova RA, and Zhivoljapina RR: Materials for the study of tick-borne encephalitis in the Ekhirit-Belegat region of Irkutsk Oblast'. Doklady Irkutskogo Protivochumnogo Instituta 8:189, 1969.

146. Krol G, Becker R, Zimmerman R, et al: In Valk J (ed): Contribution of MRI to the diagnosis of intracranial complications of acquired immune deficiency syndrome. Neuroradiology 1985/1986.

147. Krupp LB, Lipton RB, Swerdlow ML, Leeds NE, and Llena J: Progressive multifocal leukoencephalopathy: Clinical and radiographic features. Ann Neurol 17:344–349, 1985.

148. LaFrance N, Pearlson GD, Schaerf

FW, et al: I 123 IMP-SPECT in HIV-related dementia. Advances in Functional Imaging 1:9–15, 1988.

149. Lampert PW: Autoimmune and virus-induced demyelinating diseases. Am J Pathol 92:176–197, 1978.

150. Lampert PW, Gajdusek DC, and Gibbs CJ Jr: Subacute spongiform virus encephalopathies. Scrapie, kuru and Creutzfeldt-Jakob disease: A review. Am J Pathol 68:626–652, 1972.

151. Lampert PW, Gajdusek DC, and Gibbs DJ Jr: Pathology of dendrites in subacute spongiform virus encephalopathies. In Kreutzberg GW (ed): Advances in Neurology, Vol 12. Raven Press, New York, 1975.

152. Lebon P and Lyon G: Non-congenital rubella encephalitis. Lancet 2:468, 1974.

153. Levy JA, Shimabukuro J, Hollander H, Mills J, and Kaminsky L: Isolation of AIDS-associated retroviruses in cerebrospinal fluid and brain of patients with neurological symptoms. Lancet 2:586–588, 1985.

154. Levy RM, Bredesen DE, and Rosenblum ML: Neurological manifestations of the acquired immunodeficiency syndrome (AIDS): Experience at UCSF and review of the literature. J Neurosurg 62:475–495, 1985.

155. Levy RM, Rosenbloom S, and Perrett LV: Neuroradiologic findings in AIDS: A review of 200 cases. Am J Roentgenol 147:977–983, 1986.

156. Manuelidis EE: Transmission of Creutzfeldt-Jakob disease from man to the guinea pig. Science 190:571–572, 1975.

157. Manuelidis EE, Kim JH, Mericangas Jr, and Manuelidis L: Transmission to animals of Creutzfeldt-Jakob disease from human blood (letter). Lancet 2:896–897, 1985.

158. Manz HJ: Progressive multifocal leukoencephalopathy after renal transplantation. Ann Intern Med 75:77–81, 1971.

159. Markand ON and Panszi JG: The electroencephalogram in subacute sclerosing panencephalitis. Arch Neurol 32:719–726, 1975.

160. Masters CL, Harris JO, Gajdusek DC, Gibbs CJ Jr, Bernoulli C, and Asher DM: Creutzfeldt-Jakob disease: Patterns of worldwide occurrence and the significance of familial and sporadic clustering. Ann Neurol 5:177–188, 1979.

161. Matthews WB: Epidemiology of Creutzfeldt-Jakob disease in England and Wales. J Neurol Neurosurg Psychiatry 38:210–213, 1975.

162. McArthur JC: Neurologic manifestations of AIDS. Medicine (Baltimore) 66:407–437, 1987.

163. McArthur JC, Cohen BA, Farzedegan H, et al: Cerebrospinal fluid abnormalities in homosexual men with and without neuropsychiatric findings. Ann Neurol (Suppl)23:S34–S37, 1988.

164. McArthur JC, Cohen BA, Selnes OA, et al: Low prevalence of neurological and neuropsychological abnormalities in healthy HIV-1 infected individuals: Results from the Multicenter AIDS Cohort Study. Ann Neurol 26:601–611, 1989.

165. McArthur JC, Kumar AJ, Johnson DW, et al: Multicenter AIDS Cohort Study: Magnetic resonance findings in HIV-1 infection. Journal of AIDS 3:252–259, 1990.

166. McArthur JC, Sipos E, Cornblath DR, et al: Identification of mononuclear cells in CSF of patients with HIV infection. Neurology 39:66–70, 1989.

167. McFarland HF: The effect of measles virus infection on T and B lymphocytes in the mouse. I. Suppression of helper cell activity. J Immunol 113:1978–1983, 1974.

168. McKinney RE and Katz SL: Chronic enteroviral meningoencephalitis in agammaglobulinemic patients. Rev Infect Dis 9:334–356, 1987.

169. Meyer A, Leigh D, and Bagg CE: A rare presenile dementia associated with cortical blindness (Heidenhain's syndrome). J Neurol Neurosurg Psychiatry 17:129–133, 1954.

170. Meyer HM Jr, Johnson RT, Crawford IP, Dascomb HE, and Rogers NG: Central nervous system syndromes of "viral" etiology. A study of 713 cases. Am J Med 29:334–347, 1960.

171. Miller JK, Hesser F, and Tompkins VN: Herpes simplex encephalitis: Report of 20 cases. Ann Intern Med 64:92–103, 1966.

172. Modlin JF, Halsey NA, Eddins DL, et al: Epidemiology of subacute sclerosing panencephalitis. J Pediatr 94: 231–236, 1979.

173. Modlin JF, Jabbour JT, Witte JJ, and Halsey NA: Epidemiologic studies of measles, measles vaccine, and subacute sclerosing panencephalitis. Pediatrics 59:505–512, 1977.

174. Moench TR, Griffin DE, Obriecht CR, Vaisburg A, and Johnson RT: Distribution of measles virus antigen and RNA in acute measles with and without neurologic involvement. J Infect Dis 158:433–442, 1988.

175. Nahmias AJ, Whitley RJ, Visintine AN, Takei Y, and Alford CA Jr: Herpes simplex virus encephalitis: Laboratory evaluations and their diagnostic significance. J Infect Dis 145:829–836, 1982.

176. Narayan O and Cork LC: Lentiviral diseases of sheep and goats: Chronic pneumonia, leukoencephalomyelitis and arthritis. Rev Infect Dis 7:89–98, 1985.

177. Narayan O, Penney JB Jr, Johnson RT, Herndon RM, and Weiner LP: Etiology of progressive multifocal leukoencephalopathy. N Engl J Med 289:1278–1282, 1973.

178. Nathanson N, Georgsson G, Palsson PA, Najjar JA, Lutley R, and Petursson G: Experimental visna in Icelandic sheep: The prototype lentivirus infection. Rev Infect Dis 7:75–82, 1985.

179. Navia BA, Cho ES, Petito CK, and Price RW: The AIDS dementia complex: II. Neuropathology. Ann Neurol 19:525–535, 1986.

180. Navia BA, Jordan BD, and Price RW: The AIDS dementia complex: I. Clinical features. Ann Neurol 19:517–524, 1986.

181. Navia BA and Price RW. The acquired immunodeficiency syndrome dementia complex as the presenting or sole manifestation of human immunodeficiency virus infection. Arch Neurol 44:65–69, 1987.

182. Nelson DA, Weiner A, Yanoff M, and DePeralta J: Retinal lesions in subacute sclerosing panencephalitis. Arch Ophthalmol 84:613–621, 1970.

183. Nielsen SL, Petito CK, Urmacher CD, and Posner JB: Subacute encephalitis in acquired immune deficiency syndrome: A post mortem study. Am J Clin Pathol 82:678–682, 1984.

184. Norrby E, Kristensson K, Brzosko WJ, and Kapsenberg JG: Measles virus matrix protein detected by immune fluorescence with monoclonal antibodies in the brain of patients with subacute sclerosing panencephalitis. J Virol 56:337–340, 1985.

185. Oesch B, Westaway D, Walchi M, et al: A cellular gene encodes scrapie PrP 27-30 protein. Cell 40:735–746, 1985.

186. Oldstone MBA: Viruses can alter cell function without causing cell pathology: Disordered function leads to imbalance of homeostasis and disease. In Notkins AL and Oldstone MBA (eds): Concepts in viral pathogenesis. Springer-Verlag, New York, 1984.

187. Padgett BL and Walker DL: Prevalence of antibodies in human sera against JC virus, an isolate from a case of progressive multifocal leukoencephalopathy. J Infect Dis 127: 467–470, 1973.

188. Padgett BL, Walker DL, ZuRhein GM, Eckroade RJ, and Dessel BH: Cultivation of papova-like virus from human brain with progressive multifocal leukoencephalopathy. Lancet 1:1257–1260, 1971.

189. Panitch HS, Gomez-Plascencia J, Norris FH, Cantell K, and Smith RA: Subacute sclerosing panencephalitis: Remission after treatment with intraventricular interferon. Neurology 36:562–566, 1986.

190. Pattison IH, Hoare MN, Jebbett JN, and Watson WA: Spread of scrapie to sheep and goats by oral dosing with fetal membranes from scrapie affected sheep. Vet Rec 90:465–468, 1972.

191. Payne FE, Baublis JV, and Itabashi HH: Isolation of measles virus from

cell cultures of brain from a patient with subacute sclerosing panencephalitis. N Engl J Med 281:585–589, 1969.

192. Pert CB, Hill JH, Ruff MR, et al: Octapeptides deduced from the neuropeptide receptor-like pattern of antigen T4 in brain potently inhibit human immunodeficiency virus receptor binding and T-cell infectivity. Proc Natl Acad Sci U S A 83:9254–9258, 1986.

193. Petito CK, Navia BA, Cho ES, Jordan BD, George DC, and Price RW: Vacuolar myelopathy pathologically resembling subacute combined degeneration in patients with the acquired immunodeficiency syndrome. N Engl J Med 312:874–879, 1985.

194. Petrov PA: Vilyuisk encephalitis in the Yakut republic (USSR). Am J Trop Med Hyg 19:146–150, 1970.

195. Pette H and Doring G: Über einheimische Panencephalomyelitis vom Charakter der Encephalitis japonica. Deutsch Z Nervenheilk 149:7–44, 1939.

196. Pomerantz RJ, Kuritzkes DR, de la Monte SM, et al: Infection of the retina by human immunodeficiency virus type 1. N Engl J Med 317:1643–1647, 1987.

197. Portegies P, deGans J, Lange JM, et al: Declining incidence of AIDS dementia complex after introduction of zidovudine treatment [published erratum appears in BMJ 299(6708):1141, 1989]. BMJ 299:819–821, 1989.

198. Powell-Jackson J, Weller RO, Kennedy P, Preece MA, Whitcombe EM, and Newsom-Davis J: Creutzfeldt-Jakob disease following human growth hormone administration. Lancet 2:244–246, 1985.

199. Price RW and Brew BJ: The AIDS dementia complex. J Infect Dis 158:1079–1083, 1988.

200. Price RW and Navia BA: Infections in AIDS and in other immunosuppressed patients. In Kennedy PGE and Johnson RT (eds): Infections of the Nervous System. Butterworth & Co, London, 1987.

201. Price RW, Sidtis J, and Rosenblum M: AIDS dementia complex: Some current questions. Ann Neurol (Suppl)23:S27–S33, 1988.

202. Prusiner SB: Novel proteinaceous infectious particles cause scrapie. Science 216:136–144, 1982.

203. Prusiner SB: Prions and neurodegenerative diseases. N Engl J Med 317:1571–1581, 1987.

204. Pumarola-Sune T, Navia BA, Cordon-Cardo C, Cho E-S, and Price RW: HIV antigen in the brains of patients with the AIDS dementia complex. Ann Neurol 21:490–496, 1987.

205. Rasmussen T and McCann W: Clinical studies of patients with focal epilepsy due to "chronic encephalitis." Transactions of the American Neurological Association 93:89–94, 1968.

206. Resnick L, diMarzo-Veronese F, Schupbach J, et al: Intra-blood-brain-barrier synthesis of HTLV-III–specific IgG in patients with neurologic symptoms associated with AIDS or AIDS-related complex. N Engl J Med 313:1498–1504, 1985.

207. Rhodes RH: Histopathology of the central nervous system in the acquired immunodeficiency syndrome. Hum Pathol 18:636–643, 1987.

208. Richardson EP Jr: Our evolving understanding of progressive multifocal leukoencephalopathy. Ann N Y Acad Sci 230:358–364, 1974.

209. Riehl J-L and Andrews JM: The uveomeningoencephalitic syndrome. Neurology 16:603–609, 1966.

210. Robb RN and Watters GV: Ophthalmic manifestations of subacute sclerosing panencephalitis. Arch Ophthalmol 83:426–435, 1970.

211. Roos RP: Viruses and demyelinating disease of the central nervous system. Neurol Clin 1:681–700, 1983.

212. Roos RP, Chou SM, Rogers NG, Basnight M, and Gajdusek DC: Isolation of an adenovirus 32 strain from human brain in a case of subacute encephalitis. Proc Soc Exp Biol Med 139:636–640, 1972.

213. Roos RP, Gajdusek DC, and Gibbs CJ Jr: The clinical characteristics of

transmissible Creutzfeldt-Jakob disease. Brain 96:1–20, 1973.

214. Roos RP, Graves MC, Wollmann RL, Chilcote RR, and Nixon J: Immunologic and virologic studies of measles inclusion body encephalitis in an immunosuppressed host: The relationship to subacute sclerosing panencephalitis. Neurology 31:1263–1270, 1981.

215. Rottenberg DA, Moeller JR, Strother SC, et al: The metabolic pathology of the AIDS dementia complex. Ann Neurol 22:700–706, 1987.

216. Rowley AH, Whitley RJ, Lakeman FD, and Wolinsky SM: Rapid detection of herpes-simplex-virus in cerebrospinal fluid from patients with herpes simplex encephalitis. Lancet 335:440–441, 1990.

217. Sawyer J, Ellner J, and Ransohoff DF: To biopsy or not to biopsy in suspected herpes simplex encephalitis. Med Decis Making 8:95–101, 1988.

218. Schmitt FA: Cognitive and emotional changes associated with retrovir treatment. Paper presented at Spectrum of Dementing Illnesses Conference, Columbia, SC, November 14, 1987.

218a. Schrott G, Gawahn J, Thron A, et al: Early diagnosis of herpes simplex encephalitis by MRI. Neurology 37:179–183, 1987.

219. Scott GB, Buck BE, Leterman JG, Bloom FL, and Parks WP: Acquired immunodeficiency syndrome in infants. N Engl J Med 310:76–81, 1984.

220. Scott M, Foster D, Mirenda C, et al: Transgenic mice expressing hamster prion protein produce species-specific scrapie infectivity and amyloid plaques. Cell 59:847–857, 1989.

221. Sells CJ, Carpenter RL, and Ray CG: Sequelae of central nervous system enterovirus infections. N Engl J Med 293:1–4, 1975.

222. Shah KV: Evidence for an SV40-related papovavirus infection of man. Am J Epidemiol 95:199–206, 1972.

223. Shah KV, Daniel RW, and Strandberg JD: Sarcoma in a hamster inoculated with BK virus, a human papovavirus. J Natl Cancer Inst 54:945–950, 1975.

224. Shah KV, Daniel RW, and Warszawski RN: High prevalence of antibodies to BK virus, an SV40-related papovavirus in residents of Maryland. J Infect Dis 128:784–787, 1973.

225. Shapoval AN: Chronic forms of tick-borne encephalitis in the Far East. Zh Nevropatol Psikhiatr 14:59–61, 1945.

226. Sharer LR, Cho ES, and Epstein LG: Multinucleated giant cells and HTLV-III in AIDS encephalopathy. Hum Pathol 16:760, 1985.

227. Sharer LR and Kapila R: Neuropathologic observations in acquired immunodeficiency syndrome (AIDS). Acta Neuropathol (Berl) 66:188–198, 1985.

228. Shaw GM, Harper ME, Hahn BH, et al: HTLV-III infection in brains of children and adults with AIDS encephalopathy. Science 227:177–182, 1985.

229. Sheppard RD, Raine CS, Bornstein MB, and Udem SA: Rapid degradation restricts measles virus matrix protein expression in a subacute sclerosing panencephalitis cell line. Proc Natl Acad Sci U S A 83:7913–7917, 1986.

230. Sigurdsson B: Rida, a chronic encephalitis of sheep, with general remarks on infections which develop slowly and some of their special characteristics. Br Vet J 110:341–354, 1954.

231. Silberstein CH, McKegney FP, O'Dowd MA, et al: A prospective longitudinal study of neuropsychological and psychosocial factors in asymptomatic individuals at risk for HTLV-III/LAV infection in a methadone program: preliminary findings. Int J Neurosci 32:669–676, 1987.

232. Silverman L and Rubenstein LJ: Electron microscopic observations on a case of progressive multifocal leukoencephalopathy. Acta Neuropathol (Berl) 5:215–224, 1965.

233. Skoldenberg B, Forsgren M, Alestig

K, Bergstrom T, Burman L, and Dahl-quist E: Acyclovir versus vidarabine in herpes simplex encephalitis. Randomised multicenter study in consecutive Swedish patients. Lancet 2: 707–711, 1984.

234. Small JA, Scangos GA, Cork L, Jay G, and Khoury G: The early region of human papovavirus JC induces dysmyelination in transgenic mice. Cell 46:13–18, 1986.

235. Smith JB, Westmoreland BF, Reagan TJ, and Sandok BA: A distinctive clinical EEG profile in herpes simplex encephalitis. Mayo Clin Proc 50:469–474, 1975.

236. Smith JE: St. Louis encephalitis: Sequelae. Neurology 8:884, 1958.

237. Snider WD, Simpson DM, Nielson G, Gold JWM, Metroka CE, and Posner JB: Neurological complications of acquired immune deficiency syndrome: Analysis of 50 patients. Ann Neurol 14:403–418, 1983.

238. Sodroski J, Kowalski M, Dorfman T, Basiripour L, Rosen C, and Haseltine W: HIV envelope-CD4 interaction not inhibited by synthetic octapeptides. Lancet 1:1428–1429, 1987.

239. Spillane JC and Wells CEC: The neurology of Jennerian vaccination. Brain 87:1–44, 1964.

240. Stam FC: Multifocal leukoencephalopathy with slow progression and very long survival. Psychiatr Neurol Neurochir 69:453–459, 1966.

241. Stoler MH, Eskin TA, Benn S, Angerer RC, and Angerer LM: Human T-cell lymphotropic virus type III infection of the central nervous system. JAMA 256:2360–2364, 1986.

242. Sutton RNP: Slow viruses and chronic disease of the central nervous system. Postgrad Med J 55: 143–149, 1979.

243. Tateishi J, Kitamato T, and Hiratani H: Creutzfeldt-Jakob disease pathogen in growth hormone preparation is eliminatable (letter). Lancet 2: 1299–1300, 1985.

244. Tateishi J, Sato Y, Koga M, Doi H, and Ohta M: Experimental transmission of human subacute spongiform encephalopathy to small rodents. I.

Clinical and histological observations. Acta Neuropathol (Berl)51: 127–134, 1980.

245. Tellez-Nagel I and Harter DH: Subacute sclerosing leukoencephalitis. I. Clinico-pathological, electron microscopic, and virologic observations. J Neuropathol Exp Neurol 25:560–581, 1966.

246. Townsend JJ, Baringer JR, Wolinsky JS, et al: Progressive rubella panencephalitis: Late onset after congenital rubella. N Engl J Med 292:990–993, 1975.

247. Trapp BD, Small JA, Pulley M, Khoury G, and Scangos GA: Dysmyelination in transgenic mice containing JC virus early region. Ann Nuerol 28:38–48, 1988.

248. Traub RD, Gajdusek DC, and Gibbs CJ Jr: Transmissible dementia. The relation of transmissible spongiform encephalopathy to Creutzfeldt-Jakob disease. In Kinsbourne M and Smith L (eds): Aging, Dementia and Cerebral Function. Spectrum Publishing, Flushing, NY, 1977.

249. Tyler HR: Neurological complications of rubeola (measles). Medicine (Baltimore) 36:147–167, 1957.

250. Van Bogaert L: Une leuco-encéphalite sclérosante subaigue. J Neurol Neurosurg Psychiatry 8:101–120, 1945.

251. Von Pirquet C: Das verhalten der kutanen Tuberkulinreaktion wahrende der Masern. Dtsch Med Wochenschr 34:1297–1300, 1908.

252. Van Rossum A: Spastic pseudosclerosis (Creutzfeldt-Jakob disease). In Vinken PJ and Bruyn GW (eds): Handbook of Clinical Neurology, Vol 6. Elsevier, Amsterdam, 1968.

253. Van Wielink G, McArthur JC, Moench T, et al: Intrathecal synthesis of anti-HIV IgG: Correlation with increasing duration of HIV-1 infection. Neurology 40:816–819, 1990.

254. Vazeux R, Brousse N, Jarry A, et al: AIDS subacute encephalitis: Identification of HIV-infected cells. Am J Pathol 126:403–410, 1987.

255. Walker DL, Padgett BL, ZuRhein GM, Albert AE, and Marsh RF: Human

papovavirus (JC): Induction of brain tumor in hamsters. Science 181:674–676, 1973.

256. Ward JM, O'Leary TJ, Baskin GB, et al: Immunohistochemical localization of human and simian immunodeficiency viral antigens in fixed tissue sections. Am J Pathol 127:199, 1987.

257. Wechsler SL, Weiner HL, and Fields BN: Immune response in subacute sclerosing panencephalitis: Reduced antibody response to the matrix protein of measles virus. J Immunol 123:884–889, 1979.

258. Weil M, Itabashi H, Cremer NE, Oshiro L, Lennette EH, and Carnay L: Chronic progressive panencephalitis due to rubella virus simulating subacute sclerosing panencephalitis. N Engl J Med 292:994–998, 1975.

259. Weiner LP, Herndon RM, Narayan O, et al: Isolation of virus related to SV40 from patients with progressive multifocal leukoencephalopathy. N Engl J Med 286:385–390, 1972.

260. Westaway P, Goodman PA, Mirenda CA, McKinley MP, Carlson GA, and Prusiner SB: Distinct prion proteins in short and long scrapie incubation period mice. Cell 51:651–662, 1987.

261. Whitley RJ, Alford CA, Hirsch MS, et al: Vidarabine versus acyclovir therapy in herpes simplex encephalitis. N Engl J Med 314:144–149, 1986.

262. Whitley RJ, Soong S-J, Hirsch MS, et al: Herpes simplex encephalitis. Vidarabine therapy and diagnostic problems. N Engl J Med 304:313–318, 1981.

263. Wiley CA and Nelson JA: Role of human immunodeficiency virus and cytomegalovirus in AIDS encephalitis. Am J Pathol 133:73–81, 1988.

264. Wiley CA, Schrier RD, Nelson JA, Lampert PW, and Oldstone MB: Cellular localization of human immunodeficiency virus infection within the brains of acquired immune deficiency syndrome patients. Proc Natl Acad Sci U S A 83:7089–7093, 1986.

265. Wisniewski HM, Bruce ME, and Fraser H: Infectious etiology of neuritic (senile) plaques in mice. Science 190:1108–1110, 1975.

266. Wolinsky JS, Berg BO, and Maitland CJ: Progressive rubella panencephalitis. Arch Neurol 33:722–723, 1976.

267. Yarchoan R, Berg G, Brouwers P, et al: Response of human immunodeficiency-virus-associated neurological disease to 3'-azido-3'-deoxythymidie. Lancet 1:132–135, 1987.

268. ZuRhein GM and Chou SM: Particles resembling papova viruses in human cerebral demyelinating disease. Science 148:1477–1497, 1965.

Chapter 9

BACTERIAL, FUNGAL, AND PARASITIC CAUSES OF DEMENTIA

James Ashe, M.B., M.R.C.P.I.,
Steven A. Rosen, M.D.,
Justin C. McArthur, M.B., B.S.,
  M.P.H., and
Larry E. Davis, M.D., F.A.C.P.

DEMENTIA AS A SEQUELA OF
  BACTERIAL MENINGITIS
BACTERIAL INFECTIONS CAUSING
  PROGRESSIVE DEMENTIA
FUNGAL INFECTIONS CAUSING
  PROGRESSIVE DEMENTIA
PROTOZOAL AND PARASITIC
  INFECTIONS CAUSING
  PROGRESSIVE DEMENTIA

Making a diagnosis of bacterial, fungal, or parasitic infections of the central nervous system (CNS) in a patient with a progressive dementia is especially important because effective treatment will arrest and often reverse the dementing process. Insofar as CNS infections account for about only 1% of all cases of dementia,[*] however, one should be selective about performing uncomfortable and expensive tests on any patient with dementia.

Certain historical features should raise the suspicion of a CNS infection in a dementing patient. First, the rate of intellectual decline should be considered. If the process is occurring over weeks to a few months, the cause is more likely a CNS infection than if the dementia has been present for years. Second, a history of fevers or night sweats suggests a possible CNS infection. The fevers are often low-grade and intermittent. Third, delirium, rather than only dementia, may be a prominent early feature, and both delirium and dementia may be present as the disease progresses. Fourth, headaches, nausea, vomiting, focal neurologic deficits, or seizures should suggest the possibility of an intracranial infection. Fifth, CNS infections should be considered in patients who are debilitated or immunosuppressed from either an underlying disease or drugs. Finally, young patients are less likely to have dementia due to degenerative or vascular causes, and are somewhat more likely to have cognitive impairment as part of a CNS infection.

The physical examination may also provide clues to a possible infection. Fever or meningismus is often present. Focal neurologic signs, particularly cra-

---

[*]References 50, 63, 67, 83, 88, 90, 145, 170, 171.

nial nerve palsies, aphasia, hemiparesis, and visual field defects, may be present in CNS infections that cause cognitive decline. Any patient with a rapidly progressive mental deterioration and focal neurologic deficits requires an aggressive evaluation to rule out a CNS infection.

If a CNS infection is suspected, several laboratory tests may aid in the diagnosis. A computed tomographic (CT) scan with and without contrast, or magnetic resonance imaging (MRI) may demonstrate meningeal inflammation, cerebral edema, or parenchymal damage due to meningitis or encephalitis. Focal masses that are ring enhancing may suggest a brain abscess. Elevated white blood cell counts or elevated erythrocyte sedimentation rates suggest an infectious process. A rapid plasma reagin test that is reactive suggests active systemic syphilis and possible neurosyphilis. A positive tuberculin skin test indicates prior or active infection with *Mycobacterium tuberculosis*. A chest roentgenogram may show pulmonary tuberculosis or fungal infections that have disseminated to the brain.

Lumbar puncture may establish the diagnosis of a CNS infection.[7,49] The opening pressure should be measured. The cerebrospinal fluid (CSF) should be examined for a cell count, and differential, protein, glucose, immunoglobulin G level, oligoclonal bands, and CSF venereal disease research laboratory (VDRL) tests should be performed. Bacteriologic, fungal, and tuberculosis cultures should be done, particularly when there is a CSF pleocytosis. Cryptococcal antigen test and fungal antibody titers may also be performed. Although a mononuclear pleocytosis is common in many CNS infections, it is not diagnostic. CSF pleocytosis may also be seen in noninfectious processes such as CNS neoplasms, vasculitis of cranial vessels, and CNS sarcoidosis.[175]

Several pathophysiologic processes may cause dementia in the patient with a CNS infection. Chronic encephalitis may destroy neurons in the frontal, temporal, and parietal lobes and damage structures crucial to memory, learning, motivation, and affect. Chronic meningitis may cause vasculitis with subsequent arterial or venous occlusions leading to brain infarctions. Chronic meningitis may also obstruct normal CSF pathways, leading to communicating or noncommunicating hydrocephalus and raised intracranial pressure, which impairs cognitive function. Brain granulomas and abscesses, in addition to behaving as space-occupying lesions and increasing intracranial pressure, may destroy regional areas of the brain. Neurotoxic substances may also be released by the infectious agent or produced by an immunologic reactive process.

Chapter 8 reviewed dementias resulting from viral infections. A comprehensive review of other infections of the CNS is beyond the scope of this chapter. Many detailed publications are available.[13,32,76,94] The organisms discussed in this chapter have been chosen because cognitive impairment is an important aspect of their clinical manifestations. Some bacterial infections can cause an acute or chronic encephalitis and present with progressive dementia (Table 9–1).

Table 9–1 Bacteria Causing Acute or Chronic Encephalitis

Borrelia burgdorferi (Lyme disease)[22,117]
Leptospira species[43,73]
Borrelia species (Relapsing fever)[150]
Listeria monocytogenes[65,172,173]
Brucella species[14,47]
Mycoplasma pneumoniae[48,114,123]
Legionella species[71]
Treponema pallidum[91]

DEMENTIA AS A SEQUELA OF BACTERIAL MENINGITIS

In the preantibiotic era, more than 95% of individuals with bacterial meningitis died within 1 to 6 months of onset. With the advent of antibiotics, more than 90% of adults and more than 95% of children survive bacterial meningitis.[39] Unfortunately, as many as 50% of survivors of meningitis have some sequelae from their disease.[78]

Clinical Features

Most studies of survivors of bacterial meningitis have found that about 10% of children are left with significant mental retardation.[78,85,134,135,153] One study of 56 patients who were observed after surviving bacterial meningitis found 29% to have significant neurologic sequelae including dementia (IQ below 60), epilepsy, or marked hearing loss.[135] In another study, 4% of 82 surviving children with *Haemophilus influenzae* meningitis were left with marked mental retardation.[134] Some of these surviving children also demonstrated abnormal behavior in school, hyperactivity, poor impulse control, and an inability to learn in school.[136] If they were young, delayed language development occurred in about 15%. Complicating the mental retardation, some children also had visual impairment (5%) or hearing loss (10%) as a sequela of the meningitis.[40,78] The hearing loss was often profound, was unilateral or bilateral, and was usually sensorineural in type.[10]

In addition, most studies of surviving children with bacterial meningitis have found that about 5% are left with motor sequelae such as hemiparesis, quadriparesis, spasticity, or poor coordination.[78] Three percent of children are left with a permanent seizure disorder.[2]

Adults surviving bacterial meningitis frequently are left with cognitive impairments or hearing loss. In one study, adults aged 15 to 49 years who survived bacterial meningitis had a 41% incidence of neurologic complications. In the elderly (above age 65), the rate of neurologic complications rose to 85%.[55] Some of these complications were minor, but some patients were left with sensorineural deafness, optic neuritis, or cognitive impairments.[55] The impact of bacterial meningitis in causing dementia is more difficult to assess in the elderly, many of whom had preexisting problems of higher cortical function.

Laboratory Findings

Children and adults with mental retardation or dementia following bacterial meningitis frequently have abnormalities on CT or MRI.[21,28a] These scans may demonstrate cerebral or cerebellar infarctions, focal areas of brain necrosis, or mild to moderate ventricular dilation. Hydrocephalus, marked subdural effusions, subdural empyemas, and brain abscesses may occur but are less common. Electroencephalograms usually show mild to moderate slowing which may be somewhat asymmetrical. Occasionally, spikes may be seen. The audiogram may show sensorineural hearing loss, and auditory evoked potentials may be abnormal.[107]

Pathophysiology

Bacteria in the meninges and subarachnoid space promptly give rise to an intense, inflammatory reaction. The combination of bacterial products (such as endotoxin) and lymphokines from inflammatory cells may directly or indirectly damage the underlying cerebral cortex.[32,165] Thrombosis of cerebral vessels may occur, leading to focal areas of cerebral infarction. Large infarctions of the brain can occur from arteritis with secondary stenosis or occlusion of the supraclinoid portion of the internal carotid artery, the proximal portion of the middle cerebral artery, the proximal anterior carotid artery, or their medium-sized branches.[68] Stenosis or occlusion of small, penetrating meningeal arteries or draining veins may cause smaller areas of infarction. In most cases the infarction is bland, but occasionally hemorrhagic infarctions develop. Bacterial toxins may cause cerebral necrosis.[41,146] During the course of bacterial meningitis, ventriculomegaly is common. This presumably results from impairment of CSF absorption at the superior sagittal sinus, or flow past the tentorium, giving rise to a communicating hydrocephalus. If the meningitis progresses long enough untreated, bacteria eventually invade the brain to cause a bacterial encephalitis or multiple brain abscesses.

Neurologic complications may also develop as a consequence of increased intracranial pressure. This increased pressure results from cerebral edema and impaired CSF reabsorption, and may cause a sufficient fall in cerebral blood perfusion to cause secondary neuronal hypoxia.[41] If shock develops in the course of the bacterial meningitis, cerebral blood flow may rapidly diminish, adding to the cerebral ischemia.

Hearing loss may be the result of bacterial invasion into the inner ear from CSF via the perilymphatic canal or internal auditory canal, or be caused by a vasculitis of the eighth cranial nerve.[78,134]

Therapy

Prompt treatment of bacterial meningitis with appropriate broad-spectrum antibiotics has been shown to decrease, but not eliminate, neurologic sequelae. Marked delays in antibiotic treatment worsen the sequelae. Whether the frequency of neurologic complications may be diminished by the addition of corticosteroids to the treatment program is controversial. The use of corticosteroids is based on the argument that the intense inflammation in the meninges and inner ear is what causes secondary damage to the underlying brain and cochlea.[144] Anti-inflammatory drugs such as corticosteroids would then reduce the degree of inflam-

mation and lower the incidence of brain and ear damage. Two major clinical trials in humans have demonstrated efficacy for corticosteroids,[84,104] but other studies have failed to demonstrate benefit.[8,35] Once damage to the cerebral cortex has occurred, use of corticosteroids will not reverse the process.

Prognosis

Children surviving bacterial meningitis should be carefully observed for signs of mental retardation, visual impairment, or sensorineural hearing loss. It is advised that all young children be tested for hearing, as hearing impairment will impede school performance.[40] Special-education classes may be necessary for children with moderate to severe mental retardation. One study also found that surviving children who appeared to have recovered completely still functioned less well in school than their peers.[136] On the other hand, many neurologic sequelae following bacterial meningitis may continue to improve spontaneously months to years after the acute event.

BACTERIAL INFECTIONS CAUSING PROGRESSIVE DEMENTIA

Neurosyphilis

Syphilis is the third most frequently reported communicable disease in the United States, and the incidence is increasing.[26] Untreated or inadequately treated primary syphilis leads to symptomatic neurosyphilis in 5% to 10% of cases.[52] Because an estimated 50,000 cases of syphilis remain undetected each year,[18,137] the incidence of untreated neurosyphilis may be as high as 2 to 5 per 100,000 of the adult population. Of the various syphilitic syndromes, general paresis and, occasionally, meningovascular syphilis are the most likely to cause dementia. The signs and symptoms of the other stages

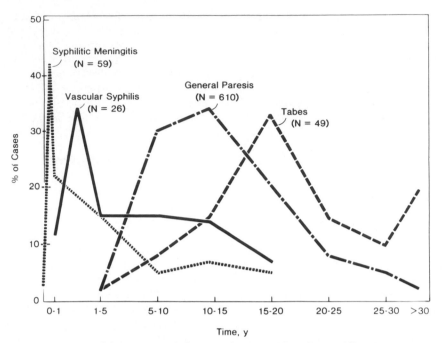

Figure 9–1. Time course of the neurosyphilitic syndromes. (From Simon,[142] p. 607, with permission.)

of neurosyphilis are discussed in several monographs[32,92,142] and will not be covered in detail here.

PATHOGENESIS

Syphilis is caused by the spirochete *Treponema pallidum*, which was first isolated in 1905.[131] In patients with primary syphilis who are untreated, 25% to 30% will subsequently have a spirochetal infection of the meninges and brain. CNS infection usually occurs during secondary syphilis, which develops one to several months after the primary infection (Fig. 9–1). The initial meningeal infection is usually asymptomatic,[95] but occasional patients may develop the clinical picture of an acute aseptic meningitis (acute syphilitic meningitis).[93]

Spirochetes usually persist in the meninges, causing a very low-grade meningitis, but patients often remain asymptomatic for years. Two to 10 years later, some patients develop meningovascular syphilis.[92] These patients present with one or more strokes involving the brainstem and cerebral cortex.[142] Pathologically there is an endarteritis with vessel thrombosis leading to focal areas of encephalomalacia (Fig. 9–2).

In addition to the chronic meningitis, spirochetes may invade the brain, giving rise to a low-grade bacterial encephalitis. Parenchymatous neurosyphilis or general paresis usually becomes manifest 8 to 25 years after the primary infection. The final stage of neurosyphilis develops from a chronic arachnoiditis of the meninges of the base of the brain and spinal cord, which causes tabes dorsalis.[92] Tabes dorsalis usually develops about 10 to 30 years after the primary infection. The chronic arachnoiditis appears to cause ischemic damage to the spinal cord, particularly the dorsal columns, and to the optic nerves. Clinically this gives rise to ataxia, sensory losses, lightning abdominal or leg pains, optic atrophy, and pupil abnormalities, particularly the Argyll Robertson pupil (see below).[91]

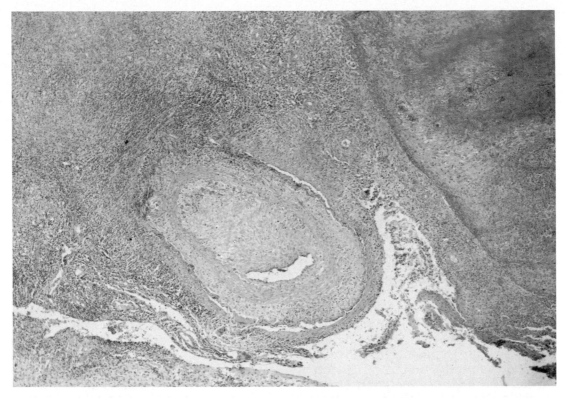

Figure 9-2. Meningovascular syphilis. Narrowing of the arterial lumen with extensive intimal proliferation; disruption of the muscularis layer; and mononuclear cell infiltration of the vessel wall, brain parenchyma, and subarachnoid space are seen.

CLINICAL FEATURES OF PARENCHYMATOUS NEUROSYPHILIS

General paresis starts insidiously with neuropsychiatric symptoms[92] including irritability, forgetfulness, nervousness, impaired concentration, carelessness in appearance, insomnia, and personality changes.[92] As the disease progresses over weeks to months, patients lose insight, have impaired recent memory, and display periods of confusion and disorientation. They often have difficulties in judgment and may develop changes in affect, with periods of elation or depression. Psychoses may appear and present as agitated depression, mania, or paranoia. "Delusions of grandeur" have been reported in 20% of patients with neurosyphilis.[72]

Early in the illness, focal neurologic signs are uncommon unless the patient has coexistent meningovascular syphilis with small strokes. Occasionally, however, patients will develop seizures, tremors, or muscular spasticity. Pupillary abnormalities are common, particularly a slow constriction to light shown in the eyes. Some patients develop the classic Argyll Robertson pupil: (1) the pupils are small, fixed, and do not react to light; (2) the pupils react normally to accommodation; (3) mydriatics (atropine) fail to dilate pupils fully; and (4) visual loss does not occur. About half the patients with general paresis will manifest some of these pupillary findings.

LABORATORY FINDINGS

Early in general paresis, the CT scan often shows few changes. Cerebral atrophy and ventricular dilation develop later.[51] Syphilitic gummata may appear as localized, 1 to 2 cm, contrast-enhancing lesions.[53] The electroencephalogram is abnormal in 80% of cases and usually demonstrates slowing of background activity.[159]

CEREBROSPINAL FLUID FINDINGS

The CSF in all stages of neurosyphilis usually shows a low-grade lymphocytic pleocytosis with a cell count ranging from 10 to 700 lymphocytes/mm³. CSF protein is typically elevated above 40 mg/dL, but is seldom greater than 200 mg/dL. There is usually an increased synthesis of CSF immunoglobulin G.[79] Electrophoresis of CSF often shows an increase in the percentage of γ-globulin. Acrylamide gel electrophoresis typically shows several oligoclonal bands in the γ-globulin region. CSF glucose is typically normal. The CSF-VDRL test is usually positive or reactive in general paresis. In addition, the blood fluorescent treponemal antibody absorption test (FTA-ABS) and the blood rapid plasma reagin (RPR) are reactive. Other treponemal tests such as the microhemagglutination assay for *T pallidum* (MHA-TP) and the *T pallidum* hemagglutination assay (TPHA) are also reactive.[82]

DIAGNOSIS

A firm diagnosis of neurosyphilis can be made when the CSF demonstrates typical findings and the CSF-VDRL test is reactive.[69] Recently there has been some concern that occasional patients may have active neurosyphilis in the absence of a reactive CSF-VDRL test.[33] Neurosyphilis is extremely unlikely if the serum FTA-ABS test is nonreactive.[69]

THERAPY

Penicillin is the drug of choice for treatment of neurosyphilis. To date, no penicillin-resistant *T pallidum* strains have been recognized. To achieve adequate antibiotic levels in the brain and CSF following systemic therapy, the blood-brain barrier must be overcome. The Centers for Disease Control[27] currently recommend two treatment regimens, shown on Table 9−2. Because *T pallidum* spirochetes replicate at a slow rate, it is essential for the penicillin treatment to be continued for 2 to 4 weeks. Occasional patients may develop a Jarisch-Herxheimer reaction in the first 24 hours after starting penicillin treatment. These patients develop a fever with transient worsening of their psychosis or neurologic signs; 2 to 3 days of prednisone 5 mg four times daily, with gradual reduction of dosage, may be beneficial.

Patients who are seriously allergic to penicillin may be treated with high doses of ceftriaxone for several weeks. Ceftriaxone has been shown to cross the blood-brain barrier. Although it is effective in secondary syphilis, experience has been limited in treatment of tertiary syphilis.[66] Tetracycline or doxycycline may also be used as an alternative.[26]

Over 90% of patients with neurosyphilis that are treated with full doses of penicillin are cured. Nevertheless, the patient should be followed for 1 to 2 years to ensure that the treatment was

Table 9−2 Penicillin Treatment Regimens for Neurosyphilis

1. Aqueous crystalline penicillin G: 12−24 million units IV per day for 10−14 days, followed by benzathine penicillin G, 2.4 million units IM weekly for three doses.
2. Aqueous procaine penicillin G: 2.4 million units IM daily, plus probenicid (500 mg PO q.i.d.), both for 10−14 days, followed by benzathine penicillin G, 2.4 million units IM weeky for three doses.

Source: From Centers for Disease Control,[27] p. 9, with permission.

effective. A lumbar puncture should be repeated at 4 weeks, 6 months, and 1 year after therapy.[26] With effective therapy the CSF pleocytosis should return to normal within the first 6 months. The CSF protein should fall to normal or near normal by 6 months to 1 year. The CSF-VDRL titer should fall toward zero but may not always become nonreactive. The CSF-FTA-ABS test usually remains positive.

Patients with immunosuppressive diseases, such as HIV infection, appear to experience an accelerated and more atypical course of neurosyphilis.[70] In these patients the time course to general paresis may be truncated and the clinical manifestations become more florid. These patients may also develop syphilitic retinitis and otitic syphilis.

PROGNOSIS

The prognosis for clinical recovery in patients with general paresis depends on how long the signs and symptoms have been present. If treated within the first 6 months to 1 year, patients often experience considerable improvement in their cognitive function. Unfortunately, if the general paresis has been present for 1 to 2 years, patients seldom clinically improve, even though progression of the dementia may be halted.

Tuberculous Meningitis

CLINICAL FEATURES

Infection of the CNS by *Mycobacterium tuberculosis* is uncommon in developed countries. In underdeveloped nations it remains an endemic disorder, particularly in children, in whom it comprises 1% to 5% of all hospital admissions.[138,168] Tuberculous meningitis complicates pulmonary tuberculosis in 20% to 40% of pediatric cases, but in only 3% to 6% of adult cases.

Tuberculous meningitis begins insidiously with fever, malaise, anorexia, and intermittent headache, followed by more prominent neurologic symptoms and signs including worsening headache, meningismus, nausea, vomiting, cranial nerve palsies, hemiplegia, seizures, and altered mental state. Most patients will have been ill for only 1 to 4 weeks. Almost 25% of patients develop symptoms over several months, however, making the diagnosis less obvious. Death usually occurs in 1 to 2 months in untreated cases. Atypical presentations include acute meningitis, strokelike hemiparesis, and epilepsy. Acute increased intracranial pressure is more common in children.

While cognitive deterioration is present in more than two thirds of cases of tuberculous meningitis, the presence of dementia without clinical evidence of a subacute delirium, meningitis, or focal neurologic process is extremely rare.[75,158,163,169] Yet elderly patients with tuberculous meningitis may not have fever or meningismus; progressive confusion may be the sole presenting complaint.[80] Dixon and colleagues[38] reported on tuberculous meningitis in six elderly patients. A short prodromal illness of less than 2 weeks was followed by restlessness, irritability, and delirium. Headache, fever, meningismus, or evidence of active tuberculosis were not uniformly present in all cases. Cognitive decline was characterized by the fairly abrupt onset of disorientation, lassitude, drowsiness, and incontinence. Recovery occurred gradually over several weeks and was often incomplete.

The majority of long-term follow-up studies of tuberculous meningitis focus on pediatric populations or antedate the diagnostic use of CT and the therapeutic use of isoniazid.[45,111,161,168] More recent studies include smaller numbers of patients with relatively short follow-up.[38,75,158] Some studies are directed at a single aspect of tuberculous meningitis, such as the use of CT[77] and shunting for hydrocephalus.[100] Taken together, these studies indicate that, among patients with tuberculous meningitis who were previously healthy, a good prognosis can be expected in those who are over 2 years of age, who present with a brief illness, and who are alert without focal neurologic signs. Following treatment, more than 75% have normal or above-normal intelligence on formal psychometric testing and are working or attending school.

Patients who present with altered consciousness (particularly stupor or coma) and who have focal neurologic deficits have a much worse prognosis, however. Of those who survive, 50% have epilepsy or mild to moderate focal neurologic deficits. Severely disabled patients often have a "chronic brain syndrome" characterized by mental deterioration involving impairment of intellect, judgment, and skill.[45] In fact, dementia or impairment of mental development severe enough to require institutionalization occurs in 25% of the survivors.[111]

LABORATORY FINDINGS

Laboratory diagnosis of tuberculous meningitis is often difficult. A high incidence of falsely negative paraphenylenediamine (PPD) skin tests occurs in the chronically ill. Routine blood studies are nondiagnostic, although hyponatremia secondary to the syndrome of inappropriate antidiuretic hormone (SIADH) can occur. This in itself can contribute to mental status changes. A cavitary lesion on chest roentgenogram is suggestive of tuberculosis but is nonspecific. Demonstration of mycobacteria in pathologic specimens from the lung and other sources suggests a similar process intracranially. CSF examination reveals an elevated protein (100 to 500 mg/dL), a lymphocytic pleocytosis (100 to 500 cells/mm³) and hypoglycorrhachia. However, atypical CSF findings are seen in a significant minority of cases. Acid-fast staining and microscopic examination of large volumes of CSF are crucial to the diagnosis. Kennedy and Fallon[75] reported that four serial spinal taps revealed a diagnosis in 87% of cases when centrifuged sediment from 10 mL of CSF was examined microscopically. Cultures take several weeks. Some 15% to 20% of proven cases of tuberculous meningitis will have repeatedly negative microscopic and culture results. Head CT scanning may show hydrocephalus, tuberculomas, or infarctions.[5] Contrast enhancement may demonstrate basilar arachnoiditis. Whether MRI (particularly with paramagnetic contrast agents) has greater utility remains to be determined.

PATHOPHYSIOLOGY

Tuberculous meningitis results from rupture of a tubercle (Rich focus) into the subarachnoid space. These juxtaependymal foci arise following hematogenous dissemination from foci of chronic tuberculous infection in the lungs and other organs. In children, however, meningitis may accompany primary or miliary tuberculosis. The meningitis may progress to a thick, gelatinous basal arachnoiditis extending from the pons to the optic nerves, with a predilection for the optic chiasm (Fig. 9–3). Cranial nerve palsies and hypothalamic dysfunction are common. Border-zone encephalitis (consisting of edema, perivascular inflammatory cells, microglial reaction, and gliosis) occurs within brain parenchyma wherever it comes in contact with the tuberculous exudate. Vasculitis with inflammation, spasm, and thrombosis occurs as the vessels penetrate the basal exudate. This leads to multiple infarcts, especially of subcortical gray matter. Communicating hydrocephalus is common early in the course of tuberculous meningitis. Noncommunicating hydrocephalus secondary to aqueductal obstruction is less frequently seen. CT and MRI have demonstrated a greater incidence of CNS tuberculomas than was previously appreciated.[140]

A postinfectious encephalitis known as tuberculous encephalopathy was described by Dastur and Udani[31,167] in the 1960s. Their pathologic studies revealed diffuse brain damage characterized by edema and perivascular myelin loss. Some cases showed a hemorrhagic or necrotizing leukoencephalopathy. This condition, which occurs mainly in

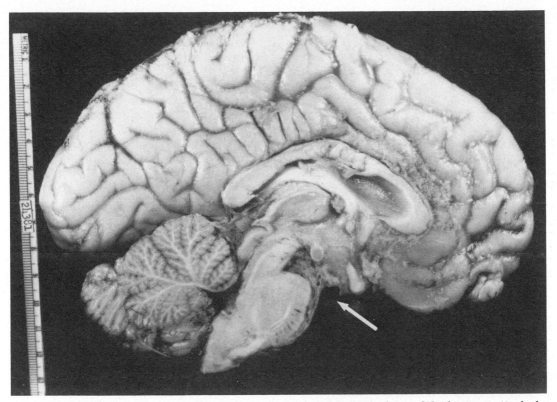

Figure 9–3. Tuberculous meningitis. A thick exudate surrounds the base of the brain, particularly from the rostral brainstem to the optic chiasm (*arrow*). Numerous small tuberculomas can be seen throughout the frontal region.

children, is characterized by the abrupt or insidious onset of convulsions and altered mental state, with or without signs of meningitis.

THERAPY

Isoniazid, rifampin, pyrazinamide, and streptomycin are effective antibiotics in combination. Ethambutol, cycloserine, and ethionamide are second-line agents. The use of corticosteroids in tuberculous meningitis remains controversial despite more than 30 years of use. Steroids are generally recommended in proven cases of tuberculous meningitis when there is early and increasing hydrocephalus, a contrast-enhancing basal exudate seen on CT scan, significant edema surrounding a tuberculoma, or clinical evidence of spinal cord compression.[80] Ventriculoperitoneal shunting for hydrocephalus is often necessary, despite the risk of infection and other complications, although the neurologic outcome does not always improve following shunt placement.[169] In many cases shunting has come late in the course of the illness, when considerable neuronal damage may have already occurred. Newman, Cumming, and Foster[100] suggest that hydrocephalus should be actively sought and that, if found, early ventricular decompression should be combined with standard antituberculous chemotherapy.

Neurobrucellosis

Four strains of brucellae cause disease in humans. Cattle, which harbor *Brucella abortus*, are the most common animal reservoir associated with neurobrucellosis in the United States.[24] Abattoir workers account for almost half of those affected; farmers, dairy workers, and veterinary surgeons are also at relatively high risk.

Infection may be subclinical, acute, chronic, or relapsing. The acute syndrome consists of high fever and nonspecific symptoms of systemic infection (malaise, chills, sweats, weakness, arthralgia, headache, and weight loss).[19] Nervous system involvement, which is seen in less than 5% of cases, may occur during the acute phase or with subsequent relapses.[119,174] Meningitis is the most common manifestation and is the presenting feature of the disease in one third of those with neurologic involvement,[15] although encephalitis, myelitis, radiculitis, and neuritis have all been described.[47,101] Cranial nerves are frequently affected, particularly the eighth, seventh, and sixth.[125,176] Mental status changes ranging from dementia to coma have been reported.[4,19,22,125]

The diagnosis is made through culture of the organism or by indirect methods that suggest infection. *Brucella* species are rarely detected in the CSF, and blood culture is positive in only 7% of those with nervous system involvement.[101] The most common indirect method is the standard tube agglutination (STA) test. A fourfold rise in antibody titer or a single agglutination titer greater than 1 : 160 is indicative of infection.[23] Other methods include a complement fixation (CF) test and a Coombs test. Radioimmunoassay (RIA) and enzyme-linked immunoabsorbent assay (ELISA) are better techniques than the STA or CF.[110,143]

The treatment of brucellosis is controversial. Tetracyclines, sulfonamides, streptomycin, and rifampin have all been used. One group with considerable experience in treating brucellosis of the nervous system favors the use of rifampin, doxycycline, and streptomycin.[14] Response to treatment was assessed by CSF examination and fall in antibody titers. The mean length of treatment was 8.5 months.

Lyme Disease

Lyme disease or Lyme borreliosis was proven to be caused by the spirochete *Borrelia burgdorferi* in 1983.[156] Lyme disease has been recognized in the United States only since 1975. A true increase in the incidence of Lyme disease is occurring throughout the United States. At present it is endemic throughout much of the Northeast and has been recognized on the West Coast, as well as parts of the South.[25]

PATHOPHYSIOLOGY

B burgdorferi is a spiral bacteria that is transmitted primarily by *Ixodes* species of ticks (*I dammini*, *I pacificus*, *I scapularis*, *I ricinus*, and *I persulcatus*).[155] Humans are only an accidental host in the normal zoonosis of *B burgdorferi*. The normal life cycle involves several vertebrates, including mice and deer.[154] Human infection is usually acquired when nymphal ticks feed between May and July. Approximately 10% to 50% of individuals become infected following the tick bite. The initial spirochetal replication occurs locally in the skin. If untreated, spirochetes then disseminate to infect multiple organs including the lymphatic system, joints, and the nervous system.[154] There is strong evidence that most manifestations of Lyme disease are due to spirochete infection of the target organ. There is some evidence, however, that the immune system may contribute to some of the neurologic signs and symptoms.[1,141]

CLINICAL FEATURES

It has been estimated that about 15% of untreated patients will develop neurologic involvement, including radiculoneuritis, aseptic meningitis, and cranial neuritis.[109] In Europe this syndrome is called Bannwarth's syndrome. These patients often experience attacks of headache and meningismus; up to one half may develop some degree of facial nerve involvement.

Occasional patients may develop a late persistent CNS infection. In these individuals the spirochete infection appears to persist and produce a variety of CNS signs and symptoms that develop years after the primary infection. Most reports have described these patients as having a progressive meningoencephalitis. Patients may develop lethargy, poor concentration, fatigue, memory loss, irritability, episodes of confusion, depression, or even frank psychosis with hallucinations.[61,62,86,108,118] These patients have difficulty remembering things, often having to make lists to remember appointments; others have trouble in finding words and are unusually irritable.[86] The encephalopathy is severe enough to interfere with work. Many patients also have a polyneuropathy.[86] Occasional patients also may experience spastic paraparesis, hemiparesis, or transversal myelitis. Many of these patients also have a chronic arthritis characterized by episodes of joint swelling that last months to years. Large joints are more commonly involved than small joints.

LABORATORY FINDINGS

In patients with late persistent infections, laboratory findings have varied. Patients have demonstrated objective abnormalities on memory testing but usually have had normal values on intelligence tests. MRI of the brain may show small foci of increased signals, usually within the white matter on T_2-weighted images.[61,86,117] CT and visual evoked responses have yielded nonspecific findings. CSF abnormalities have been noted in fewer than one half of patients, usually a CSF pleocytosis and elevated protein. Oligoclonal bands in the CSF have seldom been found. A limited number of brain biopsies have demonstrated an increase in lymphocytes and microglial cells in the brain parenchyma. In one patient, spirochetes compatible with B burgdorferi were identified in the biopsy specimen.[108]

DIAGNOSIS

In patients with a dementia from the late persistent stage of B burgdorferi infection, the diagnosis of Lyme disease may be difficult. No pathognomonic lab test is yet available. Patients typically have serum antibodies against B burgdorferi. Presently, the ELISA antibody test for Lyme disease is felt to be more specific than the immunofluorescent tests. The immunoblot or Western blot test for B burgdorferi appears to be the most specific of the available tests, but it is not widely available.[57] Demonstration of intrathecal production of specific antibody to B burgdorferi has been reported in 50% to 90% of patients with meningitis (early disseminated stage), and in about 50% of patients with late neurologic involvement of the CNS.[64,154] Because serologic testing for Lyme disease is not fully standardized, both false-negative and false-positive tests may occur. Thus serologic results must always be interpreted along with the patient's history and examination.

THERAPY

Patients with disseminated infection with neurologic disease have shown clinical improvement following parenteral courses of penicillin[157] and ceftriaxone.[34] In one study, 89% of patients with neuropathy, meningitis, or encephalitis improved following ceftriaxone treatment.[34] The usual dose of ceftriaxone is 2 g/day intravenously for 14 to 28 days. (D45.)[34]

PROGNOSIS

Most patients with early disseminated infection and neurologic disease respond well to treatment and make an excellent recovery.[61] The outcome in patients with late persistent infection and CNS involvement is variable. In those patients who show clinical improvement, it often occurs over several months but may not lead to a complete recovery.[86]

Brain Abscess

PATHOGENESIS

Cerebral pyogenic brain abscess generally occurs in specific clinical settings. A contiguous, suppurative focus such as otitis media or mastoiditis is found in 20% to 40% of cases. There is a bimodel distribution in the age of presentation of otogenic brain abscess. Almost 25% of brain abscesses occur in children under age 15, often along with acute otitis media.[102] An older group consists of adults with chronic otitis media, in whom the lateral sinus and temporal lobes are most commonly affected. Paranasal sinus infections are the source in 15% to 25% of brain abscesses; in this situation involvement is limited almost exclusively to the cavernous sinus and frontal lobes. Dental and facial infections and meningitis are rare causes of bacterial brain abscess.

Hematogenous spread from distant foci, including infections of the lung, skin, pelvis, abdomen, and bone, may cause brain abscesses in up to 50% of patients. *Actinomyces, Norcardia,* and the more common anaerobic organisms are the main causative agents. Abscesses may be polymicrobial. Bacteremia in the setting of a normal blood-brain barrier rarely results in brain abscess formation. For example, brain abscess rarely complicates systemic infections such as subacute bacterial endocarditis unless septic emboli occur.[16,96,116] Regardless of the source, brain abscesses secondary to hematogeneous spread typically are in the distribution of the middle cerebral artery, are multiple and multiloculated, and are located at the gray-white junction.[177] Head trauma with open fracture or penetrating wound is the third clinical setting in which brain abscesses are seen. Finally, cryptogenic abscess, in which no source for infection can be found, comprises almost 20% of all cases.[106] These are felt to have a hematogenous origin.

CLINICAL FEATURES

Symptoms usually develop over a few weeks to a month.[96] The clinical features of brain abscess usually suggest a mass lesion rather than infection. Focal deficits, nausea, vomiting, and papilledema are noted in 30% to 60% of cases. Headache occurs in 60% to 80%, nuchal rigidity in 20% to 30%, and fever in only 50%. The classic triad of headache, fever, and focal neurologic deficits is present in less than 50% of cases. Seizures are a feature in 30% to 40% of cases, particularly with frontal lobe involvement.

Mental status changes occur in 30% to 70% of cases. Patients often develop psychomotor slowing with apathy, a slowing of mentation, and slowness to respond, especially when they have increased intracranial pressure. If the abscess is located in the frontal lobe, the patient may also have drowsiness, inattention, and general impairment of cognition. If the abscess is in the dominant parietal lobe, the patient may develop parietal lobe syndromes, including the inability to perform learned motor skills on command and the development of a disturbed appreciation of self in relation to the environment. If the abscess is in the dominant temporal lobe, speech and language difficulties are common, and the patient may develop a Wernicke's aphasia.[72,96,102,106,177,178] As the abscess expands, the signs and symptoms progress and worsen. If untreated, patients may become comatose and die because of brain herniation.

PATHOLOGY AND LABORATORY FINDINGS

The pathologic evolution of a brain abscess may be divided into several stages, which correlate with CT findings. During the first 3 days of early cerebritis there is a marked perivascular inflammatory infiltrate surrounding a developing necrotic center, along with profound white-matter edema. As the necrotic center reaches its maximum

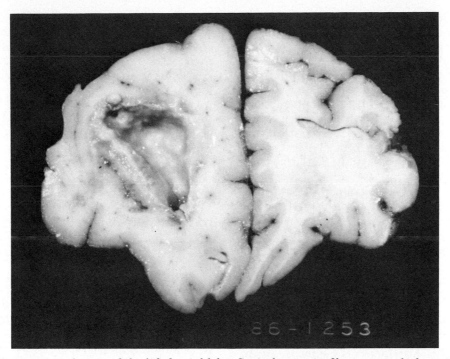

Figure 9-4. Brain abscess of the left frontal lobe. Central necrosis, fibrous capsule formation, and edema are present.

size in 4 to 9 days, fibroblast proliferation and neovascularization at the periphery increase, surrounded by persistence edema and ongoing gliosis. By 10 to 13 days the necrotic center begins to shrink, as a fibrous capsule is formed. The final stage is characterized by a thick, fibrous capsule, gliosis, and decreasing edema (Fig. 9-4). Without the use of contrast media, CT reveals areas of low density corresponding to early stages of abscess formation (cerebritis), whereas a high-density rim indicates the capsular stages. With contrast media, ring enhancement with surrounding edema is indicative of capsule formation and neovascularization (Fig. 9-5), whereas the lack of enhancement, or diffuse or nodular enhancement, tends to represent early cerebritis.[17] Steroids markedly diminish inflammation and edema and delay capsule formation, thereby altering early CT findings. A healed abscess may appear as an area of nodular con-

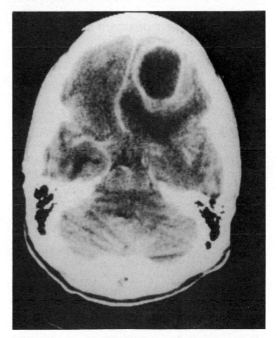

Figure 9-5. Contrast-enhanced CT scan of the brain demonstrates a left frontal-lobe abscess with characteristic ring enhancement and edema with mass effect.

trast enhancement for 1 to 4 months after therapy, but ultimately it will not enhance.[17]

The classic finding of a thin, ring-enhancing lesion surrounded by edema is common but not always seen. The radiographic differential diagnosis includes tumor, infarction, resolving hematoma, granuloma, radiation necrosis, and recent surgery. MRI or radionuclide scanning is more sensitive than CT in detecting the early cerebritis stage of abscess formation. Examination of the CSF is contraindicated if one suspects a brain abscess, because of the potential for herniation. Additionally, the findings, although often abnormal, are rarely diagnostic, as specific organisms are infrequently cultured from CSF.

THERAPY

Optimal antibiotic therapy in brain abscess is based on identification of the organism(s) involved. Empiric broad-spectrum coverage with penicillin and chloramphenicol is commonly used while awaiting culture results. Metronidazole and cefotaxime offer several theoretical advantages but have not been systematically compared. The empiric drug regimen should be altered in certain clinical settings. Antistaphylococcal agents (e.g., nafcillin) plus cefotaxime are indicated following surgery or trauma. Antipseudomonal drugs are often needed in patients with lung or ear infections. The duration of intravenous therapy is controversial, but is usually 4 to 8 weeks, depending on confirmation of abscess resolution by CT. Some authorities advocate an oral regimen for an additional 2 to 6 months. The use of steroids is reserved for those patients with enough edema to produce clinically significant increased intracranial pressure or mass effect. Anticonvulsant therapy may also be appropriate.

Although success using antibiotics alone has been documented,[12,122] most patients with brain abscess require surgery. No prospective randomized trial has compared burr-hole placement with drainage versus craniotomy with resection. Some new data suggest, however, that surgical resection reduces mortality but results in greater neurologic morbidity, particularly severe focal deficits and epilepsy.[124] Exceptions to surgery include medical conditions that increase the risk of surgery; multiple abscesses; a deep or dominant-hemispheric location of the abscess; concomitant ependymitis or meningitis; or a clear response to antibiotic therapy.[12,122] Urgent surgery may be needed in the event of herniation.

PROGNOSIS

The incidence of permanent neurologic sequelae ranges from 30% to 50%.[28a,72,103,128] Long-term cognitive impairment occurs in 15% to 20% of patients. Many of these have associated neurologic deficits or seizures. Nielsen and colleagues[103] suggest that brain abscess during childhood results in permanent intellectual impairment more commonly (33%) than in adulthood (13%).

The mortality rate of patients with brain abscess is less than 30%. The significant reduction in mortality seen in the past decade is mostly a result of improved early diagnosis by CT. The single most important predictor of outcome remains the clinical state of the patient prior to initiation of therapy.

FUNGAL INFECTIONS CAUSING PROGRESSIVE DEMENTIA

Cryptococcal meningitis is the archetypal, as well as the most common, cause of fungal meningitis. The general characteristics of the clinical syndrome apply equally well to the other fungal meningitides (Table 9–3).

Cryptococcal Meningitis

Cryptococcus neoformans is a ubiquitous yeastlike fungus. The organism

Table 9-3 Chronic Fungal Infections

Infection	CSF	Serology	Culture	Other Features
Cryptococcosis	Often increased pressure Lymphocytic pleocytosis <150 WBC/mm^3 Low glucose, high protein Cell count, glucose, protein may be normal in AIDS India ink stain Lumbar puncture for cryptococcal antigen	Not helpful	CSF Blood (especially in AIDS)	Most often associated with AIDS and other immuno-suppressed states Systemic involvement is rare
Candidiasis	Lymphocytic pleocytosis ≤600 WBC/mm^3 Low glucose, high protein Organisms seen on wet stain (40%)	Not helpful	Blood CSF	Hydrocephalus common Disseminated infection in 50% Particularly associated with immuno-suppression
Histoplasmosis	Pleocytosis (monocytic or polymorpho-nuclear) 100–300 WBC/mm^3 Low glucose, high protein Immunologic tests unreliable Low glucose, high protein	CF titers ≥1 : 32 or a fourfold rise is highly suggestive of active infection Immunologic tests unreliable	Blood — low yield in chronic disease CSF + <50%	Infection is usually asymptomatic, almost universal in endemic areas Painful oropharyngeal ulceration common Affects otherwise healthy persons
Coccidioidomycosis	Lymphocytic pleocytosis ≤3500 WBC/mm^3 Low glucose, high protein	Titer in serum ≥1 : 32 suggestive of active infection	Blood — low yield CSF + in 33%	Endemic in southwest U.S. Pathology resembles tuberculosis
Aspergillosis	Monocytic or poly-morphonuclear pleocytosis ≥600 WBC/mm^3 High protein, glucose often normal	Not helpful	Blood and CSF — low yield	CNS infection often directly from paranasal sinuses or lung Associated with immunosuppression
Blastomycosis	Lymphocytic pleocytosis ≤1200 WBC/mm^3 High protein, glucose low or normal	Not helpful	CSF — low yield	Affects otherwise healthy persons

enters the body through inhalation, but clinical pulmonary infection is quite rare. The most common manifestation of disease is a chronic meningoencephalitis. This predilection for infection of the CNS may be related to the virtual absence of an inflammatory response against the fungus at that site.

Men are infected three times more commonly than women. In the pre-AIDS era, as many as half the cases of CNS cryptococcosis occurred in those with predisposing conditions: leukemia, lymphoma, corticosteroid therapy, or sarcoidosis.[20,37] Now the majority of cases are associated with HIV infection.

CLINICAL FEATURES

The course of the illness is subacute, often extending over weeks to months, with spontaneous partial remission and relapses. Mental status changes are common, vary from lethargy to frank dementia, and are frequent presenting features. Chronic low-grade headaches occur in up to 87%[20,36]; fever is noted in more than half. Nausea and vomiting are common, particularly as the disease progresses. Complaints of double vision and poor visual acuity are the most common cranial-nerve symptoms.

The clinical signs are often few, never pathognomonic, and may be limited to abnormal cognitive function. It is common for patients to develop progressive confusion, disorientation, memory loss, and lethargy. Meningismus is mild or absent. Papilledema has been noted in one third of cases. Cryptococcal granulomas may cause focal neurologic signs, depending on their location.

PATHOLOGY

The major CNS changes are those of a chronic meningoencephalitis. The meninges at the base of the brain are the most severely affected. Cryptococci form cystic clusters within the brain, particularly in the cortical gray matter and the basal ganglia. These clusters elicit a minimal inflammatory response. Large cryptococcal granulomata occasionally occur.

DIAGNOSIS

Because the symptoms of chronic fungal meningitis are nonspecific, one must rely heavily on CSF tests to make the diagnosis. The opening CSF pressure is elevated in more than half the patients. CSF examination shows a lymphocytic pleocytosis, with the white cell count generally less than 150 white blood cells.[20] CSF glucose is usually decreased[36,152] and the protein level is usually elevated.[20,36,152] In HIV infection, however, cell count, protein, and glucose may all be normal.[81]

Isolation of the yeast from CSF is the most specific method of making the diagnosis. The fungus can be grown from CSF after repeated cultures in 90% to 100% of infected patients.[16,26,59] Cryptococci may be visualized in CSF on India ink preparation in 40%[126] to 82%[81] of patients. The yield of these direct methods may be increased by examining large volumes of CSF and, in some cases, by doing cisternal puncture. The most sensitive indirect way to make the diagnosis is by using the latex agglutination test for cryptococcal antigen in CSF. The sensitivity of this test has been reported to be as high as 100%.[81] Blood culture in HIV-positive patients suspected of having cryptococcal meningitis also gives relatively high yields.[126]

THERAPY

The standard therapy for cryptococcal meningitis is amphotericin B, which when given alone (1 to 1.5 mg/kg per day intravenously) affects a cure in up to 70% of patients.[20,152] There is no conclusive evidence that the addition of 5-fluorocytosine improves the outcome, but it does allow a reduction in the dose of amphotericin, which may diminish the overall drug toxicity.[126] Duration of therapy should be 6 weeks. CSF should be reexamined at 3, 6, and 12 months following treatment, or when symptoms recur.

The outlook for HIV-infected patients is less sanguine; most are still infected with cryptococcus at the time of death. In patients with AIDS, the response to initial treatment is 58%, and in only 20% is improvement sustained. Fluconazole is a superior maintenance drug that prevents recurrence of cryptococcal meningitis. The median survival from the time of diagnosis with HIV-related cryptococcal meningitis is 9 months.[133]

More detailed discussions on the treatment of cryptococcal meningitis should be consulted.[9,81,179] Other fungi[32,127] such as *Candida albicans*,[6] *Histoplasma capsulatum*,[54] and *Coccidioides immitis*[15,74] also can cause a chronic meningitis and a dementialike syndrome.

PROTOZOAL AND PARASITIC INFECTIONS CAUSING PROGRESSIVE DEMENTIA

Toxoplasmosis

Toxoplasma gondii is an obligate intracellular protozoan that infects species throughout the animal kingdom. In humans, CNS infection may be congenital or acquired. Transplacental infection of the fetus during an acute infection of the mother results in congenital toxoplasmosis. A discussion of congenital toxoplasmosis is beyond the scope of this chapter, and the reader is referred to many excellent reviews in the literature.[29,30] In acquired cerebral toxoplasmosis, infection most commonly occurs through ingestion of infected meats. Infection via blood products or following laboratory accidents has also been reported. Prior to the AIDS epidemic, acquired CNS toxoplasmosis was rare, and at least half of reported cases were among immunosuppressed patients with a malignancy (especially hematologic malignancy), with a chronic ill-

ness,[59] or in patients who were on immunosuppressive drugs.[87,164a]

CLINICAL FEATURES

There are three major presentations of acquired CNS toxoplasmosis.[164a] The most common clinical presentation is a subacute encephalitis. The patient develops a slowly progressive confusion, disorientation, recent memory difficulties, and eventually obtundation. The disease progresses over a period of days to weeks. The patient may have a mild headache but may not be febrile. Seizures occur in about half of patients.

A second clinical form is that of meningoencephalitis. These patients often have headaches and a stiff neck along with signs of an encephalitis.

The third form is that of single or multiple progressive mass lesions. These patients may present with severe headaches, papilledema, and several focal neurologic signs. CNS toxoplasmosis is common in AIDS patients and may present as a space-occupying lesion or as a subacute dementia similar to HIV dementia.[97-99]

PATHOLOGY

The severity of CNS dysfunction correlates with the pathologic changes. Even in asymptomatic cases, toxoplasma organisms disseminate throughout the body. Cysts may persist in all tissues, although muscle and brain are particularly susceptible. Within brain, the basal ganglia are commonly involved. Most lesions are microscopic, with small areas of necrosis and infiltration of a few granulocytes, mononuclear cells, and microglia.[164a] Microglial nodules are occasionally seen. As the intensity of infection increases, perivascular inflammation, necrotizing vasculitis, and larger areas of gray-matter coagulation necrosis (occasionally extending into the white matter) occur. Toxoplasma-filled cysts and numerous free and intracellular organisms can be seen at the periphery of the necrosis. A moderate reactive astrocytosis surrounds the necrotic abscess.[30,46,99] A fluid-filled cystic cavity surrounded by gliosis typifies the final pathologic stage.

LABORATORY FINDINGS

The diagnosis of CNS toxoplasmosis relies on a combination of clinical features, radiographic and laboratory tests, histologic confirmation, and often response to empiric treatment. In the immunocompetent host, a fourfold rise in serum IgG is indicative of infection. None of the serologic tests are completely reliable, however, in the immunocompromised host. Immunodiagnostic tests can be performed on CSF, although they are often falsely negative.[46,145] An elevated CSF antitoxoplasma IgG antibody titer, compared with the serum antitoxoplasma IgG antibody titer, if present, is considered presumptive evidence of toxoplasma infection of the CNS. Other CSF findings are generally nonspecific. Pleocytosis may or may not be present. The protein may be modestly elevated, whereas the glucose is usually normal. On occasion, toxoplasma organisms can be demonstrated in CSF. Head CT reveals single or multiple hypodense, rounded lesions surrounded by edema, which ring-enhance or diffusively enhance with use of a contrast agent. MRI may have heightened sensitivity compared with CT, particularly early in the course of the illness. The radiographic differential diagnosis includes (1) other infections giving rise to abscess formation, particularly fungal infections in the immunocompromised host; (2) metastatic tumor; and in AIDS patients, (3) primary CNS lymphoma and (4) progressive multifocal leukoencephalopathy, although this rarely causes edema or shows contrast enhancement. Often, biopsy of the lesion provides a definitive diagnosis. Many authorities feel that biopsy presents undue risk to the patient and that it should be reserved for those who fail to respond to empiric therapy or are otherwise atypical.[115]

THERAPY

Treatment of cerebral toxoplasmosis is fairly successful, although in AIDS and other immunocompromised states, relapses occur with cessation of therapy. Pyrimethamine and sulfadiazine plus folinic acid supplementation should result in clinical improvement within 1 to 2 weeks. Adverse reactions to sulfa drugs necessitate the substitution of clindamycin for sulfadiazine. Corticosteroids are not usually indicated unless there is marked cerebral edema.

Neurocysticercosis

As a result of changing immigration patterns, neurocysticercosis, once limited to the endemic areas of South and Central America, southern Africa, and Asia, is now seen worldwide. It is increasingly common in the Hispanic-American population of the southwestern United States.[130] The encysted larvae of the cestode *Taenia solium*, or pork tapeworm, gain access to the host human intestine following ingestion of contaminated food. The cysts hatch into embryos, penetrate the intestinal wall to reach the bloodstream, and eventually lodge in the brain to form cysts, or in the meninges to produce abortive cysts and a chronic meningitis.

CLINICAL FEATURES

As brain cysts degenerate 2 to 4 years later, they leak antigens into the brain, producing inflammation and symptoms. Seizures occur in more than half of patients.[32] Cerebral edema often develops surrounding the cysts and gives rise to focal neurologic signs in 10%. Altered mental status develops in about 15%.[148,164] Patients may develop episodes of confusion, apathy, emotional lability, amnesia, or even a dementia. Dementia as the initial presentation occurs in about 3%.[130] These patients often demonstrate multiple CNS cysts or have a hydrocephalus from the chronic meningitis or ventriculitis.[129,132] Meningitis is often complicated by cranial nerve palsies or hydrocephalus, which is seen in 25% to 30% of cases.

PATHOLOGY

The pathologic features of neurocysticercosis are extremely varied and account for the wide range of neurologic signs and symptoms.[11,139,147,148,164] Within brain parenchyma the extent of inflammatory reaction varies from little or no reaction to a severe mononuclear infiltrate with gliosis and edema surrounding single or multiple cysts. Neurologic dysfunction depends on this inflammatory reaction as well as on the location, size, and number of cysts. Ventriculitis occurs if the larvae reach the ventricular system. Extension into the subarachnoid space causes a severe fibrosing arachnoiditis in about 50% of autopsied cases. Cranial nerve injury, communicating or noncommunicating hydrocephalus, and vasculitis with consequent parenchymal infarction may result.[11,44,139,147,148] Chronic cysts in which the larvae have died undergo granulomatous reaction and may ultimately calcify.

LABORATORY FINDINGS AND DIAGNOSIS

The diagnosis of neurocysticercosis should be considered if there has been travel to endemic areas. Head CT or MRI often demonstrates typical cysts. The cysts are 5 to 20 mm in diameter and are often located near the gray-white junctions of the cerebral cortex. The cyst wall tends to be smooth and thin and may show surrounding cerebral edema. Dead cysts collapse to become isodense with brain or may calcify into nodules 2 to 6 mm in diameter.[89,120,121] CT or MRI may also show hydrocephalus resulting from the chronic meningitis or ventriculitis.

The CSF is abnormal in 50% of cases. It commonly contains a mild lymphocytic pleocytosis, but in 15% of patients it also contains eosinophils. Protein is elevated in 40%. The ELISA test for CSF antibodies to cysticerci is positive in 80% to 95%.[147] A new cysticercosis immunoblot test is both highly sensitive and specific (about 98%) in both CSF and serum.[164a]

THERAPY

Because neurocysticercosis can cause clinical signs by several mechanisms,[148] treatment must be individualized. Patients with active parenchymal cysts often respond to praziquantel at a dose of 50 mg/kg/per day (in three divided doses orally) for 15 days.[147] This drug has few side effects. Albendazole is another drug that has been shown to kill parenchymal cysts.[147] Surgical removal of ventricular cysts often is indicated, as they may otherwise dislodge and cause obstructive hydrocephalus. If obstructive hydrocephalus is present, ventriculoperitoneal shunting is needed.

PROGNOSIS

Marked clinical improvement has been reported after praziquantel therapy in 90% of patients with parenchymal cysts, but in only 50% of patients with arachnoiditis.[149] Ventriculoperitoneal shunting of patients with obstructive hydrocephalus often dramatically improves their mental status.

African Trypanosomiasis

African trypanosomiasis or African sleeping sickness are infections caused by subspecies of the hemoflagellate *Trypanosoma brucei* known as *T brucei gambiense* and *T brucei rhodesiense*. These infections are transmitted to humans through the bite of the tsetse fly of the genus *Glossina*. The normal habitat of this fly is in the middle of Africa, between latitudes 15 degrees north and 15 degrees south.[58] In parts of Tanzania, Kenya, Uganda, Zaire, Congo, Gabon, and Cameroon, African sleeping sickness is an important cause of chronic, progressive nervous system deterioration. Because it takes months after the primary infection before neurologic symptoms begin, occasional visitors to endemic areas of Africa return to the United States or Europe before developing the neurologic disease.

CLINICAL FEATURES

A chancre typically develops at the site of the bite 5 to 15 days after the bite of an infected tsetse fly.[3] The chancre subsides spontaneously within 3 weeks, leaving a residual scar. About this time, the hemolymphatic stage develops, characterized by periodic fevers, malaise, arthralgias, and headaches. There is usually moderate splenomegaly and hepatomegaly, as well as generalized lymphadenopathy. This stage typically lasts several weeks to a few months. Occasional patients develop deep hyperesthesia in the legs and feet.[3] This is usually described as delayed, painful sensation following a mild blow to soft tissues of the feet and lower legs.

In the more common Gambian form of the disease, a meningoencephalitic stage of the illness begins months after the primary infection with subacute mental deterioration.[3,58,151] Personality deterioration, mental dullness, apathy, lethargy, and indifference to surroundings slowly progress. Emotional lability is common, with laughter, crying, or outbursts of rage frequent. Episodes of manic or outright confusional behavior often develop, with hallucinations. As the mental deterioration progresses, patients experience abnormalities in their sleep pattern, giving rise to the name of this disease. Patients develop progressive daytime somnolence and eventually sleep most of the day. Loss of weight and wasting typically accompany this phase of the disease. Eventu-

ally the conscious level declines until the patient becomes stuporous and lapses into a progressive, fatal coma.

In addition to the mental deterioration, patients often develop extrapyramidal signs, with chorea or athetotic movements; stiff, shuffling gait; ataxia, and general tremors. Hyperreflexia is common. Patients typically have a constant bifrontal headache. Patients may have a mild carditis and a pleural effusion, presenting as persistent tachycardia. Patients also show evidence of endocrine dysfunction, with impotence and often arrested menstruation.

LABORATORY FINDINGS

Patients usually have a moderately severe anemia. Erythrocyte sedimentation rate is markedly elevated (usually above 100 mm/h by the Westergren method). Characteristic for African trypanosomiasis is a markedly elevated serum immunoglobulin M (IgM) level, typically greater than five times normal values.[58,151] CSF usually shows a lymphocytic pleocytosis with elevated total protein and IgM levels. CSF glucose is usually normal. Occasionally trypanosomes can be seen in centrifuged CSF sediment. The electroencephalograph usually shows diffuse slowing but at times may show bilateral, synchronous bursts of delta waves.

DIAGNOSIS

African trypanosomiasis should be suspected in individuals from endemic areas who develop a progressive neurologic deterioration and have elevated serum IgM levels. The diagnosis can be confirmed by detection of trypanosomes in blood, lymph-node aspirates, or CSF sediment. Fresh, heparinized blood should be examined for the presence of motile trypanosomes under a 400X microscopic lens.[3] In addition, Geisma-stained blood smears will often reveal trypanosomes. Complement fixation and ELISA serologic tests for trypanosomiasis are available. Most serologic tests are directed against the variable surface glycoprotein (VSG) of the trypanosome. Because trypanosomes show marked antigenic variation in this protein, however, current serologic tests are not highly sensitive.

PATHOLOGY

The brain usually shows signs of a chronic meningoencephalitis. The parenchyma typically shows spotty areas of perivascular infiltration accompanied by inflammation and increased gliosis.[56,105,113] In the later stages of the illness, brain atrophy develops. Trypanosomes are difficult to find in brain parenchyma.

PATHOPHYSIOLOGY

The life cycle of trypanosomes is between the tsetse fly and humans. The trypanosome undergoes several major morphologic and metabolic changes as it travels from fly to human.[58,105,151] In the fly, the procyclic form lacks the dense surface coat composed of the VSG. The procyclic form eventually matures in the fly to a metacyclic form that is infectious to humans. Following the insect bite, metacyclic trypanosomes enter the subcutaneous tissue, where they replicate, forming a chancre. Weeks later, trypanosomes invade the lymphatic system, causing a generalized lymphadenopathy. Invasion of the meninges and brain occurs late in this stage.

It is now recognized that the persistence of trypanosomes in humans despite an intense humoral and cellular immune response is the result of antigenic variation, which is expressed through changes in the VSG.[166] This glycoprotein forms the surface of the bloodstream trypanosome and functions to shield the subsurface molecules from attack by host antibodies. Through the process of antigenic variation, trypanosomes frequently express different VSGs during the course of the infection. The process of frequent antigenic variation develops as a consequence of changes in VSG gene expres-

sion. A given trypanosome has as many as 1000 different VSG genes but only expresses one at a time. Hence the intensity of the parasitemia shows a cyclic nature. As one population of trypanosomes with a given VSG coat is disappearing as the result of the host antibody process, another population with a new VSG is emerging. This frequent antigenic variation of VSG not only results in persistence of the infection but also prohibits the use of vaccines to protect populations.

THERAPY

Standard treatment for the meningoencephalitic stage of the disease is melarsoprol.[58] Melarsoprol is a 3.6% solution of melarson oxide and dimercaprol in propylene glycol. Melarson contains arsenic as its active ingredient. The maximal dose is 3.6 mg/kg, or 5 mL for a 50-kg adult, administered through intravenous injection. In general, groups of three daily injections are separated by a rest period of 1 week. The total dose is usually 35 to 37 mL. Most regimens start with low doses and slowly increase the dosage to the maximum.

Melarsoprol unfortunately has serious side effects. Thrombophlebitis is common, and severe tissue damage may result from an extravascular injection. In addition, a Jarisch-Herxheimer reaction may develop early in the course of treatment. Hepatic damage and an exfoliative dermatitis may also develop. The most serious complication, however, is a reactive or arsenical encephalopathy, which occurs in up to 5% of treated patients[60] and is fatal in up to 75% of those affected. Acute signs usually develop about 10 days after the start of treatment and include sudden neurologic deterioration, deepening coma, seizures, and often frank psychotic reactions. Pathologically there are severe cerebral edema and multiple hemorrhages of the brainstem.[60] Present evidence suggests that this is a drug-related, delayed immune response.

Because of the occasional but often severe toxicity of melarsoprol, a new drug, eflornithine, is being experimentally tried. This drug appears effective for the Gambian form of the disease.[42,112,160] Eflornithine is a polyamine biosynthesis inhibitor that crosses the blood-brain barrier. Limited use of the drug in Africa and in the United States suggests that it has considerably less toxicity but just as much therapeutic efficacy as melarsoprol.

PROGNOSIS

Use of melarsoprol or eflornithine usually halts progression of the neurologic deterioration. If treatment is given early in the course of the meningoencephalitic stage, marked improvement of the mental status often occurs. Untreated patients with the Gambian form usually relentlessly progress to coma and death over 1 to 3 years; the Rhodesian form progresses faster, and death occurs in 6 to 9 months.

SUMMARY

Bacterial, fungal, and parasitic infections of the CNS that cause dementia are often reversible with appropriate treatment. An acute or subacute process associated with fever, delirium, headaches, nausea, vomiting, other neurologic deficits, or seizures should raise the clinician's suspicion of the possibility of an intracranial infection. Examination of CSF is critical in establishing the diagnosis and appropriate treatment for nonviral infection.

Static dementia is not an infrequent sequela of bacterial meningitis, whereas other infections, most notably neurosyphilis, cause a progressive dementia. Another infectious disease that, like syphilis, may once again become a threat to our society is tuberculosis, which can cause dementia in association with meningitis. Neurobrucellosis and Lyme disease, if the history suggests possible exposure to the appropriate agent, need to be consid-

ered in a patient with cognitive impairment. Brain abscesses often present as a slowly developing structural lesion in the CNS. Thus a variety of fungal, protozoal, and parasitic infections also need to be considered in individuals with dementia and with appropriate risk factors. Immunosuppression, either iatrogenic or HIV-related, renders a large group of patients more susceptible to such infections, particularly of the fungal and protozoal types.

ACKNOWLEDGMENTS

Preparation of this chapter was supported in part by the Research Service of the Department of Veterans Affairs. We thank Ms. Verna Lee for her editorial assistance.

REFERENCES

1. Aberer E, Brunner C, Suchanek G, et al: Molecular mimicry and Lyme borreliosis: A shared antigenic determinant between Borrelia burgdorferi and human tissue. Ann Neurol 26:732–737, 1989.
2. Annegers JF, Hauser WA, Beghi E, et al: The risk of unprovoked seizures after encephalitis and meningitis. Neurology 38:1407–1410, 1988.
3. Apted FIC: Signs and symptoms of sleeping sickness. In Mulligan HW, Potts WH, and Kershaw WE (eds): The African Trypanosomiases. John Wiley & Sons, New York, 1970, pp 661–683.
4. Ariza Cardenal J: Brucellosis. MTA Medicine Interna 2:113–164, 1984.
5. Bargava S, Gupta AK, and Tandon PN: Tuberculous meningitis—a CT study. Br J Radiol 55:189–196, 1982.
6. Bayer AS, Edwards JE Jr, Seidel JS, and Guze LB: Candida meningitis. Report of seven cases and review of the English language literature. Medicine (Baltimore) 55:477, 1976.
7. Becker PM, Fensoner JR, Mulrow CD, Williams BC, and Vokaty KA:

The role of lumbar puncture in the evaluation of dementia: The Veterans Association/Duke University Study. J Am Geriatr Soc 33:392, 1985.

8. Belsey MA, Hoffpauir CW, and Smith MHD: Dexamethasone in the treatment of acute bacterial meningitis: The effect of study design on the interpretation of results. Pediatrics 44:503–513, 1969.

9. Bennett JE, Dismukes WE, Dumas RJ, et al.: A comparison of amphotericin B alone and combined with fluorocytosine in the treatment of cryptococcal meningitis. N Engl J Med 301:126–131, 1979.

10. Berlow SJ, Caldarelli DD, Matz GJ, et al: Bacterial meningitis: A prospective investigation. Laryngoscope 90: 1445–1452, 1980.

11. Bia FJ and Barry M: Parasitic infections of the central nervous system. In Booss J and Thornton GF (eds): Infectious Diseases of the Central Nervous System. Neurol Clin 4(1):182–187, 1986.

12. Boom WH and Tuazon CU: Successful treatment of multiple brain abscesses with antibiotics alone. Rev Infect Dis 7(2):189–199, 1985.

13. Booss J and Thornton GF (eds.): Infectious Diseases of the Central Nervous System. Neurol Clin, 4(1):1986.

14. Bouza E, de la Torre Parras F, et al: Brucellar meningitis. Rev Infect Dis 9:810–822, 1987.

15. Bouza E, Dreyer JS, Hewitt WL, et al: Coccidioidal meningitis. An analysis of 31 cases and review of the literature. Medicine (Baltimore) 60:139, 1981.

16. Brewer NS, MacCarty CS, and Wellman WE: Brain abscess: A review of recent experience. Ann Intern Med 82:571–576, 1975.

17. Britt RH and Enzmann DR: Clinical stages of human brain abscess on serial CT scans with contrast infusion. J Neurosurg 59:972–989, 1983.

18. Brown WJ: Status and control of syphilis in the United States. J Infect Dis 124(4):428–433, 1971.

19. Buchanan TM, Faber LC, Feldman RA, et al: Brucellosis in the United States 1960–1972. An abattoir-associated disease. I, II, III. Medicine (Baltimore) 53:403–409, 1974.

20. Butler WT, Alling DW, Spickard A, et al: Diagnostic and prognostic value of clinical and laboratory findings in cryptococcal meningitis. N Engl J Med 270:59, 1964.

21. Cabral DA, Flodmark O, Farrell K, and Speert DP: Prospective study of computed tomography in acute bacterial meningitis. J Pediatr 111:201–205, 1987.

22. Carlsson M and Malmvall B-E: Borrelia infection as a cause of presenile dementia. Lancet 2:798, 1987.

23. Centers for Disease Control: Brucellosis Surveillance: Annual Summary, 1977. Centers for Disease Control, Atlanta, GA, 1978.

24. Centers for Disease Control: Brucellosis surveillance annual survey, 1978. Centers for Disease Control, Atlanta, GA, 1979.

25. Centers for Disease Control: Lyme disease. MMWR 37:1–3, 1988.

26. Centers for Disease Control: Continuing increase in infectious syphilis —United States. JAMA 259:975–977, 1988.

27. Centers for Disease Control: Sexually transmitted diseases treatment guidelines. MMWR 38:(Suppl S-8):5–15, 1989.

28. Chun CH, Johnsond JD, Hofstetter M, and Raff MJ: Brain abscess. A study of 45 consecutive cases. Medicine (Baltimore) 65:415–431, 1986.

28a. Cockrill HH, Dreisbach J, Lowe B, and Yamauchi T: Computed tomography in leptomeningeal infections. Am J Roentgenol 130:511–515, 1978.

29. Couvreur J and Desmonts G: Congenital and maternal toxoplasmosis. A review of 300 congenital cases. Dev Med Child Neurol 4:519–530, 1962.

30. Couvreur J and Desmonts G: Toxoplasmosis. In Vinken PJ, Bruyn GW, and Klawans HL (eds): Handbook of Clinical Neurology, Vol 35. Elsevier, Amsterdam, 1978, pp 115–144.

31. Dastur DK and Udani PM: The pa-

thology and pathogenesis of tuberculous encephalopathy. Acta Neuropathol (Berl) 6:311–326, 1966.

32. Davis LE and Reed WP: Infections of the central nervous system. In Rosenberg RN (ed): Comprehensive Neurology. Raven Press, New York, 1991, pp 215–287.

33. Davis LE and Schmidt JW: Clinical significance of cerebrospinal fluid tests for neurosyphilis. Ann Neurol 25:50–55, 1989.

34. Dattweiler RJ, Halperin JJ, Volkman DJ, et al: Treatment of late Lyme borelliosis — randomized comparison of ceftriaxone and penicillin. Lancet 1:1191–1194, 1988.

35. DeLemos RA and Haggerty RJ: Corticosteroids as an adjunct to treatment in bacterial meningitis. Pediatrics 44:30–34, 1969.

36. Dewitt CN, Dickson PL, and Wolt GW: Cryptococcal meningitis: A review of 32 years' experience. J Neurol Sci 53:283, 1982.

37. Diamond RD and Bennett JE: Prognostic factors in cryptococcal meningitis: A study in 111 cases. Ann Intern Med 80:176, 1974.

38. Dixon PE, Cayley ACD, and Hoey C: Tuberculous meningitis in the elderly. Postgrad Med J 6:586–588, 1984.

39. Dodge PR: Sequelae of bacterial meningitis. Pediatr Infect Dis J 5:618–620, 1986.

40. Dodge PR, Davis H, Feegin RD, et al: Prospective evaluation of hearing impairment as a sequela of acute bacterial meningitis. N Engl J Med 311:869–874, 1984.

41. Dodge PR and Swartz MN: Bacterial meningitis: A review of selected aspects: II. Special neurologic problems, postmeningitic complications and clinicopathological correlations. N Engl J Med 272:1003–1010, 1965.

42. Doua F, Boa FY, Schechter PJ, et al: Treatment of human late stage gambiense trypanosomiasis with α-difluoromethylornithine (eflornithine): Efficacy and tolerance in 14 cases in Côte D'Ivoire. Am J Trop Med Hyg 37:525–533, 1987.

43. Edward GA and Domm BM: Human leptosporosis. Medicine (Baltimore) 39:177, 1960.

44. Estanol B, Klerrga E, Loyo M, et al: Mechanisms of hydrocephalus in cerebral cysticercosis: Implications for therapy. Neurosurgery 13:119–122, 1983.

45. Falk A: US Veterans Administration —Armed Forces Cooperative Study of the Chemotherapy of Tuberculosis. Part XIII. Tuberculous meningitis in adults with special reference to survival, neurologic, residuals, and work status. Am Rev Respir Dis 91:823–831, 1965.

46. Farkash AE, MacCabe PJ, Sher JH, Landesman SH, and Hotson G: CNS toxoplasmosis in acquired immune deficiency syndrome: A clinical-pathological-radiological review of 12 cases. J Neurol Neurosurg Psych 49:744–748, 1986.

47. Fincham RW, Sachs AL, and Joynt RJ: Protean manifestations of nervous system brucellosis. JAMA 184:269, 1963.

48. Fisher RS, Clark AW, Wolinsky JS, et al: Postinfectious leukoencephalitis complicating mycoplasma pneumoniae infection. Arch Neurol 40:109, 1983.

49. Fishman RA: Cerebrospinal Fluid in Diseases of the Nervous System. Philadelphia, WB Saunders, 1980, pp 225–285.

50. Freemon FR: Evaluation of patients with progressive intellectual deterioration. Arch Neurol 33:658–659, 1976.

51. Gante SR, Cohen M, Sane P, and Hilal SK: Computed tomography in cerebral syphilis. J Comput Assist Tomogr 5:345–347, 1981.

52. Gjestland T: The Oslo study of untreated syphilis. Acta Derm Venereol (Suppl 34)35:1–368, 1955.

53. Godt P, Stoeppler L, Wischer V, et al: The value of computed tomography in cerebral syphilis. Neuroradiology 18:197–200, 1979.

54. Goodwin RA, Shapiro JL, Thurman GH, et al: Disseminated histoplasmosis. Clinical and pathological cor-

relation. Medicine (Baltimore) 59:1, 1980.

55. Gorse GJ, Thrupp LD, Nudleman KL, et al: Bacterial meningitis in the elderly. Arch Intern Med 144:1603–1607, 1984.

56. Greenwood BM and Whittle HC: The pathogenesis of sleeping sickness. Trans R Soc Trop Med Hyg 74:716–725, 1980.

57. Grodzicki RL and Steere AC: Comparison of immunoblotting and indirect enzyme-linked immunosorbent assay using different antigen preparations for diagnosing early Lyme disease. J Infect Dis 157:790–797, 1988.

58. Hajduk SL, Englund PT, and Smith DH: African trypanosomiasis. In Warren KS and Mahmoud AAF (eds): Tropical and Geographical Medicine, Ed 2. McGraw-Hill, New York, 1990, pp 268–281.

59. Hakes TB and Armstrong D: Toxoplasmosis: Problems in diagnosis and treatment. Cancer 52:1535–1540, 1983.

60. Haller L, Adams H, Merouze F, and Dago A: Clinical and pathological aspects of human African trypanosomiasis (T.b. gambiense) with particular reference to reactive arsenical encephalopathy. Am J Trop Med Hyg 35:94–99, 1986.

61. Halperin JJ: Abnormalities of the nervous system in Lyme disease response to antimicrobial therapy. Rev Infect Dis (Suppl 6):11:1499–1504, 1989.

62. Halperin JJ, Krupp LB, Golightly MG, et al: Lyme borreliosis–associated encephalopathy. Neurology 40:1340–1343, 1990.

63. Hammerstrom DC and Zimmer B: The role of lumbar puncture in the evaluation of dementia: The University of Pittsburgh Study. J Am Geriatr Soc 33:397, 1985.

64. Hansen K, Cruz M, and Link H: Oligoclonal Borrelia burgdorferi-specific IgG antibodies in cerebrospinal fluid in Lyme neuroborelliosis. J Infect Dis 161:1194–1202, 1990.

65. Heck AF, Hameroff SB, and Hornick RB: Chronic listeria monocytogenes meningitis and normotensive hydrocephalus. Neurology 28:263–270, 1971.

66. Hook EW, Roddy RE, and Hansfield HH: Ceftriaxone therapy for incubating and early syphilis. J Infect Dis 158:881–884, 1988.

67. Hutton JT: Results of clinical assessment for the dementia syndrome: Implications for epidemiologic studies. In Mortimer JA and Schuman LM (eds): The Epidemiology of Dementia. Oxford University Press, New York, 1981, pp 62–69.

68. Igarashi M, Gilmartin RC, Gerald B, et al: Cerebral arteritis and bacterial meningitis. Arch Neurol 41:531–535, 1984.

69. Jaffe HW and Robins SA: Cerebrospinal fluid examinations in patients with syphilis. Rev Infect Dis 4:842–847, 1982.

70. Johns DR, Tierney M, and Felsenstein D: Alteration in the natural history of neurosyphilis by concurrent infection with the human immunodeficiency virus. N Engl J Med 316:1569–1572, 1987.

71. Johnson JD, Raff MJ, and Van Arsdall JA: Neurologic manifestations of Legionnaire's disease. Medicine (Baltimore) 63:303–310, 1984.

72. Kaplan K: Brain Abscess. In Molavi A and LeFrock JL (eds): Infections of the Central Nervous System. Med Clin North Am 69(2):354–359, 1985.

73. Kaufman AF: Epidemiologic trends of leptospirosis in the United States 1965–1974. In Johnson RC (ed): The Biology of Parasitic Spirochetes. Academic Press, New York, 1976.

74. Kelly PC: Coccidioidal meningitis. In Stevens DA (ed): Coccidioidomycosis. Plenum, New York, 1980, p 163.

75. Kennedy DH and Fallon RJ. Tuberculous meningitis. JAMA 241(3):264–268, 1979.

76. Kennedy PGE and Johnson RT (eds): Infections of the Nervous System. Butterworth & Co, London, 1987.

77. Kingsley DPE, Hendrickse WA, Kendall BE, Swash M, and Singh V: Tuberculous meningitis: The role of CT

in management and prognosis. J Neurol Neurosurg Psychiatry 50:30–36, 1987.

78. Klein JO, Feigin RD, and McCracken GH: Report of the task force on diagnosis and management of meningitis. Pediatrics (Suppl)78:955–982, 1986.

79. Kobat EA, Moore DH, and Landow W: An electrophoretic study of the protein components in cerebrospinal fluid and their relationship to the serum proteins. J Clin Invest 21:571–580, 1942.

80. Kocen RS: Tuberculosis of the nervous system. In Kennedy PGE and Johnson RT (eds): Infections of the Nervous System. Butterworth & Co, London, 1987, pp 23–42.

81. Kovacs JA, Kovacs AA, Polis M, et al: Cryptococcosis in the acquired immunodeficiency syndrome. Ann Intern Med 103:533–538, 1985.

82. Larsen SA, Hambie EA, Peltidge DE, et al: Specificity, sensitivity and reproducibility among the fluorescent treponemal antibody absorption test, the microhemagglutination assay for Treponema pallidum and the hemagglutination treponemal test for syphilis. J Clin Microbiol 14:441–445, 1981.

83. Larson EB, Reifler BV, Sumi SM, Canfield CG, and Chinn NM: Diagnostic tests in the evaluation of dementia. A prospective study of 200 elderly outpatients. Arch Intern Med 146:1917–1922, 1984.

84. Lebel MH, Freij BJ, Syrogiannopoulos GA, et al: Dexamethasone therapy for bacterial meningitis. N Engl J Med 319:964–971, 1988.

85. Lindberg J, Rosenhall U, Nylen O, and Ringner A: Long-term outcome of Haemophilus influenzae meningitis related to antibiotic treatment. Pediatrics 60:1–6, 1977.

86. Logigian EL, Kaplan RF, and Steere AC: Chronic neurologic manifestations of Lyme disease. N Engl J Med 323:1438–1444, 1990.

87. Luft BJ, Brook RG, Conley FK, McCabe RE, and Remington JS: Toxoplasma encephalitis in patients with acquired immune deficiency syndrome. JAMA 252:913–917, 1984.

88. Maletta GJ, Pirozzolo FR, Thompson G, and Mortimer JA: Organic mental disorders in a geriatric outpatient population. Am J Psychiatry 139:521–523, 1982.

89. Mancuso P, Guarnera F, Augello G, Chiarmonte I, Daliberti G, and Tropea R: Computed axial tomography versus NMR on the diagnosis of neurocysticercosis. Neurochirurgia (Stuttgart) 30:152–153, 1987.

90. Marsden CD and Harrison MJG: Outcome of investigation of patients with presenile dementia. BMJ 2:249–252, 1972.

91. Merritt HH: A Textbook of Neurology. Lea & Febiger, Philadelphia, 1973.

92. Merritt HH, Adams RD, and Solomon HC: Neurosyphilis. Oxford University Press, New York, 1946.

93. Merritt HH and Moore M: Acute syphilitic meningitis. Medicine (Baltimore) 14:119–183, 1935.

94. Molavi A and LeFrock JL: Tuberculous meningitis. Med Clin North Am, 69(2):315–332, 1985.

95. Moore JE: The modern treatment of syphilis, Ed 2. Charles C Thomas, Springfield, IL, 1943.

96. Morgan H, Wood M, and Murphy F: Experience with 88 cases of brain abscess. J Neurosurg 38:698–704, 1973.

97. Navia BA, Cho ES, Petito CK, and Price RW: The AIDS dementia complex II. Neuropathology. Ann Neurol 19:525–535, 1986.

98. Navia BA, Jordan BD, Price RW: The AIDS dementia complex. I. Clinical features. Ann Neurol 19:517–524, 1986.

99. Navia BA, Petito CK, Gold JWM, Cho ES, Jordan BD, and Price RW: Cerebral toxoplasmosis complicating acquired immune deficiency syndrome: Clinical and neuropathologic findings in 27 patients. Ann Neurol 19:224–238, 1986.

100. Newman PK, Cumming WJK, and Foster JB: Hydrocephalus and tuberculous meningitis in adults. J Neurol

Neurosurg Psychiatry 43:188–190, 1980.

101. Nichols E: Meningoencephalitis due to brucellosis with a report of a case in which B abortus was recovered from the cerebrospinal fluid and a review of the literature. Ann Intern Med 35:673, 1951.

102. Nielsen H, Gyldensted C, and Harmsen A: Cerebral abscess: Aetiology and pathogenesis, symptoms, diagnosis, and therapy. A review of 200 cases from 1935–1976. Acta Neurol Scand 65:609–622, 1982.

103. Nielsen H, Harmsen A, and Glydensted C: Cerebral abscess: A long term follow-up. Acta Neurol Scand 67:330–337, 1983.

104. Odio CM, Faingezicht I, Paris M, et al: The beneficial effects of early dexamethasone administration in infants and children with bacterial meningitis. N Engl J Med 324:1525–1531, 1991.

105. Ormerod WE: Pathogenesis and pathology of trypanosomiasis in man. In Mulligan HW, Potts WH, and Kershaw WE (eds): The African Trypanosomiases. John Wiley & Sons, New York, 1970, pp 587–601.

106. Overturf GD: Pyogenic bacterial infections of the CNS. In Booss J and Thornton GF (eds): Infectious Diseases of the Central Nervous System. Neurol Clin: 4(1):84–88, 1986.

107. Ozdamar O, Kraus N, and Stein L: Auditory brainstem responses in H influenzae meningitis: Prospective evaluation. Dev Med Child Neurol 24:338–343, 1982.

108. Pachner AR, Duray P, and Steere AC: Central nervous system manifestations of Lyme disease. Arch Neurol 46:790–795, 1989.

109. Pachner AR and Steere AC: The triad of neurological manifestations of Lyme disease: Meningitis, cranial neuritis, and radiculoneuritis. Neurology 35:47–53, 1985.

110. Parrot D, Nieken KH, White RG, et al: Radioimmunoassay of IgM, IgG, and IgA brucella antibodies. Lancet 1:1075, 1977.

111. Pentti R, Donner M, Valanne E, and Wasz-Hockert O: Late psychological and psychiatric sequelae of tuberculous meningitis. Acta Paediatr Hung 51(Suppl)141:65–77, 1962.

112. Peplin J, Milord F, Guern C, and Schechter PJ: Difluoromethylornithine for arseno-resistant Trypanosoma brucei gambiense sleeping sickness. Lancet 2:1431–1433, 1987.

113. Poltera AA: Pathology of human African trypanosomiasis with reference to experimental African trypanosomiasis and infections of the central nervous system. Br Med Bull 41:169–174, 1985.

114. Ponka A: Central nervous system manifestations associated with serologically verified Mycoplasma pneumoniae infection. Scand J Infect Dis 12:175–184, 1980.

115. Price RW and Navia BA: Infections in AIDS and other immunosuppressed patients. In Kennedy PGE and Johnson RT (eds): Infections of the Nervous System. Butterworth & Co, London, 1987, pp 266–268.

116. Pruitt AA, Rubin RHJ, Karchmer AW, and Duncan GW: Neurologic complications of bacterial endocarditis. Medicine (Baltimore) 57:329–343, 1978.

117. Reik L, Smith L, Khan A, et al: Demyelinating encephalopathy in Lyme disease. Neurology 35:267–269, 1985.

118. Reik L, Steere AC, Bartenhagen NH, Shope RE, and Malawista SE: Neurologic abnormalities of Lyme disease. Medicine (Baltimore) 58:281–294, 1979.

119. Rico Irles J, Juarez Fernandez C, Pena Angulo JF, and Torres Velasco F: Nuestra experiencia personal sobre la fiebre de malte. Rev Clin Esp 126:113–124, 1972.

120. Rodriguez-Carbajal J, Boleaga-Duran B, and Dorfsman J: The role of computed tomography (CT) in the diagnosis of neurocysticercosis. Childs Nerv Syst 3:199–202, 1987.

121. Rodriguez-Carbajal J, Salgado P, Gutierrez R, Escobar A, Aruff D, and Palacios E: The acute encephalitic

phase of neurocysticercosis: Computed tomography manifestations. AJNR 4:51–55, 1983.

122. Rosenbloom ML, Hoff JT, Norman D, et al: Non-operative therapy of brain abscess in selected high risk patients. J Neurosurg 52:217–225, 1980.

123. Rothstein TL and Kerny GE: Cranial neuropathy, myeloradiculopathy and myositis: Complications of Mycoplasma pneumoniae infection. Arch Neurol 36:476–477, 1979.

124. Rousseaux M, Lesoin F, Destee A, Jomin M, and Petit H: Long term sequelae of hemispheric abscesses as a function of treatment. Acta Neurochir (Wien) 74:61–67, 1985.

125. Roux J: Épidémiologie et prévention de la brucellose. Bull World Health Organ 57:179–194, 1979.

126. Sabetta JR and Andriole VT: Cryptococcal infections of the nervous system. Med Clin North Am 69:333–344, 1985.

127. Salaki JS, Louria DB, and Chmel H: Fungal and yeast infection of the central nervous sytem. Medicine (Baltimore) 63:108, 1984.

128. Sampson DS and Clark K: A current review of brain abscess. Am J Med 54:201–210, 1973.

129. Sandyk R, Bamford C, Iacono RP, and Gillman MA: Cerebral cysticercosis presenting as progressive dementia. Int J Neurosci 35:251–254, 1987.

130. Scharf D: Neurocysticercosis — 238 cases from a California hospital. Arch Neurol 45:777–780, 1988.

131. Schaudinn FR and Hoffman E: Vorlaufiger bericht uber das vorkommen von spirochaeten in syphilitischen krankheitsproducken und bei papillomen arbeine aus dem K Gesundkeitsamte 22:527, 1905.

132. Schnur JA: Case record of Massachusetts General Hospital. N Engl J Med 297:773–780, 1977.

133. Schuster M, Zuger A, Simberkoff MS, Rahal JJ, and Holzman RS: Maintenance therapy of cryptococcal meningitis in patients with AIDS (abstr). Presented at 2nd International Conference on AIDS, Paris, June 1986.

134. Sell SHW: Long-term sequelae of bacterial meningitis in children. Pediatr Infect Dis J 2:90–93, 1983.

135. Sell SHW, Merrill RE, Doyne EO, and Zimsky EP: Long-term sequelae of Haemophilus influenzae meningitis. Pediatrics 49:206–211, 1972.

136. Sell SHW, Webb WW, Pate JE, and Doyne EO: Psychological sequelae to bacterial meningitis: Two controlled studies. Pediatrics 49:212–217, 1972.

137. Sexually transmitted disease fact sheet, Ed 24. HEW Publication No (CDC) 79-8195, US Department of Health, Education, and Welfare, 1980.

138. Shah AK and Gandhi VK: Prognosis of tubercular meningitis. Indian J Pediatr 21:791–795, 1984.

139. Shanley JD and Jordan MC: Clinical aspects of CNS cysticercosis. Arch Intern Med 140:1309–1313, 1980.

140. Sheller JR and DesPrez RM: CNS tuberculosis. In Booss J and Thornton GF (eds): Infectious Diseases of the Central Nervous System. Neurol Clin 4(1):143–158, 1986.

141. Sigal LH and Tatum AH: Lyme disease patients' serum contains IgM antibodies to Borrelia burgdorferi that cross react with neuronal antigens. Neurology 38:1439–1442, 1988.

142. Simon RP: Neurosyphilis. Arch Neurol 42:606–613, 1985.

143. Sippel JE, El-Masry NA, and Farid Z: Diagnosis of human brucellosis with ELISA. Lancet 2:19, 1982.

144. Smith AL: Neurologic sequelae of meningitis. N Engl J Med 319:1012–1014, 1988.

145. Smith JS and Kiloh LG: The investigation of dementia: Results in 200 consecutive cases. Lancet 1:824–827, 1981.

146. Snyder RD, Stovring J, Cushing AH, et al: Cerebral infarction in childhood bacterial meningitis. J Neurol Neurosurg Psychiatry 44:581–585, 1981.

147. Sotelo J: Neurocysticercosis. In Kennedy PGE and Johnson RT (eds): Infections of the Nervous System. Butterworth & Co, London, 1987, pp 145–155.

148. Sotelo J, Guerrero V, and Rubio F:

Neurocysticercosis: A new classification based on active and inactive forms. A study of 753 cases. Arch Intern Med 145:442–445, 1985.

149. Sotelo J, Torres B, Rubio-Donnadieu F, et al: Praziquantel in the treatment of neurocysticercosis: Long term follow-up. Neurology 35:752–755, 1985.

150. Southern PM Jr and Sanford JP: Relapsing fever. A clinical and microbiological review. Medicine (Baltimore) 48:129, 1969.

151. Spencer HC Jr, Gibson JJ Jr, Brodsky RE, and Schultz MG: Imported African trypanosomiasis in the United States. Ann Intern Med 82:633–638, 1975.

152. Spickard A, Butler WT, Andriole VT, et al: The improved prognosis of cryptococcal meningitis with amphotericin B therapy. Ann Intern Med 58:66, 1963.

153. Sproles ET, Azerrad J, Williamson C, and Merrill RE: Meningitis due to Haemophilus influenzae: Long-term sequelae. Pediatrics 75:782–788, 1969.

154. Steere AC: Lyme disease. N Engl J Med 321:586–596, 1989.

155. Steere AC, Broderick TF, and Malawista SE: Erythema chronicum migrans and Lyme disease: Epidemiological evidence for a tick vector. Am J Epidemiol 108:312–321, 1978.

156. Steere AC, Grodzicki RL, Kornblatt AN, et al: The spirochetal etiology of Lyme disease. N Engl J Med 308:733–738, 1983.

157. Steere AC, Pachner AR, and Malawista SE: Neurologic abnormalities of Lyme disease: Successful treatments with high dose IV penicillin. Ann Intern Med 99:767–772, 1983.

158. Stockstill MT and Kauffman CA: Comparison of cryptococcal and tuberculous meningitis. Arch Neurol 40:81–85, 1983.

159. Swartz MN: Neurosyphilis. In Holmes KK, Mardh P-A, Sparling PF, and Wiesner PJ (eds): Sexually Transmitted Diseases, McGraw-Hill, New York, 1990, pp 231–246.

160. Taelman H, Schechter PJ, Marcelis L, et al: Difluoromethylornithine, an effective new treatment of Gambian trypanosomiasis. Am J Med 82:607–614, 1987.

161. Tondon PN: Tuberculous meningitis. In Vinken PJ, Bruyn GW, and Klawans HL (eds): Handbook of Clinical Neurology, Vol 33. Elsevier, Amsterdam, 1978, pp 195–267.

162. Townsend JJ, Wolinsky JS, Baringer JR, and Johnson PC: Acquired toxoplasmosis. Arch Neurol 32:335–343,1975.

163. Traub M, Colchester ACF, Kingsley DPE, and Swash M: Tuberculosis of the central nervous system. Q J Med 209:81–100, 1984.

164. Trelles J and Trelles L: Cysticercosis of the nervous system. In Vinken PJ, Bruyn GW, and Klawans HL (eds): Handbook of Clinical Neurology, Vol 35. Elsevier, Amsterdam, 1978, pp 291–320.

164a. Tsang VCW, Brand JA, and Boyer AE: An enzyme-linked immunoelectrotransfer blot assay and glycoprotein antigens for diagnosing human cysticercosis (Taenia solium). J Infect Dis 159:50–59, 1989.

165. Tunkel AR, Wispelwey B, and Scheld WM: Bacterial meningitis: Recent advances in pathophysiology and treatment. Ann Intern Med 112:610–623, 1990.

166. Turner MJ: The biochemistry of the surface antigens of the African trypanosomes. Br Med Bull 41:137–143, 1985.

167. Udani PM and Dastur DK: Tuberculous encephalopathy with and without meningitis. Clinical features and pathological correlations. J Neurol Sci 10:541–561, 1970.

168. Udani PM, Parekh UC, and Dastur DK: Neurological and related syndromes in CNS tuberculosis. Clinical features and pathogenesis. J Neurol Sci 14:341–57, 1971.

169. VanBeusekon GT: Complications in hydrocephalus shunting procedure. In Willenbur R, Brock M, and Klinger M (eds): Advances in Neurosurgery, Ed 6. Springer-Verlag, New York, 1978, pp 28–30.

170. Vandam LD and Dripps RD: Long term follow-up of patients who re-

ceived 10,098 spinal anesthetics. JAMA 161:586, 1956.

171. Victoratos GC, Leumau JAR, and Herzberg L: Neurological investigation of dementia. Br J Psychiatry 130:131–133, 1977.

172. Watson GW, Fuller TJ, Elms J, and Klug RM: Listeria cerebritis: Relapse of infection to renal transplant patients. Arch Intern Med 138:83–87, 1978.

173. Whitty CWM and Macauley JD: Listeria monocytogenes meningoencephalitis in an adult. BMJ 1:634, 1965.

174. Wick HM: Brucella meningoencephalitis in childhood. Neuropediatrics 12:330–336, 1981.

175. Wilhelm C and Ellner JJ: Chronic meningitis. In Booss J and Thornton GF (eds): Infectious Diseases of the Central Nervous System. Neurol Clin 4(1):115–141, 1986.

176. Williams E: Brucellosis. BMJ 1:791–793, 1973.

177. Wispelwey B and Scheld WM: Brain abscess. Clin Neuropharmacol 10 (6):483–510, 1987.

178. Yang S: Brain abscess: A review of 400 cases. J Neurosurg 55:794–797, 1981.

179. Zuger A, Louie E, and Holzman RS: Cryptococcal disease in patients with the acquired immunodeficiency syndrome. Ann Intern Med 104:234–240, 1986.

Chapter 10

METABOLIC DEMENTIA

Edward Feldmann, M.D., and
Fred Plum, M.D.

Metabolic dementia describes a global, sustained impairment of intellectual capacity due to diffuse dysfunction of the brain at the molecular-chemical level. The cause can be either a systemic deficiency or exogenous intoxication. Metabolic dementia must be distinguished from *primary dementia*, the result of an intrinsic failure of the brain cells, as well as from *acute metabolic encephalopathy*, an abrupt and usually short-lived condition that is marked by an acute confusional state, prominent impairment of arousal, and alteration of the sleep-wake cycle. *Progressive metabolic dementia* usually begins insidiously, advances gradually over weeks or months, and wreaks widespread damage on cognitive mechanisms without impairing arousal. *Fixed metabolic dementia* is a nearly constant state of mental decline due to a single severe metabolic insult that, when ended, no longer damages the brain. Patients who have survived a single episode of acute Wernicke's encephalopathy or severe hypoxia, for example, suffer little or no additional intellectual change over months and years. By contrast, those suffering from untreated hypothyroidism or toxic drug ingestion, deteriorate steadily with the passage of time.

The concept that a metabolic disorder can produce dementia does not imply that the brain has remained free of structural damage or that the dementia is reversible. Hepatic encephalopathy, for example, can temporarily alter brain astrocyte structure yet respond to therapy, whereas cyanocobalamin deficiency can persist undetected for years, eventually causing cerebral structural abnormalities and permanent intellectual impairment.

EPIDEMIOLOGY

An increasingly aging population suffering from reduced cerebral reserves, a high susceptibility to systemic illness, and a tendency to medicate for every complaint has produced a considerable incidence of metabolic dementia. Chronic systemic illness affects 86% of all hospital outpatients over age 65,[21] and more than 70% of the demented elderly suffer from systemic disorders that contribute to mental impairment.[21,45] Despite these high risks, many physicians and nurses fail to recognize cognitive impairment in their patients.

The prevalence of metabolic dementia varies not only with the physician's index of suspicion, but also with the pa-

Table 10–1 FINAL DIAGNOSIS IN PATIENTS REFERRED TO EIGHT DIFFERENT SPECIALTY CENTERS WITH THE SUSPICION OF DEMENTIA (n = 808 PATIENTS)

Alzheimer's disease	39%
Multi-Infarct dementia	13%
Alcoholism*	7%
Metabolic abnormalities*	4%
Tumor	3%
Hydrocephalus	3%
Huntington's disease	2%
Drug reactions*	1%
Parkinson's disease	1%
Infection	1%
Miscellaneous	8%
Pseudodementia	18%

*Potential metabolic dementias.
Source: From van Horn,[94] p. 105, with permission.

tient's age, socioeconomic status, and the referral bias of the study population. Metabolic dementia is relatively common among indigent, elderly medical outpatients, but is underrepresented on neurologic and other inpatient services where primary and structural causes dominate. Estimates of the condition's prevalence vary from 1% to 18% of elderly patients,[21,94,51] (Table 10–1) with medications the most frequent cause[51] (Table 10–2). Anxiolytics, sedatives, and antihypertensives are the major offenders.[50]

The potential reversibility of a drug-induced metabolic dementia places a premium on recognizing it. The key to diagnosis lies in obtaining a history of longstanding cognitive difficulties in tasks requiring sustained mental effort, coupled with an apathetic mood, slowing of responses, poor memory, inattention, and intermittent confusion. Most cases show few specific, abnormal motor signs, although many patients move slowly and have an increased resistance to passive limb movement (gegenhalten). Aphasia and agnosia are

Table 10–2 CAUSES OF METABOLIC DEMENTIA IN ELDERLY PATIENTS WITH SYMPTOMS FOR AT LEAST 3 MONTHS

Medications	9.5%*
Hypothyroidism	3.0%
Hyperparathyroidism	1.0%
Hypoglycemia†	1.0%
Hyponatremia‡	1.0%

*Percentages of 200 patients evaluated with dementia. The remainder of the 200 patients had other causes of dementia.
†Due to insulin.
‡Due to diuretics.
Source: Adapted from Larson et al,[51] p. 490.

Table 10–3 DISTINGUISHING IRREVERSIBLE FROM POTENTIALLY REVERSIBLE CAUSES OF DEMENTIA*

	Irreversible (n = 77)	Reversible (n = 15)
Duration (months)	52	29
Severity (Mini-Mental State score)	15	20
Prescription drugs (number)	1.4	2.5

*All variables shown are means and are significantly different between the groups.
Source: Adapted from Larson et al,[51] p. 490.

uncommon. Several conditions can resemble metabolic dementia, including psychological depression, a mild and prolonged subacute metabolic encephalopathy, primary dementia, and the AIDS-dementia complex. In most instances reduced alertness provides a strong clue to the existence of acute metabolic or structural encephalopathy rather than a true dementia. Features that best distinguish metabolic from primary dementias include a shorter duration of illness and a greater intake of prescription drugs (Table 10–3). Also, few metabolic insults by themselves produce a profound degree of dementia.

Although many agree on the clinical importance of metabolic dementia, diagnostic strategies differ greatly. Some testing batteries exhaust both patient and pocketbook and include procedures that offer little specific diagnostic usefulness. Among these are isotope cisternography, angiography, and brain biopsy (Table 10–4). Nevertheless, a few uncomplicated tests are helpful for establishing a diagnosis and guiding treatment in most cases: thyroid screen, vitamin B_{12} determination, complete blood count, and screening chemistries.[50] Even without considering the current medicolegal climate, a single computed tomography (CT) or

Table 10–4 AN EXTENSIVE POTENTIAL TESTING BATTERY FOR THE EVALUATION OF THE DEMENTED PATIENT

CT scan or MRI
Thyroid screen
Serum and urine drug screen
SMA-16
Complete blood count and differential
Arterial blood gas
Syphilis serology
Vitamin B_1, B_{12}, and folate levels
EEG
Lumbar puncture
Isotope cisternography
Erythrocyte sedimentation rate
Antinuclear antibody (ANA); lupus
   anticoagulant
Cerebral angiography
Brain biopsy
Positron emission tomography (PET)
HIV titer

Source: From van Horn,[94] p. 106, with permission.

**Table 10–5 EXHAUSTIVE VERSUS EQUALLY
EFFECTIVE SELECTIVE TEST-ORDERING STRATEGIES
IN 200 DEMENTED OUTPATIENTS**

	Exhaustive	*Selective*
Complete blood count	X	X
ESR	X	X
VDRL or FTA-Abs	X	X
Serum folate	X	X
Serum B_{12}[a]	X	X′ (15%)
SMS-12	X	X
Aspartate aminotransferase	X	—
Serum phosphate	X	—
Thyroid screen[b]	X	X′ (19%)
Urinalysis	X	—
TSH	X	X
Corticotropin stimulation	X	—
Chest roentgenogram	X	—
Skull roentgenogram	X	—
CT[c]	X	X′ (16%)
EEG (standard)	X	—
ECG	X	—

— = Not used at all.
X = Used 100% of the time.
X′ = Selectively used.
a = Used only if blood count abnormal.
b = Used only if TSH abnormal.
c = Used only if mild symptoms, recent onset, sudden deterioration, atypical features, or for diagnostic reassurance.
Source: Adapted from Larson et al.[52]

magnetic resonance imaging (MRI) head scan is desirable in most instances, especially whenever symptoms have had a recent onset, if there have been sudden deteriorations or atypical features, or when family or physician need diagnostic reassurance. Head scanning, however, rarely offers any help if symptoms are severe (Mini-Mental State score <15), have lasted longer than 36 months, and are unaccompanied by motor signs.[50]

Selective testing strategies can minimize patient discomfort, reduce cost, and cut down the risk of major diagnostic errors. When the selective strategy illustrated in Table 10–5 was retrospectively applied to 200 patients with dementia, substantial cost savings were realized and no important diagnoses were overlooked. No strategy, however, can succeed in the absence of a careful clinical evaluation in experienced hands.

PATHOPHYSIOLOGY

Metabolic disorders produce widespread changes in brain biochemistry and physiology (Table 10–6). Electroencephalographic (EEG) tracings typically reveal diffuse, nonspecific, relatively symmetrical background slowing, which can precede or outlast symptoms. Cerebral blood flow or positron emission tomography (PET) studies commonly demonstrate a diffuse reduction in cerebral blood flow and about a 20% reduction in oxygen metabolism. Many of the cellular and subcellular abnormalities responsible for these global dysfunctions can be illustrated by reviewing the myriad effects of oxygen deprivation on the nervous system.

When brain hypoxia is produced by levels of cerebral blood flow (CBF) <16–20 mL/100 g per minute, synaptic failure occurs and neurons cease firing. Ionic membrane pumps and mem-

Table 10-6 SUMMARY OF METABOLIC PERTURBATIONS IN BRAIN ASSOCIATED WITH VARIOUS INSULTS

Aging	Parallel decrease of blood flow and metabolic rate,[11] diminished activity of choline acetyltransferase, tryosine hydroxylase, dopa decarboxylase, and glutamate decarboxylase.[11]
Hyperammonemia	Interferes with postsynaptic inhibition, alters blood-brain carrier mechanisms, may affect neurotransmitter activity, alters astrocyte function.[20]
Alcohol	Diminished choline acetyltransferase activity,[3] diminished muscarinic binding sites,[68] chronic endoneurial edema,[77] impaired membrane function and acetylcholine synthesis and release, fluctuations in concentration of GABA, altered metabolism of glutamate and glutamine.[77]
Thiamine deficit	Impaired synthesis of neurotransmitter amino acids,[9,11] impaired acetylcholine turnover and transynaptic transmission,[11] spongy and split myelin lamellae, altered decarboxylation of branched chain keto acids.[9]
Carbon monoxide	Dilation and fragmentation of endoplasmic reticulum in oligodendroglia.[29]
Lithium	Impaired potassium uptake into astrocytes and cortical neurons,[32,39] impaired dopamine synthesis, increased norepinephrine and serotonin uptake, enhanced acetylcholine release, increased opiate binding, decreased GABA binding.[32]
Barbiturate	Impaired presynaptic calcium entry,[40] augmented postsynaptic GABA-mediated inhibition, diminished glutamine-mediated excitation, direct increases in chloride conductance at synapse, diminished potassium uptake into astrocytes.[39]
Addison's disease	Increased intracellular sodium, brain excitability, protein synthesis, and carbohydrate utilization; no change in Na-K pump; diminished GABA levels and calcium release into CSF.[7]
Steroids (exogenous)	Decreased intracellular sodium, ribonucleotide, fat and protein synthesis, carbohydrate utilization and GABA levels; increased serotonin levels.[7]
Phenothiazines	Impaired membrane permeability, respiratory enzymes; uncoupling of oxidative phosphorylation; altered monoamine and lipid metabolism; serotonin antagonism, α-adrenergic blockade; increased acetylcholine release and turnover.[56]
Tricyclic antidepressants	Anticholinergic effects, altered catecholamine and serotonin metabolism,[11,82] impaired deamination and uptake of norepinephrine; may block postsynaptic norepinephrine receptors.[82]
Metachromatic leukodystrophy	Increased sulfatide depletes other white-matter lipids and disrupts myelin.[30]
Lead	Endothelial, perivascular damage with edema[77]; inclusions in astrocytes; myelin swelling and disruption via impaired mitochondrial calcium transport.[14]
Copper	Distention of myelin loops, altered dopamine synthesis, binding to sulfhydryl groups.[98]
Mercury	Inhibition of glucose, amino acid passage across blood-brain barrier[44]; endothelial injury with edema; perivascular hemorrhage.[77]
Triethyl tin	Myelin sheath edema.[77]
DDT	Prolonged depolarizing presynaptic afterpotential.[66]
Organophosphate	Impaired oxidative metabolism and protein synthesis.[76]
Cyanide	Complexing with cytochrome oxidase, depression of acetyl-COA synthesis.[29]

brane integrity fail with CBF < 6 – 10 mL/100 g per minute. Severe oxygen deprivation promotes the accumulation of lactic acid, which, if extreme, produces profound lowering of extracellular pH and necrosis of most of the brain's cellular elements.[74] Thus, prolonged, severe hypoxia ultimately leads to cellular energy failure and cell death. The exact degree and duration of hypoxia that distinguishes reversible injury from that causing death only of neurons, the brain's most vulnerable cells, or that causing death of all cellular elements, remains unclear.[74]

Most clinical situations involve milder degrees of temporary brain hypoxia. Under these conditions, multiple mechanisms exist whereby the cellular elements of the brain are damaged.

Hypoxia can profoundly affect several brain neurotransmitter systems. Mild selective hypoxia (15% inspired O_2) reduces brain acetylcholine synthesis by 40%.[9,11,84] In humans the abrupt application of this degree of hypoxia impairs higher cognitive function.[11] Further evidence of the harmful effects of cholinergic deficiency in severe hypoxia comes from the experimental evidence that the administration of cholinergic agonists and cholinesterase inhibitors delays seizures and death in this state. Hypoxia impairs monoamine systems as well: in rats, inspiration of 5.6% O_2 for 30 minutes decreases catecholamine turnover by 10% and serotonin turnover by 30%.[23] Mild hypoxia in the mouse also decreases the synthesis of numerous amino acids by 3% to 25%.[31]

Hypoxia does not damage brain only by *impairing* the synthesis of neurotransmitters. Excitatory neurotransmitters are *released* during or after hypoxia and can have profound cytotoxic effects. Ischemia-induced neuronal depolarization, coupled with impaired transmitter uptake, leads to the accumulation of large quantities of glutamate, an excitatory neurotransmitter. Glutamate acts at three receptors: N-methyl-D-aspartate (NMDA), alpha-amino - 3 - hydroxy - 5 - methyl - 4 - isoxasole propionic acid (AMPA), and me-tabotropic. Glutamate leads to abnormal fluxes of sodium (AMPA- and NMDA-receptor – gated channels) and calcium (NMDA-receptor – gated channel only), and the formation of inositol triphosphate and diacylglycerol. These initial ion fluxes activate transport and channel mechanisms that promote the excessive intracellular accumulation of calcium, which is augmented by the inositol-triphosphate – induced release of intracellular calcium. These preliminary events amplify into a cascade as the initial calcium buildup sensitizes cells to the effects of glutamate and leads to further glutamate release.[18]

Intracellular calcium activates multiple processes and, in excessive amounts, releases enzymes that destroy structural and genetic elements, ultimately leading to cell death. Calcium promotes phospholipid and subsequent arachidonic acid release from membranes, leading to the formation of free radicals that produce peroxidative damage to mitochondria and cellular membranes. Phospholipid breakdown also promotes the release and activation of substances such as platelet activating factor, which intensify and enlarge the ischemic process by impairing blood flow in previously uninvolved vessels.[18] Elevations of intracellular calcium can also directly impair mitochondrial function, leading to cellular energy failure. The process spreads to initially uninvolved neurons via the release of potassium from damaged cells, leading to depolarization of the neighboring cells and reinitiation of the entire sequence. However, the mechanism of hypoxic neuronal death may not be this complicated or prolonged. In certain situations, passage of sodium via NMDA- or AMPA-receptor – gated channels leads to massive intracellular edema and rapid cell death.[81]

The cascade of biochemical damage to hypoxic neurons can outlast the episode of hypoxia and take many hours to evolve, providing a window for intervention. Recent studies have focused on the development of drugs that block excitatory neurotransmission at the

NMDA[2] or AMPA receptors,[57] and the identification of agents such as GABA-ergic, purinergic, and noradrenergic inhibitors of neurotransmission that antagonize the overall excitatory process.[2,18] GM1 gangliosides putatively maintain injured plasma membrane structure and antagonize the disordered intracellular calcium homeostasis that follows the excitatory cascade. Cyclooxygenase inhibitors may reduce the toxic degree of phospholipid and arachidonic acid release from membranes. Drugs such as dimethylthiourea, 21-aminosteroids, and allopurinol are believed either to prevent the formation of free radicals or to scavenge them.[18]

Oxygen deprivation can damage the brain in several other ways. Mild hypoxia limits the synthesis of lipids, proteins, and nucleic acids even when it spares energy production and ATP levels.[11] Postischemic rabbit brain slices demonstrate a 15% to 60% reduction in RNA polymerase activity, and protein synthesis fails for at least 3 hours following recovery.[102] Moreover, following ischemia in rat brain, synthesis and maintenance of proteins, nucleotides, and lipids are persistently impaired.

Metabolic brain disease not only attacks neurons but also can damage glial elements. Among other functions, glial cells maintain tight control over a variety of substances in the cerebral interstitial microenvironment. Astrocytic extensions envelop both capillaries and neurons, oligodendroglia generate myelin, and both types of cells may provide structural support, with the astrocytes and microglia removing much of the debris that follows neuronal injury. Astrocytes buffer extracellular potassium, detoxify ammonia, stabilize the brain's acid-base balance, help remove chemical transmitters, and exchange glucose and amino acids between the cellular and interstitial microenvironments.[46] Astrocytic nuclei enlarge in hypoxia, water intoxication, and hepatocerebral degeneration. Ouabain, by blocking the Na^+K^+-ATPase pump, also swells the astrocytes. Experimental lead poisoning produces electron-dense, intranuclear astrocytic inclusions. Ouabain, lithium, and barbiturates all impair astrocytic potassium uptake.[39]

Exactly which of the above biochemical and structural abnormalities causes the symptoms of metabolic dementia is not known. All evidence, however, indicates that the synapse is the anatomic site most vulnerable to metabolic disequilibrium. Thus the brain's neuronal dendritic arborization decreases with aging,[11] prominent changes in cholinergic neurotransmitter metabolism develop with hypoxia and other metabolic injuries, and barbiturates mediate their sedative action at the synapse.[40] The common alterations that affect astrocytes in several of the metabolic encephalopathies suggest that progressive damage to this compartment or deterioration of its function also contributes to the chronic cognitive impairment of many permanent metabolic brain diseases. A detectable failure of energy metabolism, however, is not directly implicated in the etiology of metabolic dementia.[59]

Few patients recover from a purely metabolic dementia (see section on Prognosis at the end of this chapter), implying that most insults eventually cause permanent cell damage. The absence of currently satisfactory morphometric techniques makes it difficult to confirm this suggestion anatomically. In some metabolic dementias such as Korsakoff's psychosis (see page 328) or posthypoxic amnesia,[103] neuronal cell loss adequately explains the functional impairment, but these are exceptions.

SPECIFIC CAUSES OF METABOLIC DEMENTIA

Exogenous Toxins

The wide prevalence in modern society of potentially harmful pharmaceuticals, industrial compounds, and beverages has raised the incidence of toxic metabolic delirium and dementia to near-epidemic proportions. The elderly are particularly at risk because of their diminished body mass and reduced availability of proteins for binding these agents. Moreover, an average decrease in hepatic and renal function of nearly 40% between the ages of 30 and 90 years materially impairs the metabolism of harmful drugs and chemicals.[11] Reduced heart and lung function further limits the reserve margin of blood and oxygen supply for the brain. Because the elderly have a diminished neuropil and a reduced number of synaptic connections, any additional exogenous insult threatens their baseline capacities.

MEDICATIONS

Drugs are the most common cause of metabolic dementia in the elderly. In one cohort of 242 elderly outpatients (mean age 73), only 8% were not ingesting potentially harmful neuroactive medications.[45] Although a large number of drugs in excess can impair cognitive function, many older patients suffer from an idiosyncratic susceptibility to even subtherapeutic doses. The resulting deficits may be reversible but hard to recognize.

Sedatives. Sedative hypnotics, especially long-acting benzodiazepines such as diazepam, flurazepam, oxazepam, and clonazepam, are the agents most frequently responsible for medication-related dementia. Benzodiazepines, for example, were the responsible agents in 16 of 35 such cases in one study.[49] Cognitive impairment developed either soon after medication was begun or insidiously over years. Symptoms included global cognitive impairment without significant alterations in the level of consciousness. In all 16 patients, cognition improved upon withdrawal of the offending agent. No patient developed withdrawal symptoms. Full recovery, however, occurred only in one third, and long-term follow-up resulted in the diagnosis of primary dementia in the remaining patients. The

example illustrates how these drugs can exacerbate an underlying dementia. Nevertheless, it appears possible that, just as an excess of alcohol or phenytoin can lead sooner or later to direct neuronal injury, persistent deficits following chronic sedative abuse need not always imply a preexisting primary dementia. In one study nearly 40% of patients abusing both barbiturates and analgesics were found to have persistent cognitive and EEG abnormalities 3 to 5 months after drug cessation. The degree of permanent abnormalities correlated directly with the amount of drug previously used.[21]

Alcohol. Fallaice[26] has suggested that one out of every eight adults in the United States drinks escessively, and it is estimated that alcohol may be a major contributor to nearly 7% of all dementias. Clinically obvious dementia is apparent in 3% of alcoholics.[21]

Nearly 50% of persons consuming excessive alcohol, defined as two bottles of wine, seven pints of beer, or one half bottle of distilled spirits daily, show neuropsychological impairment. The changes appear more commonly in the elderly and earlier in women.[21] Intellectual deficits include impaired performance, intelligence, and memory quotient. Subtle and insidious memory deficits, psychomotor retardation, perseveration, circumstantiality, inattention, and disorientation are characteristic.[15] Often, CT scans reveal cortical atrophy, disproportionate for age and independent of hepatic dysfunction. The degree of dementia and atrophy are not closely related: cognitive symptoms account for only 30% of the variance seen in atrophy revealed by CT. Moreover, brain atrophy may appear abnormally early in life for the alcoholic, predisposing to a future risk of functional cerebral impairment.[15] Abstinence has been reported to result in partial reversal of atrophy in two thirds of young alcoholics, and 75% concurrently experienced improved cognition.[15,16,26] In demented alcoholics over age 60, EEG studies have shown background slowing and temporal slow-wave transients in five of seven patients, although CT revealed atrophy in only three of seven.[67] Reportedly, EEG abnormalities also improve with abstinence.[15]

The precise cellular changes responsible for the clinical, radiologic, and electrophysiologic abnormalities of alcoholism are unknown. Nutritional deficiency plays a large but not exclusive role, since alcoholic dementia in so many ways recapitulates the symptoms of acute drunkenness. Neuropathologic studies are almost always confined to patients who died following debilitating systemic illness, aspiration, or repeated seizures. Some patients have shown limited lesions of the Wernicke-Korsakoff variety,[94] whereas the brains of others have contained cortical gliosis, neuronal loss, and ventriculomegaly secondary to generalized cerebral and thalamic atrophy.[66] Although the evidence suggests that chronic alcoholics may have distinct intellectual deficits, no thorough studies describe the anatomic substrate of any of the alcoholic dementias other than the Wernicke-Korsakoff syndrome. Until the morphology is correlated with radiologic and EEG changes, the mechanism of non-Korsakovian alcoholic dementia will remain controversial.

Marchiafava-Bignami disease is a rare and possibly obsolete disorder consisting principally of demyelination of the corpus callosum and adjacent cerebral white matter. Virtually confined to male alcoholics,[72] the condition can follow many forms of severe alcoholism and no longer is linked exclusively to drinking red wine. The symmetric demyelination of corpus callosum and other commissural structures in this disorder seems insufficient to explain all the findings of a profound chronic dementia. The demyelination may be an epiphenomenon, related in its pathogenesis to the systemic water and electrolyte complications that plague the severe alcoholic and sometimes produce central pontine myelinolysis.[89]

Symptoms of alcoholic dementia sometimes appear as a late, severe complication of a prolonged drinking bout or after an episode of stupor resolves. Signs in severe cases include amnesia, aphasia, disorientation, personality change, seizures and, often, a broad-based ataxia. More subtle and more common, however, is the empty personality and loss of productivity that occur in previously successful chronic heavy drinkers derived from every social stratum.

Psychotropics. Antidepressant drugs are said to produce chronic cognitive impairment in 10% to 15% of all ingestors,[21] and in perhaps as many as 35% of those over 40 years of age.[41] In most instances anticholinergic effects account for the cognitive effects of the antidepressants, but impairment in gastric motility also can contribute to malabsorption of dietary nutrients.[21] Amitriptyline has the greatest anticholinergic effect of the antidepressants.[59] Symptoms include difficulty concentrating, increased amnesia, feelings of depersonalization, and giddiness. Anticholinergic signs that provide clues to the diagnosis include agitation, mydriasis, warm dry skin, urinary retention, and constipation. All improve with lowering the dose or discontinuing the drug.

Lithium in toxic doses (blood levels of 2.5 to 3.0 mEq/L) can cause a prominent acute delirium coupled with extrapyramidal motor signs including dysarthria, tremor, chorea, and cerebellar ataxia. A few patients become hypokinetic and rigid. Acutely, disorientation and mental withdrawal are prominent. Many patients are left with permanent mental deficits after lithium is discontinued. Lithium also has been associated with global cognitive impairment in a few patients receiving therapeutic doses with normal blood levels, but such reports are neither recent nor confirmed.[86] EEG slowing occurs with therapeutic levels of lithium and worsens with symptom severity during intoxication. Prognostic data with long-term follow-up are not available in these patients. In combination with haloperidol, lithium has been reported to cause an irreversible dementia.[19,21] Hyperthermia, agitation, leukocytosis, elevated creatine kinase, and other liver enzymes are said to be followed by chronic cognitive impairment, incontinence, dysarthria, masked facies, ocular dyskinesia, limb and truncal ataxia, and persistent EEG slowing.

Phenothiazines can produce chronic cognitive impairment that must be distinguished both from the sedation these agents produce and the patient's underlying psychosis. Mental symptoms in patients receiving phenothiazines stem from their anticholinergic effects, and the physician must beware of exacerbating such impairment by inappropriately coprescribing anticholinergic antiparkinsonian agents. Two such antiparkinsonian drugs, trihexyphenidyl and benztropine, produce in as many as half their recipients anticholinergic effects and a pattern of mental impairment akin to that seen with antidepressants.[62]

Glycosides and Antihypertensives. Digitalis is prescribed in some form to between 5% and 25% of elderly persons. Their diminished lean body mass, reduced volume of distribution, and declining renal function greatly increase the risk of toxicity.[24] Typically, premonitory gastrointestinal and cardiac side effects occur, but in about 10%, neurologic toxicity represents the earliest and most severe complication. The digitalis dose need not climb above mid "therapeutic" range for such symptoms to appear. At a minimally toxic level, the drug produces inattention and indifference; more severe symptoms include disorientation, vivid paranoia, complex and frightening hallucinations, visual disturbances, headache, and rarely, seizures.[24] Most disappear within 1 week of drug withdrawal, but rarely, a subtle postdrug delirium can persist for many weeks.

Antihypertensive agents may impair higher brain functions as well as reduce blood pressure. Drugs that affect central adrenergic synapses alter seroton-ergic, cholinergic, and GABA transmission as well. Chronic mental symptoms, when they appear, are rarely if ever associated with bringing the blood pressure down, although sudden reductions of more than 40 to 50 mm Hg during acute treatment of chronic hypertension occasionally can reduce cerebral blood flow enough to cause cerebral symptoms.[35]

Clonidine, a central α-adrenergic agonist, produces in up to 50% of patients diminished concentration, memory, and calculating ability.[35] Those affected may appear either lethargic and depressed or aggressive. Variably, they complain of incontinence, dry mouth, hallucinations, delusions, dizziness, fatigue, headache, and anorexia. The EEG can be normal despite prominent symptoms. Recovery usually occurs within 2 weeks of discontinuing the drugs.[53]

Alphamethyl-dopa (Aldomet) is converted to α-methyl norepinephrine and acts on brainstem receptors.[35] Toxicity consists of impaired concentration, memory, and ability to make calculations.[1,21,35] Nasal congestion, dry mouth, and feelings of depression are reported to affect 10% to 50% of patients.[35] Symptoms can improve in as little as 4 days after drug removal.[53]

Propranolol (Inderal) inhibits central sympathetic activity, perhaps via adrenergic antagonism in the posterior hypothalamus.[35] Semichronic side effects can include depression or cognitive impairments, the latter including fatigue, impotence, nightmares, sleep disorder, hallucinations, and generalized weakness.[21,35] Symptoms improve with drug discontinuation.

Antineoplastic Agents. Methotrexate, a folic acid antagonist, inhibits the enzyme dihydrofolate reductase[90] and is used to treat leukemia, choriocarcinoma, and solid tumors. Because its hydrophobic nature limits penetration of the blood-brain barrier, it is administered intrathecally for meningeal leukemia, lymphoma, and metastatic carcinoma. Toxicity can occur when intrathecal methotrexate is combined with radiotherapy to treat meningeal disease, appearing when more than 2000 rads and more than 50 mg of intrathecal or 40 to 80 mg/m^2 of systemic methotrexate are given per week. Dementia develops insidiously and advances inexorably, often in parallel with signs of bilateral corticospinal dysfunction, meningeal irritation, or transverse myelopathy. CT scanning reveals diffuse, hypodense, white-matter lesions. Postmortem examination reveals gliosis, demyelination, axonal degeneration[90] and white-matter infarctions secondary to fibrinoid degeneration and thrombosis of small vessels.[101]

Radiotherapy alone, when delivered in excess of approximately 5000 to 6000 rads, can damage the brain's microvasculature, leading to a delayed white-matter degeneration.[21] The risk following lower radiation doses is controversial, as few reports include satisfactory data about portal volume, time-dose fractionation, and clinical factors. The threshold for damage correlates best with total dose and daily fraction size.[101] Postradiation brain necrosis presents as a solitary mass or as multifocal lesions, either of which may produce a dementia. The onset commonly is delayed for months to years after treatment and comes on insidiously and progressively. CT scans typically reveal a low-density, variably enhancing mass or diffuse, small, white-matter hypodensities coupled with cerebral atrophy. Pathologic studies describe a hemorrhagic necrosis of white matter with preservation of overlying cortex, plump astrocytes, demyelination, reactive blood vessels, swollen endothelium, and perivascular inflammation.[79]

L-Asparaginase has been used with some success to treat leukemia and some solid tumors. In 25% to 40% of patients[101] it can cause an acute encephalopathy or an insidious dementia starting about a week after the onset of treatment and lasting months.[21,101] Because L-asparaginase does not cross the blood-brain barrier, the mental symptoms may stem from a systemic effect releasing ammonia or aspartic acid. Alternatively, reduced availability of L-asparagine for normal brain protein synthesis may be responsible. Symptoms and associated EEG slowing are dose related. Reduction of treatment dose often suffices to eliminate or reduce the neurologic symptoms.[101]

Mustards are powerful alkylating agents used to treat lymphoma. They can cause a chronic dementia when given in high doses, especially by intracarotid and regional perfusion techniques.[21,90]

Anticonvulsants. Anticonvulsants, with the exception of phenobarbital in children, rarely cause either a chronic delirium or dementia when maintained at therapeutic concentrations and with seizures under good control. Phenytoin in certain cases can produce chronic and permanent mental impairment associated with nystagmus, ataxia, chorea, ophthalmoplegia, peripheral neuropathy, and asterixis. Barbiturates, mephenytoin, and ethosuximide possess a similar acute toxicity.[94] Idiosyncratic responses to valproate can cause intoxicating hyperammonemia or even stupor and coma with rapid initial administration. EEG demonstrates high-voltage slow waves, which correlate with mental impairment but may persist after clinical improvement occurs. Also, inattention and slowed learning in children have been linked to phenobarbital given in therapeutic doses. Except in high doses, however, little other evidence suggests that anticonvulsants independently contribute to permanent intellectual decline. A few papers in the older literature that claimed such an association failed to acknowledge persistent seizures as an equally likely cause.

HEAVY METALS

Prolonged moderate or acute high-level exposure to a variety of metals can interfere with the brain's cellular metabolism and produce dementia. The

Table 10-7 FEATURES OF DEMENTIA ASSOCIATED WITH HEAVY METAL EXPOSURE

	Arsenic[21,27]	*Bismuth*[11,21]	*Gold*[21,61]
Setting	Exposure to illicitly manufactured alcohol, wood preservatives, insecticide spray, animal disinfectant, enamels, chronic organic ingestion; byproduct of lead and copper smelting.	Therapy of syphilis or gastrointestinal complaints, at levels of 5–20 g/day for 2 months to 6 years.	Idiosyncratic response during therapy for arthritis.
Clinical Features	Somnolence, inattention, poor memory, disorientation, agitation, paranoia. Perhaps myelopathy or peripheral and optic neuropathy. Associated skin hyperpigmentation, Mees lines, gastrointestinal, cardiac, and respiratory abnormalities.	Dementia associated with hallucinations, anxiety, delusions, and, if severe, seizures, myoclonus, dysarthria, unsteady gait.	Headache, apathy, disorientation, poor memory, hallucinations, depression, and associated pruritus, exfoliative dermatitis. Neurologic symptoms often isolated. May also have polyneuritis or meningitis, seizures, focal signs, movement disorder.
Diagnosis	Blood level >0.01 mg/100 mL; hair, nail level >0.1 mg/100 g. Pathology: punctate white-matter hemorrhage and neuronal chromatolysis.	Bismuth levels in blood, urine, and CSF. EEG: diffuse beta waves and temporal slowing. CT may show reversible cortical hyperdensity and white-matter hypodensity. Pathology: bismuth in neurons with no necrosis, no bleeding, and no alterations in blood-brain barrier.	Eosinophilia, CSF, and urine gold levels somewhat unreliable. EEG slow. CSF protein increased.
Treatment	Dimercaprol and decreased exposure.	Decrease exposure.	Penicillamine, steroids, decreased exposure.
Prognosis	Anywhere from partial response to permanent deficits.	Usually reversible in 3–12 weeks.	Usually good recovery over weeks.

(continued)

clinical setting, features of the illness, diagnosis, treatment, and prognosis are summarized in Table 10–7.

INDUSTRIAL COMPOUNDS

Many industrial compounds, especially the organic solvents, can induce permanent cerebral damage. Table 10–8 summarizes the details.

System Dysfunction

ENDOCRINE DYSFUNCTION

Endocrine disease occasionally produces chronic mental impairment, but a failure to apply strict diagnostic criteria and rigorously exclude other factors plagues the literature on the subject. The following paragraphs sum-

Table 10–7 FEATURES OF DEMENTIA ASSOCIATED WITH HEAVY METAL EXPOSURE—*Continued*

	Lead[17,21,47,94,99]	Manganese[21]	Mercury[17,21]
Setting	Occupational exposure to exhaust fumes, lead fumes, lead dust, smelters, storage batteries, paint pigments, auto repair. Ingestion of contaminated moonshine, gasoline sniffing.	Occupational exposure in mines, chlorine gas manufacture, storage batteries, paint, colored glass, soaps—after 6–24 months of exposure.	More acute in organic poisoning, delayed years with inorganic. Occupational inhalation or gastrointestinal absorption with electrical apparatus, paint, paper, thermometers, pulp manufacture.
Clinical Features	Adults get neuropathy more often than chronic memory impairment, inattention, hallucinations, agitation, ataxia, and tremor seen in children. Associated anemia, pallor, gingival lead line, weight loss, constipation, headache.	Abrupt or insidious memory loss, compulsivity, euphoria, hallucinations, irritability. Associated extrapyramidal dysarthria, tremor, rigidity, masked facies, bradykinesia.	More common and severe with organic poisoning: impaired memory, agitation, hallucinations with sensory neuropathy, diminished visual fields, cerebellar ataxia, and tremor.
Diagnosis	Blood level > 80 μg/dL, 24-hr urine delta-aminolevulinic acid, increased free erythroporphyrin. Pathology: scattered necrosis, astrocytic proliferation, congestion, endothelial swelling, petechiae.	Clinical history. Pathology: damage to substantia nigra, globus pallidus, subthalamic nucleus, caudate, and putamen.	Increased erythrocyte to plasma mercury ratio, mercury in hair, blood, or saliva, EEG slow. Pathology: occipital, insular and cerebellar atrophy, reactive astrocytes.
Treatment	Chelation with EDTA, penicillamine, and avoid exposure.	Chelation with EDTA; levodopa, and decreased exposure.	Chelation with penicillamine and avoid exposure.
Prognosis	10%–50% have subsequent seizures and permanent mental impairment.	Anywhere from partial response to dramatic recovery.	Only partial response seen with treatment.

(continued)

marize the best available information.

Thyroid Disease.   Only drug intoxication exceeds thyroid disorders as a cause of metabolic dementia. Mental change may dominate the clinical presentation, warranting a high index of clinical suspicion. The clinical features of *hyperthyroidism* depend on the patient's age. Thyrotoxicosis occurring at ages less than 40 affects predominantly women. Its causes include toxic nodule, multinodular goiter, thyroid cancer, a thyrotropin-secreting pituitary tumor, ectopic thyrotropin secretion by an unrelated carcinoma, Graves' disease, or idiopathic hyperthyroidism. Weight

Table 10–7 FEATURES OF DEMENTIA ASSOCIATED WITH HEAVY METAL EXPOSURE —*Continued*

	Organotin[21,99]	*Thallium*[5,21]
Setting	Occupational exposure with skin and gastrointestinal absorption in polyvinyl chloride work, polyurethane, biocidal chemicals.	Exposure to rodenticides, insecticides, glass catalysts, imitation jewelry, fireworks.
Clinical Features	Progressive insomnia, inattention, poor memory, and apathy; perhaps headache, myelopathy, or pseudotumor cerebri.	Gastrointestinal and neurologic symptoms first, followed in weeks by characteristic alopecia. Ataxic painful neuropathy, seizures, vomiting, abdominal pain, muscle tenderness, chorea, tremor, psychosis. Dementia may follow coma or as an insidious decline in memory, irritability, hallucinations.
Diagnosis	Generalized slowing and epileptiform discharge on EEG. Known exposure $> 100 \ \mu g/m^3$.	Alopecia, serum thallium level. Pathology: edema, vascular engorgement, chromatolysis predominantly in motor cortex.
Treatment	Decrease exposure.	Chelation or hemodialysis and decreased exposure.
Prognosis		

loss, anxiety, tremor, heat intolerance, palpitations, tachycardia, and irritable hyperkinetic behavior are prominent. Emotional irritability often overshadows subtle impairments of attention, memory, and calculation.[72] Corticospinal signs, optic neuropathy, retinopathy, exophthalmos, and ophthalmoplegia occasionally coexist.

Elderly thyrotoxic patients differ. They rarely demonstrate hyperkinetic symptoms but suffer an "apathetic" toxicity with psychomotor retardation accompanied by weight loss, atrial fibrillation, congestive heart failure, myopathy, peripheral neuropathy, and blepharoptosis.[60,92] Thyromegaly and laboratory evidence of excessive thyroid function confirm the diagnosis.

The EEG is abnormal in 60% of thyrotoxic patients, revealing slow waves, paroxysms of sharp waves and spikes, and large-amplitude, fast, triphasic and delta activity.[92] These nonspecific changes correlate poorly with symptom severity or effect of treatment. Paroxysmal fast activity on EEG persists despite successful therapy in nearly half the patients.[69] Regrettably, clinical reports rarely quantify the intellectual response to treatment. Most patients "improve greatly" with therapy,[21] with only a "minority" suffering permanent impairment.[60] The percentage of elderly patients who return to their former level of functioning after therapy is unknown.

Hypothyroidism more commonly leads to dementia, which affects about 5% of such patients.[21] Clues to diagnosis include weight gain, cold intolerance, coarse hair, thick skin, absence of perspiration, deafness, constipation, myopathy, and ataxia. Laboratory data are definitive. The manifestations of dementia can vary widely. Some patients have simply a mild impairment of memory, abstractions, orientation, and attention. Others may display a florid psychosis ("myxedema madness"), sarcasm or anger, or express paranoid ideas and auditory hallucinations.[92] Still others become hypersomnolent to the point of stupor or coma. Hypoventilation producing hypoxemia and hypercarbia are late and serious manifestations that must be treated promptly. Additional physical signs include hypothermia, mild resistance to passive stretch of the extremities, and delayed muscle relaxation time following elicitation of deep tendon reflexes. Spinalfluid protein is mildly increased in most patients. EEG changes are nonspecific and correlate poorly with symptom severity. They include background slowing, low amplitude, and diminished drive to photic stimulation.[21,92] Therapy helps most patients in a gratifying way, but few chronically hypothyroid patients over age 50 return to fully active lives.

Addison's Disease. Addison's disease produces mild, chronic mental impairment. Etiologies include idiopathic adrenal cortical atrophy, granuloma, tuberculosis, fungus infection, amyloidosis, or metastases.

Patients with hypoadrenalism are languid and apathetic, with anorexia, weight loss, low blood pressure, reduced blood volume, and hyperpigmented skin. Mental impairment is universal and includes irritability, paranoia, agitation, poor memory, blunted initiative, and disorientation.[60] Laboratory confirmation requires low morning cortisol levels, abnormal adrenal cortical stimulation tests, and elevated serum corticotropin levels.[21] EEG reveals diffuse, high-amplitude slow activity.[60] Therapy requires glucocorticoids; mineralocorticoid replacement alone is insufficient. Even profound mental disturbances can recover completely, but mild apathy and personality difficulties often persist and few patients resume all former activities.[21,60]

Cushing's Syndrome. Cushing's syndrome, whether endogenous or iatrogenic, produces mental impairment in nearly 40% of affected patients.[33] The most common cause is chronic steroid administration; endogenous overproduction by the adrenal medulla is less frequent. The remainder of cases are caused by adrenal overstimulation by the pituitary, and, rarely, by paraneoplastic glucocorticoid secretion.

Florid examples exhibit obesity, a round face, thick supraclavicular fat pads, abdominal panniculus, delicate bruisable skin, abdominal striae, hirsutism, acne, oligomemorrhea, osteoporosis, hypertension, and glucose intolerance. Chronic mental impairment expresses itself as fatigue (97%), irritability (86%), poor concentration and memory (83%), depression (79%), anxiety (63%), sleep disturbance (57%), psychosis (20%), and delusions and hallucinations.[60,88] Mental symptoms may precede the physical stigmata[60] and are proportional to the degree of cortisol or corticotropin elevation. Severe symptoms accompany cortisol secretion over 60 mg/d (equivalent to 40 mg/d of exogenous prednisone), the presence of 8 AM plasma cortisol levels of 30 μg/dL, urinary free cortisol levels in excess of 600 μg/d, and 8 AM plasma corticotropin levels greater than 200 pg/mL.[21,88] Diagnosis is confirmed by elevation of morning and evening blood cortisol, an increase in 24-hour urinary corticosteroids, and failure to suppress cortisol release with dexamethasone.[60] Reducing steroid levels will often alleviate the

Table 10–8 FEATURES OF DEMENTIA ASSOCIATED

	Acrylamide[55]	Carbon disulfide[85]	Carbon tetrachloride[75]
Setting	Occupational skin exposure to polymers in mining, waste, water purification, paper, and cardboard manufacture.	Occupational inhalation in rayon and cellophane manufacture.	Exposure to fire extinguishers or dry cleaning, oil solvents, insecticides.
Clinical Features	Confusion, ataxia, impaired memory, mild peripheral neuropathy later. Associated weight loss, excess sweating, skin exfoliation.	Global impairment, muscle pain, sensorimotor neuropathy usually earliest symptom, pseudobulbar palsy. Associated mucous blisters, cough, dyspepsia, coronary and renal vascular disease, retinal microaneurysms, impotence.	Dementia consequent to liver damage.
Diagnosis	Clinical syndrome and increased CSF protein, decreased sensorimotor action, potential amplitude. No CNS pathologic data.	EEG slowing in 40%, EMG slowing of nerve conduction, delayed peripapillary filling in eye vessels. Pathology: scattered foci of necrosis.	Clinical syndrome, hepatic dysfunction.
Treatment	Decrease exposure.	Decrease exposure.	Decrease exposure.
Prognosis	Mental and peripheral symptoms may abate or remain permanent, dependent on severity.	Progresses for months after exposure stops, then about 5% return to normal while nearly 50% continue to progress for years. About 40% stabilize.	

acute mental changes,[88] but well-documented follow-up is sparse, especially in long-lasting cases.

Parathyroid Disease and Other Causes of Altered Serum Calcium Levels. Mental impairment in parathyroid disease stems from abnormalities in serum calcium. Hypercalcemia accompanies several conditions, including hyperparathyroidism, myeloma, sarcoidosis, metastatic cancer, milk-alkali syndrome, vitamin D intoxication, acute adrenal insufficiency, body immobilization, and hypophosphatemia.[21,72] Mental symptoms may progress unrecognized over a period of years. Nearly half of all severely hypercalcemic patients develop diminished initiative, irritability, and emotional explosiveness. Memory and concentration become impaired, and if untreated, the disorder can cause paranoia, hallucinations, and coma. An isolated chronic dementia occurs in about 12% of patients. Diagnostic clues include anorexia, nausea, vomiting, weight loss, constipation, abdominal pain, arthralgias, polyuria, muscle weakness, and headache.[28,60,72] Diagnosis requires an elevated serum calcium (>12 mEq/L), low phosphorus, hypercalciuria, and an identification of their cause. The EEG may be normal or

WITH EXPOSURE TO INDUSTRIAL COMPOUNDS

Methyl chloride[75]	Organophosphates[21,63]	Toluene[75]	Trichloroethylene[75]
Occupational exposure to plastics and synthetic rubber.	Insecticides, pesticide exposure.	Exposure to paint solvent, lacquers, explosives, and in dye manufacture.	Exposure to dry cleaning, paints, rubber production, degreasing.
Poor memory, ataxic gait, tremor, weakness, paresthesias, and blurred vision.	Poor memory, irritability, anxiety, poor sleep, muscle aches.	Tremor, ataxic gait, bizarre behavior with emotional lability and poor memory.	Restless, impaired memory, trigeminal neuropathy, visual symptoms, tremor, neuropathy.
Clinical syndrome.	Clinical syndrome, EEG slowing.	Clinical syndrome and >100–400 ppm exposure for weeks.	Clinical syndrome, chronic exposure >100 ppm.
Decrease exposure.	Decrease exposure.	Decrease exposure.	Decrease exposure.
Symptoms abate in about 10 weeks.	Partially reversible or permanent.		

reveal background slowing with excess theta, delta, and high-voltage, synchronous frontal delta activity. In most instances, reduction of calcium levels reverses the mental impairment.[21,28]

Chronic hypocalcemia produces mild mental impairment without signs of neuromuscular irritability. The usual causes are idiopathic or postoperative hypoparathyroidism, or pseudohypoparathyroidism with tissue receptors unresponsive to the hormone.[21] Patients suffer poor concentration and memory, disorientation, apathy, and hallucinations.[21,87] Accompanying features include parkinsonism, chorea, corticospinal tract signs, seizures, agitation, papilledema, cataracts, coarse skin, and tetany with Chvostek's and Trousseau's signs.[87] Serum and spinal-

fluid calcium are low, and phosphorus levels can be evaluated.[21,87] CT often reveals calcification of the basal ganglia. This finding, however, is inconsistent and nonspecific. Similar calcification can be idiopathic or due to toxoplasmosis, cysticercosis, trichinosis, abscess, tuberculosis, tuberous sclerosis, arteriovenous malformation, aneurysm, or tumor. Effective treatment of prolonged hypoparathyroidism is difficult. In one series, only 20 of 50 patients approached their former level of functioning.[60]

Pituitary Disease. Most patients with panhypopituitarism have thyroid, adrenal, and gonadal failure in combination and suffer from intellectual impairment. In one series, only 6 of 78 patients had normal mental function.[60] Pituitary dysfunction may arise from adenoma, craniopharyngioma, postpartum necrosis, granuloma, syphilis, tuberculosis, surgery, or cavernous sinus thrombosis.[21] Symptoms include apathy, lethargy, poor concentration and memory, delusions, hallucinations, fatigue, impotence, paranoia, and seizures.[36,60] The EEG is slow.[36] Replacement therapy reverses the dementia in about 8 weeks.[36] Cortisone appears to be more important than thyroxine in this regard.[36,60]

CARDIOVASCULAR AND PULMONARY FAILURE

Impaired oxygen delivery to brain alters cerebral metabolism and intellectual function. Either a decrease in blood oxygenation, a loss of oxygen-carrying capacity of the blood, or a decline in cerebral perfusion can cause tissue hypoxia.

Transient Severe Hypoxia. Although precise figures are hard to obtain, asystole for longer than 1 or 2 minutes appears capable of producing at least some permanent damage to the brain.[72] More sustained exposure to severe hypoxia increases the risk proportionally. Causes include cardiopulmonary arrest, carbon monoxide intoxication, strangulation, hanging, recurrent severe syncope, or sustained generalized (and possibly, complex partial) status epilepticus. Damage to cognitive functions can range from the barely discernible to the extremes of a permanent vegetative state or brain death. Higher brain functions are especially vulnerable.

Following transient, severe hypoxia, damage to the brain may occur immediately or can be delayed for several days or more. Three patterns of delayed injury are possible. Two of these particularly affect victims of carbon monoxide poisoning or prolonged exposure to partial hypoxemia such as occurs with sudden ascent to high terrestrial altitudes. One of the latter, relatively uncommon, affects cerebral white matter selectively and can begin within 1 to 10 days or more following the acute insult. Symptoms include agitation and confusion progressing into stupor, coma, and even tetraplegia and death.[73] Some patients recover from such delayed demyelination; others are left with permanent dysfunction.

A second variant includes delayed necrosis of the globus pallidus, sometimes accompanied by similar areas of ischemic infarction involving "watershed" parasagittal areas of the cerebral hemispheres. Characteristically, such patients develop chorea, sometimes accompanied by mild symptoms and motor signs of frontal-lobe dysfunction consisting of apathy, paratonic resistance of the extremities, and occasionally memory impairment. These abnormalities subside in many such patients but some suffer permanent cognitive impairment.

The third, more common, delayed syndrome is well defined in experimental animals but less certainly identified in humans.[71,78] Degeneration of large pyramidal neurons of the CA1 zone of the hippocampus occurs 48 to 72 hours after acute severe global ischemia such as occurs during cardiac arrest. In humans the lesion underlies an amnesic dementia of variable, but often great, severity.[97]

Pathologic changes following hypoxia are well described, but systematic clinicopathologic correlation is lacking. Delayed postanoxic demyelination affects white matter diffusely, sparing subcortical U-fibers, as well as, in most instances, cortical neurons and the entire brainstem.[73] Oligodendroglia are conspicuously absent in light microscopic sections. Patients with selective amnesia show severe hypoxic damage in the hippocampi. Diffuse laminar cortical necrosis or thalamic infarction can result from hypoxic damage in severely affected cases.[97]

Chronic Hypercapnia-Hypoxia. Intellectual deficits are common in patients suffering from severe chronic obstructive pulmonary disease (COPD). Krop and co-workers[48] reported neuropsychiatric deficits in 10 patients with severe COPD having PAO_2 values below 55 mm Hg. As pulmonary function fails, patients insidiously become inattentive, forgetful, drowsy, irritable, and confused.[4,34] Diagnostic clues include tremulousness, asterixis, multifocal myoclonus, dull headache, papilledema, and specific signs of cardiopulmonary failure.[4,34] Impaired short-term memory and defects in attention and speed of calculation appear with $PaCO_2$ values of 50 to 55 mm Hg[11,48] and become more pronounced when $PaCO_2$ rises above 55 to 60.[4] EEG reveals background slowing with prominent theta and delta waves, which may outlast blood gas correction by a week or more. Spinal fluid pressure is increased, and its pH often falls below 7.25.[4]

Dementia seldom accompanies isolated COPD but can result when hypercapnia, hypoxia, congestive heart failure, or infection occur in combination. In order to improve mentation, all abnormalities need not be reversed. In the demented patients studied by Krop and colleagues,[48] mean scores on 8 of 10 neuropsychiatric tests improved to normal after 4 weeks of oxygen therapy alone. Oxygen therapy can impair ventilatory drive, however, and in such cases increasing $PaCO_2$ levels reduce arousal and increase motor system abnormalities.[4] Nevertheless, most intensively treated patients have a reasonable chance for mental recovery.[34,48]

Congestive Heart Failure. Chronic congestive heart failure occasionally produces short-lived mental impairment.[21,22] but seldom a dementia. The approximate hemodynamic deficit required to impair cognition is a 25% decrease in cardiac index, perhaps less in older patients.[11,22] In 21 confused subjects with congestive heart failure, Eisenberg and co-workers[25] found that cerebral blood flow was decreased by 50%, oxygen metabolism by 13%, and glucose metabolism by 25%. More re-

cent studies are unavailable. Patients with severe heart failure exhibit weight loss, irritability, disorientation, impaired memory, and somnolence.[22] Deficits are said to reverse themselves within 72 hours after cardiac function improves.[21,22] Brain MRI in patients with idiopathic dilated cardiomyopathy has revealed atrophy and ventricular enlargement. The morphologic abnormalities were associated with impaired cognitive test performance.[83]

Anemia. Low hemoglobin impairs mentation by limiting the oxygen-carrying capacity of the blood. Etiologies include chronic low-grade bleeding, hemoglobinopathy, failure of normal erythropoiesis, and excessive red cell destruction. Symptoms occur when blood oxygen-carrying capacity is reduced by more than half,[72] but milder reductions may add to symptoms in the elderly. Intellectual impairment, inattention, emotional lability, restlessness, and myoclonus ensue. Correction of anemia usually reverses the deficit.[21]

Hyperviscosity Syndromes. Viscous blood congests the microvasculature and promotes the development of medium- and large-artery thrombosis. Dangerously viscous states include Waldenstrom's macroglobulinemia, polycythemia vera, and 5% to 10% of IgG or IgA in myeloma.[21,65] Hyperlipidemia probably does not increase viscosity but makes blood more coagulable.[38] Symptoms of hyperviscosity include generalized weakness, fatigue, headache, anorexia, and global cognitive impairment,[100] associated with dysarthria, paratonia, and grasp reflexes.[65] Symptoms usually appear when relative serum viscosity exceeds 4, and nearly always with values over 8. Modifying factors include the state of the primary disease, the presence of atherosclerosis, the hematocrit, and the degree of congestive heart failure.[12] EEG occasionally shows background slowing. Patients that have recovered fully after treatment with plasmapheresis or phlebotomy had relative serum viscosities that decreased from 4.1 to

2.1 (normal = 1.4 to 1.8).[65] One patient with hyperlipidemia is described as clearing mentally with a decrease in cholesterol from 768 to 303 mg/dL, and in triglycerides from 7102 to 950 mg/dL.[38] Neurologic data from large series are not available.

HEPATIC DYSFUNCTION

Portosystemic   Encephalopathy. Mental impairment may follow hepatic dysfunction of any cause. Nearly 5% of patients with advanced alcoholic cirrhosis develop portosystemic encephalopathy.[20] Half have had surgical shunting. Intellectual function is particularly sensitive to fluctuations in gastrointestinal protein content. Symptoms develop insidiously, may fluctuate from hour to hour, and include euphoria or depression, poor concentration, attention, and memory, constructional abnormalities, and motor impersistence. Physical clues to the diagnosis include asterixis, hypertonus and hyperreflexia, gait ataxia, postural tremor, and fetor hepaticus.

Hepatic encephalopathy (HE) probably has several direct causes, acting either alone or in concert. The most frequent offender in chronic HE is ammonia, but mercaptans, short-chain fatty acids, false neurotransmitter amines, and altered GABA transmission also have been implicated.[20] In fulminating hepatic failure, HE precedes a serious rise in blood ammonia. Recent work has explored the role of benzodiazepines in the genesis of HE.[6] A recent autopsy study compared the brain content of substances inhibiting binding of a radiolabeled imidazobenzodiazepine to its receptors in patients dying of fulminant hepatic failure with that in patients dying of other causes. More than half of the patients dying with liver failure had elevated amounts of benzodiazepines detected in the frontal cortex. The origin of the substances was unknown,[6] and the significance of the finding remains uncertain. Concentrations thus far found in the brain and other tissues have been less than those

found necessary to produce severe narcosis or coma in otherwise healthy persons.

Arterial ammonia levels correlate best with clinical symptoms and range from 100 to 300 μg/dL (normal <50 μg/dL) in impaired patients. At the clinically significant concentrations, ammonia interferes with inhibitory postsynaptic potentials.[20] EEGs contain disorganized background slowing, generalized slow waves, and 2-Hz synchronous triphasic waves with frontal predominance. Symptoms and concurrent blood ammonia levels do not correlate closely with the EEG changes. Microscopic examination of brain in chronic HE reveals hyperplasia of protoplasmic astrocytes, a small decrease in number of neurons, and altered brain capillaries with increased transmembrane transport.[20,21]

Therapy is directed at decreasing gut protein with lactulose. Levodopa,[21] bromocriptine, and branched-chain amino acids have not been established as advantageous.[64] A sustained low-protein diet, with or without oral lactulose supplements, offers the best long-term regimen. Tremor and motor abnormalities improve less well than cognitive symptoms. Future efforts will undoubtedly be directed at studying the role of benzodiazepine receptor antagonists such as flumazenil in treating patients with cognitive dysfunction related to liver failure.[6] At present, the long-term prognosis is poor and includes recurrent encephalopathy and a life shortened by liver disease.

Chronic Acquired Hepatocerebral Degeneration. Rarely,   permanent neurologic deficits occur in patients surviving many episodes of portosystemic encephalopathy. The risk increases with each bout, but permanent neurologic deficits may occur without an antecedent episode of severe hepatic decompensation. Dementia may even precede the detection of liver disease and varies widely in severity among such cases.[95] Motor symptoms are invariable,   including   dysarthria, ataxia, dysmetria, titubation, asterixis, tremor, chorea, facial grimacing, and increased muscle tone. The EEG is slow and spinal fluid protein may be increased.[95] Neuropathology reveals an increase in the size and number of protoplasmic astrocytes, and patchy cortical laminar or pseudolaminar necrosis affecting the gray-white junction, the striatum, and the cerebellum.[95] Symptoms can remain fixed or progress insidiously. Death eventually results from hepatic failure. Treatment aimed at reducing blood ammonia levels does not completely reverse symptoms but does reduce the incidence of recurrent portosystemic encephalopathy.[21,95]

RENAL DYSFUNCTION

Uremia. Any form of chronic renal failure can cause mental impairment. Etiologies include glomerulonephritis, pyelonephritis, polycystic kidney, urinary tract obstruction, malignant hypertension, arteritis, granulomatous disease, amyloidosis, diabetes, or renal toxins.[21] Patients suffer fatigue, apathy, poor concentration and memory, disorientation, irritability, hallucinations, and paranoia. Hypertonus, asterixis, multifocal myoclonus, and tremor occur; seizures, peripheral neuropathy, and focal motor abnormalities appear late. CT reveals atrophy and ventriculomegaly in late stages. EEG abnormalities correlate with disease severity, showing a disorganized, slow background with burst of paroxysmal bilateral synchronous slow waves.[21] Therapy is directed at the cause of the renal failure, and mental symptoms improve in parallel with renal function.

Dialysis Dementia. Dialysis dementia usually develops unpredictably after several years of such treatment. Aluminum, present in both dialysis water and phosphate-binding gels taken orally, has been incriminated as the pathogenic agent. Typically, symptoms initially appear after a dialysis run, then worsen transiently after each subsequent session.[21,54] The earliest and most severe sign is a stuttering dysarthria which can progress to mutism and may be accompanied by a comprehension deficit.[21] Untreated, the illness progresses to persistent speech abnormality, global intellectual deterioration, myoclonus, agitation, apathy, perseveration, asterixis, seizures, apneic spells, and death. The spinal fluid may show slightly elevated protein levels.[54] EEGs are markedly abnormal: slow-wave bursts appear early, followed by slowing of background, sharp waves, spikes, polyspikes, and bilateral spike and waves. The latter are highly specific to the disorder but correlate poorly with clinical symptoms.[21,42,54] Severe slowing appears at end-stage. The CT scan may be normal or reveal atrophy. Neuropathology is nonspecific, although an increase in gray-matter aluminum has been documented. Patients rarely survive more than 2 years.[54] Diazepam improves mentation but only temporarily. Strategies to chelate aluminum are now being studied. Rarely, the syndrome occurs in undialyzed patients with exposure to high aluminum sources resulting in elevated serum aluminum levels. They may improve with dialysis.[80]

Deficiency States

Alcoholics, as noted earlier, commonly suffer the mental effects of dietary deprivation. Physicians must also beware of nutritional deficiency in those who are socially isolated, elderly, or anorexic, or who suffer from chronic illness, psychological depression, or food faddism.

GLUCOSE

Recurrent hypoglycemia sufficient to injure the brain may be reactive or due to glucose overutilization or underproduction.[60] Reactive hypoglycemia can accompany early diabetes, subtotal gastrectomy, or the ingestion of galactose, fructose, or amino acids in hyperalimentation diets. Glucose overutilization can occur with exogenous insulin, insulinoma, thyrotoxicosis, or massive sarcoma. Overutilization also may occur with chlorpropamide therapy, since tissue levels continue to rise for a week or more after starting the drug. Underproduction of glucose occurs with glycogen storage disease, hepatic failure, adrenocorticoid deficit, or insulin overdose. The longer hypoglycemia lasts, the greater the danger of irreversible neuronal loss. An insidious and progressive dementia was observed some years ago in zealously controlled diabetics suffering recurrent minor hypoglycemia, and in about 5% of patients after gastrectomy.[72] Current approaches to the treatment of diabetes, however, appear to have minimized this risk. The elderly are particularly susceptible to hypoglycemia because of erratic food intake, decreased hepatic glycogen stores, marginal hepatic and renal function, and sensitivity to the hypoglycemic effects of alcohol.

Mental symptoms of hypoglycemia usually parallel the rate and degree of decline in serum glucose. Since slowly falling or chronically low levels of blood sugar may not stimulate catecholamine secretion, brain injury can develop unaccompanied by tachycardia, sweating, anxiety, or pallor.[60] Most hypoglycemic patients complain of headache, confusion, restlessness, and irritability. If hypoglycemia is prolonged and cerebral recovery is incomplete, personality changes, aggressiveness, apathy, and emotional lability follow. Poor memory, impaired motor performance, and diminished spontaneous activity are the predominant mental signs. Some patients develop focal motor deficits or peripheral neuropathy.[60]

The existence of hypoglycemia can be difficult to diagnose in subtle cases (some insulinomas) and rests on the history, a 5-hour glucose tolerance test, a 3-day fast, and perhaps pancreatic imaging.[60] Recent data suggest that abnormal blood glucose measurements during spontaneously occurring symptomatic episodes are more accurate in diagnosis than measurements made after oral glucose tolerance testing.[70] Pathology in advanced cases reveals patchy neuronal loss in cortex, basal ganglia, and cerebellum, with proliferation of microglia, astrocytes, and blood vessels.[21] Postgastrectomy hypoglycemia responds to a high-protein, low-carbohydrate diet. In other instances, an alteration of diet and medication suffice as treatment. Therapy halts progression of symptoms but cerebral recovery is often incomplete. Symptoms present for more than several months rarely disappear.[21,60]

THIAMINE

Thiamine deficiency causes the Wernicke-Korsakoff syndrome, especially in alcoholics with poor dietary intake; in renal patients receiving hemodialysis; in cancer patients; or after gastrointestinal surgery. The overall degree of dementia depends on the extent of other nutritional deficiencies, and often, on the coincidence of repeated head trauma or seizures. Amnesia is the major mental deficit, but even in mild cases, neuropsychological testing reveals impairment in learning ability, concentration, spatial organization, and verbal and visual abstraction. Amnesia becomes prominent with repeated or severe attacks and may be overlooked until after the delirium, acute oculomotor abnormalities, and gait ataxia abate. In as many as 20% of cases, amnesia can develop insidiously without a history of acute encephalopathy.[96] Korsakoff's amnesia consists of severe anterograde and retrograde losses, often with relatively intact remote memory. Patients are typically unconcerned, apathetic, placid, and congenial. Moreover, nystagmus, ataxia, and peripheral neuropathy may persist chronically after treatment of acute encephalopathy. Pathologically, neuronal loss, gliosis, vascular proliferation, and petechial hemorrhages affect the mamillary bodies, the periventricular gray matter of the third and fourth ventricles, and the dorsal medial nucleus of the thalamus.[96]

Certain findings suggest a genetic predisposition to Wernicke-Korsakoff dementia. Despite the wide prevalence of heavy alcoholism and poor diet, relatively few alcoholics get the disease,[96] and it has a higher incidence among Europeans than among non-Europeans with similarly deficient diets. An inherited abnormality of transketolase, a thiamine-dependent enzyme, may predispose to the syndrome.[10] Permanent mental symptoms may be prevented by prompt recognition and treatment of patients with acute ocular or cerebral symptoms. Chronic thiamine therapy can prevent recurrent bouts of encephalopathy. Unfortunately, established memory deficits usually fail to recover, although they improve in as many as 75% of cases.[96] Most improvement occurs within several months of onset, but some may continue for up to 2 years.

NIACIN

Niacin deficiency is rare in the United States, because the vitamin is supplemented in wheat flour. Deficiency occurs in alcoholics, the underprivileged, and in persons subsisting on maize diets. In most instances, dermatitis and diarrhea precede the dementia, but occasionally, neither skin nor gastrointestinal symptoms have time to evolve. In one series of 18 patients, 4 had all three symptoms, 6 had only the typical sunburn-like rash on the dorsum of the hands, 3 had dermatitis and diarrhea, and 5 had only dementia.[43] Mental symptoms include confusion, disorientation, delusions, and poor memory, with associated extrapyramidal rigidity, gait ataxia, incontinence, myelopathy, and peripheral neuropathy. The neuropathy may be due to other nutritional deficiencies and worsens if only niacin is replaced. Constitutional signs include gingivitis, stomatitis, glossitis, enteritis, abdominal pain, diarrhea, red scrotum, perioral eczema, and vesicles or bullae over the extremities. Diagnosis requires finding less than 0.5 mg of N-methylnicotinamide per gram of creatinine in a random

urine sample.[43] Postmortem studies of the brain reveal chromatolysis of Betz cells and pontine nuclei.[21] Replacement therapy includes daily doses of 300 to 500 mg nicotinic acid until initial improvement occurs, followed by a lower dose and an adequate diet. Obtunded patients should also receive thiamine. All but a few severely demented patients recover completely within several weeks.[21]

CYANOCOBALAMIN

Despite suggestions to the contrary, true vitamin B_{12} deficiency causing dementia is nowadays rare. The most common cause is pernicious anemia;[37] other possibilities include total gastrectomy, gastrointestinal cancer, esophageal stricture, gastrointestinal fistulae, diverticula, tuberculosis, ileitis, sprue, vegetarian diets, and atrophic gastritis. Nearly 40% of patients with neurologic symptoms present before the age of 60. In nearly 25% of patients, the earliest predominant symptoms are neurologic, with no signs of dementia. Conversely, approximately 25% of patients who ultimately develop neurologic symptoms present with non-neurologic gastrointestinal and hematologic symptoms.[37]

Some reports suggest that dementia may precede spinal-cord, peripheral-nerve, optic-nerve, or hematologic changes by months or years.[58] This is probably not the case. A large retrospective study of 143 patients with 153 episodes of cobalamin deficiency associated with neurologic symptoms, found only 17 patients with dementia. It was the sole manifestation of the disease in only one patient. Mental symptoms fluctuate and include a mild disorder of mood, mental slowness, poor memory, agitation, depression, delusions, paranoia, and hallucinations.[37] Myelopathy and peripheral neuropathy combined are the most common neurologic manifestations, producing vibratory sense impairment, limb weakness, spasticity, hyperreflexia or hyporeflexia, and extensor plantar responses. Patients complain of paresthesias, tenderness, distal weakness, ataxia, and memory loss, which may precede clinical signs.[21,37]

Most patients eventually develop hematologic abnormalities, including megaloblastic anemia, macrocytosis, leukopenia with hypersegmentation, and mild thrombocytopenia.[100] Bone marrow studies usually reveal a megaloblastic pattern. An abnormally low serum B_{12} level (<175 pg/mL) establishes the diagnosis.[37] A Schilling test helps elucidate the cause. Patients with borderline B_{12} levels can be diagnosed by elevation in methylmalonic-acid and homocysteine levels.[58] The EEG shows diffuse slowing but its abnormalities correlate poorly with neurologic symptoms. The spinal fluid is usually normal. Head CT may show diffuse cerebral atrophy in patients with mental impairment.[37] Patients with spinal cord signs may have intramedullary high-signal lesions detected on T_2-weighted MR images of the spinal cord.[8]

Cerebral pathology includes perivascular foci of demyelination with relatively little axonal destruction or reactive gliosis. Similar changes affect the cord, especially at the thoracic level, and the peripheral nerves.[69] Therapy starts with daily parenteral administration of at least 100 μg B_{12} for 1 week. A 1000-μg injection is administered monthly thereafter,[37] especially if gastrointestinal absorption is poor. Improvement is usually evident in days, but its rate slows after 1 month.[21] Nearly half the patients, including those with dementia, make a full recovery. The remainder experience partial (usually greater than 50%) improvement. Not surprisingly, the degree of improvement is related to the initial severity and duration of symptoms.[37]

FOLIC ACID

The relationship of folate deficit to mental impairment is controversial.[69,100] Folic acid deficiency follows inadequate intake[100]; malabsorption due to jejunal resection, gastrectomy or Crohn's disease; and chronic phenytoin or primidone treatment.[21] Reports describe folate deficiency in nearly 80% of demented nursing home patients, but also in 30% of psychiatric patients and 50% of normals.[100] Moreover, folate deficit frequently coexists with other nutritional deficiencies, and treatment typically provides multiple supplements. The strongest evidence for a specific effect of folate on brain function comes from cases of congenital specific folate malabsorption, in which progressive mental retardation occurs with ataxia, seizures, dysarthria, and athetosis. Symptoms and signs sometimes attributed to folate deficit include insomnia, memory loss, disorientation, poor concentration, irritability, pallor, fatigue, hyporeflexia, and extensor plantar responses.[91,100] Folate levels less than 3 ng/mL are considered low. No characteristic neuropathology has been described. Megaloblastic anemia may be present. EEG slowing may occur and normalize with treatment.[91] Therapy is recommended for deficient patients. Some authors recommend that B_{12} be given simultaneously.[100] Neurologic symptoms may take many months to normalize,[21,91] but the anemia corrects rapidly.[91]

TREATMENT AND PROGNOSIS IN METABOLIC DEMENTIA — A SUMMING UP

This chapter has identified three principal categories of metabolic dementia. One, a state of chronic, fixed mental impairment, can follow acute, severe metabolic perturbations such as occur with hypoxemia or asystole, hypoglycemia, or thiamine deprivation. Once the acute injury has passed, these patients suffer the results of more-or-less irreversible brain damage.

A second category of metabolic dementia consists of a reversible toxic metabolic disorder such as nutritional deprivation, which reduces the capacity of a potentially healthy brain to function normally. Although often consid-

**Table 10–9 PREVIOUSLY UNRECOGNIZED BUT
TREATABLE ILLNESSES IN 307 OUTPATIENTS
EVALUATED FOR DEMENTIA**

	n	(%)
Depression	87	(28)
Folate deficit	19	(6)
Arthritis	14	(5)
Urinary infection	12	(4)
Chronic obstructive pulmonary disease	9	(3)
Congestive heart failure	7	(2)
Anemia	5	(2)
Peptic ulcer	4	(1)
Miscellaneous	44	(14)

Source: Adapted from Larson et al,[51] p. 491.

ered in differential diagnosis, such conditions are actually rare except in undernourished countries or local populations, or among religious or dietary zealots. The long clinical experience of the senior author of this chapter includes many patients with nutritional failure and a good number of all ages who were slowed down by drug abuse. In barely a handful was a chronic, previously unrecognized, metabolic dementia such as B_{12} deficiency or myxedema both conclusively diagnosed and successfully treated. One finds many conditions to treat in patients with dementia (Table 10–9), but those who improve mentally are distressingly few. A study by Larson and colleagues[50] underscores the problem: a 2-year follow-up of 13 patients with potentially "reversible" dementia found that 8 continued to decline intellectually despite all therapeutic efforts.

This brings us to the third group of patients, in whom drugs or systemic metabolic derangements curtail the residual mental capacities of an already ailing brain, leading to social and behavioral decompensation. Here, reducing duplicating drugs, stopping self-medication as well as alcohol intake, and repairing systemic bodily insufficiencies such as heart failure can make a difference. The adverse, reversible effect of phenobarbital on the school performance of epileptic children vividly illustrates that age is not the only predisposing risk factor in iatrogenic overdose. Nevertheless, elderly persons with early dementia often accelerate the progress of the disease by ingesting what sometimes seems like tiny amounts of antidepressants, benzodiazepines, antihypertensives, anticholinergics, digitalis, or beta-blockers. Wise medical care for this increasingly large population can make a difference. It requires repeated reviews of what the patient is taking and frequent educational intervention by the physician. The result of such care may add months or even years to an individual's independence and sense of well-being.

REFERENCES

1. Adler S: Methyldopa-induced decrease in mental activity. JAMA 230:1428–1429, 1974.
2. Allain H, Decombe R, Saiag B, Bentue-Ferrer D, and Guez G: Mechanistic basis for the development of anti-ischemic drugs. Cerebrovascular Diseases (Suppl 1)1:83–92, 1991.
3. Antuono P, Sorbi S, Bracco L, Fusco T, and Amaducci L: A discrete sampling technique in senile dementia of the Alzheimer type and alcoholic dementia: Study of the cholinergic system. In Amaducci L, Davison AN, and Antuono P (eds): Aging of the Brain and Dementia. Raven Press, New York, 1980, pp 155–159.

4. Austen FK, Carmichael MW, and Adams RD: Neurologic abnormalities of chronic pulmonary insufficiency. N Engl J Med 257:579–590, 1967.

5. Bank WJ: Thallium. In Spencer PS and Schaumburg HH (eds): Experimental and Clinical Neurotoxicology. Williams & Wilkins, Baltimore, MD, 1980, pp 570–571.

6. Basile AS, Hughes RD, Harrison PM, et al: Elevated brain concentrations of 1,4-benzodiazepines in fulminant hepatic failure. N Engl J Med 325:473–478, 1991.

7. Battistin L and Dam M: Metabolic encephalopathies. In Lajtha A (ed): Handbook of Neurochemistry, Vol 10. Plenum Press, New York, 1985, pp 693–670.

8. Berger JR and Quencer R: Reversible myelopathy with pernicious anemia: Clinical/MR correlation. Neurology 41:947–948, 1991.

9. Blass JP: Metabolic dementias. In Amaducci L, Davison AN, and Antuono P (eds): Aging of the Brain and Dementia. Raven Press, New York, 1980, pp 265–289.

10. Blass JP and Gibson GE: Abnormality of a thiamine-requiring enzyme in patients with Wernicke-Korsakoff syndrome. N Engl J Med 297:1367–1370, 1977.

11. Blass JP and Plum F: Metabolic encephalopathies in older adults. In Katzman R and Terry R (eds): Neurology of Aging. FA Davis, Philadelphia, 1983, pp 189–214.

12. Bloch KJ and Maki DG: Hyperviscosity syndromes associated with immunoglobulin abnormalities. Semin Hematol 10:113–124, 1973.

13. Buge A, Supino-Viterbo V, Rancurel G, and Pontes C: Epileptic phenomena in bismuth encephalopathy. J Neurol Neurosurg Psychiatry 44:62–67, 1981.

14. Crammer W: Toxic demyelination. In Spencer PS and Schaumburg HH (eds): Experimental and Clinical Neurotoxicology. Williams & Wilkins, Baltimore, MD, 1980, pp 239–246.

15. Carlen PL, Wilkinson A, Wortzman G, et al: Cerebral atrophy and functional deficits in alcoholics with clinically apparent liver disease. Neurology 31:377–385, 1981.

16. Carlen PL, Wortzman G, Holgate RC, Wilkinson DA, and Rankin JG: Reversible cerebral atrophy in recently abstinent chronic alcoholics measured by computed tomography scans. Science 200:1076–1078, 1978.

17. Chang LW: Mercury. In Spencer PS and Schaumburg HH (eds): Experimental and Clinical Neurotoxicology. Williams & Wilkins, Baltimore, MD, 1980, pp 508–511.

18. Choi D: Cerebral hypoxia: Some new approaches and unanswered questions. J Neurosci 10:2493–2501, 1990.

19. Cohen WJ and Cohen NH: Lithium carbonate, haloperidol and irreversible brain damage. JAMA 230:1283–1287, 1974.

20. Cooper AJL and Plum F: Biochemistry and physiology of brain ammonia. Physiol Rev 67:440–519, 1987.

21. Cummings JL and Benson DF: Dementia: A Clinical Approach. Butterworth & Co, Boston, 1983.

22. Dalessio DJ, Beuchimol A, and Dimond EG: Chronic encephalopathy related to heart block: Its correction by permanent cardiac pacemaker. Neurology 15:499–503, 1965.

23. Davis JN and Carlson A: The effect of hypoxia on monoamine synthesis, levels and metabolism in rat brain. J Neurochem 21:783–790, 1973.

24. Doherty JE, deSoyza N, and Kange JJ: Cardiac glycoside. In Levinson AJ: Neuropsychiatric Side Effects of Drugs in the Elderly. Raven Press, New York, 1979, pp 39–43.

25. Eisenberg S, Madison L, and Sensenbach W: Cerebral hemodynamics and metabolic studies in patients with congestive heart failure. II. Observations in confused subjects. Circulation 21:704–799, 1960.

26. Fallaice LA: Ethyl alcohol. In Levinson AJ: Neuropsychiatric Side Effects of Drugs in the Elderly. Raven Press, New York, 1979, p 39.

27. Freeman JW and Couch JR: Prolonged encephalopathy with arsenic poisoning. Neurology 28:853–855, 1978.

28. Gatewood JW, Ocgan CH, and Mead BT: Mental changes associated with hyperparathyroidism. Am J Psychiatry 132:129–132, 1975.

29. Gerstl B: Biochemistry of demyelination and demyelinating diseases. In Cummings JN (ed): Biochemical Aspects of Nervous Disease. Plenum Press, New York, 1972, pp 72–81.

30. Gerstl B: Biochemistry of demyelination and demyelinating diseases. In Cummings JN (ed): Biochemical Aspects of Nervous Disease. Plenum Press, New York, 1972, pp 89–102.

31. Gibson GE, Peterson C, and Sanson J: Decreases in amino acid and acetylcholine metabolism during hypoxia. J Neurochem 37:192–201, 1981.

32. Goodnick PJ and Gershon S: Lithium. In Lajtha A (ed): Handbook of Neurochemistry, ed 2, Vol 9. Plenum Press, New York, 1985, pp 103–149.

33. Guynn RF: Steroidal drugs. In Levinson AJ: Neuropsychiatric Side Effects of Drugs in the Elderly. Raven Press, New York, 1979, pp 123–128.

34. Hall WJ: Psychiatric problems in the elderly related to organic pulmonary disease. In Levinson AJ and Hall RCW (eds): Neuropsychiatric Manifestations of Physical Disease in the Elderly. Raven Press, New York, 1981, pp 41–46.

35. Hammond JJ and Kirkendall WM: Antihypertensive agents. In Levinson AJ: Neuropsychiatric Side Effects of Drugs in the Elderly. Raven Press, New York, 1979, pp 48–52.

36. Hanna SM: Hypopituitarism (Sheehan's syndrome) presenting with organic psychosis. J Neurol Neurosurg Psychiatry 33:192–193, 1970.

37. Healton EB, Savage DG, Brust JCM, Garrett TJ, and Lindebaum J: Neurologic aspects of cobalamin deficiency. Medicine (Baltimore) 70:229–245, 1991.

38. Heilman KM and Fisher WR: Hyperlipidemic dementia. Arch Neurol 31:67–68, 1974.

39. Hertz L: Potassium transport in astrocytes and neurons in primary cultures. Ann N Y Acad Sci 481:318, 1986.

40. Heyer EJ and Macdonald RL: Barbitu-
rate reduction of calcium-dependent action potentials: Correlation with anesthetic action. Brain Res 236:157–171, 1982.

41. Hollister LE: Psychotherapeutic drugs. In Levinson AJ: Neuropsychiatric Side Effects of Drugs in the Elderly. Raven Press, New York, 1979, p 79.

42. Hughes JR and Schreeder MT: EEG in dialysis encephalopathy. Neurology 30:1148–1154, 1980.

43. Ishii N and Nishihara Y: Pellagra among chronic alcoholics: Clinical and pathological study of 20 necropsy cases. J Neurol Neurosurg Psychiatry 44:209–215, 1981.

44. Jacobs JM: Vascular permeability and neuronal injury. In Spencer PS and Schaumburg HH (eds): Experimental and Clinical Neurotoxicology. Williams & Wilkins, Baltimore, MD, 1980, pp 102–104.

45. Jarvik LF and Perl M: Overview of physiologic dysfunction related to psychiatric problems in the elderly. In Levinson AJ and Hall RCW (eds): Neuropsychiatric Manifestations of Physical Disease in the Elderly. Raven Press, New York, 1981, pp 7–11.

46. Kandel ER: Nerve cells and behavior. In Kandel ER and Schwartz JH (eds): Principles of Neural Science, Ed 2. Elsevier, New York, 1985, pp 13–24.

47. Krigman MR, Bouldin TW, and Mushalk P: Lead. In Spencer PS and Schaumburg HH (eds): Experimental and Clinical Neurotoxicology. Williams & Wilkins, Baltimore, MD, 1980, pp 490–492.

48. Krop HD, Block AJ, and Cohen E: Neuropsychologic effects of continuous oxygen therapy in chronic obstructive pulmonary disease. Chest 64:317–322, 1973.

49. Larson EB, Kukull WA, Buchner D, and Reifler BV: Adverse drug reactions associated with global cognitive impairment in elderly persons. Ann Intern Med 107:169–173, 1987.

50. Larson EB, Reifler BV, Featherstone HJ, and English DB: Dementia in elderly outpatients: A prospective study. Ann Intern Med 100:417–423, 1984.

51. Larson EB, Reifler BV, Suni SM, Can-

field CG, and Chinn NM: Features of potentially reversible dementia in elderly outpatients. West J Med 145: 488–492, 1986.

52. Larson EB, Reifler BV, Suni SM, Canfield CG, and Chinn NM: Diagnostic tests in evaluation of dementia: A prospective study of 200 elderly outpatients. Arch Intern Med 146:1917–1922, 1986.

53. Lavin P and Alexander CP: Dementia associated with clonidine therapy. BMJ 1:628, 1975.

54. Lederman RJ and Henry LE: Progressive dialysis encephalopathy. Ann Neurol 4:199–204, 1978.

55. LeQuesne PM: Acrylamide. In Spencer PS and Schaumburg HH (eds): Experimental and Clinical Neurotoxicology. Williams & Wilkins, Baltimore, MD, 1980, pp 309–310.

56. Leysen JE and Niemegeers CJE: Neuroleptics. In Lajtha A (ed): Handbook of Neurochemistry, ed 2, Vol 10. Plenum Press, New York, 1985, pp 331–362.

57. Li H, Lesiuk H, and Buchan AM: Postischemic treatment with AMPA, but not NMDA, antagonists prevents CA1 neuronal injury. Stroke 23:14, 1992.

58. Lindenbaum J, Healton EB, Savage DG, et al: Neuropsychiatric disorders caused by cobalamin deficiency in the absence of anemia or macrocytosis. N Engl J Med 318:1720–1728, 1988.

59. Lipowski ZL: Delirium: Acute Confusional States. Oxford University Press, New York, 1990.

60. Martin JB and Reichlin S: Clinical Neuroendocrinology, Ed 2. FA Davis, Philadelphia, 1987.

61. McAuley DLF, Lecky BRF, and Earl CJ: Gold encephalopathy. J Neurol Neurosurg Psychiatry 40:1021–1022, 1977.

62. McEvoy GK: American Hospital Formulary Service. American Society of Hospital Pharmacists, Bethesda, MD, 1988, pp 581–587.

63. Metcalf DR and Holmes JH: EEG, psychological and neurological alterations in humans with organophosphorus exposure. Ann N Y Acad Sci 160:357–365, 1969.

64. Morgan MY, Jakobovits A, Elithorn A, James IM, and Sherlock S: Successful use of bromocriptine in the treatment of a patient with chronic portosystemic encephalopathy. N Engl J Med 296:793–794, 1974.

65. Mueller J, Hotson JR, and Langston JW: Hyperviscosity-induced dementia. Neurology 33:101–103, 1983.

66. Narahashi T: Nerve membrane as a target of environmental toxicants. In Spencer PS and Schaumburg HH (eds): Experimental and Clinical Neurotoxicology. Williams & Wilkins, Baltimore, MD, 1980, pp 225–231.

67. Newman SE: The EEG manifestations of chronic ethanol abuse: Relation to cerebral cortical atrophy. Ann Neurol 3:299–304, 1978.

68. Nordberg A, Aldofsso R, Aquilonius SM, Maukwad S, Oreland L, and Winbland B: Brain enzymes and acetylcholine receptors in dementia of the Alzheimer type and chronic alcohol abuse. In Amaducci L, Davison AN, and Antuono P (eds): Aging of the Brain and Dementia. Raven Press, New York, 1980, pp 169–173.

69. Olsen RZ, Stoier M, Siersbak-Nielsen K, Hansen JM, Schioler M, and Kristensen M: Electroencephalographic findings in hyperthyroidism. Electroencephalogr Clin Neurophysiol 32:171–177, 1972.

70. Palardy J, Havrankova J, Lepage R, et al: Blood glucose measurements during symptomatic episodes in patients with suspected postprandial hypoglycemia. N Engl J Med 321:1421–1425, 1989.

71. Petito CK, Feldmann E, Pulsinelli WA, and Plum F: Delayed hippocampal damage in humans following cardiorespiratory arrest. Neurology 37: 1281–1286, 1987.

72. Plum F and Posner JB: Diagnosis of Stupor and Coma, Ed 3. FA Davis, Philadelphia, 1982.

73. Plum F, Posner JB and Hain RF: Delayed neurological deterioration after anoxia. Arch Intern Med 110:56–63, 1962.

74. Plum F and Pulsinelli WA: Cerebral metabolism and hypoxic ischemic brain injury. In Asbury AK, McKhann

GM, and McDonald WI (eds): Disease of the Nervous System. Clinical Neurobiology, Vol 2. WB Saunders, Philadelphia, 1992, pp 1002–1015.

75. Politis MJ: Neurotoxicity of selected chemicals. In Spencer PS and Schaumburg HH (eds): Experimental and Clinical Neurotoxicology. Williams & Wilkins, Baltimore, MD, 1980, pp 613–619.

76. Porcellati G: Demyelinating cholinerterase inhibition: Lipid and protein metabolism. In Lajtha A (ed): Handbook of Neurochemistry. Plenum Press, New York, 1972, pp 457–466.

77. Powers HC, Myers RR, and Lampert PW: Edema in neurotoxic injury. In Spencer PS and Schaumburg HH (eds): Experimental and Clinical Neurotoxicology. Williams & Wilkins, Baltimore, MD, 1980, pp 124–131.

78. Pulsinelli WA, Brierley JB, and Plum F: Temporal profile of neuronal damage in a model of transient forebrain ischemia. Ann Neurol 11:491–499, 1982.

79. Rottenberg DA, Horten B, Kim J-H, and Posner JB: Progressive white matter destruction following irradiation of an extracranial neoplasm. Ann Neurol 8:76–78, 1980.

80. Russo LS, Beale G, and Sandroni S: Dialysis dementia in undialyzed chronic renal failure. Neurology (Suppl 1)40:253, 1990.

81. Scatton B, Carter C, Benavides J, and Giroux C: N-methyl-D-aspartate receptor antagonists: A novel therapeutic perspective for the treatment of ischemic brain injury. Cerebrovascular Diseases 1:121–135, 1991.

82. Schildkraut JJ: Antidepressants and related drugs. In Lajtha A (ed): Handbook of Neurochemistry. Plenum Press, New York, 1972, pp 363–369.

83. Schmidt R, Fazekas F, Offenbacher H, Dusleag J, and Lechner H: Brain magnetic resonance imaging and neuropsychologic evaluation of patients with idiopathic dilated cardiomyopathy. Stroke 22:195–199, 1991.

84. Scremin OU and Jenden DJ: Time-dependent changes in cerebral choline and acetylcholine induced by transient global ischemia in rats. Stroke 22:643–647, 1991.

85. Seppalainen AM and Haltia M: Carbon disulfide. In Spencer PS and Schaumburg HH (eds): Experimental and Clinical Neurotoxicology. Williams & Wilkins, Baltimore, MD, 1980, pp 356–357.

86. Shopsin B, Johnson G, and Gershon S: Neurotoxicity with lithium: Differential drug responsiveness. International Pharmacopsychiatry 5:170–182, 1970.

87. Slyter H: Idiopathic hypoparathyroidism presenting as dementia. Neurology 29:393–394, 1979.

88. Starkman MN and Schteingart DE: Neuropsychiatric manifestations of patients with Cushing's syndrome. Arch Intern Med 141:215–219, 1981.

89. Sterns RH, Riggs JE, and Schochet SS: Osmotic demyelination syndrome following correction of hyponatremia. N Engl J Med 314:1535–1542, 1986.

90. Stewart DJ and Benjamin RS: Cancer chemotherapeutic agents. In Levinson AJ: Neuropsychiatric Side Effects of Drugs in the Elderly. Raven Press, New York, 1979, pp 191–202.

91. Strachan RW and Henderson JG: Dementia and folate deficiency. Q J Med 36:189–204, 1967.

92. Swanson JW, Kelly JJ, and McConahey WM: Neurologic aspects of thyroid dysfunction. Mayo Clin Proc 56:504–512, 1981.

93. Valpey R, Sumi M, Copass MD, and Goble GJ: Acute and chronic progressive encephalopathy due to gasoline sniffing. Neurology 28:507–510, 1978.

94. van Horn G: Dementia. Am J Med 83:101–110, 1987.

95. Victor M, Adams RD, and Cole M: The acquired (non-wilsonian) type of chronic hepatocerebral degeneration. Medicine (Baltimore) 44:345–396, 1965.

96. Victor M, Adams RD, and Collins GH: The Wernicke-Korsakoff Syndrome, Ed 2. FA Davis, Philadelphia, 1989.

97. Volpe BT and Petito CK: Dementia with bilateral medial temporal lobe

ischemia. Neurology 35:1793–1797, 1985.

98. Walshe JM: The biochemistry of copper in man and its role in the pathogenesis of Wilson's disease. In Cumings JN (ed): Biochemical Aspects of Nervous Disease. Plenum Press, New York, 1972, pp 140–147.

99. Watanabe I: Organotins. In Spencer PS and Schaumburg HH (eds): Experimental and Clinical Neurotoxicology. Williams & Wilkins, Baltimore, MD, 1980, pp 545–546.

100. Weinger RS: Psychiatric manifestations of hematopoietic system disease. In Levinson AJ and Hall RCW (eds): Neuropsychiatric Manifestations of Physical Disease in the Elderly. Raven Press, New York, 1981, pp 83–91.

101. Weiss HD, Wallin MD, and Wiernik PH: Neurotoxicity of commonly used antineoplastic agents. N Engl J Med 281:75–81, 1974.

102. Yanagahira T: Cerebral anoxia: Effect on transcription and translation. J Neurochem 22:113–117, 1974.

103. Zola-Morgan S, Squire LR, and Amaral DG: Human amnesia and the medial temporal region: Enduring memory impairment following a bilateral lesion limited to field CA1 of the hippocampus. J Neurosci 6:2950–2967, 1986.

Chapter 11

MISCELLANEOUS CAUSES OF DEMENTIA

Mario F. Mendez, M.D., Ph.D.

HYDROCEPHALUS
TRAUMA
NEOPLASIA
MULTIPLE SCLEROSIS
EPILEPSY

Several causes of dementia do not readily fall into the categories discussed in previous chapters. The "miscellaneous" dementing disorders discussed here include hydrocephalus, trauma, neoplasm, multiple sclerosis, and epilepsy. This chapter is concerned with cognitive declines sufficient to constitute dementia in these five disorders rather than in isolated cognitive impairments that may occur in some of these diseases. The dementias in these disorders are not as frequent or as well characterized as they are in the more common dementing illnesses discussed in previous chapters. Similarly, the specific mechanisms by which the disease produces cognitive impairment often are not known.

HYDROCEPHALUS

Physicians have long recognized that mental retardation and acute confusional states could result from obstructive hydrocephalus. A more recent discovery was that dementia also occurs from an acquired chronic form of obstructive hydrocephalus with normal cerebrospinal fluid (CSF) pressure. In 1965, Hakim[60] and Adams[2] described normal-pressure hydrocephalus (NPH) in several patients with a characteristic triad of dementia, gait disturbance, and urinary incontinence. Their patients responded to CSF shunting, and NPH became one of the most important potentially reversible causes of dementia.

Epidemiology

NPH occurs in 1.6% to 7% of all cases of dementia and in as many as a quarter of all those with a reversible etiology.[21,69,72] Approximately 67% of NPH cases have a discoverable cause; the two most common known causes are prior subarachnoid hemorrhage and head trauma.[10,72] Patients diagnosed with NPH are usually 50 to 70 years old,[69] although in one series, 80% of patients with NPH were over 70 years old.[44] Furthermore, a more latent form of this disorder may be a common cause of abnormal gait in the elderly.[44]

Clinical Features

The clinical triad of NPH is nonspecific. Only about 12% of patients presenting with the complete triad prove to have NPH,[91] and the diagnosis of NPH requires a high index of suspicion in the presence of only one or two

337

symptoms of the triad. Gait disturbance is often the most prominent symptom and usually precedes urinary incontinence and cognitive decline.[43] Because of the prominence of gait disturbance in NPH, the differential diagnosis of this disorder primarily includes movement disorders such as Parkinson's disease and the normal gait changes of the elderly.

The gait disorder is commonly referred to as apraxia of gait, magnetic gait, or frontal ataxia. Patients complain of weak legs, feelings of unsteadiness, difficulty getting started, and problems changing direction.[115] Besides the nonspecific finding of short steps, low speed, and a broader base, patients have difficulty initially lifting the feet off the ground, decreased clearance, and variable force of steppage.[114] Patients with NPH also have a more general postural instability, with a tendency to fall and difficulty turning over in bed in advanced stages.[114,119] Furthermore, electromyography of the lower extremities shows co-contraction of agonist and antagonist muscles and continuous activity in antigravity muscles throughout the gait.[75,119]

Patients with NPH may have other neurologic features. In the lower extremities they frequently have spasticity and extensor plantar responses, and in the upper extremities they occasionally show decreased coordination of fine finger movements, deterioration in handwriting, and a fine action tremor.[114] Early symptoms of urinary urgency and frequency may progress to incontinence, and there is a relative lack of concern for the loss of bladder control, despite the presence of excessively strong bladder contractions on cystometrograms.[43,72] Fecal incontinence may also occur late in the course.

Neuropsychology

The dementia of NPH has prominent disturbances in attention, initiation, and frontal executive functions.[41] NPH patients are often inattentive and easily distractible. They are psychomotor slowed and lethargic, lack spontaneity and initiative, have little spontaneous speech, and may appear withdrawn and depressed.[30,41,44,58] Some patients progress to an abulic or an apathetic mute state in advanced stages.[115] These patients may also show a lack of goal-directed behaviors, poor judgment, and disinhibition.[103] On neuropsychological testing, attention and recent memory are impaired, writing and drawing are disorganized, and the performance subtests of the Wechsler Adult Intelligence Scale (WAIS) are decreased in comparison with the verbal subtests.[30,58,71] Finally, when compared with patients with Alzheimer's disease (AD), patients with NPH have more impairments in subcortical-frontal systems of behavior but lack deficits attributable to cortical association areas, such as focal aphasias, agnosias, and apraxias.[58]

Neuroimaging and Special Tests

Diagnostic tests are of special importance in the evaluation of NPH and are emphasized here. The diagnosis of hydrocephalus begins with the finding of enlarged ventricles on cranial neuroimaging studies such as computed tomography (CT) or magnetic resonance imaging (MRI) (Fig. 11–1). Obstructive hydrocephalus such as NPH must then be differentiated from hydrocephalus ex vacuo, ventricular enlargement from loss of brain tissue.[79] On CT scans, NPH is suggested by large ventricles with relative absence of cortical atrophy. The frontal and temporal horns may expand disproportionately: The width of the frontal horns is usually greater than 30% of that of the cranial cavity, and the temporal horns are 2 mm or greater in width.[79] The best CT predictors of shunt responsiveness may be a large ventricle-to-brain ratio (VBR) and periventricular hypolucencies spreading out from the frontal horns in a "handlike" fashion.[14,124] On MRI, in addition to ventricular enlargement and cerebral atrophy, there is periventricular hyper-

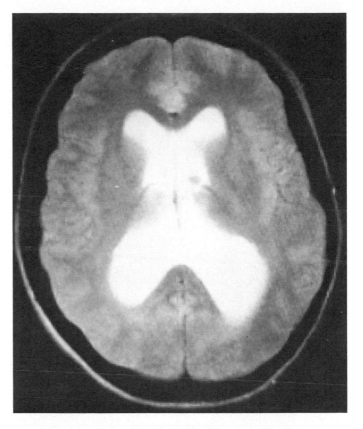

Figure 11–1. MRI (horizontal view) in obstructive hydrocephalus showing enlarged ventricles and decreased prominence of gyral pattern.

intensity and decreased attenuation through the aqueduct of Sylvius (signal-void phenomenon, SVP) (Fig. 11–2).[16,94] SVP in NPH probably reflects more rapid flow of CSF through the aqueduct owing to decreased capacity of the ventricular canal to buffer pressure changes.[94] Future work may prove that the SVP is a sensitive measure for differentiating NPH from hydrocephalus ex vacuo, but none of the other neuro-imaging techniques consistently predict the presence of NPH.[100]

Radioisotope cisternography, a measure of CSF dynamics, was introduced with the hope that it would be a better predictor of the presence of NPH and of improvement following shunting. In this technique a radioisotope such as RISA (radio-iodinated serum albumin) is introduced into the lumbar space and its course is plotted with brain scans at various intervals, usually 6, 24, and 48 hours. Normally the isotope circulates over the cerebral convexities, becomes concentrated in the parasagittal area, and disappears by 48 hours. In NPH there may be failure of the radioisotope to be concentrated at the parasagittal area at 24 or more hours, with reflux into the ventricles and failure of reabsorption at 48 hours.[122] This pattern correlates best with a positive shunt response, but there are frequent false positives and negatives.[12,67,122,135] Other studies, which have not proven superior to isotope cisternography, include electroencephalography (EEG), pneumoencephalography (PEG), the metrizimide CT scan, cerebral blood flow determinations, measures of the absorption of isotope from the CSF into the blood, single photon emission computed tomography (SPECT), and positron emission tomography (PET), which shows decreased glucose metabolism, especially in frontal areas.[67,68,71,92,122]

Because of the limitations of cranial neuroimaging and isotope cisternography in the evaluation of NPH, investi-

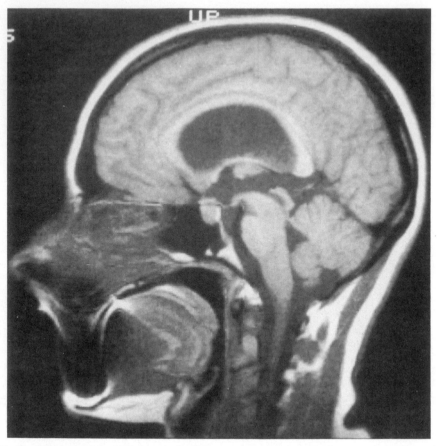

Figure 11–2. MRI (sagittal view) demonstrating noncommunicating obstructive hydrocephalus with aqueductal stenosis.

gators have proposed the use of more invasive physiologic techniques in patients suspected of this disorder. Infusion manometric techniques have assessed CSF dynamics by the instillation of saline solution or artificial CSF into the lumbar CSF at a constant rate.[72] Simple measurements of the rate of rise of CSF pressure were not reliable in predicting response to shunting, and this has led to various modifications of this technique.[14,63] Measurement of resistance to CSF outflow (R_{out}) compensated for differences in baseline pressure by comparing the rate of rise at two different infusion rates.[63] Measurement of conductance to CSF outflow (C_{out}) also compensated for the distention of the ventricular canal by determining the rate of CSF exiting the ventricles per change in infusion pressure.[14] This lumboventricular infusion technique accurately predicted shunt responsiveness in 80% of patients suspected of having NPH; however, this technique required an intraventricular monitor for measurement of CSF outflow.[124] Intraventricular pressure monitoring in NPH patients has revealed plateau waves and spike-shaped waves (Lundberg B waves) occurring as intermittent pressure deviations, particularly during periods of REM sleep. Good shunt responsiveness resulted if B waves occurred for 2 hours or more during a 48-hour monitoring period,[25,52] indicating that NPH is not "normal" but "intermittent high"–pressure hydrocephalus.

Finally, one important procedure is

the "Fisher test" or the CSF tap-test, the removal of CSF during a spinal tap.[43,138] In some patients with NPH, an improvement in gait, psychometric functions, or both starts 30 to 60 minutes after removal of 20 to 50 mL of CSF and has a positive correlation with response to shunting.[138] The improvement in gait can last for months and may be consequent to a decrease in pressure sufficient to improve the blood supply.[43] Importantly, a lack of response to CSF removal does not preclude a positive response to shunt placement. Further investigation of the sensitivity of this test is needed, particularly of its effects on the dementia and the urinary incontinence elements of the NPH triad.

Neurobiology

The basic physiologic disturbance in NPH is an abnormal balance between CSF production and absorption.[50,71] CSF production occurs at the choroid plexus as an energy-requiring secretory process. Normally, most CSF circulates out of the ventricles, into the subarachnoid space, and over the convexities, where it is reabsorbed into the venous sinuses at the arachnoid villae. This absorption process depends on the differential pressure across these structures, as well as on their normal patency. NPH is a type of obstructive hydrocephalus in which there is either disturbed CSF absorption at the arachnoid villae or impeded CSF flow from the choroid plexus to its absorption sites. These two forms of obstructive hydrocephalus are referred to as communicating or noncommunicating, respectively, depending on whether there is free passage of CSF from the ventricles out to the arachnoid space. Communicating NPH may be due to scarring of the arachnoid villae or to abnormal CSF viscosity, and noncommunicating NPH to partial or intermittent obstruction in the ventricles, foramina of Monro, aqueduct of Sylvius, or the foramina of Magende and Lushka.

Hakim and Adams[60] explained the physics of normal CSF pressure in obstructive hydrocephalus by invoking Pascal's law: force is equal to the product of pressure and surface area. Because less pressure is required with a constant force applied to a larger surface area, "normal" pressure in the face of enlarged ventricles is actually abnormal. They believed that the abnormal production-absorption balance resulted in an initial force and pressure elevation; as a new balance developed over time, the pressure returned to normal in the face of ventricular enlargement. Studies of CSF dynamics in obstructive hydrocephalus corroborate an initial phase of increased CSF pressure followed by normal pressure but persistently elevated R_{out}.[52,77]

In NPH there is a decrease in the compliance of the enlarged ventricular system, as reflected by the intermittent B waves of increased pressure.[25,85] There is a higher-than-expected incidence of stroke in NPH,[78] and infarcts and other degenerative changes in the periventricular white matter promote decreased tensile strength and compliance of the ventricular wall.[4,55,78] The incidence of hypertension in NPH is also higher than expected,[55] and hypertension contributes to the increased CSF pulse pressure which, in the face of the weakened ventricular wall, results in periventricular edema and destruction and loss of protein and lipids, particularly around the vulnerable frontal horns.[43,71]

Many of the symptoms of NPH may result from deep frontal pathology or microvascular changes. The disruption around the frontal horns is consistent with disturbed frontal behavior, lower extremity motor involvement from stretching of frontal periventricular fibers, "disinhibited" urinary incontinence, and the occasional grasp reflex and other primitive reflexes. The decreased initiation and disturbed executive abilities reflect this frontal dysfunction, and the gait disorder may represent a release of frontal grasp reflexes from the feet or of the postural righting reflexes normally elicited by weight bearing.[39] Other aspects of the dementia of NPH, such as the attentional deficits, may be due to the white-matter disease with decreased conduction velocities in pathways running from attention-mediating structures in subcortical regions to higher cognitive centers in cortical regions.[41]

Etiology

The causes of NPH can be divided into communicating, noncommunicating, and idiopathic. Communicating NPH occurs from decreased CSF absorption at the arachnoid villae owing to prior subarachnoid hemorrhage, head trauma, infectious meningitis, or carcinomatous meningitis[71]; from blockage at the arachnoid villae by a sagittal sinus meningioma or other lesion; or from blockage at the incisura by tentorial or cerebellar mass lesions. Spinal tumors also may result in communicating hydrocephalus, although the mechanism is not clear.[40] Noncommunicating NPH occurs from aqueductal stenosis, intraventricular neoplasms, ependymitis, colloid cysts of the third ventricle, fourth-ventricular outflow obstruction consequent to Arnold-Chiari malformations and similar disorders, or displacement of an atherosclerotic basilar artery upward into the third ventricle.[36] Furthermore, lateral ventricular enlargement from communicating hydrocephalus may result in downward displacement of the third ventricle, stretching and obstruction at the aqueduct, and a self-perpetuating obstructive hydrocephalus.[93] Finally, approximately one third of cases have no identifiable cause.[71] Most of this idiopathic group appears to be communicating, but recent evidence suggests that many have occult stenosis of the aqueduct of Sylvius.[134] (See Fig. 11–2.)

Specific Management

Surgical shunting of the CSF remains the primary therapy for NPH.[115] Shunt success ranges from 33% to 80% depending on the surgical team and the patient selection criteria.[11,58,65,101,124,130] Although not totally reliable, positive prognostic factors for shunt responsiveness include (1) illness of no more than 2 years' duration and preferably less than 6 months with minimal or no dementia[56,101,124]; (2) presence of a gait disturbance, particularly preceding any dementia[11,56,67]; (3) a known etiology[124]; (4) CT scan findings of periventricular lucencies, large frontal horn span, minimal atrophy or sulcal enlargement, and large temporal horns[17,124]; (5) CSF dynamics showing opening pressures over 100 or 110 mm H_2O, improvement following CSF removal, obstructive pattern on cisternogram, and an abnormal CSF infusion test (particularly C_{out})[14,17,125,138]; and (6) the presence of significant intermittent high pressure waves on intracranial pressure monitoring.[25,56,122] Newer suggested measures for assessing shunt responsiveness include temporary external CSF drainage and urodynamic testing in connection with a lumbar puncture.[3,59]

The initial high enthusiasm for CSF shunting in NPH has subsided because of shunt-related morbidity, particularly in elderly patients, and a lack of a consistently effective way of predicting shunt responsiveness.[65,101] Significant long-term improvement after shunting occurs in about 21% of all NPH patients and only 15% of those without a known etiology.[136] Shunt complications occur in 20% to 44%, often necessitate reoperation and shunt revision, and include problems with maintenance of shunt patency, regulation of ventricular pressure, subdural hematomas, infections, emboli, intracerebral hemorrhage, and epilepsy.[11,65,66,101,130] Shunt complications with serious morbidity occur in about 7%, so that, for every three or four successfully shunted NPH patients, there is one serious shunt complication.[136] Subdural hematomas are the most serious complications and result from tearing of bridging veins from the siphoning of CSF.[122] Ventriculoatrial shunts have resulted in pulmonary emboli, superior vena caval dissections, sepsis, and cardiac tamponade.[47] Ventriculoperitoneal shunts have resulted in CSF ascites, loculated cysts, abdominal visceral perforation, and intestinal volvulus.[12,98,111] Lumboperitoneal shunts avoid the problems of intraventricular placement, but regulation of shunt pressure may be difficult and patients may experience low CSF pressures on standing if the valve pressure is too low.[12,46]

In sum, CSF shunting should be considered if there is recent onset of a characteristic gait disturbance, CT or MRI evidence of hydrocephalus and periventricular lucencies, and confirmation of diagnosis by either CSF removal, cisternography, or one of the more invasive techniques. The decision to shunt those who do not fit these criteria is difficult. Ultimately, the risks of shunt placement must be weighed against the potential benefits of an improvement in gait and the less-frequent improvement in cognition. Palliative medical therapy for NPH is also a consideration and includes the use of acetazolamide (a carbonic anhydrase inhibitor), digitalis, monoamine oxidase inhibitors, and osmotic diuretics. Ultimately, we need further delineation of the natural history of NPH and follow-up studies on the long-term effectiveness of shunting.

TRAUMA

Head injury is the most common cause of neurologic illness in young people, and dementia is the most debilitating consequence of head trauma.[13,45] The behavioral consequences of head trauma discussed here refer to the residual damage after the acute head injury has subsided and can be divided into the postconcussive syndrome, focal deficits from penetrating or closed head injury (CHI), more global residual cognitive compromise after a single severe CHI, and the cumulative effects of repeated blows to the head. Only the last two result in "traumatic dementia"; they have similar clinical findings and are discussed together in this section.

Epidemiology

Several million head injuries occur annually in the United States, including about 240 severe and 22 to 23 fatal CHIs per hundred thousand population.[13] CHI accounts for about 2% of cases of dementia,[13,45,112] and the cognitive impairment may progressively worsen during the first months or years after the head injury.[13,45] Cognitive impairments are more likely to develop after CHI if the injuries are severe or multiple and if there is a history of alcoholism, cerebrovascular disease, or a low premorbid IQ.[137] In severe CHI, about 40% die within the first 48 hours and 35% are left with considerable cognitive impairments. Only about 25% have a better recovery.[13]

A special group are those who sustain repeated blows to the head, the most salient examples of which are boxers.[131] Boxers who develop the progressive cognitive compromise referred to as dementia pugilistica or "punch-drunk syndrome" have usually started fighting at a young age, had over 10 years of boxing, and accumulated over 150 fights.[22,131] The dementia begins near the end of their boxing careers or shortly after retirement, but can be delayed in onset.[22] This syndrome is not associated with the number of knockouts or episodes of loss of consciousness, but more with the total number and type of blows to the head, particularly if the angle of impact or failure to stabilize the head results in rotational movement of the brain (Fig. 11-3).[131]

In addition, epidemiologic reports have debated a higher-than-average incidence of head injury in the history of patients with AD,[90,110,120] suggesting that head trauma provides a provocative or permissive role in the development of AD. (See Chapters 1 and 6.)

Clinical Features

The immediate consequences of CHI range from minor postconcussive changes in attention, memory, and personality to a severe global encephalopa-

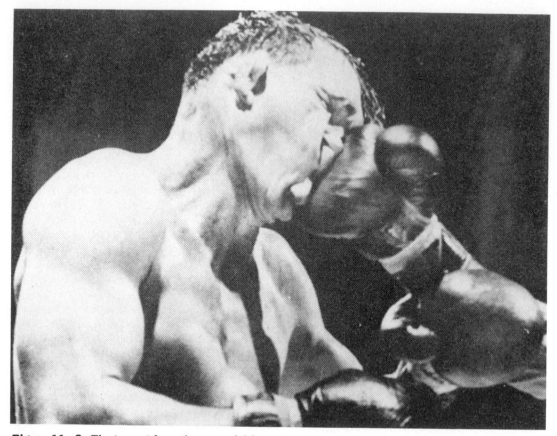

Figure 11–3. The impact from the powerful force of a boxer's blow can cause visible facial distortion. This force is transduced to the brain as linear acceleration-deceleration injury and rotation of the brain within the skull. (From the Bettman Archive, New York, NY, with permission.)

thy.[13,45] Residual cognitive impairment is almost assured if the period of post-traumatic amnesia (PTA) is greater than or equal to 4 weeks or the period of coma (< 8 on the Glasgow Coma Scale)[70] is more than 24 hours.[13] About half the survivors have a poor recovery if the PTA is more than 1 week or the period of coma is 6 hours or more.[13] The residual cognitive deficits are established within 6 to 9 months of the head injury, after which they persist with little change except for some secondary recovery owing to compensatory adaptation.[13,19] Finally, a delayed decline in cognition may result from obstructive hydrocephalus, subdural hematomas, or traumatic vascular occlusions.[10]

The clinical picture of repeated blows to the head has some unique neurologic features. Besides the usual cognitive and behavioral changes of severe CHI, there is often dysarthria and scanning speech, ataxia and decreased coordination, extrapyramidal deficits and parkinsonism, occasional pyramidal tract signs, alcohol intolerance, and belligerence.

Neuropsychology

The most prominent cognitive disturbances in severe CHI and dementia pugilistica are in attention, memory, speed of information processing, and frontal systems.[13,19,137] Some deficits, such as the attentional and memory impairment, are more universal, whereas others vary with the focal locations of the brain injuries. Attention deficits result in concentration problems and difficulty filtering out irrelevant information. Unlike NPH, memory problems are disproportionately prominent, with difficulties in new learning and relative preservation of old memories except for a short period of residual retrograde amnesia for the time immediately preceding the head injury. Other disabilities in these patients occur in frontal executive abilities such as judgment, abstraction, reasoning, planning, and organization. Frontal injury may cause patients to manifest inappropriate behavior, to be disinhibited, irritable and often explosive and prone to psychosis and violence.[82] Conversely, they are occasionally withdrawn and apathetic, have an exacerbation of their premorbid personality traits, or manifest a reactive depression. Other deficits include mental and motor slowing and a greater decline of performance IQ than of verbal IQ. Finally, without focal injury there are no aphasias, agnosias, or other related disturbances of higher cortical functioning.[81]

Neuroimaging

CT scanning and other neuroimaging may show the effects of contusion located under the place of impact (coup) or near the opposite pole (contrecoup). Acutely, there may be edema, hypodensities, or intracranial bleeding. Late sequelae include atrophy, ventricular enlargement, porencephalic cysts, and chronic subdural collections. Additionally, a common finding on head scans of boxers is a cavity (cavum) in the septum pellucidum[22] (Fig. 11–4), although this can be a normal variant.

Neurobiology

In general, the more severe the injury, the greater the structural damage and the cognitive deficits. Injuries with linear acceleration may result in cortical gray-matter coup-contrecoup contusions but generally cause less severe brain damage than rotational acceleration of the brain within the cranial cavity.[131] Rotational movement results in shearing of nerve fibers in the subcorti-

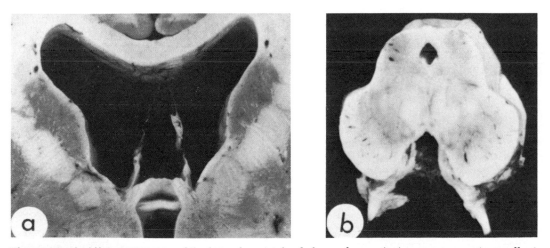

Figure 11–4. (A) Anterior view of the lateral ventricle of a boxer demonstrates a cavum septum pellucidum separated by a cavity. (B) Midbrain of a boxer demonstrates loss of the normal dark bands that comprise the substantia nigra.

cal white matter, as well as damage to corpus callosum and brainstem.[1,118,125] Atrophy and ventricular enlargement ensue from the diffuse neuronal atrophy. Linear and rotational movement also damage the brain wherever it abuts nonsmooth bony surfaces, such as in the orbitofrontal region and the temporal poles. Subdural hematomas, obstructive hydrocephalus, cerebral edema, cerebral hypoxia, traumatic vascular injury, disseminated intravascular coagulation, and systemic fat emboli may also contribute to the brain damage.

Minor rotational injuries from repeated blows to the head can result in cumulative brain damage.[57,97] Corsellis[22] studied the brains of boxers and showed an increased prevalence of changes: cavum septum pellucidum with rupture and fenestration; ventricular enlargement and loss of white matter from axonal shearing; neurofibrillary tangles with β-amyloid deposition but without classical neuritic plaques,[108] concentrated in temporal horn areas; cerebellar tonsillar injury and Purkinje cell loss, probably from transient tonsillar herniation; and loss of pigment in the substantia nigra (see Fig. 11–4B). In addition, Payne[99] found microscars in the gray matter, possibly from petechial and direct contusional injury.

The cognitive deficits from head trauma reflect the individual location of the brain damage, but certain brain areas are particularly susceptible to traumatic injury. Hippocampal damage in the temporal poles is associated with memory impairment, orbitofrontal damage is associated with disinhibition and executive disturbances, and deep white-matter damage is associated with impaired attention. Finally, the development of residual damage from head injury also is affected by the context in which the injury occurs, such as the age of the patient, the momentum of the lesion, and whether a single head injury or multiple sequential injuries occurred.

Prevention and Management

Management efforts include the prevention of head injuries and the rehabilitation of patients. Educational efforts should stress the value of protective headgear and seat belts in reducing the risk of severe head injury, as well as the dangers of the use of alcohol when driving. Strict regulations must cover activities in which there are repeated blows to the head, such as boxing. Active rehabilitation results in modest gains in neuropsychological functions and significant gains in emotional status and interpersonal skills.[104] No single rehabilitative approach is best for all patients or types of injury. It is too soon to assess the value of the new field of cognitive rehabilitation therapy, but older therapeutic interventions, such as speech, physical, and occupational therapy, help in maximizing recovery in posttraumatically impaired patients. Early rehabilitative intervention may increase the probability of a more successful outcome.

NEOPLASIA

Tumors are one of the potentially treatable causes of dementia. They cause changes in mentation by localized effects in areas such as the frontal or temporal lobes, by diffuse tumor involvement such as from multiple metastasis, and by secondary effects such as paraneoplasia and the cognitive effects of cancer therapy.

Epidemiology

About 1% of all cases of dementia are due to tumors.[112] About 80% of brain tumors cause behavioral changes; the exact prevalence is unclear, however, because of the different behavioral methodologies used. The most common type of tumors causing dementia are located in the frontal lobes or the temporal lobes or involve diffuse CNS metastases.[73,117]

Clinical Features and Neuropsychology

Many cognitive changes from tumors are missed because they are subtle and vary with the location of the tumor.[28] Most patients have attentional disturbances with impairments of arousal and timing, headaches, other neurologic findings on examination, and a slow EEG.[28]

Direct effects of frontal lobe tumors include apathy and decreased psychomotor activity, euphoria and facetiousness, impaired executive abilities, and, especially if bilateral, dementia. In one group of patients with frontal tumors, 62% had impaired intellect, 57.5% had decreased memory and orientation, and 42% had retardation of speech, thought, and action.[117] One special case of frontal pathology is the "butterfly glioma" of the anterior corpus callosum,[62] which additionally includes subtle signs of hemispheric disconnection and a lack of elementary neurologic findings.

In a large series of patients with temporal lobe involvement, 56% had intellectual impairment and 50% had decreased memory and orientation.[73] These patients were often described as irritable, depressed, and prone to hallucinations. Language disturbances occurred if the lesions were in the left hemisphere. As in the case of frontal lobe tumors, behavioral changes were frequently the first and only symptoms in these patients and occurred in the absence of other focal neurologic deficits.

A third localized region for neoplastic dementia is the diencephalon. Memory loss and other cognitive impairments have been reported with tumors of the third ventricular area, hypothalamus, and thalamus. These tumors produce obstructive hydrocephalus or alter behavior by affecting local structures. For example, many of the cognitive changes due to colloid cysts of the third ventricle occur from compression or vascular compromise of diencephalic limbic structures.[83] In addition, hypothalamic involvement, such as with gangliocytomas, can result in dementia with hyperphagia and hypersomnolence,[7] and thalamic tumors can alter cognition by affecting the medial thalamic nuclei, which project to the frontal cortex.[20]

Dementia from diffuse tumor involvement results from metastatic disease, either multiple tumor nodules or diffuse infiltration of tumor cells into parenchyma, perivascular spaces, and meninges.[84] These patients frequently have seizures, headache, meningeal irritation, cranial nerve dysfunction, other focal neurologic findings, and abnormal CSF cytology. Dementia may result from insidious infiltrates, as from chronic lymphocytic leukemia,[77] and from meningeal carcinomatosis from breast, lung, malignant melanoma, and other tumors.[123] Gliomatosis cerebri is a brain tumor in which mental deterioration results from diffuse overgrowth and infiltration of neoplastic glial elements.[24] A rare cause of dementia is neoplastic angioendotheliosis, a CNS tumor that produces multiple CNS infarcts by lymphomatous proliferating in the lumina of blood vessels.[35,74] Finally, dementia may accompany primary intracranial arachnoid cysts in the elderly.[139]

The secondary effects of tumors on the nervous system include limbic encephalitis, ectopic hormone production, and progressive multifocal leukoencephalopathy (PML). Limbic encephalitis is most frequently associated with oat cell carcinoma of the lung, and presents with disturbed affect, anxiety or depression, prominent recent memory loss, other cognitive deficits, and possible hallucinations or seizures.[53] There are increased lymphocytes and immunoglobulin G (IgG) in the CSF, and lymphocytic infiltrates and perivascular cuffing in the hippocampus, amygdala, and the cingulate and orbital cortex. Limbic encephalitis is part of the spectrum of paraneoplastic encephalomyelitis that also includes bulbar encephalitis from involvement of the lower brainstem, myelitis with damage of the anterior horn cells at varying levels, ganglioradiculitis with destruction of posterior root ganglia, and Wallerian degeneration of posterior columns and peripheral nerves. Systemic carcinomas can produce ectopic hormones such as antidiuretic hormone and parathormone, and these may also compromise cognition by altering the fluid, electrolyte, and endocrine balance.[27] Furthermore, dementia may be a manifestation of opportunistic CNS infections such as papovavirus (the organism of progressive multifocal leukoencephalopathy), which occur with immunosuppression. (See Chapter 8.)

In cancer therapy a delayed leukoencephalopathy with apathy, abulia, and memory loss results from whole-brain irradiation, especially in patients who have also received chemotherapy.[29,109,113] Demyelination can occur months or years after combination therapy with cranial radiation of more than 20 Gy, particularly if delivered in high daily fractions.[29] This leukoencephalopathy can occur from whole brain radiation alone, but is facilitated by chemotherapy such as intrathecal methotrexate greater than 50 mg or 40 to 80 mg/m² per week.[54] In one series, radiation-induced brain atrophy with dementia occurred in 49% of patients radiated for brain tumors. The dementia appeared 2 to 3 months after the completion of radiation therapy.[6]

Neurobiology

Direct tumor effects are more likely to alter cognition if the tumor involves both sides of the brain, is located supratentorially, and involves frontal or temporal lobes.[73,117] Behavioral effects are more likely with increased tumor malignancy because of rapid growth and local

tissue destruction, central tumor necrosis, increased parenchymal infiltration, and cerebral edema. There may also be evidence of vascular compromise or ventricular obstruction and hydrocephalus. Tumor-induced increased intracranial pressure, which usually results in prominent deficits in attention and consciousness, should be distinguished from a more chronic dementia and managed with measures to reduce cerebral edema. Therapy is otherwise directed at the individual tumor.

MULTIPLE SCLEROSIS

Dementia may result from primary white-matter diseases. These disorders are either myelinoclastic, with myelin destruction, or dysmyelinating, with abnormal myelin formation. Myelinoclastic diseases include multiple sclerosis (MS) and its variants such as Schilder's disease. Dysmyelinating diseases include the leukodystrophies: metachromatic leukodystrophy (MLD), adrenal leukodystrophy, and lipomembranous polycystic osteodystrophy. MS is discussed here; the leukodystrophies and the secondary demyelinating conditions that may cause dementia are discussed in Chapter 6.

Epidemiology

After trauma, MS is the most prevalent neurologic disease of young people.[87] It occurs in 50 to 60 individuals per 100,000, with onset in their 20s or 30s in most cases.[87] The majority of patients with MS have a mild loss of memory and abstract reasoning abilities[61,121]; 50% have some measurable deficits on neuropsychological tests[102]; 17 to 28% have an isolated significant cognitive impairment[61,64]; and 2 to 6.7% have multiple significant cognitive impairments sufficient to constitute dementia.[9,23,61,89] Variations in the prevalence estimates for cognitive changes in MS reflect the difficulties in detecting the often-subtle cognitive deficits with insensitive bedside mental status tests.[49] More rigorous neuropsychological investigations yield higher rates of cognitive dysfunction in MS.[49] (See Chapter 5.)

Clinical Features and Neuropsychology

MS results in demyelination through acute recurrent episodes or a slowly progressive decline, with an eventual accumulation of neurologic deficits, including deficits in cognition. The cognitive changes do not correlate consistently with the presence of other neurologic findings,[133] but there are small positive correlations with overall length and severity of illness.[8,41,49,61,106]

The dementia of MS has a relatively specific neuropsychological profile and occurs most commonly in chronic progressive MS but may also be seen as a relapsing-remitting feature.[9,61,137] Like NPH, trauma, and other disorders involving the white matter, MS may result in slowed information processing speed.[42,108] Significant deficits also follow a pattern of frontal behavioral change, that is, carelessness and slovenliness, lack of judgment, perseveration, decreased conceptual efficiency, difficulty shifting sets, and lack of response to environmental feedback.[105] In cognitively impaired MS patients,[42] frontal release signs in the lower extremities are common, such as gait apraxia similar to that of NPH.[49] MS patients can also develop prominent memory problems, and recall memory may be more severely impaired than recognition memory, suggesting retrieval problems.[105] Many MS patients have a relative euphoria and are unable to recognize the severity of their illness.[121] In some MS patients, average performance IQ scores are 7 to 14 points lower than verbal IQ scores, with the lowest subtest scores on the digit symbol test and the best on the picture completion test.[105] Finally, some patients have signs of interhemispheric disconnections, major affective disturbances, visuospatial difficulties, and occasionally, aphasia with decreased spontaneous speech and paraphasias.[8,96,102]

Neuroimaging

CT and MRI scans in the myelinoclastic diseases show areas of white-matter lucency (Fig. 11–5). MS lesions are multiple, prominent in the periventricular region, and, when acute, may enhance with the use of a contrast medium. On MRI scans in chronic progressive patients, the total lesion area correlates with cognitive impairment,[48,106] and the size of the corpus callosum may be particularly associated with decreased sustained attention.[48,106]

Neurobiology

Cognitive and behavioral changes in MS may be associated with frontal periventricular plaques, plaques located in the gray matter, or the presence of widespread disease. The disturbed fundamental functions such as mental speed, attention, timing, and activation probably reflect cortical-subcortical disconnection from demyelination, particularly of white matter pathways emanating from prefrontal cortex.[41,89] MS plaques tend to be strategically located in the frontal lateral periventricular white matter.[41,42,48,49,89] There may be disconnection of white-matter pathways between prefrontal and posterior cortex.[41] Finally, the emotional disturbances could result from demyelination affecting the limbic system and its connections.

Management

Currently there is no curative treatment for MS, but immunosuppressive

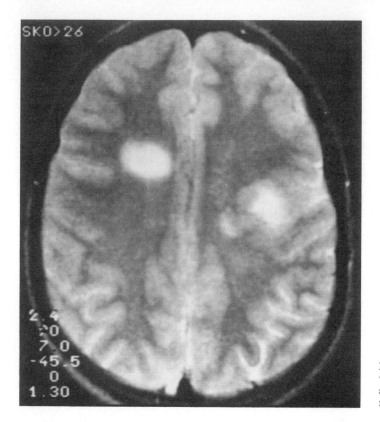

Figure 11–5. MRI (horizontal view) of a patient with multiple sclerosis and cognitive impairment.

therapies may help the patient over an acute relapse or possibly delay the progression of the disease.[87] The cognitive disturbances may be the most serious consequences of MS and could respond to immunosuppressive therapy. Remission of cognitive symptoms in patients with relapsing-remitting MS has been reported.[48]

EPILEPSY

In the 19th century a number of writers claimed that epileptics suffered from impaired memory and intellect.[80,129] It was subsequently recognized, however, that such impressions were based on institutionalized epileptics, a highly biased sample.[129] Although many epileptics have isolated cognitive deficits, the majority have little or no cognitive deterioration, and only a small minority could be described as having dementia.[80]

Epidemiology

Epileptics comprise 1% to 2% of the United States population and have an average IQ slightly less than normal.[97] The markedly impaired cognition seen in about 1.5% of these patients is primarily due to preexisting brain damage and secondarily to the seizures themselves.[80,126,129] Genetic epilepsies are often associated with dementia. One example is Lafora's disease, an autosomal-recessive myoclonic epilepsy that usually occurs in patients before the second decade but has been reported in individuals as old as 63 years.[116] In addition, seizures may occur as part of multi-infarct dementia, Creutzfeldt-Jakob disease, posttraumatic dementia, and, more rarely, AD.[126]

Clinical Features

Seizure variables that may bear on cognitive deterioration include the presence of "symptomatic" epilepsy from known brain disease, type of seizures, age of onset, the severity and frequency of seizures, and the effects of medications.[5,15,80,128] In one series the average IQ of symptomatic epileptics was lower than those with idiopathic disease (89.1 versus 102.5), and follow-up of symptomatic epileptics shows a greater average deterioration in IQ.[15] Generalized-seizure patients have more attentional difficulties and lower WAIS IQ and Halstead Battery results than partial seizure patients. Temporal-lobe epileptics, however, have more memory impairment.[100,127,129] Seizures with onset before age 5 probably augur of a lower IQ.[32,95] Other studies show a positive correlation between high seizure frequency and lower IQ,[31] and decreased IQ scores are associated with a larger number and extent of epileptiform discharges and depth electrode activity.[33,107] Many of these cognitive effects of seizures are at least partially reversible with the attainment of good seizure control.[51] Cognitive impairment is characteristic of active seizure states such as spike-wave stupor or absence status epilepticus.

At therapeutic levels most anticonvulsant medications cause only minimal cognitive slowing[34]; however, the barbiturates frequently adversely affect cognition.[86,127,129] (See Chapter 4.) Phenobarbital may decrease brain glucose utilization by 30% or more.[37] In addition, phenytoin may result in folate deficiency,[127] and a few patients on phenytoin have developed a severe encephalopathy termed "Dilantin dementia."[132] Patients who develop this dementia have generally been mentally retarded children with frequent seizures, increased CSF protein, and evidence of cerebellar atrophy.

Neuropsychology

Epileptics vary in their neuropsychologic profiles owing to the location of the epileptic foci and other areas of damage.[129] Some epileptics, particularly those with temporal lobe seizures, have a decrease in memory. There is evidence that verbal memory is affected more with left-sided temporal foci, and visual memory more with right-sided foci.[107,129] Part of the apparent decrease in verbal memory could be due to an anomia.[88] Other epileptics have decreased perceptuomotor skills, slowed information processing, and mood and personality alterations.[129] Finally, therapeutic levels of phenobarbital can cause decreases in attention, concentration, learning, memory, and motor speed; and toxic levels of all anticonvulsant drugs can impair mental speed, and cause an encephalopathy.[34,80,86,126]

Neurobiology

Preexisting brain damage does not completely explain the neuropsychological deficits, which may also result from the seizure activity itself, the anticonvulsant therapy, or a combination of both.[129] Subclinical seizures may result in memory impairment and other cognitive deficits, and the memory disturbances correlate with increased spike discharges in the hippocampal regions.[18] PET studies reveal decreased metabolism in a broader area of brain than is reflected in the seizure focus itself.[38] Animal studies link brain disturbance to seizures by showing that the induction of a single seizure interferes with maze-solving ability at a later age, that neuronal degeneration is associated with repeated seizures, and that seizures have inhibitory effects on brain protein synthesis and growth.[26,80] Finally, cognitive deterioration severe enough to call "epileptic dementia" is more likely in those with early-onset seizures and brain damage, tonic-clonic and multiple types of seizures, and a high seizure frequency.

Management

Seizure management must balance the potentially harmful effects of uncontrolled seizures with those due to anticonvulsant medications.[128] In general, it is best to prevent seizures but to achieve this control using the fewest possible anticonvulsant drugs in the lowest effective dosage, particularly because any cognitive effects from anticonvulsant medications may be additive.[128] Episodes of anticonvulsant drug toxicity also may be detrimental to normal cognitive development in children and should be avoided.[15]

SUMMARY

Several causes of dementia that do not fit into well-defined categories have been reviewed in this chapter, including hydrocephalus, trauma, neoplasia, demyelinating disease, and epilepsy.

Different forms of hydrocephalus can cause dementia, but the most difficult, conceptually and clinically, is normal-pressure hydrocephalus, which is characterized by the triad of dementia, gait disturbance, and urinary incontinence. A variety of laboratory techniques have been developed to try to improve diagnostic accuracy and to predict the effects of ventricular shunting, with mixed results.

Head injury is an exceedingly common cause of neurologic illness in young people; the clinical picture can vary considerably depending on the nature and site of injury.

Similarly, tumors can present in different ways, depending on the rate of growth and location. Both primary and secondary tumors affect the nervous system, as do several conditions that occur as a consequence of cancer therapy, such as leukoencephalopathy.

White-matter disease includes myelinoclastic (normal myelin is destroyed) and dysmyelinating (abnormal myelin is formed) disorders. MS is the most common illness causing destruction of normal myelin and is frequently associated with slowed mental speed, memory retrieval difficulties, and executive disturbances.

The relationship between epilepsy and dementia is controversial. The pattern of cognitive impairment clearly depends on the nature of the seizures and their underlying cause.

The features of these dementias associated with normal-pressure hydrocephalus, trauma, tumor, MS and epilepsy are not as well defined as those of the degenerative or vascular dementias, but these are increasingly recognized as dementing disorders. More investigation needs to be done on the clinical phenomenology, underlying pathophysiologic mechanisms, and potential management strategies of dementias in patients with these disorders.

REFERENCES

1. Adams JH, Mitchell DE, Graham DI, and Doyle D: Diffuse brain damage of immediate impact type. Its relationship to primary brain-stem damage in head injury. Brain 100:489–502, 1977.
2. Adams RD, Fisher CM, Hakim S, Ojemann RG, and Sweet WH: Symptomatic occult hydrocephalus with "normal" cerebrospinal fluid pressure. N Engl J Med 273:117–126, 1965.
3. Ahlberg J, Norlen L, Blomstrand C, and Wikkelso C: Outcome of shunt operation on urinary incontinence in normal pressure hydrocephalus predicted by lumbar puncture. J Neurol Neurosurg Psychiatry 51:105–108, 1988.
4. Akai K, Vchigasaki S, Tanaka V, and Komatsu A: Normal pressure hydrocephalus: Neuropathological study. Acta Pathol Jpn 37:97–110, 1987.
5. Arieff AJ and Yacorzynski GK: Deterioration of patients with organic epilepsy. J Nerv Ment Dis 96:49–55, 1942.
6. Asai A, Matsutani M, and Takakura K: Subacute brain atrophy induced by radiation therapy of malignant brain tumors. Gan No Rinsho 33:753–761, 1987.
7. Beal MF, Kleinman GM, Ojemann RG,

and Hochberg FH: Gangliocytoma of third ventricle: Hyperphagia, somnolence, and dementia. Neurology 31: 1224–1228, 1981.

8. Beatty PA and Gange JJ: Neuropsychological aspects of multiple sclerosis. J Nerv Ment Dis 164:42–50, 1977.

9. Bergin JD: Rapidly progressing dementia in disseminated sclerosis. J Neurol Neurosurg Psychiatry 20:285–292, 1957.

10. Beyerl B and Black PM: Posttraumatic hydrocephalus. Neurosurgery 15: 257–261, 1984.

11. Black PM: Idiopathic normal-pressure hydrocephalus. J Neurosurg 52:371–377, 1980.

12. Black PM, Ojemann RG, and Tzouras A: CSF shunts for dementia, incontinence and gait disturbance. Clin Neurosurg 32:632–651, 1985.

13. Bond MR: Neurobehavioral sequelae of closed head injury. In Grant I and Adams KH (eds): Neuropsychological Assessment of Neuropsychiatric Disorders. Oxford University Press, New York, 1986, pp 348–373.

14. Borgesen SE and Gjerris F: The predictive value of conductance to outflow of CSF in normal pressure hydrocephalus. Brain 105:65–86, 1982.

15. Bourgeois BFD, Prensky AL, Palkes HS, Talent BK, and Busch SG: Intelligence in epilepsy: A prospective study in children. Ann Neurol 14:438–444, 1983.

16. Bradley WG, Whittemore AR, Kortman KE, et al: Marked cerebrospinal fluid void: indicator of successful shunt in patients with suspected normal-pressure hydrocephalus. Radiology 178:459–466, 1991.

17. Brasey DL, Fankhauser H, and de Tribolet N: Normal pressure hydrocephalus in adults. Analysis of results and complications following ventriculocardiac derivation. Schweiz Med Wochenschr 118:919–923, 1988.

18. Bridgman PA, Malanut BL, Sperling MR, Saykin AJ, and O'Connor MJ: Memory during subclinical hippocampal seizures. Neurology 39:853–856, 1989.

19. Brooks DN: Wechsler memory scale performance and its relationship to brain damage after severe closed head injury. J Neurol Neurosurg Psychiatry 39:593–601, 1976.

20. Cheek WR and Taveras JM: Thalamic tumors. J Neurosurg 24:505–512, 1966.

21. Clarfield AM and Davis MB: Normal-pressure hydrocephalus: Saga or swamp? JAMA 262:2592–2593, 1989.

22. Corsellis JAN, Bruton CJ, and Browne DF: The aftermatch of boxing. Psychol Med 3:270–303, 1973.

23. Cotrell SS and Wilson SAK: The affective symptomatology of disseminated sclerosis. Neurology and Psychopathology 7:1–30, 1926.

24. Couch JR and Weiss SA: Gliomatosis cerebri. Neurology 24:504–511, 1974.

25. Crockard HA, Hanlon K, Duda EE, and Mullan JF: Hydrocephalus as a cause of dementia: Evaluation by computerized tomography and intracranial pressure monitoring. J Neurol Neurosurg Psychiatry 40:736–740, 1977.

26. Dam AM: Epilepsy and neuron loss in the hippocampus. Epilepsia 21:617–629, 1980.

27. Daniels AR, Chokroverty S, and Barron KD: Thalamic degeneration, dementia, and seizures. Inappropriate ADH secretion associated with bronchogenic carcinoma. Arch Neurol 21:15–24, 1969.

28. Davis BD, Fernandez F, Adams F, et al: Diagnosis of dementia in cancer patients. Psychosomatics 28:175–179, 1987.

29. DeAngelis L, Delattre J-Y, and Posner JB: Radiation-induced dementia in patients cured of brain metastases. Neurology 39:789–796, 1989.

30. DeMol J: Neuropsychological symptomatology in normal pressure hydrocephalus. Schweiz Arch Neurol Psychiatr 137:33–45, 1986.

31. Dikmen S and Matthews CG: Effect of major motor seizure frequency upon cognitive-intellectual functions in adults. Epilepsia 18:21–29, 1977.

32. Dikmen S, Matthews CG, and Harley

JP: Effect of early versus late onset of major motor epilepsy on cognitive-intellectual performance: Further considerations. Epilepsia 18:31–36, 1977.

33. Dodrill CB and Wilkus RJ: Relationships between intelligence and electroencephalographic epileptiform activity in adult epileptics. Neurology 26:525–531, 1976.

34. Dodrill CB and Wilensky AJ: Neuropsychological abilities before and after 5 years of stable antiepileptic drug therapy. Epilepsia 33:327–334, 1992.

35. Drlicek M, Grisold W, Liszka U, Hitzenberger P, and Machacek E: Angiotropic lymphoma (malignant angioendotheliomatosis) presenting with rapidly progressive dementia. Acta Neuropathol (Berl) 82:533–535, 1991.

36. Ekbon K, Greitz T, and Kugelberg E: Hydrocephalus due to ectasia of the basilar artery. J Neurol Sci 8:465–477, 1969.

37. Engel J Jr, Kuhl DE, Phelps ME, and Mazziotta JC: Interictal cerebral glucose metabolism in partial epilepsy and its relation to EEG changes. Ann Neurol 12:510–517, 1982.

38. Engel J Jr: Pathological correlates of focal temporal lobe hypometabolism in man. Epilepsia 22:236, 1981.

39. Estanol BV: Gait apraxia in communicating hydrocephalus. J Neurol Neurosurg Psychiatry 44:305–308, 1981.

40. Feldman E, Bromfield E, Naria B, Pasternak GW, and Posner JB: Hydrocephalic dementia and spinal cord tumor. Report of a case and review of the literature. Arch Neurol 43:714–718, 1986.

41. Filley CM, Franklin GM, Heaton RK, and Rosenberg NL: White matter dementia. Clinical disorders and implications. Neuropsychiatry Neuropsychol Behav Neurol 1:239–254, 1989.

42. Filley CM, Heaton RK, Nelson LM, Burks JS, and Franklin GM: A comparison of dementia in Alzheimer's disease and multiple sclerosis. Arch Neurol 46:157–161, 1989.

43. Fisher CM: The clinical picture in occult hydrocephalus. Clin Neurosurg 24:270–284, 1977.

44. Fisher CM: Hydrocephalus as a cause of disturbances of gait in the elderly. Neurology 32:1358–1363, 1982.

45. Fisher JM: Cognitive and behavioral consequences of closed head injury. Semin Neurol 5:197–201, 1985.

46. Foltz EL and Blanks JP: Symptomatic low intracranial pressure in shunted hydrocephalus. J Neurosurg 68:401–408, 1988.

47. Forrest DM and Cooper DGW: Complications of ventriculoatrial shunts. J Neurol 29:506–512, 1968.

48. Franklin GM, Heston RK, Nelson LM, Filley CM, and Seibert C: Correlation of neuropsychological and MRI findings in chronic/progressive multiple sclerosis. Neurology 38:1826–1829, 1988.

49. Franklin GM, Nelson LM, Filley CM, and Heston RK: Cognitive loss in multiple sclerosis. Case reports and review of the literature. Arch Neurol 46:162–167, 1989.

50. Geschwind N: The mechanism of normal pressure hydrocephalus. J Neurol Sci 7:481–493, 1968.

51. Giordani B, Sackellares JC, Miller S, et al: Improvement in neuropsychological performance in patients with refractory seizures after intensive diagnostic and therapeutic intervention. Neurology 33:489–493, 1983.

52. Gjerris F, Borgesen SE, Sorensen PS, et al: Resistance to cerebrospinal outflow and intracranial pressure in patients with hydrocephalus after subarachnoid hemorrhage. Acta Neurochir (Wien) 88:79–86, 1987.

53. Glaser GH and Pincus JH: Limbic encephalitis. J Nerv Ment Dis 149:59–67, 1969.

54. Goldberg ID, Bloomer WD, and Dawson DM: Nervous system toxic effects of cancer therapy. JAMA 247:1437–1441, 1982.

55. Graff-Radford NR, and Godersky JC: Idiopathic normal pressure hydrocephalus and systemic hypertension. Neurology 36:868–871, 1987.

56. Graff-Radford NR, Godersky JC, and Jones MP: Variables predicting surgi-

cal outcome in symptomatic hydro-cephalus in the elderly. Neurology 39:1601–1604, 1989.

57. Gronwall D and Wrightson P: Cumulative effect of concussion. Lancet 2:995–997, 1975.

58. Gustafson L and Hagberg B: Recovery in hydrocephalic dementia after shunt operation. J Neurol Neurosurg Psychiatry 41:940–947, 1978.

59. Haan J and Thomeer RT: Predictive value of temporary external lumbar drainage in normal pressure hydrocephalus. Neurosurgery 22:388–391, 1988.

60. Hakim S and Adams RD: The special clinical problem of symptomatic hydrocephalus with normal cerebrospinal fluid pressure. Observations on cerebrospinal fluid hydrodynamics. J Neurol Sci 2:307, 1965.

61. Halligan FR, Reznikoff M, Friedman HP, and LaRocca NG: Cognitive dysfunction and change in multiple sclerosis. J Clin Psychol 44:540–548, 1988.

62. Harrison MJG: Dementia due to tumors of the corpus callosum. Postgrad Med J 60:321–323, 1984.

63. Hartmann A and Alberti E: Differentiation of communicating hydrocephalus and presenile dementia by continuous recording of cerebrospinal fluid pressure. J Neurol Neurosurg Psychiatry 40:630–640, 1977.

64. Huber SJ, Paulson GW, Shuttleworth EC, et al: Magnetic resonance imaging correlates of dementia in multiple sclerosis. Arch Neurol 44:732–736, 1987.

65. Hughes CP, Siegel BA, Coxe WS, et al: Adult idiopathic communicating hydrocephalus with and without shunting. J Neurol Neurosurg Psychiatry 41:961–971, 1978.

66. Ines DF and Markand ON: Epileptic seizures and abnormal electroencephalographic findings in hydrocephalus and their relation to the shunting procedures. Electroencephalogr Clin Neurophysiol 42:761–768, 1977.

67. Jacobs L, Conti D, Kinkel WR, and Manning EJ: Normal-pressure hydrocephalus. JAMA 235:510–512, 1976.

68. Jagust WJ, Friedland RP, and Budinger TF: Positron emission tomography with fluoro-deoxyglucose differentiates normal pressure hydrocephalus from Alzheimer-type dementia. J Neurol Neurosurg Psychiatry 48:1091, 1985.

69. Jellinger K: Neuropathological aspects of dementia resulting from abnormal blood and cerebrospinal fluid dynamics. Acta Neurol Belg 76:83–90, 1976.

70. Jennett B: Assessment of the severity of head injury. J Neurol Neurosurg Psychiatry 39:647–655, 1976.

71. Katzman R: Normal pressure hydrocephalus. In Wells CE (ed): Dementia, Ed 2. FA Davis, Philadelphia, 1977, pp 69–92.

72. Katzman R and Hussey F: A simple constant-infusion manometric test for measurement of CSF absorption. Neurology 20:534–544, 1970.

73. Keschner M, Bender M, and Strauss I: Mental symptoms in cases of tumor of the temporal lobe. Arch Neurol Psychiatry 35:572–596, 1936.

74. Knight RSG, Anslow P, and Theaker JM: Neoplastic angioendotheliosis: A case of subacute dementia with unusual cerebral CT appearances and a review of the literature. J Neurol Neurosurg Psychiatry 50:1022–1028, 1987.

75. Knutsson E and Lying-Tunnell U: Gait apraxia in normal pressure hydrocephalus. Neurology 35:155, 1985.

76. Korsager S, Laursen B, and Mortensen TM: Dementia and central nervous system involvement in chronic lymphocytic leukaemia. Scandinavian Journal of Haematology 29:283–286, 1982.

77. Kosteljanetz M: CSF dynamics and pressure-volume relationships in communicating hydrocephalus. J Neurosurg 64:45–52, 1986.

78. Koto A, Rosenberg G, Zingesser LH, Horoupian D, and Katzman R: Syndrome of normal pressure hydrocephalus: Possible relation to hypertensive and arteriosclerotic vasculopathy. J Neurol Neurosurg Psychiatry 40:73–79, 1977.

79. LeMay M and Hochberg FH: Ventricular differences between hydrostatic hydrocephalus and hydrocephalus *ex vacuo* by computed tomography. Neuroradiology 17:191–195, 1979.

80. Lesser RP, Lüders H, Wyllie E, Dinner DS, and Morris HH III: Mental deterioration in epilepsy. Epilepsia (Suppl 2)27:S105–S123, 1986.

81. Levin HS, Grossman RG, and Kelly PJ: Aphasic disorder in patients with closed head injury. J Neurol Neurosurg Psychiatry 39:1062–1070, 1976.

82. Lishman WA: The psychiatric sequelae of head injury: A review. Psychol Med 3:304–318, 1973.

83. Lobosky JM, Vangilder JC, and Damasio AR: Behavioral manifestations of third ventricular colloid cysts. J Neurol Neurosurg Psychiatry 47:1075–1080, 1984.

84. Madow L and Alpers BJ: Encephalitic form of metastatic carcinoma. Archives of Neurology and Psychiatry 65:161–173, 1951.

85. Matsumoto T, Nagai H, Kasuga Y, and Kamiya K: Changes in intracranial pressure (ICP) pulse wave following hydrocephalus. Acta Neurochir (Wien) 82:50–56, 1986.

86. Matthews CG and Harley JP: Cognitive and motor-sensory performances in toxic and nontoxic epileptic subjects. Neurology 25:184–188, 1975.

87. Matthews WB, Acheson ED, Batchelor JR, and Weller RO: McAlpine's Multiple Sclerosis. Churchill Livingstone, New York, 1985, pp 233–278.

88. Mayeux R, Brandy J, Rosen J, and Benson FD: Interictal memory and language impairment in temporal lobe epilepsy. Neurology 30:120–125, 1980.

89. Mendez MF and Frey WH II: Multiple sclerosis dementia. Neurology 42:696, 1992.

90. Mendez MF, Underwood KL, Zander BA, Mastri AR, Sung JH, and Frey WH II: Risk factors in Alzheimer's disease: A clinicopathological study. Neurology 42:770–775, 1992.

91. Mulrow CD, Feussner JR, Williams BC, and Volcaty KA: The value of clinical findings in the detection of normal pressure hydrocephalus. J Gerontol 42:277–279, 1987.

92. Norstrup S, Christensen J, Gjerris F, et al: Cerebral blood flow in patients with normal-pressure hydrocephalus before and after shunting. J Neurosurg 66:379–387, 1987.

93. Nugent GR, Al-Mefty O, and Chou S: Communicating hydrocephalus as a cause of aqueductal stenosis. J Neurosurg 51:812–818, 1979.

94. Ohara S, Nagai H, Matsumoto T, and Banno T: MR imaging of CSF pulsatory flow and its relation to intracranial pressure. J Neurosurg 69:675–682, 1988.

95. O'Leary DS, Seidenberg M, Berent S, and Boll TJ: Effects of age of onset of tonic-clonic seizures on neuropsychological performance in children. Epilepsia 22:197–204, 1981.

96. Olmos-Lau N, Ginsberg MD, and Geller JB: Aphasia in multiple sclerosis. Neurology 27:623–626, 1977.

97. Oppenheimer DR: Microscopic lesions in the brain following head injury. J Neurol Neurosurg Psychiatry 31:299–306, 1968.

98. Parry SW, Schuhmacher JF, and Llewellyn RC: Abdominal pseudocysts and ascites formation after ventriculoperitoneal shunt procedures. J Neurosurg 43:476–480, 1975.

99. Payne EE: Brains of boxers. Neurochirurgia (Stuttg) 14:173–188, 1968.

100. Petersen B and Dam M: Memory disturbances in epileptic patients. Acta Neurol Scand (Suppl 109)74:11–14, 1986.

101. Petersen RC, Mokri B, and Laws ER Jr: Surgical treatment of idiopathic hydrocephalus in elderly patients. Neurology 35:307–311, 1985.

102. Peyser JM, Edwards KR, Poser CM, and Filskov SB: Cognitive function in patients with multiple sclerosis. Arch Neurol 37:577–579, 1980.

103. Price TRP and Tucker GJ: Psychiatric and behavioral manifestations of normal pressure hydrocephalus. J Nerv Ment Dis 164:51–55, 1977.

104. Prigatano G, Fordyce D, Zeiner H, et al: Neuropsychological rehabilitation after closed head injury in young

adults. J Neurol Neurosurg Psychiatry 217:505–513, 1984.

105. Rao SM, Leo GJ, Bernandin L, and Unverzagt F: Cognitive dysfunction in multiple sclerosis: I. Frequency, patterns, and prediction. Neurology 41:685–691, 1991.

106. Rao SM, Leo GJ, Haughton VM, St. Aubin-Faubert P, and Bernardin BS: Correlation of magnetic resonance imaging with neuropsychological testing in multiple sclerosis. Neurology 39:161–166, 1989.

107. Rausch R, Lieb JP, and Crandall PH: Neuropsychologic correlates of depth spike activity in epileptic patients. Arch Neurol 35:699–705, 1978.

108. Roberts GW, Allsop D, and Bruton C: The occult aftermath of boxing. J Neurol Neurosurg Psychiatry 53:373–378, 1990.

109. Rottenberg DA, Horten B, Kim JH, and Posner JB: Progressive white matter destruction following irradiation of an extracranial neoplasm. Ann Neurol 8:76–78, 1979.

110. Rudelli R, Strom JO, Welch PT, and Ambler MW: Posttraumatic premature Alzheimer's disease. Neuropathologic findings and pathogenetic considerations. Arch Neurol 39:570–575, 1982.

111. Sakoda TH, Maxwell JA, and Brackett CE: Intestinal volvulus secondary to a ventriculoperitoneal shunt. J Neurosurg 35:95–96, 1971.

112. Smith JS and Kiloh LG: The investigation of dementia: Results in 200 consecutive admissions. Lancet 2:824–827, 1981.

113. So NK, O'Neill BP, Frytak S, Eagan RT, Earnest F, and Lee RE: Delayed leukoencephalopathy in survivors with small cell lung cancer. Neurology 37:1198–1201, 1987.

114. Soelberg, Sorensen S, Jansen EC, and Gjerris F: Motor disturbances in normal-pressure hydrocephalus. Arch Neurol 43:34–38, 1986.

115. St-Laurent M: Normal pressure hydrocephalus in geriatric medicine: A challenge. J Geriatr Psychiatry Neurol 1:163–168, 1988.

116. Stam FC, Wigboldus JM, and Botts G Th A M: Presenile dementia—a form of Lafora disease. J Am Geriatr Soc 28:237–240, 1980.

117. Strauss I and Keschner M: Mental symptoms in cases of tumor of the frontal lobe. Archives of Neurology and Psychiatry 33:986–1007, 1935.

118. Strich SJ and Oxon DM: Shearing of nerve fibers as a cause of brain damage due to head injury. Lancet 2:443–448, 1961.

119. Sudarsky L and Simon S: Gait disorder in late-life hydrocephalus. Arch Neurol 44:263–267, 1987.

120. Sullivan P, Petti D, and Barbaccia J: Head trauma and age of onset of dementia of the Alzheimer type. JAMA 257:2289–2290, 1987.

121. Surridge D: An investigation into some psychiatric aspects of multiple sclerosis. Br J Psychiatry 115:749–764, 1969.

122. Symon L and Hinzpeter T: The enigma of normal pressure hydrocephalus: Tests to select patients for surgery and to predict shunt function. Clin Neurosurg 24:285–315, 1977.

123. Theodore WH and Gendelman S: Meningeal carcinomatosis. Arch Neurol 38:696–699, 1981.

124. Thomsen AM, Borgesen SE, Bruhn P, and Gjerris F: Prognosis of dementia in normal-pressure hydrocephalus after a shunt operation. Ann Neurol 20:304–310, 1986.

125. Thomsen IV: Late outcome of very severe blunt head trauma: A 10–15 year second follow-up. J Neurol Neurosurg Psychiatry 47:260–268, 1984.

126. Trimble MR: Dementia in epilepsy. Acta Neurol Scand (Suppl)99:99–104, 1984.

127. Trimble MR: Anticonvulsant drugs and cognitive function: A review of the literature. Epilepsia (Suppl 3)28:537–545, 1987.

128. Trimble MR: Cognitive hazards of seizure disorders. Epilepsia (Suppl 1)29:519–524, 1988.

129. Trimble MR and Thompson PJ: Neuropsychological aspects of epilepsy. In Grant I and Adams KH (eds): Neuropsychological Assessment of Neuropsychiatric Disorders. Oxford Uni-

versity, New York, 1986, pp 321–346.

130. Udvarhelyi GB, Wood JH, James AE Jr, and Bartelt D: Results and complications in 55 shunted patients with normal pressure hydrocephalus. Surg Neurol 3:271–275, 1975.

131. Unterharnscheidt, FJ: Injuries due to boxing and other sports. In Vinken PJ and Bruyn GW (eds): Handbook of Clinical Neurology, Vol 23. Elsevier, New York, 1975, pp 531–567.

132. Vallarta JM, Bell DB, and Reichart A: Progressive encephalopathy due to chronic hydantoin intoxication. Am J Dis Child 128:27–34, 1974.

133. Van den Burg W, Van Zomeren AH, Minderhoud JM, Prange AJ, and Meijer NSA: Cognitive impairment in patients with multiple sclerosis and mild physical disability. Arch Neurol 4:494–501, 1987.

134. Vanneste J and Hyman R: Non-tumoral aqueduct stenosis and normal pressure hydrocephalus in the elderly. J Neurol Neurosurg Psychiatry 49:529–535, 1986.

135. Vanneste J, Augustijn P, Davies GAG, Dirven C, and Tan WF: Normal-pressure hydrocephalus: Is cysternography still useful in selecting patients for a shunt? Arch Neurol 49:366–370, 1992.

136. Vanneste J, Augustijn P, Dirven C, Tan WF, and Goednart ZD: Shunting normal-pressure hydrocephalus: Do the benefits outweigh the risks? A multicenter study and literature review. Neurology 42:54–59, 1992.

137. Violon A and DeMol J: Psychological sequelae after head traumas in adults. Acta Neurochir (Wien) 85:96–102, 1987.

138. Wikkelso C, Andersson H, Blomstrand C, Lingquist G, and Svendsen P: Normal pressure hydrocephalus. Predictive value of the cerebrospinal fluid tap-test. Acta Neurol Scand 73:566–573, 1986.

139. Yamakawa H, Ohkuma A, Hattori T, Niikawa S, and Kobayashi H: Primary intracranial arachnoid cyst in the elderly: A survey of 39 cases. Acta Neurochir (Wien) 113:42–47, 1991.

Chapter 12

COGNITIVE IMPAIRMENT IN PSYCHIATRIC SYNDROMES

Peter V. Rabins, M.D., M.P.H.,
Godfrey D. Pearlson, M.B.,
  B.S., and
Milton E. Strauss, Ph.D.

FUNCTIONAL MENTAL ILLNESSES WITH COGNITIVE IMPAIRMENT CONDITIONS WITH COGNITIVE SYMPTOMS WITHOUT FRANK DEMENTIA

Emil Kraepelin[31] established a hierarchical diagnostic tradition 80 years ago that still persists in modern classification systems such as DSM-III and ICD-9. This approach posits a distinction between "organic" and "functional" psychiatric disorders and places the organic disorders above the functional in the hierarchy. It implies absolute dissociations between these two categories, suggests that functional disorders are not caused by structural brain abnormalities, and excludes the possibility that disorders at these two levels can exist simultaneously.

The distinction between the "organic" and the "functional" continues to have clinical use. It emphasizes the treatable nature of disorders that are characterized as functional, for example, and pushes the clinician to find such disorders. Nonetheless, many lines of evidence now suggest that the major mental illnesses are associated with an altered brain physiology and structure. It should not be surprising,

therefore, that disorders in the organic and functional realms sometimes coexist and confound the clinician who demands a dichotomy between them.

The concept of "pseudodementia" illustrates the strengths and weaknesses of the hierarchical approach. The concept has the strength of alerting clinicians to the fact that some patients who complain of difficulty in thinking or who have symptoms of dementia may suffer from a disorder that can be treated with currently available somatic or psychotherapeutic techniques. On the other hand, the name implies an imitation of dementia and suggests that when an apparent dementia is found in the setting of a functional or hysterical psychiatric condition, the disorder of cognition is bogus.

The term pseudodementia was first used by Madden and colleagues[35] in 1952 to describe a group of elderly individuals with depression and other psychiatric illnesses who had complaints and symptoms of cognitive impairment but who responded to treatment for depression. The term was popularized by Kiloh[29] in an influential paper entitled "Pseudo-dementia." He noted that a variety of psychiatric disorders could present with symptoms or signs of cognitive impairment. He presented 11 case examples of patients who suffered from depression, mania, schizophrenia, and hysteria/malingering, showing that several different psychiatric disorders could be associated with poor cognitive functioning or complaints of cognitive difficulty, and that a careful clinical examination could identify such patients.

The concept that depression and other psychiatric disorders are important in the differential diagnosis of dementia was furthered by the landmark study of Marsden and Harrison.[36] These authors demonstrated that 20% of patients presenting for evaluation of cognitive difficulties suffered from a potentially treatable disorder and that depression and other psychiatric disorders were very common among these individuals with complaints of cognitive impairment. Other studies[45,61] highlighted the clinical relevance of this observation, demonstrating that patients were being misdiagnosed as irreversibly demented, when, in fact, they were suffering from a functional "psychiatric disorder." Similar findings have been reported by others, although the rates of "reversible" or incorrectly diagnosed dementia have declined in recent years. (See Rabins[52] for a review of this literature.)

The most influential and clearest presentation of the view that functional disorder can *mimic* dementia is contained in the work of Wells.[72,73] He, too, emphasized that a variety of psychiatric disorders could present as cognitive impairment and conceptualized these as "imitations" of cognitive disorder rather than true dementias. His listing of symptoms that identify individuals with pseudodementia[72] has been widely cited.

This chapter examines two groupings of syndromes in which cognitive impairment or complaints thereof coexist with symptoms usually conceptualized as psychiatric: (1) diseases traditionally seen as functional mental illness, that is, affective disorder and schizophrenia; and (2) conditions in which the complaint of cognitive impairment is present but signs of dementia are not present or are imitated. The chapter also discusses in passing disorders in which brain pathology is clearly present, such as Alzheimer's disease (AD) and Huntington's disease (HD)[39] and in which depressive symptoms are seen as secondary to this primary process. The allocation of attention to these different conditions will match the frequency and difficulty of the problems faced by clinicians. Thus more attention will be devoted to affect, less to schizophrenia, and even less to hysteria.

FUNCTIONAL MENTAL ILLNESSES WITH COGNITIVE IMPAIRMENT

Affective Disorder

Interactions between mood and cognitive functioning have been noted since the 10th century, when the Arabic physician Ibn Imran[25] noted that some depressives had difficulty thinking clearly. Similar observations were made in 1621 by Burton,[9] in 1883 by Mairet,[2] and at the beginning of this century by Kraepelin.[31]

In the late 1970s, the view that pseudodementia was a treatable form of dementia was challenged in two provocatively titled articles by Liston[34] ("Occult Presenile Dementia") and Shraberg[54] ("The Myth of Pseudo-Dementia"). Liston demonstrated that some patients who presented in late life with depressive symptoms were found at follow-up to be suffering from irreversible progressive dementia. Shraberg presented the case of an individual who was found to have both depressive symptoms and cognitive disorder and who showed no improvement in cognition despite successful treatment of her affective disorder. Both these authors suggested that depression presenting with cognitive impairment could be an early manifestation of a progressive irreversible dementia.

Others[37,38,57,58] have suggested that

there may be two distinct explanations for coexisting depression and dementia. According to this view, coexisting depression and cognitive impairment can occur when (1) depression is a symptom of AD, in which case the depression would respond to treatment, but the cognitive disorder would not; or (2) the cognitive disorder is a symptom of depression, in which case both the depression and the cognitive disorder would respond to antidepressant therapy.

Several groups have proposed criteria to identify patients in the second group, the reversible dementia of depression, and to distinguish them from patients with irreversible cognitive deficits. Both treatment response[52,57] and long-term follow-up[32,52,55] have been used to validate these criteria. One group[49] reported that 50% of 16 inpatients with concurrent depression and cognitive disorder responded to treatment for depression, whereas others[53] found that 80% of patients diagnosed as having depression-induced cognitive disorder were cognitively normal at 2-year follow-up (three subjects had died). These findings demonstrate that patients with reversible dementia of depression

do exist, at least when normal cognition at short-term follow-up is used as the validating criterion. In contrast, another researcher[32] reported that 20 of 22 individuals with coexisting dementia and depression were irreversibly demented at 7- to 15-year follow-up. These data suggest that long-term (greater than 5 years) follow-up studies will be necessary to determine whether most patients with concomitant depression and dementia are manifesting very early irreversible dementia at first presentation (that is, whether most patients fall into group 1).

The work of Reding and co-workers[56] presents the clearest data base upon which to determine the frequency (prevalence) of reversible dementia due to depression and its short-term outcome. The results of their 1985 report are presented in Figure 12–1. They first evaluated 225 individuals who presented to a memory disorder clinic. Forty-four patients (20%) were found not to be demented, a majority of whom were thought to be depressed. On 30-month (mean) follow-up, however, more than half of this depressed group had developed an irreversible dementia. The researchers retrospectively identified the

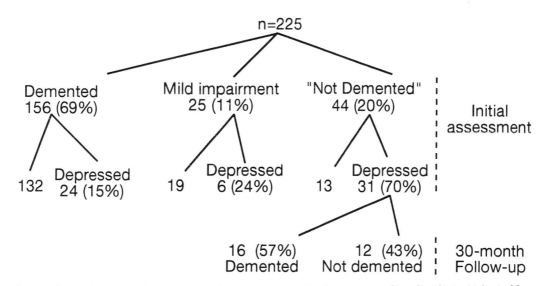

Figure 12–1. Outcome of evaluations of patients presenting to a memory disorder clinic. (Adapted from Reding et al,[56] p. 895.)

presence of focal neurologic findings, low scores on cognitive testing, the presence of cerebrovascular disease, and becoming delirious from tricyclic antidepressants as predictors of irreversible dementia. The 57% rate of dementia they found in outpatients was similar to the rate reported by Reynolds and associates[60] in psychiatric inpatients.

PATHOPHYSIOLOGY

The pathophysiology of the cognitive disorder in individuals with the reversible dementia syndrome of depression is unclear, and opinions are divided. Quantitative features of performance on neuropsychological tests suggest a physiologic basis, in that the patterns of failure are different in the depressed and the dementia group.[55,74] One useful schema subdivides information processing into effortful and automatic processing; effortful cognition involves concentration and attention, whereas automatic information processing proceeds without conscious effort.[70] Weingartner and colleagues[14] have reported that abnormalities of "effortful cognition," rather than of automatic cognitive processes, underlie the memory impairments of depression, whereas the memory disorder of AD is more generalized and includes disruption of both kinds of processes.[70,71]

Complaints of memory impairment are common among depressed persons, but objective memory deficits are found principally in the severely depressed.[26] Because severely depressed patients may not be fully engaged in psychological testing, the appearance of deficits on memory testing may reflect unwillingness to report the recall or recognition of a test item. Patients with irreversible dementia may occasionally produce irrelevant errors, but this does not seem to occur in reversible dementias associated with depression.[74] Examination of memory using methods of signal detection theory generally suggests that the pure memory functions of depressed patients are intact, but that depressives do poorly on formal testing because they are overly cautious.[20,26,42] A true recognition-memory deficit can be demonstrated among depressives under some testing conditions, however.[68]

It has also been proposed that cognitive disorder in depressives can be conceptualized as a "subcortical dementia."[10,19,40] This hypothesis rests on the demonstration in depression of disordered performance in tests of memory, concept formation, motor speed, and persistence, with preserved language function and praxis. Similar patterns of dysfunction are found in HD, Parkinson's disease, and normal-pressure hydrocephalus, disorders in which subcortical neuropathology predominates and in which frontal subcortical pathways are known to be interrupted.[18,40]

Support for the hypothesis that structural brain dysfunction underlies the reversible dementia syndrome of depression is offered by recent work of Pearlson and associates,[49] which demonstrated that depressed elderly patients with cognitive disorder fully responsive to treatment with tricyclic antidepressants or electroconvulsive therapy have enlarged ventricles and lower CT-scan attenuation numbers, compared with age-matched normals. These CT-attenuation-number abnormalities were more marked in cognitively impaired depressives than in cognitively normal depressives. Because cognitively impaired depressives tended to have lower education levels than the age-matched cognitively intact depressives and age-matched normals, Pearlson and colleagues were unable to distinguish between the hypotheses that the cognitive disorder was a lifelong problem unmasked by the depression, or that it was a late-life problem caused or predisposed to by poor education.

The etiology of depression manifesting for the first time in AD is likewise unknown. Recent preliminary studies demonstrating that depressed AD patients are more likely to have a family history of affective disorder[50] suggest links with the etiology of idiopathic affective disorder.

Several studies[62,76,77] have suggested the patients with AD who are depressed in life may demonstrate, at autopsy, greater cell loss in the locus ceruleus. Changes in raphe nuclei and substantia nigra may also occur. Such studies should be considered preliminary, particularly insofar as sample sizes are limited, but they support notions of a bioaminergic basis for depression, as has been suggested for affective disorders not associated with cognitive impairment. The most effective antidepressants, tricyclics and monoamine oxidase inhibitors, probably act by increasing bioamine levels in the brain.

DIAGNOSIS

Inasmuch as both depression-induced cognitive disorder and depression secondary to irreversible dementia are common, how can the clinician distinguish them? Several studies have examined this question. Wells[72] listed a total of 22 criteria that he thought differentiated pseudodementia from true dementia. McHugh and Folstein[39] also listed clinical criteria that they suggested would distinguish between the two. Neither presented empirical validation of their suggestions, however.

To validate the criteria proposed by Wells,[72] Rabins and Moberg (unpublished data) devised a 17-item questionnaire that operationalized the items Wells proposed. A trained psychometrician, blind to the hypothesis of the study and to the patients' diagnoses, examined 35 patients with depression and cognitive disorder and 25 patients with clinically diagnosed irreversible dementia. Rabins assigned the patients to these groups using previously published criteria.[52] Table 12–1 also lists the criteria proposed by various other authors. They suggest that a careful clinical assessment should be able to distinguish, with acceptable sensitivity and specificity, between patients likely to have remission of both affective and cognitive symptoms, and patients who will remain demented in spite of adequate treatment for depression.

The first column of Table 12–1 lists the four criteria proposed by Wells[72] that were validated by Rabins and Moberg's study to distinguish between reversible dementia of depression and irreversible dementia. The dexamethasone suppression test is not included because it lacks specificity.[65] Sleep electroencephalographic (EEG) studies may prove to be useful in the future,[80] in that shortened rapid-eye-movement (REM) latency discriminates affective disorder patients from those with primary dementia, but such studies remain a research tool at present.

In summary, coexisting depression

Table 12–1 VALIDATED CRITERIA IDENTIFYING REVERSIBLE DEMENTIA DUE TO DEPRESSION

Wells[72] (1979)	Rabins[53] (1984)	Reding[56] (1985)	Reynolds[60] (1986)
Patient complains frequently of memory loss	Past history of depression	Lack of cerebrovascular, extrapyramidal, or spinocerebellar disease	MMSE >21
Patient ephasizes disability	Subacute onset (<6 months)	Modified HIS <4	HDRS >21
Memory loss for recent and remote events is equally severe	Delusions of guilt, self-blame, hopelessness	MSQ >8	Sleep efficiency <75%
Memory loss for specific period or events	Appetite loss	Haycox <7	
	Reports depressed mood	Not delirious on tricyclic antidepressants	

IIIS = Hachinski Ischemic Score; MSQ = Mental Status Questionnaire; MMS = Mini-Mental State Examination; HDRS = Hamilton Depression Rating Scale.

and cognitive disorder can be seen as resulting from three distinct syndromes: (1) secondary major depression that complicates an irreversible structural dementia, (2) major depression with secondary reversible cognitive difficulties that improve with the treatment of depression and that do not progress, and (3) an imitation of dementia, either a hysterical dementia (discussed later in this chapter) or a hypochondriacal delusional depression in which the patient is convinced that he or she is demented, but is cognitively normal when examined. Preliminary data suggest that the second group has structural brain abnormalities that are unmasked by normal age-associated brain changes and by the depression. A similar hypothesis was suggested by Mairet a century ago (see Berrios[2]).

Recognizing that coexisting depression and dementia can have several etiologies is important, because treatment differs depending on the underlying syndrome. It is also important at a conceptual level: the relative frequency of coexisting dementia and depression in late life suggests that the neuromechanisms underlying emotion and cognition interact directly in the brain. Thus, further study of individuals in whom both cognitive and "functional" disorders exist is one research strategy by which these interrelationships within the brain can be identified. Our knowledge is too limited to permit the use of a simple algorithm for differential diagnosis, but the key conceptual and practical issues reviewed here should be considered in caring for patients with these conditions.

Schizophrenia

The schizophrenic syndrome is of unknown etiology and mechanism, is generally chronic, and is found in all cultures. It lacks a defining pathognomonic symptom and is currently defined only on the basis of cross-sectional symptoms and course. Inclusionary and exclusionary criteria are now the object of greater consensus than in the past.

The schizophrenic syndrome can begin at any age but often has its onset in adolescence or early adulthood. Population prevalence is approximately 1%. Schizophrenic symptoms are often spoken of as belonging to two broad classes: "positive" symptoms (delusions, hallucinations, thought disorder), which represent the addition of new features to mental life, and "negative" symptoms, which represent a loss or diminution of normal psychological capabilities, including goal-directedness, close emotional involvement with others, or range of emotional expression. Positive symptoms may emerge suddenly in apparently normal individuals or evolve more slowly. None of the above symptoms is exclusive to schizophrenia, however; they can occur in delirium, dementia, or major affective disorder.

Negative symptoms generally emerge in the course of recurrent acute episodes. They can lead to chronic disability, the state of deterioration to which Kraepelin[31] drew attention in distinguishing schizophrenia from affective disorder.

Older textbooks on schizophrenia frequently refer to a "deficit state," "residual state," or "state of psychological deterioration." These terms probably refer to a combination of two phenomena, negative symptoms and cognitive impairment (to which may be added the effects of institutionalization). Cognitive impairment occurring in schizophrenia was formerly explained as an artifact of reduced concentration and attention due to distraction by hallucinations, or as a generalized deficit due to reduced motivation and cooperation.[66] Among the mental abnormalities present in patients with schizophrenia that produce behaviors seen in demented individuals are concrete thinking, perseveration, and what Lishman[33] refers to as a "buffoonery syndrome," that is, inappropriate and facile behavior. After possible effects of neuroleptics and the distraction by positive symptoms are accounted for, however, deficits on a wide range of neuropsychological tests can be demonstrated. These deficits are especially prominent on conceptual tasks and with procedures that require shifts of attention of cognitive "set."

The degree of "generalized deficit"[11] in schizophrenia is related to the premorbid adjustment of patients and is greater in those with a history of poor psychosocial adaptive skills and chronic illness. Indeed, schizophrenics, particularly chronic patients, perform much like patients with structural brain lesions on standard neuropsychological test batteries.[21-23] Recently, more direct evidence (as discussed below) has emerged to support the contention that the negative symptoms and mild dementia of the schizophrenic syndrome are biologically rooted in underlying structural and functional cortical and subcortical abnormalities.

The negative symptoms of schizophrenia may be progressive and are likely to be present between episodes of florid illness. The extent to which the cognitive deficits of schizophrenia are progressive is unclear, principally because there are few well-controlled longitudinal studies.[24,66] The available data suggest that the cognitive deficits are partially reversible in some patients and stable in others,[13] although a small but significant proportion of patients with schizophrenia undergo severe deterioration and require long-term institutionalization.[3]

Recent years have seen an upsurge of interest in the negative symptoms of schizophrenia.[15] It is now thought that the negative-symptom complex in schizophrenia may be a part of the genetically inherited component of the disease.[15] Negative symptoms frequently fail to respond to treatment with neuroleptics to the same extent as do positive ones. Preliminary data, however, suggest that negative symptoms may be diminished by social intervention.

PATHOPHYSIOLOGY

Several studies suggest that negative symptoms may be associated with structural brain disease.[1,47] Andreasen and colleagues[1] found that increased ventricle-to-brain ratio (VBR) on CT scans in schizophrenics was associated with lower Mini-Mental State scores and a tendency to more negative symptoms. Other investigators have reported an association between cognitive deficit and VBR.[22] Pearlson and co-workers[47] found these ventricular measures to be associated with a greater number of negative symptoms and earlier onset of disease. Johnstone and colleagues[27] found that institutionalization had a relatively minor effect on negative symptoms and concluded that such deficits were an integral feature of schizophrenia. VBR abnormalities appear to be integral components of schizophrenia in a large proportion of cases; they are unaffected by the duration of the illness.[75] The links between structural brain abnormalities, negative symptoms, and cognitive impairments in schizophrenia are reinforced by the observation of poorer premorbid functioning and educational difficulties prior to first hospitalization in patients with negative symptoms.[51]

Recent research and theoretical analyses of the dementia of schizophrenia have focused on specific brain regions, especially frontal and temporal cortex.[30,69] Several lines of evidence suggest that frontal cortical dysfunction is a significant component of schizophrenia; these include neuropsychological examination,[30] CT studies,[63] EEG,[44] positron emission tomography (PET) deoxyglucose studies,[9] and cerebral blood flow studies with xenon 133.[69] Using the Wisconsin Card Sort Test (WCST) as an activating task for dorsolateral prefrontal cortex, researchers found that poor task performance in schizophrenics was correlated with reduced frontal blood flow.[69] Neuroleptic drug administration did not significantly affect flow or test performance.

The WCST is an abstract-reasoning and problem-solving task that is particularly sensitive to dorsolateral prefrontal lesions. (See Chapter 5.) Goldberg and co-workers[21] argued that the inability of the chronic schizophrenics they studied to learn the WCST even with direct instruction strongly implicated specific frontal deficits, because the individuals studied were able to learn a word list and were not demented as judged by Mini-Mental State scores. Mild memory deficits also have been identified on neuropsychological testing of schizophrenics, however.[11,30] The neurobehavioral significance of these deficits is supported by recent postmortem studies in schizophrenics,[4,76] which show abnormalities in temporolimbic areas that, in animals, have major connections to the prefrontal cortex.

DIAGNOSIS

Schizophrenic patients with marked negative symptoms may resemble individuals with frontal lobe disease or advanced dementia. A clinical presentation of blunted emotions, inappropriate behavior, lack of self-care, social breakdown, and poverty of ideas, combined with reduced motivation, inattention, and poor cooperation, can be compatible with any of these three syndromes.[33] A thorough history and examination should distinguish among them, however. In AD, for example, first-rank symptoms, such as thought broadcasting,[41] are rare, and visual hallucinations more common than auditory hallucinations, the reverse of the situation in schizophrenia. When delusional beliefs occur in AD, they are generally vague, unorganized, short-lived, and changeable, whereas those seen in schizophrenia are fixed and tend to be complex.[18]

As noted above, schizophrenia begins in the second or third decade in a majority of cases. Whether it can begin in late life has been a controversial issue. Kraepelin[31] accepted the possibility that a classic schizophrenic syndrome can begin in late life, and a long European research tradition[28] has supported this belief, as have more recent American[43,48,54] and European[6] studies. The late-onset condition is similar to early-onset schizophrenia in symptom profile, treatment response, and course, but late-onset cases have less thought disorder and less personality deterioration than do early-onset cases.

There is little information in the literature about the neuropsychological characteristics of late-onset schizophrenics. Cullom and associates[16,17] found no gross neuropsychological differences between late-onset schizophrenics and age-matched normals. This suggests that the conceptual abilities of late-onset schizophrenics may be more robust than those of early-onset cases, as would be expected given the previously discussed correlations between early age of onset, negative symptoms, and cognitive deficits. The patient's history is critical in the differential diagnosis of schizophrenia, particularly in the case of elderly patients, in whom identifiable central nervous system disease often presents with psychiatric symptomatology.[67] The history of cognitive deficit prior to the onset of hallucinations and/or delusions should alert the clinician to search for a neurologic disease causing the symptoms.

CONDITIONS WITH COGNITIVE SYMPTOMS WITHOUT FRANK DEMENTIA

Hysterical Dementia

Hysteria is defined as the imitation of a medical or psychiatric condition without conscious awareness. Hypochondriasis, in contrast, is defined as a persistent overconcern with bodily or psychological ill-health. Both can be conceptually distinguished from feigned or malingered disorders by virtue of the absence of conscious intention, although the determination of "intent" can be an exceedingly difficult matter.

According to Lishman,[33] "Of all the forms of pseudodementia, there is probably least difficulty in distinguishing the typical case of hysterical pseudodementia from true organic dementia. On occasion, however, there may be protracted difficulty." The diagnosis of a hysterical condition should be suspected when there is no medical or psychiatric condition (e.g., brain injury or depression) to explain the degree of cognitive impairment, and when the patient's expressed inabilities do not match his behavior. Inconsistency and fluctuation in disability also are common in hysterical dementia. The Ganser state, sometimes called "hysterical pseudostupidity," is an example: Answers are often patently absurd (e.g., denying knowledge of self or saying two plus two equals five). The syndrome, first described in prisoners, generally occurs in a setting in which the primary gain is evident.

The diagnosis of a psychogenic cognitive disorder may be confounded by the fact that patients with hysterical symptoms can have coexisting structural disease. For example, hysterical dementia is sometimes seen in individuals with mental retardation or a known brain injury. In such cases the previously identified deficits persist while the superimposed hysterical symptoms fluctuate, are "nonphysiologic," and can improve with suggestion.

Empirical investigations in imitated disorders of memory are rare. The verification of memory complaints as well as of suspicious sensory-perceptual symptoms can be approached through neuropsychological and psychophysical testing methods.[5,46] Qualitative differences between the memory failures of patients with amnesias associated with brain disease and those amnesias of apparently psychogenic origin are characterized by the preservation of "islands" of excellent memory in the latter and the limited temporal grading of anterograde memory deficits that they show. Careful neuropsychological evaluation can be particularly helpful in the differential diagnosis of such patients because of the heterogeneity in forms of memory failure in the dementias associated with brain disease.[5]

Age-Associated Memory Impairment

Age-associated memory impairment[60] (or benign senescent forgetfulness) is a term proposed to categorize individuals who complain about the mild changes in memory and cognition that occur with normal aging. (See also Chapters 1 and 4.) It does not progress to dementia in most individuals. Although self-reports of poor memory are common (and probably accurate) in late life, few individuals with normal memory changes present to clinicians for an assessment of it. Those who persist in identifying it as a problem once dementia has been ruled out might best be diagnosed as suffering from hypochondriasis. To our knowledge, no study has identified which individuals with complaints of memory disorder but no clinical or historical evidence of decline will go on to have dementia and which will not.

SUMMARY

This chapter has reviewed several syndromes traditionally seen as psychiatric in which cognitive disorder is present or imitated. The distinction between functional and structurally based cognitive impairments is not easily maintained for two of these disorders, schizophrenia and major depression. In schizophrenia, in which cognitive disorder may be an inherent feature of the disease, symptoms of dementia may be relatively enduring, whereas in major depression the dementia may be reversible. It is increasingly clear, though, that some patients with coexisting depression and dementia suffer from an irreversible progressive dementia in which depression is a secondary symptom.

A number of factors can influence cognitive performance in elderly or demented patients. In addition to depression, these include levels of premorbid social competence, intelligence, and education; socioeconomic status; and social history, especially of institutional care.[70] Careful neuropsychological evaluation can be helpful in difficult cases because of the qualitative differences in the forms of memory failure seen among the dementias and pseudodementias, but the difficulty of these differential diagnoses is epistemologic as well as clinical. (See Chapter 5.) The studies reviewed compare patients already assigned clinically to different diagnostic categories. In contrast, the clinician is faced with the task of categorizing (diagnosing) patients by presenting signs and symptoms. Unfortunately, these approaches are not complementary. Thus, the clinical use of these studies must be demonstrated by prospective studies of symptomatically diverse populations. The clinician must still rely on multiple sources of data (including past history, careful elucidation of current symptoms, neuropsychological testing, and appropriate laboratory tests) in the differential diagnosis of the conditions discussed here.

ACKNOWLEDGMENTS

Preparation of this chapter was supported in part by NIMH grants MH40843 (PR, GP), MH40391 (GP, MS), and MH40362 (MS); the American Federation for Aging Research (PR, GP); the T. Rowe and Eleanor Price Foundation; and a gift from Mrs. Samuel Hecht.

REFERENCES

1. Andreasen NC, Olsen SA, Dennert JW, and Smith MR: Ventricular enlargement in schizophrenia: Relationship to positive and negative symptoms. Am J Psychiatry 139:3, 1982.

2. Berrios G: "Depressive pseudodementia" or "melancholic dementia": A 19th century view. J Neurol Neurosurg Psychiatry 48:393–400, 1985.

3. Bleuler M: Long-term course of schizophrenic psychoses. Annual Review of the Schizophrenia Syndrome 4:435–453, 1976.

4. Bogerts B: Basal ganglia and limbic system pathology in schizophrenia. Arch Gen Psychiatry 42:784–791, 1985.

5. Brandt J: Malingering amnesia. In Rogers R (ed): Clinical Assessment of Malingering and Deception. Guilford Press, New York, 1988, pp 65–83.

6. Bridge TP and Wyatt RJ: Paraphrenia: Paranoid states of late life. I. European Research. J Am Geriatr Soc 28:193–200, 1980.

7. Brown R: Postmortem evidence of structural brain changes in schizophrenia. Arch Gen Psychiatry 43:36–42, 1986.

8. Buchsbaum MS, DeLisi LE, Holcomb HH, et al: Anterior-posterior gradients in cerebral glucose use in schizophrenia and affective disorders. Arch Gen Psychiatry 41:1159–1166, 1984.

9. Burton R: The Anatomy of Melancholy. Reprinted by Vantage Books, New York, 1977. (Originally published in 1671.)

10. Caine E: Pseudodementia: Current concepts and future directions. Arch Gen Psychiatry 38:1359–1364, 1981.

11. Calev A: Recall and recognition in chronic nondemented schizophrenia: Use of matched tasks. J Abnorm Psychol 93:172–177, 1984.

12. Chapman LJ and Chapman JP: Disordered Thought in Schizophrenia. Appleton-Century-Crofts, New York, 1973.

13. Ciompi L: Review of follow-up studies on long-term evolution and aging in schizophrenia. In Miller NE and Cohen GD (eds): Schizophrenia and Aging. Guilford Press, New York, 1987, pp 37–51.

14. Cohen RM, Weingartner H, Smallberg SA, Pickar D, and Murphy DL: Effort and cognition in depression. Arch Gen Psychiatry 39:593–597, 1982.

15. Crowe TJ: Molecular pathology of schizophrenia: More than one disease process. BMJ 280:66–68, 1980.

16. Cullom CM, Heaton RK, and Memiroff B: Neuropsychology of late life psychoses. In Jeste DV and Zisook S (eds): Psychiatr Clin North Am 11:47–59, 1988.

17. Cullom CM, Jeste DV, Harris MJ, Grant I, and Heaton RK: Neuropsychological characteristics of patients with the onset of schizophrenic symptoms after age 45 (abstr). J Clin Exp Neuropsychol 10:71, 1988.

18. Cummings JC: Organic delusions: Phenomenological and anatomical correlations. Br J Psychiatry 146:184–197, 1985.

19. Cummings JC and Benson DF: Subcortical dementia: Review of an emerging concept. Arch Neurol 41:874–879, 1984.

20. Dunbar GC and Lishman WA: Depression, recognition memory and hedonic-tone: A signal detection analysis. Br J Psychiatry 144:376–382, 1984.

21. Goldberg TE, Weinberg DE, Berman KF, Pliskin NH, and Podd MH: Further evidence for dementia of the prefrontal type in schizophrenia? A controlled study of teaching the Wisconsin Card Sorting Test. Arch Gen Psychiatry 44:1008–1014, 1987.

22. Goldstein G: The neuropsychology of schizophrenia. In Grant I and Adams K (eds): Neuropsychological Assessment of Psychiatric Disorders. Oxford University Press, New York, 1986, pp 147–171.

23. Goldstein L and Kyc F: Performance of brain-damaged, schizophrenic, and normal subjects on a visual searching task. Percept Mot Skills 46:731–734, 1978.

24. Heaton RK and Drexler M: Clinical neuropsychological findings in schizophrenia and aging. In Miller NE and Cohen GD (eds): Schizophrenia and Aging. Guildord Press, New York, 1987.

25. Jackson SW: Melancholia and Depression. Yale University Press, New Haven, 1986.

26. Johnson MH and Magaro PA: Effects of mood and severity on memory processes in depression and mania. Psychol Bull 101:28–40, 1987.

27. Johnstone EC, Cummingham-Owens DG, Gold A, Crow TJ, and Macmillan JF: Institutionalization and the defects of schizophrenia. Br J Psychiatry 139:195–203, 1981.

28. Kay DWK and Roth M: Environmental and hereditary factors in the schizophrenias of old age ("late paraphrenia") and their bearing on the general problem of causation in schizophrenia. J Ment Sci 107:649–686, 1961.

29. Kiloh LC: Pseudo-dementia. Acta Psychiatr Scan 37:336–351, 1961.

30. Kolb B and Whishaw IQ: Performance of schizophrenic patients on tests sensitive to left or right frontal, temporal or parietal function in neurological patients. J Nerv Ment Dis 171:435–443, 1983.

31. Kraepelin E: Clinical Psychiatry. Diefendorf AF (trans and ed). Macmillan, New York, 1915.

32. Kral VA: The relationship between senile dementia (Alzheimer type) and depression. Can J Psychiatry 28:304–306, 1983.

33. Lishman A: Organic Psychiatry. Blackwell Scientific UK, Oxford, 1987.

34. Liston EH: Occult presenile dementia. J Nerv Ment Dis 164:263–267, 1977.

35. Madden JJ, Lohan JA, Kaplan LA, and Manfredi HM: Nondementing psychoses in older persons. JAMA 150:1567–1570, 1952.

36. Marsden CD and Harrison MJG: Outcome of investigation of patients with prescribed dementia. BMJ 2:249–252, 1972.

37. McAllister TW: Overview: Pseudodementia. Am J Psychiatry 140:528–533, 1983.

38. McAllister TW and Price TRP: Severe depressive pseudodementia with and without dementia. Am J Psychiatry 139:626–629, 1982.

39. McHugh PR and Folstein MF: Psychiatric syndromes of Huntington's chorea: A clinical and phenomenological study. In Benson DF and Blumer D (eds): Psychiatric Aspects of Huntington's Disease. Grune & Stratton, New York, 1975.

40. McHugh PR and Folstein MF: Psychopathology of dementia: Implications for neuropathology. In Katzman R (ed): Congenital and Acquired Cognitive Disorders. Raven Press, New York, 1979.

41. Mellor CS: First rank symptoms of schizophrenia. Br J Psychiatry 117: 15–23, 1970.

42. Miller E and Lewis P: Recognition memory in elderly patients with depression and dementia. J Abnorm Psychol 86: 84–86, 1977.

43. Miller NE and Cohen GD: Schizophrenia and Aging. Guilford Press, New York, 1987.

44. Morihisa JM, Duffy F, and Wyatt RJ: Brain electrical activities mapping (BEAM) in schizophrenic patients. Arch Gen Psychiatry 40:719–728, 1983.

45. Nott PN and Fleminger JJ: Presenile dementia: The difficulties of early diagnosis. Acta Psychiatr Scand 51:210–217, 1975.

46. Pankratz L: A new technique for the assessment and modification of feigned memory deficit. Percept Mot Skills 57:367–372, 1983.

47. Pearlson GD, Garbacz DJ, Moberg PJ, Ahn HS, and DePaulo JR: Symptomatic, familial, perinatal, and social correlates of computerized axial tomography (CAT) changes in schizophrenia and bipolars. J Nerv Ment Dis 173:42–50, 1985.

48. Pearlson GD and Rabins PV: The late onset psychoses: Possible risk factors. Psychiatr Clin North Am 11:15–32, 1988.

49. Pearlson GD, Rabins PV, Kim WS, et al: Structural brain CT changes and cognitive deficits in elderly depressives with and without reversible dementia ("pseudodementia"). Psychol Med 19:573–584, 1989.

50. Pearlson GD, Ross CA, Lohr WD, Rovner BW, Chase GA, and Folstein MF: Association between family history of affective disorder and the depressive syndrome in Alzheimer's disease. Am J Psychiatry 147:452–456, 1990.

51. Pogue-Geile MF and Harrow M: Negative and positive symptoms in schizophrenia and depression: A follow-up. Schizophr Bull 10:371–387, 1984.

52. Rabins PV: Reversible dementia and the misdiagnosis of dementia: A Review. Hosp Community Psychiatry 34:830–835, 1983.

53. Rabins PV, Merchant A, and Nestadt G: Criteria for diagnosing reversible dementia caused by depression: Validation by 2-year follow-up. Br J Psychiatry 144:488–492, 1984.

54. Rabins PV, Pauker S, and Thomas J: Can schizophrenia begin after age 44? Compr Psychiatry 25:290–293, 1984.

55. Raskin A: Partialing out the effects of depression and age on cognitive functions: Experimental data and methodological issues. In Poon LW (ed): Handbook for Clinical Memory Assessment of Older Adults. American Psychological Association, Washington DC, 1986, pp 244–256.

56. Reding M, Haycox J, and Blass J: Depression in patients referred to a dementia clinic. Arch Neurol 42:894–896, 1985.

57. Reiffler BV: Mixed cognitive-affective disturbances in the elderly: A new classification. J Clin Psychiatry 47:354–356, 1986.

58. Reiffler BV, Larson E, and Hanley R: Coexistence of cognitive impairment and depression in geriatric outpatients. Am J Psychiatry 139:623–626, 1982.

59. Reisberg B: Alzheimer's disease. Free Press, New York, 1983, pp 6–7.

60. Reynolds CF, Kupfer DJ, Hoch CC, Stack JA, Houck PR, and Sewitch DE: Two-year follow-up of elderly patients with mixed depression and dementia. J Am Geriatr Soc 34:793–799, 1986.

61. Ron MA, Roone BK, Garralda ME, and Lishman WA: Diagnostic accuracy in presenile dementia. Br J Psychiatry 134:161–168, 1979.

62. Ross C: Determinants of depression in Alzheimer's disease. Paper presented at meeting of the American Psychiatric Association, Montreal, May 1988.

63. Shelton RC, Karson CN, Doran AR, Piakcer D, Bigelow LB, and Weinberger DR: Cerebral structural pathology in schizophrenia: Evidence for a selective prefrontal defect. Am J Psychiatry 145:154–163, 1988.

64. Shraberg D: The myth of pseudo-dementia: Depression and the aging brain. Am J Psychiatry 135:601–603, 1978.

65. Spar JE and Gerner R: Does the dexamethasone suppression test distinguish dementia from depression? Am J Psychiatry 139:238–240, 1982.

66. Strauss ME: Behavioral differences between acute and chronic schizophrenics. Course of psychosis, effects of institutionalization or sampling biases? In Cancro R (ed): Annual Review of the Schizophrenic Syndrome, 1976–1977. Brunner/Mazel, New York, 1978, pp 139–152.

67. Sutton S: Fact and artifact in the psychology of schizophrenia. In Hammer M, Salzinger K, and Sutton S (eds): Psychopathology: Contributions from Biological, Behavioral and Social Sciences. John Wiley & Sons, New York, 1973, pp 197–213.

68. Watts FN, Morris L, and MacLeod AK: Recognition memory in depression. J Abnorm Psychol 96:273–275, 1987.

69. Weinberger DR, Berman KF, and Zec RF: Physiological dysfunction of dorsolateral prefrontal cortex in schizophrenia: 1. Regional cerebral blood flow (rCBF) evidence. Arch Gen Psychiatry 43:114–124, 1986.

70. Weingartner H: Automatic and effort-demanding cognitive processes in depression. In Poon LW (ed): Handbook for Clinical Memory Assessment of Older Adults. American Psychological Association, Washington DC, 1986, pp 218–225.

71. Weingartner H, Grafman J, and Newhouse P: Toward a psychobiological taxonomy of cognitive impairments. In Glenner GG and Wurtman RJ (eds): Advancing Frontiers in Alzheimer's Disease Research. University of Texas Press, Austin, 1987, pp 249–262.

72. Wells CE: Pseudodementia. Am J Psychiatry 136:894–896, 1979.

73. Wells CE: Refinements in the diagnosis of dementia. Am J Psychiatry 139:621–622, 1982.

74. Whitehead A: Verbal learning and memory in elderly depressives. Br J Psychiatry 123:203–208, 1973.

75. Woods BT and Wolf J: A reconsideration of the relation of ventricular enlargement to duration of illness in schizophrenia. Am J Psychiatry 140:1564–1570, 1983.

76. Zubenko GS and Moossy J: Major depression in primary dementia. Arch Neurol 45:1182–1186, 1988.

77. Zweig RM, Ross CA, Hedreen JC, et al: The neuropathology of aminergic nuclei in Alzheimer's disease. Ann Neurol 24:233–242, 1988.

Part III

MANAGEMENT AND TREATMENT OF PATIENTS WITH DEMENTIA

Chapter 13

BIOLOGIC THERAPIES FOR ALZHEIMER'S DISEASE

John H. Growdon, M.D.

Clinical manifestations of dementing illnesses such as Alzheimer's disease (AD) are believed to result from neuronal dysfunction and death. Studies to determine the causes of neuronal death and to explain patterns of neuronal vulnerability that are characteristic for specific diseases are dominant themes of research in neurobiology. Until these fundamental issues are fully understood, curative treatment for AD will remain an elusive goal. A question related to treatment can, however, be addressed at this time: What can be done to modify the consequences of neuronal dysfunction and death? Answers to this question carry the underlying assumption that clinical features of dementia stem in part from abnormalities in the neurochemical environment of the brain, especially in the synthesis and release of specific neurotransmitters, and that neurotransmitter abnormalities are amenable to correction by drugs. Drugs already exist that affect behavior, although none reverses the dementia of AD nor slows its progression. Nonetheless, advances in identifying neurochemical abnormalities that accompany AD fuel expectations that drug therapies can be developed that will correct or bypass the neurotransmitter deficits in AD and thereby restore normal cognitive function.

This chapter considers the question of biologic therapy for AD from two perspectives, practical and theoretical. The practical perspective details palliative treatments for emergent psychiatric and behavioral symptoms associated with AD, using drugs that are currently available. The theoretical perspective outlines an approach to developing drug treatments directed toward the core cognitive deficits in AD and reviews the current state of experimental therapy in AD. The two perspectives merge in a section that describes principles for conducting and evaluating the results of investigational drug studies. The chapter concludes with a forecast of future directions in drug development.

PALLIATIVE TREATMENTS FOR ALZHEIMER'S DISEASE

Poor memory, impaired use of language and objects, and compromised visuospatial perception are the medical hallmarks of dementia, but disrupted sleep-wake cycle, restlessness, mood changes, hallucinations, and delusions are common symptoms that disturb the AD patient's home. Whereas the cognitive symptoms remain refractory to treatment, behavioral or noncognitive symptoms can be modified by administration of appropriate drugs. Some, such as agitation and sleep disturbance, are also amenable to behavioral methods of treatment, as discussed in Chapter 14. Identification and treatment of the behavioral disturbances will relieve discomfort in the patient and also diminish pressures on family members and caretakers. Guidelines for drug and dose selection for palliative treatment in AD are presented in Table 13–1. If drugs are used, one should follow good geriatric pharmacology principles such as starting at low doses, increasing doses slowly, and monitoring beneficial and harmful effects carefully.

Sleep disturbances are common in AD and may be treated with hypnotics. Drugs appropriate for use in AD include chloral hydrate and short-acting benzo-diazepines such as temazepam. Hypnotics may be expected to induce sleep, but they do not guarantee a full night of uninterrupted sleep. They should not be abused by giving a dose at each nocturnal awakening. Because most hypnotics are lipophilic, such repeated doses may accumulate in the body and cause undesirable side effects such as motor incoordination, postural instability, and additional cognitive impairments.

Agitation and minor depression often coexist in AD, and may be treated with anxiolytic drugs.[90,121] Alprazolam is an anxiolytic drug of choice because of its additional antidepressant action. Caution is advised, however, because even low doses of benzodiazepines can impair cognition.

Psychiatric symptoms are often part of true dementia; both minor and major depression are prevalent in AD. Appropriate treatment consists of conventional antidepressant drugs including tricyclic compounds such as desimipramine, monamine oxidase inhibitors such as phenelzine, and the serotonergic drug fluoxetine. Because anticholinergic drugs impair memory in both healthy subjects and AD patients, tricyclic drugs that have prominent anticholinergic side effects should be avoided. The doses and duration of treatment needed to improve mood in patients with AD are similar to those

Table 13–1 EXAMPLES OF PALLIATIVE TREATMENTS FOR ALZHEIMER'S DISEASE*

Drug	Typical Dose of Medication	Indication
Hypnotics		Sleep disruption
e.g., temazepam	15 mg h.s.	
chloral hydrate	500 mg h.s.	
Anxiolytics		Agitation, depression
e.g., alprazolam	0.25 mg t.i.d.	
Antidepressants		Depression, apathy
e.g., desimipramine	100–150 mg h.s.	
fluoxetine	20 mg daily	
Neuroleptics		Psychosis, restlessness
e.g., haloperidol	1 mg t.i.d.	

*These recommendations represent the views of the author. Individual patients may respond quite differently, and careful observation is required to monitor for positive and negative effects.

used in treating depression unaccompanied by dementia. When treatment is successful, the patient's spirits will lift and the family may report the patient's being more talkative and interested in the environment; improvement in memory or other cognitive functions is rare. Reasons for treatment failure include inadequate dose of medication, insufficient duration of treatment, or inaccurate diagnosis. The diagnosis of depression in patients with AD may be especially difficult because depression is often mistaken for apathy, and strict criteria for separating the two conditions do not exist. Families often report depression, by which they mean that the patient sits all day with a blank facial expression and lacks pep, energy, and interest in surroundings. There may be disordered sleep and appetite, but these symptoms do not necessarily indicate depression, as they are common in dementia alone. In contrast to patients with depression, patients with apathy answer "no" when asked directly whether they feel sad or despondent. Stimulants such as low doses of methylphenidate are occasionally prescribed for patients with apathy or depression.[156] Stimulants should be used with caution and under careful supervision because they may increase confusion and agitation.

Hallucinations and delusions are some of the most distressing aspects of AD and often lead to institutionalization. Psychoses may be accompanied by outbursts of verbal and physical abuse that threaten family and caretakers and disrupt home and nursing care. Neuroleptics (antipsychotic drugs) are indicated for these symptoms, as well as for severe restlessness and agitation.[122,135] Treatment should begin with low doses of antipsychotic medication; in most instances, nonsedating neuroleptics such as haloperidol are preferred. The dose of the neuroleptic is gradually increased until psychotic symptoms wane. Adequate doses of neuroleptic medication may be expected to relieve the patient's discomfort and control the disruptive behavior.

Neuroleptics should be used sparingly and for specific, targeted symptoms because of their potential side effects. Patients with AD seem especially prone to developing extrapyramidal neurologic side effects of neuroleptic treatment, including parkinsonian syndromes and tardive dyskinesia.

APPROACHES TOWARD DEVELOPING TREATMENTS IN ALZHEIMER'S DISEASE

The core cognitive symptoms of AD consist of amnesia, aphasia, apraxia, and impairments in visuospatial perception and abstract reasoning. In contrast to the array of palliative treatments for modifying emergent symptoms in AD, there are no effective treatments for these core cognitive impairments. Historically, development of treatments proposed for the core symptoms of dementia closely paralleled the changing fashion of opinion regarding the cause of AD. Thus hyperbaric oxygen was proposed to remedy a postulated decrease in cerebral oxygenation; anticoagulants were given to minimize sludged blood in the brain; and vasodilators were given to enhance cerebral blood flow. These treatments have been discarded, along with the use of psychostimulants and procaine GH_3 (Gerovitol). The rationale for administration of ergoloid mesylates (Hydergine) is less clear than that for other discarded treatments because its pharmacology is more complex. Ergoloid mesylates have been widely used for treating symptoms associated with senility for more than 30 years, and today remain widely prescribed pharmaceuticals.[70] Ergoloid mesylates may have modest alerting and antidepressant effects; there is scant evidence that their administration improves any of the core cognitive impairments of AD.

Contemporary development of drugs for treating the core cognitive impairments in AD depends on the principles of rational neuropsychopharmacology.[59] According to these tenets, drug treatments are likely to improve symptoms of disease to the extent that they correct or bypass the neurotransmitter abnormalities that result from neuronal degeneration. It therefore becomes necessary to identify the neurochemical correlates of disease with the same care taken to delineate the nature and distribution of histopathologic lesions. The goal of contemporary neuropsychopharmacology, therefore, is to uncover and then correct the underlying neurochemical lesions that account for the clinical manifestations of neurodegenerative diseases.

Evidence for neurotransmitter abnormalities in AD may come from one of four kinds of observations: (1) biochemical analyses of neurotransmitters in brain tissue obtained at autopsy or brain biopsy, (2) biochemical analyses of neurotransmitters or their metabolites in cerebrospinal fluid (CSF), (3) results of clinical pharmacologic testing, and (4) information based on relevant animal models. The implicit assumption is that the discovered neurotransmitter abnormality derived from the four sources of data is involved in the pathogenesis of AD or may actually cause its clinical manifestations.

Biochemical Analyses of Neurotransmitters in Brain Tissue

Examination of brain tissue obtained at autopsy or from brain biopsy during life constitutes the most direct evidence for neurotransmitter abnormalities in AD. The initial discovery that choline acetyltransferase (CAT) activity, a marker for neurons that synthesize and release acetylcholine (ACh), was decreased in brain tissue of patients with AD was the first neurotransmitter abnormality described.[24,38,109] Subsequent reports indicated that muscarinic receptors were largely preserved,[110] whereas nicotinic cholinergic receptors were reduced in number.[151,152] Atrophy of cholinergic cells in the ventral forebrain nuclei Ch 1–4,[97] especially the nucleus basalis of Meynert,[153] has been postulated as the cause of cholinergic reductions in cerebral cortex.[34] It is likely that deficiencies in ACh transmission are clinically important, because reduction in CAT activity and impaired ACh synthesis were significantly correlated with the extent of histopathology (senile plaques and neurofibrillary tangles) in AD, and also with clinical measures of dementia severity.[19,50,129,155] (See also Chapters 3 and 6.)

Other deficits have been described in the monoamine neurotransmitters norepinephrine,[105] dopamine,[57] and serotonin,[22] although their clinical importance is less certain than the cholinergic abnormality. Monoaminergic deficits tend to occur in early onset rather than late onset AD, whereas cholinergic lesions occur in AD cases of all ages. Of the three monoamines, the noradrenergic lesion appears to be the most important. Most of the norepinephrine (NE) in the mammalian central nervous system is synthesized by neurons within the brainstem nucleus locus ceruleus (LC). In AD, cortical levels of NE are decreased as a result of noradrenergic cell loss in the LC,[21,91] where many of the remaining neurons contain neurofibrillary tangles; cortical levels of the main NE metabolite 3-methoxy-4-hydroxyphenylethylglycol (MHPG) are variably affected. LC neurons project widely throughout the neuraxis[49]; there are major projections to regions primarily affected in AD, including neocortex, thalamus, medial septum, nucleus basalis, hippocampus, and amygdala. The α_2 adrenergic receptors that regulate NE biosynthesis and mediate NE neurotransmission are located on LC axon terminals and soma-dendritic regions, as well as on nonadrenergic neurons distal to LC axon terminals.[46,58,147] Decreased levels of serotonin (5-HT) and its main metabolite 5-hydroxyindoleacetic acid (5-HIAA), have been reported in samples of frontal and temporal cortex, and in hippocampus collected at autopsy and at brain biopsy from patients with AD[25]; the number of S_1 and S_2 serotonin receptor subtypes is decreased.[35] These biochemical abnormalities result from neurofibrillary degeneration of serotonergic neurons in the brain stem raphe nuclei.[77] Neurons in a nearby brainstem region, the substantia nigra, are affected in AD, although the extent of degeneration is variable and usually mild. Modest decreases in the levels of dopamine (DA) and its major metabolite homovanillic acid (HVA) occur in AD, usually in the end stages of this disease.[57] The number of D_2 receptors in the striatum is reduced.[120]

Neuropeptide transmitters are also affected in AD, and decreases in cortical levels of somatostatin,[37] corticotropin-releasing hormone,[16] neuropeptide Y,[11] and substance P[10] have been reported. Somatostatin receptors are decreased in the same regions where somatostatin levels are decreased.[12] Not all peptidergic neurons are affected: Concentrations of vasoactive intestinal polypeptide, cholycystokinin, thyrotropin-releasing hormone and luteinizing hormone–releasing hormone are preserved.[9,111,124,158]

Biochemical Analyses of Cerebrospinal Fluid

Examination of the cerebrospinal fluid (CSF) can provide additional information regarding neurotransmitter abnormalities in AD. This line of investigation is based on the belief that abnormalities in neurotransmitter metabolism in the brain will be reflected in the CSF. Minor abnormalities in cholinesterase activities have been detected in CSF of patients with AD[71]; decreased levels of HVA have been reported along with increased levels of MHPG, whereas levels of serotonin and its metabolites are within normal limits.[54,118] The consensus finding that levels of somatostatin are reduced in CSF of patients with AD is consistent with decreased content of this peptide in cortex,

whereas decreased levels of vasopressin are detected only in CSF.[93] Measurement of neurotransmitter markers in CSF provides indirect evidence of neurotransmitter abnormalities in brains of patients with AD; such analyses can be used to guide treatment approaches to AD and monitor drug effects during treatment but have not yet gained acceptance in diagnosis of AD because of overlaps with control values.[8,61]

Clinical Pharmacologic Testing

The results of pharmacologic testing can provide indirect evidence for neurotransmitter involvement in brain disease. Behavioral effects of sequential administration of drugs that increase or decrease transmission of a specific transmitter have been used to draw indirect inferences regarding probable underlying biochemical abnormalities in AD. For example, pharmacologic studies with cholinergic agonists and antagonists were central to the cholinergic hypothesis of memory dysfunction: Drugs that blocked cholinergic transmission, such as scopolamine, impaired memory in young healthy subjects, and this deficit was reversed by administration of physostigmine.[45] Choline, physostigmine, and arecoline were all reported to produce minor improvement in performance on memory tasks involving recall of recently learned material in young, nondemented subjects[41,130,131]; these results led to testing cholinergic agonists in AD. Pharmacologic studies also indicated that cholinergic mechanisms subserved some but not all aspects of cognitive impairment in AD: Scopolamine administration impaired fact learning and some aspects of attention in patients with AD at doses that did not impair performances in other cognitive tests, such as those that test language skills.[72,139] Scopolamine also disrupted fact learning in normal control subjects[72] but did not impair the memory system concerned with skill learning.[104] These observations indicate that cholinergic drugs may be expected to improve some aspects of memory but are unlikely to benefit all symptoms of AD.

Relevant Animal Models

Experiments in animals rarely study behaviors that exactly mimic the clinical manifestations of AD; animal models, however, permit more direct biochemical measurements and pharmacologic testing than are generally possible in humans (see also Chapter 3). Among the many preclinical experiments performed, only those involving ACh and NE are reviewed as illustrations. Young monkeys given scopolamine developed memory impairments similar to those observed in untreated aged monkeys, and physostigmine partially reversed these impairments.[5] Such studies have reinforced the cholinergic hypothesis of memory dysfunction in humans.[6] Studies that spurred the use of long-term lecithin administration in an effort to retard progression of AD[87] came from experiments in rodents that showed that declines in performance in passive avoidance tests were significantly related to increased age. When the rodents were fed diets enriched with choline, age-related decrements in performance were blunted, and aged animals performed as if they were months younger[7]; preservation of dendritic spines in hippocampal pyramidal cell neurons was proposed as a possible anatomic correlate.

Behavioral effects of alterations in monoaminergic systems have also been examined in experimental animals. Administration of clonidine, an α_2 adrenergic receptor agonist, significantly improved cognitive performance of aged monkeys in spatial delayed-response tasks.[3] Benefit from clonidine was blunted by administration of an α_2 antagonist drug, yohimbine. These preclinical pharmacologic studies, coupled with the discovery of LC degeneration in AD, evidence of decreased NE levels in brain, and altered MHPG levels in CSF,

have prompted pharmacologic investigations in humans with AD using drugs that increase NE neurotransmission.

CLASSES OF EXPERIMENTAL DRUGS PROPOSED FOR TREATING COGNITIVE IMPAIRMENTS IN ALZHEIMER'S DISEASE

Selection of experimental drugs for trials in patients with AD depends on identifying specific neurotransmitter abnormalities that produce symptoms of dementia. Although evidence linking specific neurotransmitters to particular behaviors is generally lacking, numerous deficits in transmitters are well documented; these include abnormalities in ACh, the monoamines, and the neuropeptides. This section reviews the results of experimental drug studies directed toward correcting each of these neurotransmitter abnormalities.

Cholinergic Agents

The cholinergic hypothesis of memory dysfunction in AD rests on three convergent lines of evidence: pharmacologic studies that demonstrated the importance of ACh neurotransmission in memory functions, postmortem biochemical studies of AD brains that revealed significant decreases in cortical CAT activity, and animal (and human) anatomic studies that stressed the importance of anatomic connections between the cholinergic ventral forebrain CH 1 – 4 nuclei and neocortex and hippocampus. Hopes that increasing cholinergic neurotransmission would improve memory in AD were raised by the observation that muscarinic postsynaptic receptor sites were preserved in this disorder,[110] a finding that gave rise to three treatment strategies: administration of precursors for ACh biosynthesis, such as choline and phosphatidylcholine (PC); administration of cholinomimetic drugs, such as physostigmine and arecoline; and use of a combination of precursors and ago-

Table 13–2 EXPERIMENTAL USE OF CHOLINERGIC AGENTS TO TREAT ALZHEIMER'S DISEASE*

ACETYLCHOLINE PRECURSORS
Choline
Dimethylaminoethanol
Phosphatidylcholine

CHOLINOMIMETICS
Arecoline
Bethanechol
Physostigmine
RS-86
Tetrahydroaminoacridine (THA, Tacrine)

COMBINED PRECURSORS AND CHOLINOMIMETICS
Phosphatidylcholine + physostigmine
Phosphatidylcholine + tetrahydroaminoacridine
Phosphatidylcholine + piracetam

*Although there is strong evidence supporting a cholinergic deficit in brains of patients with AD, experimental treatments with precursors, cholinomimetics and precursors combined with cholinergic agonists designed to increase ACh neurotransmission have not improved memory or other clinical manifestations of AD.

nists, such as PC plus physostigmine and PC plus tetrahydroaminoacridine (THA) (Table 13–2).

The rationale for administering choline and its naturally occurring dietary form, PC (lecithin), was based on preclinical observations that these compounds increased ACh brain levels in rats,[30] including within the presynaptic terminals of cholinergic neurons projecting to the hippocampus from the medial septum.[69] Cholinergic cells were especially sensitive to precursor availability under conditions of increased neuronal firing[15,78,88] such as may occur in the remaining neurons of the damaged ventral forebrain nuclei in AD. During the past 10 years, more than 20 studies have been conducted testing the effects of choline salts or PC in treating AD: The results are uniform in finding no significant benefit from either choline or PC.[32] A possible exception to this generalization is a subset of AD patients aged 80 years or more whose course of deterioration was believed to be slowed by administration of PC for 6 months.[87] Studies that claim that a treatment slowed the progression of illness are difficult to interpret because deterioration is not linear. Additional studies with treatment lasting at least several years will be required be-

fore accepting a beneficial effect from PC administration in old patients with AD. Chronic PC administration did not improve the condition of young patients with AD.[68,87]

Physostigmine is an acetylcholinesterase inhibitor; the net effect of its administration is to increase neurotransmission by delaying ACh hydrolysis in the synaptic cleft. Physostigmine has a theoretical limitation in treating AD because its efficacy depends on intact presynaptic ACh synthesis and release. Practical disadvantages of physostigmine include erratic absorption after oral ingestion, short duration of action, and production of widespread cholinergic side effects. Systemic side effects include tachycardia, sweating, nausea, and vomiting; toxic effects on the central nervous system can include anxiety, delirium, and seizures. At least 15 reports of physostigmine trials in AD have appeared, including double-blind, placebo-controlled studies. Of these, 7 reported statistically significant improvement in one or more aspects of memory in some patients,* whereas 8 other groups of investigators reported

*References 13, 17, 29, 40, 101, 103, 123.

no benefits from physostigmine.* In those studies reporting improved memory, the magnitude of improvement was small and transient, no patient was restored to normal function during treatment, and in most cases the putative improvement was not clinically apparent.

Muscarinic agonists have an advantage over precursors and physostigmine in that they stimulate postsynaptic receptors and therefore bypass the degenerating presynaptic cholinergic neuron completely. Despite an early encouraging report with arecoline,[29] muscarinic agonists have not achieved wide use in AD, either because they are dangerous and have intolerable side effects,[39] or because they did not improve cognitive performance.[25,150] The muscarinic agonist bethanechol has been instilled directly into the brain by means of a ventricular infusion pump in order to circumvent difficulty in crossing the blood-brain barrier and to minimize peripheral side effects. Although technically possible, infusions with bethanechol did not improve memory.[42,65]

The most optimistic reports of cholinergic treatment in AD come from trials in which improvement was reported with acetylcholinesterase inhibitors in combination with PC.[82,86,112,138,145] In the most positive study, memory improved significantly in 8 of 12 AD patients[145]; improved test performance was correlated with the extent of acetylcholinesterase inhibition in the CSF. Despite continued treatment, however, benefit was not sustained and treatment did not alter the inexorable decline in cognitive abilities. Rather more extravagant claims were made for the combination of THA plus PC,[138] in which 16 of 17 patients were reported improved, many dramatically so. The conclusions from this study are difficult to accept because of numerous methodologic flaws in areas including subject selection and cognitive testing. This report is also at odds with previous experi-

ence with THA.[28,53,82] A New Drug Application (NDA) for THA has been submitted to the Food and Drug Administration (FDA), but an advisory panel recommended not approving the drug until further data are obtained. Other drug combinations with PC, including Hydergine,[79] lithium,[117] and piracetam,[62] have been ineffective in treatment of AD.

The cholinergic hypothesis of memory dysfunction in AD has been extensively tested, but these investigations have not produced a satisfactory treatment for AD. Among the many possible reasons for the failure of cholinergic treatment to improve memory or any other aspect of cognition or activities of daily living in AD, widespread neuronal degeneration with a multiplicity of neurotransmitter abnormalities in addition to diminished ACh is paramount. Failing to discover a single treatment of neurotransmitter replacement that even palliates AD, a current neuropharmacologic approach is to dissect the neurochemical abnormalities in AD and determine whether any of these subserves specific behaviors (Table 13–3). Refinements in behavioral neuropharmacology suggest that ACh neurotransmission may be important in some aspects of memory but probably is not primarily involved in other cognitive abnormalities in AD. Thus muscarinic ACh neurotransmission apparently affects that aspect of memory concerned with fact learning and possibly attention,[72,139] but not skill learning[104] or other non-mnemonic cognitive functions. NE is postulated to be involved in some aspects of attention, memory, and mood.[89,125,159] Clinical evidence links 5-HT to arousal and mood state,[89] and DA to sensorimotor performances, spatial abilities, and sequencing.[31,60] Somatostatin may be involved in sensorimotor performance, especially by interacting with DA.

The postulated neurotransmitter-behavioral relationships outlined in Table 13-3 are speculative and may change as additional information accrues. The overall approach, however, illustrates

---

*References 4, 26, 44, 80, 126, 134, 136, 149.

**Table 13-3 HYPOTHETICAL RELATIONSHIPS
BETWEEN BRAIN NEUROTRANSMITTERS AND
COGNITIVE FUNCTIONS IN ALZHEIMER'S DISEASE**

Neurotransmitter	Cognitive Function
Acetylcholine	Memory (fact learning)
	Attention
Norepinephrine	Attention
	Memory (delayed recognition)
	Mood
Serotonin	Mood
	Arousal
Dopamine	Sensorimotor
	Spatial abilities
	Sequencing
Somatostatin	Sensorimotor

the principles of rational neuropsychopharmacology, in which there is a hypothetical framework for examining the behavioral consequences of administering drugs that increase or decrease neurotransmission within a specific system. Studies testing drugs that influence individual neurotransmitters other than ACh known to be affected in AD are just beginning. Once the behavioral effects of modifying each specific neurotransmitter have been characterized, the next logical step in drug development for AD could be combination therapy. For example, the effect of a drug that increased ACh transmission to improve memory could be supplemented by a drug given to increase serotonergic transmission to improve mood. It is also possible that combinations of drugs would act synergistically to improve memory, whereas the same drugs given individually would be ineffective. In preclinical experiments, for example, the behavioral effect of physostigmine on passive avoidance behavior was dependent on clonidine-induced increases in NE transmission in rats with combined nucleus basalis and LC lesions.[67]

Drugs That Affect Monoaminergic Transmission

There are three ways to increase monoaminergic neurotransmission: by administering precursors, direct-acting postsynaptic agonists, and inhibitors of catabolism. All three approaches have been tested for each of the major monoamines, NE, DA, and 5-HT (Table 13-4). Drugs that affect monoamines have not been as thoroughly tested in AD as cholinergic drugs because convincing evidence for impaired monoamine transmission in AD was found several years after the cholinergic deficit was discovered. Furthermore, aside from the nonspecific effects of tricyclic antidepressants, there was a lack of preexisting pharmacologic data delineating the cognitive aspects of increasing or decreasing monoaminergic tone. Tricyclic antidepressants are widely used in treating symptoms of AD; among other effects, they produce complex changes in noradrenergic and serotonergic neurotransmission. Tricyclic antidepressants can improve mood but rarely affect core cognitive symptoms of AD. Several new compounds under development as antidepressants have more specific pharmacologic actions than traditional tricyclics and offer new opportunities to influence individual monoamines. For example, zimeldine and alaproclate selectively potentiate serotonergic neurotransmission by preventing 5-HT from being inactivated by presynaptic reuptake mechanisms; in single reports, however, neither has been effective in improving symptoms in AD.[14,36] Deprenyl is a monoamine ox-

Table 13–4 DRUGS GIVEN TO AFFECT MONOAMINE NEUROTRANSMITTERS IN ALZHEIMER'S DISEASE

Drug	Neurotransmitter
L-Tyrosine*	Norepinephrine
Clonidine	
Idazoxan*	
Yohimbine	
Levodopa	Dopamine
Bromocriptine	
Pergolide	
Deprenyl	
L-5-hydroxytryptophan*	Serotonin
Alaproclate	
Zimeldine	
Fluoxetine	

*Investigational drug.

idase B inhibitor that, at low doses, selectively inhibits oxidative catabolism of DA. The single report that 10 mg/d of deprenyl improved episodic memory but not other cognitive functions in 17 patients with AD requires confirmation.[144] Increasing DA neurotransmission with the precursor levodopa[2,83,147] and with the direct D_2 receptor agonist bromocriptine did not improve symptoms of AD. In fact, high or even moderate doses of dopaminergic drugs may be detrimental, as they often cause or exacerbate confusion or hallucinations in Parkinson's disease, especially in those parkinsonians with preexisting cognitive impairments.

Despite evidence for LC damage and decreased NE transmission, drugs that affect NE have not been extensively tested in AD, except for tricyclic antidepressants and the precursor tyrosine.[98] With the advent of drugs that specifically stimulate (clonidine and guanfacine) or block (yohimbine, idazoxan) α_2 adrenoreceptors, it will be possible to test the cerebral effects of decreasing and increasing NE neurotransmission. Concern for possible cardiovascular side effects of noradrenergic drugs, including substantial changes in blood pressure, dictate caution in conducting trials in AD with these drugs.

Drugs That Affect Peptides

The rationale for considering peptides in treating AD derives from the observation that the levels of several neuropeptides in cerebral cortex are decreased in AD, including somatostatin, corticotropin releasing factor, neuropeptide Y, and substance P.[9] Preclinical studies have suggested the importance of vasopressin in animal behaviors believed to be relevant for human memory,[43] although vasopressin levels are unchanged in brains of patients with AD. Because naturally occurring peptides in the systemic circulation do not penetrate the blood-brain barrier, analogs of neuropeptides, or drugs given to influence their cerebral levels, have been tested in AD.* The initial report that naloxone, an opiate antagonist, improved cognitive function in AD[119] was premature, and numerous subsequent studies failed to confirm any beneficial effect of naloxone or naltrexone.[18,73,116,128,143] Several analogs of vasopressin have been tested despite the fact that negligible amounts cross the blood-brain barrier, even with in-

—————————

*References 8, 73, 107, 108, 116, 119, 128, 133, 143, 157.

tranasal instillation. Therapy with vasopressin analogs did not benefit patients with AD; at most, there was a mild alerting effect but no improvements in cognition or activities of daily living.[107,108] Enthusiasm for testing somatostatin or its analogs was greatly dampened by the report that the number of somatostatin receptors was decreased in regions of AD brain corresponding to the decrease in actual levels of somatostatin.[12]

Other Experimental Drugs

A new group of drugs, classed as metabolic memory enhancers, are being developed for use in AD. All are investigational drugs in the United States but several are sold commercially outside of the United States. These compounds are sometimes called nootropics (*nos* = mind, *tropin* = toward), a term proposed by Giurgia[55] in reference to the compound 2-pyrrolidone acetamide (piracetam). The nootropic concept is best defined operationally: nootropic compounds were said to have physiologic and behavioral effects in experimental animals without the side effects commonly observed following the administration of other psychoactive drugs such as the hypnotics, sedatives, neuroleptics, or antidepressants. The nootropic concept has enormous appeal because nootropics are postulated to activate mental functions, especially under experimental conditions in which they are impaired. To the extent that the multiple cognitive deficits in patients with AD stem from diffuse dysfunction of the cerebral hemispheres, metabolic enhancers that act diffusely to improve cognitive functions would have widespread application. To date, the nootropic concept has gained little scientific acceptance because the rationale for memory enhancement remains obscure, and the mechanisms whereby such improvement could occur are unknown. Furthermore, the nootropic promise re-

mains greater than its performance: in three studies, piracetam, either alone or in combination with choline or PC, did not improve cognition in AD.[51,62,132] New nootropics, such as oxiracetam and aniracetam, have been developed that are said to be severalfold more potent than piracetam in preclinical testing. Whether their greater activity in rats leads to improved cognitive function in humans with AD remains to be tested; a single report of 44 patients with AD treated for 3 months with 1 g/d of aniracetam produced no more benefit than placebo treatment.[134]

Other experimental treatments in AD have employed hormones and chelation therapy. The rationale for hormonal therapy is based on preclinical studies demonstrating estrogen receptors in brain. It was also shown that estrogen administration had behavioral effects in animals and that estrogen given to ovariectomized rats increased CAT activity in brain. In a preliminary report, low doses of estradiol improved mood and social orientation in six elderly women with AD, but there were no positive effects on cognition.[47] Chelation therapy is based on attempts to remove aluminum deposits from the senile plaques and neurofibrillary tangles in patients with AD in the hope that this will reverse or at least retard the neurodegenerative process. Desferrioxamine increases urinary excretion of aluminum, but its effect on brain aluminum content is difficult to measure. Desferrioxamine is also toxic.[27] A recent study[34a] claiming to demonstrate slowing of progression of disease with desferrioxamine has been criticized on methodologic and statistical grounds.

PRINCIPLES OF CONDUCTING A DRUG STUDY

Despite the wide variety of treatments for AD that have been tested over the past decades, none has been sufficiently effective that physicians are satisfied with available pharmacologic therapy. Many new compounds have entered clinical trials in AD and more trials with new drugs can be expected. The proliferation of clinical trials underscores the need for care in designing methods for testing drugs that may affect cognitive functions. Attention to critical issues in drug protocol design will improve the quality of clinical trials of compounds in AD; knowledge of these same principles will enable the general medical community to evaluate critically the results of these trials.

Protocol design varies depending on the stage of drug development. In phase 1 studies, early clinical trials in normal subjects test new compounds in order to study the pharmacokinetics of the drug, determine tolerance, and detect possible side effects. In phase 2 studies, one or two selected doses of the drug are administered to small numbers of subjects in the target disease population. In phase 3 studies, the drug is administered in multiple trials to a large number of subjects with the target disease in order to obtain data on safety and efficacy required by the FDA prior to releasing the drug for widespread use. Drug surveillance studies to monitor side effects and efficacy once the drug has been released constitute the final phase of drug testing (phase 4). Most drug studies currently being conducted in patients with AD are in the early phases of testing and share the principal features of drug trial protocols listed in Table 13–5.

Objectives

The goal of the study should be clearly stated. In AD, the aims can be to reverse impairments of memory and other cognitive functions, to improve behavioral symptoms, or to retard the progression of disease. The protocol should reflect these goals. A short-term study with a rapid-acting drug would be appropriate for symptomatic treatment, whereas a protocol with drug administration lasting years would be necessary to prove

Table 13–5 PRINCIPAL FEATURES OF DRUG TRIAL PROTOCOLS

OBJECTIVES OF THE STUDY
Drug phase
Protocol goal

DESIGN AND DURATION
Open label
Double blind

SUBJECT SELECTION
Symptom vs. disease
Inclusion and exclusion criteria
Number of subjects
Informed consent

VARIABLES TO BE MEASURED
Neurologic and psychiatric examinations
Neuropsychological tests
Behavioral rating scales
Laboratory tests

PROTOCOL CONDUCT
Data collection
Data analysis

efficacy in slowing the course of dementia. The same compound may be tested under both conditions: PC given for 6 months or less has been ineffective in reversing memory loss,[68,137] but a truly long-term study has not been conducted.

Design and Duration

In the early stages of a drug's development, open-label and single-blind studies to determine the optimal drug dose for the desired effect are usually the most appropriate and cost-effective protocol designs. Studies with a single drug are the most efficient way to collect information regarding tolerance and side effects in the target population. Because most drugs are tested first in normal young subjects, it is important to establish a drug's effect in older subjects because of potential differences in drug pharmacokinetics, bioavailability, and metabolism. Early phase 2 studies often guide the choice of drug dose and variables to be measured in subsequent large studies.

Drugs must be tested in double-blind protocols before they are accepted as effective. There are two principal designs: double-blind crossover and double-blind parallel studies. In a crossover design each subject receives the test drug and its placebo (or comparison drug). In parallel-design studies separate groups of subjects receive the test drug and its placebo (or comparison drug). Many studies in AD have employed a crossover design in which each subject acts as his or her own control. A crossover design avoids the practical difficulties of matching AD patients of exact dementia severity and rates of disease progression required in parallel design studies. Fewer subjects are required than in a parallel design, and it is easier to recruit subjects because all will receive active drug. Investigators testing drugs according to crossover designs must be careful to counterbalance the order of drug administration and make certain that the washout period between different treatments is sufficient for the drug to be eliminated from the body but not so long that the patient's clinical condition deteriorates. Most pharmacologists favor a parallel design, however, because these studies are free from potential confounding effects of prior treatment. Care must be taken in selecting the subject groups; careful randomization is necessary but does not ensure comparability in treatment groups.

Subject Selection

Care in selecting the target population is critical to the success of any drug study. Drug trials in which patients with signs and symptoms of dementia are lumped together would make sense if dementia were a single disorder, but dementia has many etiologies. Physicians now consider more than 50 causes of dementia whenever diagnosing a patient with acquired cognitive deficits.[63] Because the anatomic and biochemical substrates of dementia differ according to the etiology of the disease, it is unlikely that effective treatments for one condition would be useful in all dementias. Thus, antidepressant medication may help patients with the dementia of depression but will not restore memory in patients with Korsakoff's amnesia. Thyroid replacement may benefit patients with cognitive impairments associated with hypothyroidism but will not improve memory in patients with AD. Every attempt should be made, therefore, to establish the presumed etiology of dementia so as to identify patients with conditions that are responsive to standard treatments. Of course, simply knowing the cause of dementia does not guarantee success in treating it. Examples abound in which the etiology of the disease causing dementia is known, but there is limited therapeutic potential: general paresis, Wernicke-Korsakoff syndrome, Creutzfeldt-Jakob disease, and Huntington's disease, for instance. Patients with dementia disorders such as these should be excluded from experimental drug studies directed toward AD because most investigational drugs being tested in AD are selected for their potential ability to correct the presumed biochemical deficits in brains of patients with AD. Because many of these deficits, such as decreased CAT activity and decreased somatostatin levels, are relatively specific to AD, there is no rational basis for including in drug studies patients with other dementing disorders. As a general rule, the results of drug trials are most valid and convincing when the treated subjects represent a carefully selected and homogeneous diagnostic entity.

Not all patients with AD are suitable for participation in trials using experimental drugs, and most investigators establish inclusion and exclusion criteria. Examples of inclusion criteria are willingness to participate in drug research, as indicated by signing an informed consent form; good general health; stable living conditions with a responsible spouse, caretaker, or observer; a specified age range; and minimum formal education level or satisfactory work history. Subjects are generally required to meet minimal levels of cognitive test performance in order to ensure that improvements or deteriorations occurring during treatment can be detected. Scores on screening measures such as the Mini-Mental State Examination[48] and the Blessed Dementia Scale[19] are commonly used to determine the presence and severity of cognitive impairments. Subjects who are included in most studies have mild to moderate dementia and a confident clinical diagnosis of AD.[94]

Criteria for exclusion are equally important; subjects with serious underlying medical conditions such as cancer, unstable heart conditions, or organ failure should be excluded. Similarly, patients with suspected AD who also have a history of significant head trauma, alcohol abuse, or electroconvulsive therapy should be excluded because these factors may influence response to drug therapy or may independently impair cognitive test performance. Finally, subjects who require psychoactive medications such as anxiolytics, hypnotics, sedatives, analeptics, and neuroleptics should be excluded, as well as those who require drugs prescribed for medical conditions that can affect cognitive functions, such as reserpine, cimetidine, long-acting nitrates, and anticholinergic drugs.

The number of subjects tested depends on the goal of the study. In an exploratory study, substantial improvement in a single patient may be an important scientific observation and direct further drug development. To establish the efficacy of a medication as a prelude to commercial development, however, it is usually necessary to conduct several studies at different sites using 100 or more patients per study. The exact number of subjects is usually established according to the number of variables being measured, the sensitivity of the measures, and the level of statistical significance being sought in order to show a treatment effect. Patients with AD enrolled in drug studies are often stratified at the onset according to the degree of dementia (for example, a group with a Mini-Mental State

score of 13 to 17 and another group with a score of 18 to 22). Stratification increases the homogeneity of treatment groups, but it also increases the number of subjects required.

Variables To Be Measured

The FDA has established clear guidelines for determining efficacy in some drug areas but not in the field of psychogeriatrics,[85] although such guidelines are under development.[2a] Lack of guidelines reflects the fact that there is no consensus regarding the variables to be measured in studies testing drugs for AD, and there are no prototypic compounds with demonstrated efficacy that provide a standard of comparison. Ideally, drug studies should incorporate neurologic and psychiatric examinations, neuropsychological testing, behavioral observations, and laboratory tests, all administered at specified intervals during the study.

Physical examinations, including the neurologic examination, are conducted to elicit data regarding a drug's effect and to ensure its safety. Psychiatric examinations can be performed to detect mood changes or disturbances in thought that may occur during treatment. Standardized rating scales such as the Hamilton Depression Scale,[64] Montgomery-Asberg Scale,[102] Profile of Mood States,[95] and others (see Chapter 6) have been proposed for assessing mood and behavior in AD.

A wide range of neuropsychological tests have been proposed, but no single test has been universally accepted and incorporated into drug trials. A comprehensive neuropsychological assessment should include tests of verbal and nonverbal short-term and long-term memory, using multiple but equivalent forms of each test whenever possible.[33] Similar arrays of tests should be administered to assess language performance and visuospatial abilities. Practical considerations often dictate the number of cognitive tests chosen for monitoring a drug's effect, but tests selected should always be within the capabilities of the subjects being tested and relevant to their disabilities.

Behavioral observations regarding a patient's capacity for self-care, employment, work at home, communication skills, and social relationships are an integral part of assessing a drug's effect in patients with AD. Impairments in these activities of daily living (ADL) are often the most prominent disabilities in AD and contribute to its diagnosis. For a drug to be useful clinically, as opposed to causing a statistically significant effect on a cognitive test, improvement should be detected on measures of ADL. A few practical measures have been incorporated into the Blessed Dementia Scale[19]; expanded ratings of ADL have been developed by Lawton[84] and Weintraub.[148] Rating scales should offer multiple-choice responses for each area of concern in a format suitable for computer entry and analysis. Scales can be adapted for patients at home (form filled out by spouse or caretaker) or for hospitalized patients (form filled out by ward staff or physician). (See also Chapters 4 and 5.)

Laboratory tests are usually obtained during the course of a study in order to document expected physiologic effects and to detect unsuspected toxic side effects. In some instances, changes in electrophysiologic or biochemical variables related to dementia that occur during treatment provide evidence of the drug's biologic activity and possible mode of action. Thus, Thal and colleagues[145] found a significant correlation between the degree of acetylcholinesterase activity inhibition in the CSF of patients with AD and their improvement on selected memory tests during treatment with physostigmine and PC. As additional biologic markers of AD are discovered, their change during drug administration should be incorporated into experimental protocols.

FUTURE DIRECTIONS

Interpreting the neuropathologic changes and biochemical abnormalities that are discovered in brains of patients with AD gives a framework for generating ideas that may lead to effective treatments. At least four pathogenetic mechanisms are postulated to account for neuronal dysfunction in AD; each suggests fruitful neuropharmacologic approaches (Table 13–6). The first and most commonly cited pathogenetic mechanism postulates selective neuronal vulnerability and is the basis for the neurotransmitter replacement strategy highlighted in this chapter. It is unlikely, however, that damage to a single set of neurons or impaired transmission of a single transmitter will account for all of the behavioral manifestations of AD. Therefore it will be necessary to give combinations of drugs

Table 13–6 FOUR PATHOGENETIC MECHANISMS POSTULATED TO ACCOUNT FOR THE CLINICAL ABNORMALITIES IN ALZHEIMER'S DISEASE

Selective neuronal dysfunction: Disruption in the flow of information between specific cortico-cortical and cortico-subcortical nuclei
  Rx: Neurotransmitter replacement therapy

Disconnection syndrome: Isolation of the hippocampus from entorhinal cortex and medial septal nucleus
  Rx: Nerve growth factor

Generalized neuronal failure: Metabolic derangements in neuronal metabolism throughout the brain
  Rx: Phospholipids, gangliosides, nootropics

Errors of metabolism: Abnormal amyloid metabolism in the brain
  Rx: Amyloid therapy to be developed

to correct simultaneously the important neurotransmitter deficiencies known to exist in brains of patients with AD. The pace of research in this area will depend on discovering the extent to which specific behaviors result from specific neurotransmitter deficits, and whether drugs given to correct these deficiencies interact synergistically or detrimentally in affecting behavior.

Pathoanatomic disconnection of the hippocampus is a second hypothetical mechanism that could account for many of the symptoms and signs of AD. According to this view, administration of nerve growth factor is a rational strategy that should be tested in patients with AD. The hippocampus receives afferent projections from the entorhinal cortex and the medial septal nucleus; both regions are severely affected in AD.[74–76,153] The entorhinal cortex is reciprocally linked to sensory-specific and multimodal association cortices, as well as to limbic cortices. In AD, neurons in the entorhinal cortex that project to the dentate gyrus via the perforant pathway develop neurofibrillary tangles; neuritic plaques are observed in their projection termination zones. The other major projection to the hippocampus originates in the cell bodies of the cholinergic medial septal nucleus.[96] In preclinical studies, intracerebral ventricular administration of nerve growth factor (NGF) prevented degeneration of septal nuclei and induced axon regrowth of these neurons after lesions to the fimbria-fornix.[52,67] If NGF administration were to exert similar effects in humans with AD, it might rescue degenerating septal neurons and stimulate their sprouting into hippocampal regions denuded by the entorhinal lesions. Whether these effects would restore normal hippocampal function is uncertain; it is equally possible that sprouting would impair behavior and actually worsen memory. Caution has been urged in considering NGF administration to humans because of potential toxicity and uncertain side effects.[114]

Primary metabolic derangements in neurons could account for neuronal dysfunction and death, and underlie the symptoms of AD. This theory provides the rationale for ganglioside and phospholipid treatments, and an additional rationale for nootropic drugs. Support for this theory stems from new information documenting abnormal metabolism of phospholipids in the brain. Phospholipids, including phosphatidylcholine and phosphatidylethanolamine, are integral components of cell membranes, and alterations in their metabolism are likely to impair brain function. The activity of phospholipase D, the chief degradative enzyme for metabolizing phosphatidylcholine, is reduced to a level comparable to the reduction in CAT activity in brains of patients with AD.[81] Increases in levels of phospholipid precursors[113] and metabolites[20,99,100,113] have also been observed in brains of patients with AD. Identification of metabolic abnormalities such as these provide additional points of attack for developing treatments that preserve the integrity of neuronal structures.

The fourth postulated pathogenetic mechanism is based on the view of AD as an inborn error of amyloid metabolism. β-Amyloid protein forms the cores of neuritic plaques, and is deposited in cerebral blood vessels. It has been discovered recently that the β-amyloid protein is widely deposited throughout the cerebral hemispheres and cerebellum as amorphous extracellular plaques in the neuropil without surrounding neuritic dystrophy[140]; it is generally assumed that amyloid deposition is detrimental to normal brain function. It is still too early to develop treatment strategies based on this discovery because there is uncertainty regarding the exact mechanism of amyloid deposition, and even controversy whether amyloid deposition in the brain directly causes neuronal dysfunction. Under some circumstances, amyloid appears to have neuronotrophic properties.[154] What is known is that the gene encoding the β-amyloid precursor protein is located on chromosome 21 between the obligate

Down's region and the putative abnormal gene site for familial AD, and that the β-amyloid gene is not mutant or duplicated in AD.[56,141,142] It is also known that the β-amyloid gene encodes messages for at least three β-amyloid precursor proteins (APP) with different chain lengths of amino acids.[92,127] Two of them, the APP-751 and -770 amino acid variants, contain protease inhibitor domains, whereas the 695-residue sequence does not. One hypothesis for the deposition of insoluble amyloid in AD is that missing or defective protease inhibitors might allow proteolytic cleavage of the β-amyloid precursor protein and the release of self-aggregating or neurotoxic β-protein fragments. There is some support for this hypothesis. Recent in situ hybridization studies reported that neurons in the nucleus basalis of Meynert and locus ceruleus, sites of extensive cell loss and neurofibrillary tangle formation in AD, had increased message for the APP-695 (lacking the protease inhibitor domain), whereas these brain regions had normal amounts of message for the other two APPs.[107] According to these data, treatments designed to suppress the 695 message would be expected to minimize amyloid deposition. Alternatively, it is possible that a local excess of a protease inhibitor, such as the 751- and 770-residue β-APP transcripts or α-1 antichymotrypsin, might prevent a normal brain protease from clearing the abnormal product derived from the β-protein precursor.[1] This line of reasoning would suggest that treatments given to suppress the APP-751 and -770 messages would minimize amyloid deposits. (See Chapters 2 and 3.)

Surgical therapy has already begun with implantation of infusion pumps designed to deliver medication directly into the cerebral ventricles.[65] This technique permits delivery of drugs that do not easily cross the blood-brain barrier, such as the neuropeptides or NGF; it also brings drugs to the brain directly without incurring systemic toxicity. Brain implants will also be considered, especially if favorable reports from this mode of treatment in Parkinson's disease continue. Before considering implants in AD, however, it will be necessary to determine what cells to implant as well as where to place them.

Ultimately, the cure for AD in the future will come from new discoveries regarding its etiology and pathophysiology. If such insights can be gained by the concerted techniques of modern neuroscience, and the momentum of advances during the past 10 years continues, there is reason for cautious optimism in the quest for effective biologic therapies for AD.

SUMMARY

Both practical and theoretical aspects of the biologic therapy for AD have been reviewed in this chapter. The general principles considered here are also relevant for the development of treatments for other dementias. Currently, drugs are used in dementia primarily for the palliative treatment of the noncognitive symptoms, which include agitation, anxiety, depression, psychosis, and sleep disturbance.

The cognitive symptoms of AD, including amnesia, aphasia, apraxia, and visuospatial perceptual impairments, are the subjects of intense drug development research. Many approaches have been based on an understanding of the neurotransmitter abnormalities found in the brains of patients with AD. Most energy has been placed in developing cholinomimetic therapies because of the strong association between the loss of cholinergic markers and the severity of dementia. Other classes of experimental drugs proposed for the treatment of cognitive impairments in AD include drugs that affect monoamine transmission and neuropeptides. In the future we may be able to develop drugs to slow the progression of the disease based on a greater understanding of the actual pathogenesis of AD and related disorders.

The clinician should be aware of the principles of conducting a drug study, so that he or she can evaluate what will undoubtedly be a growing literature of studies of medications designed to help patients with AD and related disorders.

REFERENCES

1. Abraham CR, Selkoe JD, and Potter H: Immunochemical identification of the serine protease inhibitor alpha-1 antichymotrypsin in the brain amyloid deposits of Alzheimer's disease. Cell 52:487–501, 1988.
2. Adolfsson R, Brane G, Bucht G, et al: A double-blind study with levodopa in dementia of Alzheimer type. In Corkin S, Davis KL, Growdon JH, Usdin E, and Wurtman RJ (eds): Alzheimer's Disease: A Report of Progress in Research. Aging, Vol 19. Raven Press, New York, 1982, pp 469–473.
2a. Antidementia Drug Assessment Symposium: Meeting report of the Ad Hoc FDA Dementia Assessment Task Force. Neurobiol Aging 12:379–382, 1991.
3. Arnsten AFT and Goldman-Rakic PS: Alpha-2 adrenergic mechanisms in prefrontal cortex associated with cognitive decline in aged nonhuman primates. Science 230:1273–1276, 1985.
4. Ashford JW, Soldinger S, Schaeffer J, Cochran L, and Jarvik LF: Physostigmine and its effect on six patients with dementia. Am J Psychiatry 138:829–830, 1981.
5. Bartus RT: Physostigmine and recent memory: Effects in young and aged nonhuman primates. Science 206:1087–1089, 1979.
6. Bartus RT, Dean RL, Beer B, and Lippa AS: The cholinergic hypothesis of geriatric memory dysfunction. Science 217:408–417, 1982.
7. Bartus RT, Dean RL, Goas JA, and Lippa AS: Age-related changes in passive avoidance retention: Modulation with dietary choline. Science 209:301–303, 1980.
8. Beal MF and Growdon JH: CSF neurotransmitter markers in Alzheimer's disease. Prog Neuropsychopharmacol Biol Psychiatry 10:259–270, 1986.
9. Beal MF and Martin JB: Neuropeptides in neurological disease. Ann Neurol 20:547–565, 1986.
10. Beal MF and Mazurek MF: Substance P–like immunoreactivity is reduced in Alzheimer's disease. Neurology 37:1205–1209, 1987.
11. Beal MF, Mazurek MF, Chattha GK, Svendsen CN, Bird ED, and Martin JB: Neuropeptide Y-immunoreactivity is reduced in cerebral cortex in Alzheimer's disease. Ann Neurol 20:282–288, 1986.
12. Beal MF, Mazurek MF, Tran VT, Chattha G, Bird ED, and Martin JB: Reduced numbers of somatostatin receptors in the cerebral cortex in Alzheimer's disease. Science 229:289–291, 1985.
13. Beller SA, Oversall JE, and Swann AC: Efficacy of oral physostigmine in primary degenerative dementia. A double-blind study of response to different dose level. Psychopharmacology (Berl) 87:147–151, 1985.
14. Bergman K, Brane G, Gottfries CH, Jostell KG, Karlsson I, and Svennerholm L: Alaproclate: A pharmacokinetic and biochemical study in patients wtih dementia of Alzheimer type. Psychopharmacology (Berl) 80:279–283, 1983.
15. Bierkamper GG and Goldberg AM: Release of acetylcholine from the vascular perfused rat phrenic nerve-hemidiaphragm. Brain Res 202:234–237, 1980.
16. Bissette G, Reynolds GP, Kilts CH, Widerlow E, and Nemeroff CB: Corticotropin-releasing factor–like immunoreactivity in senile dementia of the Alzheimer type. JAMA 254:3067–3069, 1985.
17. Blackwood DH and Christie JE: The effects of physostigmine on memory and auditory P300 in Alzheimer-type dementia. Biol Psychiatry 2:557–560, 1986.
18. Blass JP, Redine MJ, Drachman D, et al: Letter to the Editor. N Engl J Med 309:556, 1983.
19. Blessed G, Tomlinson BE, and Roth M:

The association between quantitative measures of dementia and of senile change in the cerebral grey matter of elderly subjects. Br J Psychiatry 114:797–811, 1968.

20. Blusztajn JK, Gonzalez-Coviella IL, Logue M, Growdon JH, and Wurtman RJ: Levels of phospholipid catabolic intermediates, glycerophosphocholine and glycerophosphoethanolamine, are elevated in brains of Alzheimer's disease but not of Down's syndrome patients. Brain Res 536: 240–244, 1990.

21. Bondareff W, Mountjoy CQ, and Roth M: Loss of neurons of origin of the adrenergic projection of cerebral cortex (nucleus locus coeruleus) in senile dementia. Neurology 32:164–168, 1982.

22. Bowen DM: Biochemical assessment of neurotransmitter and metabolic dysfunction and cerebral atrophy in Alzheimer's disease. In Katzman R (ed): Biological Aspects of Alzheimer's Disease. Banbury Report 15. Cold Spring Harbor Laboratory, Cold Spring Harbor, NY, 1983, pp 219–230.

23. Bowen DM, Allan SH, Benton JS, et al: Biochemical assessment of serotonergic and cholinergic dysfunction and cerebral atrophy in Alzheimer's disease. J Neurochem 41:266–272, 1983.

24. Bowen DM, Smith CH, White P, and Davison AN: Neurotransmitter-related enzymes and indices of hypoxia in senile dementia and other abiotrophies. Brain 99:459–496, 1976.

25. Bruno G, Mohr E, Gillespie M, Fedio P, and Chase TN: Muscarinic agonist therapy of Alzheimer's disease. A clinical trial of RS-86. Arch Neurol 43:659–661, 1986.

26. Caltagirone C, Albanese A, Gianotti G, and Masullo C: Acute administration of individual optimal dose of physostigmine fails to improve amnesic performances in Alzheimer's presenile dementia. Int J Neurosci 18:143–147, 1983.

27. Cardelli MB, Russell M, Bagne CA, and Pomara N: Chelation therapy. Un-

proved modality in the treatment of Alzheimer-type dementia. J Am Geriatr Soc 33:548–551, 1985.

28. Chatellier G and Lacomblez L: Tacrine (tetrahydroaminoacridine; THA) and lecithin in senile dementia of the Alzheimer type: A multicentre trial. BMJ 300:495–499, 1990.

29. Christie JE, Shering A, Ferguson J, and Glen AI: Physostigmine and arecoline: Effects of intravenous infusions in Alzheimer presenile dementia. Br J Psychiatry 138: 46–50,

30. Cohen EL and Wurtman RJ: Brain acetylcholine: Increase after systemic choline administration. Life Sci 16: 1095–1102, 1975.

31. Cools AD, ven der Bercken JHL, Horstink MWI, van Spaendonck KPM, and Berger HJC: Cognitive and motor shifting aptitude disorder in Parkinson's disease. J Neurol Neurosurg Psychiatry 47:443–453, 1984.

32. Corkin S: Acetylcholine, aging and Alzheimer's disease: Implications for treatment. Trends Neurosci 4:287–290, 1981.

33. Corkin S, Growdon JH, Sullivan EV, Nissen MJ, and Huff FJ: Assessing treatment effects: A neuropsychological battery. In Poon L (ed): Handbook for Clinical Assessment of Older Adults. American Psychological Association, Washington, DC, 1986, pp 156–167.

34. Coyle JT, Price DL, and DeLong MR: Alzheimer's disease: A disorder of cortical cholinergic innervation. Science 219:1184–1190, 1983.

34a. Crapper-McLachlan DR, Dalton AJ, Druch TPA, et al. Intramuscular desferrioxamine in patients with Alzheimer's Disease. Lancet 337:1304–1308, 1991. Erratum published: Lancet 337:1618, 1991.

35. Cross AJ, Crow TJ, Ferrier IN, Johnson JA, Bloom SR, and Corsellis JAN: Serotonin receptor changes in dementia of the Alzheimer type. J Neurochem 43:1574–1581, 1984.

36. Cutler NR, Haxby J, Kay AD, et al: Evaluation of zimeldine in Alzheimer's disease. Cognitive and bio-

chemical measures. Arch Neurol 42:744–748, 1985.

37. Davies P, Katzman R, and Terry RD: Reduced somatostatin-like immuno-reactivity in cerebral cortex from cases of Alzheimer's disease and Alzheimer senile dementia. Nature 228:279–280, 1980.

38. Davies P and Maloney AJF: Selective loss of central cholinergic neurons in Alzheimer's disease. Lancet 2:1403, 1976.

39. Davis KL, Hollander E, Davidson M, Davis BM, Mohs RC, and Horvath TB: Induction of depression with oxotremorine in patients with Alzheimer's disease. Am J Psychiatry 144:468–471, 1987.

40. Davis KL and Mohs RC: Enhancement of memory in Alzheimer's disease with multiple dose intravenous physostigmine. Am J Psychiatry 139:1421–1424, 1982.

41. Davis KL, Mohs RC, Tinklenberg JR, Pfefferbaum A, Hollister LE, and Kopell BS: Physostigmine: Improvement of long-term memory processes in normal humans. Science 201:272–274, 1978.

42. Davous P and Lamour Y: Bethanechol decreases reaction time in senile dementia of the Alzheimer type. J Neurol Neurosurg Psychiatry 48:1297–1299, 1985.

43. DeWied D: The influence of the posterior and intermediate lobe of the pituitary and pituitary peptides on the maintenance of a conditioned avoidance response in rats. International Journal of Neuropharmacology 4: 157–167, 1965.

44. Drachman DA, Glosser G, Fleming P, and Longenecker G: Memory decline in the aged: Treatment wth lecithin and physostigmine. Neurology 32: 944–950, 1982.

45. Drachman DA and Leavitt J: Human memory and the cholinergic system. Arch Neurol 30:113–121, 1974.

46. Dubcovich M: Presynaptic alpha-adrenoceptors in the central nervous system. Ann N Y Acad Sci 430:7–25, 1984.

47. Fillit H, Weinreb H, Cholst I, et al: Observations in a preliminary open trial of estradiol therapy for senile dementia—Alzheimer type. Psychoneuroendocrinology 11:337–345, 1986.

48. Folstein MR, Folstein SE, and McHugh PR: Mini-Mental State. J Psychiatr Res 12:189–198, 1975.

49. Foote SL, Bloom FE, and Ashton-Jones G: Nucleus locus coeruleus: New evidence of anatomical and physiological specificity. Physiol Rev 63:844–914, 1983.

50. Francis PT, Palmer AM, Sims NR, et al: Neurochemical studies of early-onset Alzheimer's disease: Possible influence on treatment. N Engl J Med 313:7–11, 1985.

51. Friedman E, Sherman KA, Ferris SA, Reisberg B, Bartus RT, and Schneck MK: Clinical response to choline plus piracetam in senile dementia: Relation to red-cell choline levels. N Engl J Med 304:1490–1491, 1981.

52. Gage FH, Armstrong DM, Williams LR, and Varon S: Morphological response of axotomized septal neurons to nerve growth factor. J Comp Neurol 289: 147–155, 1988.

53. Gauthier S, Bouchard R, Lamontagne A, et al: Tetrahydroaminoacridine-lecithin combination treatment in patients with intermediate-stage Alzheimer's disease: Results of a Canadian double-blind, crossover, multi-center study. N Engl J Med 322:1272–1276, 1990.

54. Gibson CJ, Logue M, and Growdon JH: CSF monoamine metabolite levels in Alzheimer's disease. Arch Neurol 42:489–492, 1985.

55. Giurgea CE: Fundamentals to a Pharmacology of the Mind. Charles C Thomas, Springfield, IL, 1980.

56. Goldgaber D, Lerman MI, McBride OW, Saffiotti U, and Gajdusek DC: Characterization and chromosomal localization of cDNA encoding brain amyloid of Alzheimer's disease. Science 235: 877–880, 1987.

57. Gottfries CG, Adolfsson R, Aquilonius SM, et al: Biochemical changes in dementia disorders of Alzheimer type (AD/SDAT). Neurobiol Aging 4:261–271, 1983.

58. Grant SH and Redmond E: The neuro-

anatomy and pharmacology of the nucleus locus coeruleus. In Lal H and Fielding S (eds): Psychopharmacology of Clonidine. Alan R Liss, New York, 1981, pp 5–25.

59. Growdon JH: Neuropharmacology of degenerative diseases associated with aging. Med Res Rev 3:237–257, 1983.

60. Growdon JH and Corkin S: Cognitive impairments in Parkinson's disease. In Yahr MD and Bergman KJ (eds): Advances in Neurology, Vol 45. Raven Press, New York, 1986, pp 383–392.

61. Growdon JH, Corkin S, Buonanno F, et al: Diagnostic methods in Alzheimer's disease: Magnetic resonance brain imaging and CSF neurotransmitter markers. In Fisher A, Hanin I and Lachman C (eds): Alzheimer's and Parkinson's Disease. Plenum Publishing, New York, 1986, pp 191–204.

62. Growdon JH, Corkin S, Huff FJ, and Rosen TJ: Piracetam combined with lecithin in the treatment of Alzheimer's disease. Neurobiol Aging 7:269–276, 1986.

63. Haase GR: Diseases presenting as dementia. In Wells CE (ed): Dementia. FA Davis, Philadelphia, 1971, pp 163–207.

64. Hamilton M: A rating scale for depression. J Neurol Neurosurg Psychiatry 23:56–62, 1960.

65. Harbaugh RE, Roberts DW, Coombs DW, Saunders RL, and Reeder TM: Preliminary report: Intracranial cholinergic drug infusion in patients with Alzheimer's disease. Neurosurgery 15:514–518, 1984.

66. Hartounian V, Kanof PD, Tsuboyama G, and Davis KL: Restoration of cholinomimetic activity by clonidine in cholinergic plus noradrenergic lesioned rats. Brain Res 507:261–266, 1989.

67. Hefti F: Nerve growth factor promotes survival of septal cholinergic neurons after fimbrial transections. J Neurosci 6:2155–2162, 1986.

68. Heyman A, Schmechel D, Wilkinson W, et al: Failure of long-term high-dose lecithin to retard progression of early-onset Alzheimer's disease. In Wurtman RJ, Corkin SH, and Growdon JH (eds): Topics in the Basic and Clinical Science of Dementia. Springer-Verlag, Vienna, 1987, pp 279–286.

69. Hirsch MJ, Growdon JH, and Wurtman RJ: Increase in hippocampal acetylcholine after choline administration. Brain Res 125:383–385, 1977.

70. Hollister LE and Yesavage J: Ergoloid mesylates for senile dementias: Unanswered questions. Ann Intern Med 100:894–898, 1984.

71. Huff FH, Maire JC, Growdon JH, Corkin S, and Wurtman RJ: Cholinesterases in cerebrospinal fluid: Correlations with clinical measures in Alzheimer's disease. J Neurol Sci 72:121–129, 1986.

72. Huff FJ, Mickel SH, Corkin S, and Growdon JH: Cognitive functions affected by scopolamine in Alzheimer's disease and normal aging. Drug Development Research 12:271–278, 1988.

73. Hyman BT, Eslinger PJ, and Damasio AR: Effect of naltrexone on senile dementia of the Alzheimer type. J Neurol Neurosurg Psychiatry 48:1169–1171, 1985.

74. Hyman BT, Kromer LJ, and Van Hoesen GW: Reinnervation of the hippocampal perforant pathway zone in Alzheimer's disease. Ann Neurol 21:259–267, 1987.

75. Hyman BT, Van Hoesen GW, Damasio AR, and Barnes CL: Alzheimer's disease: Cell-specific pathology isolates the hippocampal formation. Science 225:1168–1170, 1984.

76. Hyman BT, Van Hoesen GW, Kromer LJ, and Damasio AR: Perforant pathway changes and the memory impairment of Alzheimer's disease. Ann Neurol 20:472–481, 1986.

77. Ishii T: Distribution of Alzheimer's neurofibrillary changes in the brainstem and hypothalamus of senile dementia. Acta Neuropathol 6:181–187, 1966.

78. Jenden DJ, Weiler MH, and Gundersen CB: Choline availability and acetylcholine synthesis. In Corkin S, Davis KL, Growdon JH, Usdin E, and Wurtman RJ (eds): Alzheimer's Disease: A Report of Progress in Research. Raven Press, New York, 1982, pp 315–326.

79. Jenike MA, Albert MS, Heller H, Lo-

Castro S, and Gunther J: Combination therapy with lecithin and ergoloid mesylates for Alzheimer's disease. J Clin Psychiatry 47:249–251, 1986.

80. Jotkowitz A: Lack of clinical efficacy of chronic oral physostigmine in Alzheimer's disease. Ann Neurol 14: 690–691, 1983.

81. Kanfer JN, Hattori H, and Oribel D: Reduced phospholipase D activity in brain tissue samples from Alzheimer's disease patients. Ann Neurol 20:265–267, 1986.

82. Kaye WH, Sitaram N, Weingartner H, Ebert MH, Smallberg S, and Gillin JC: Modest facilitation of memory in dementia with combined lecithin and anticholinesterase treatment. Biol Psychiatry 17:275–280, 1982.

83. Kristensen V, Olsen M, and Theilgaard A: Levodopa treatment of presenile dementia. Acta Psychiatr Scand 55:41–51, 1977.

84. Lawton MP and Brody EM: Assessment of older people: Self-maintaining instrumental activities of daily living. Gerontologist 9:179–186, 1969.

85. Leber P: Establishing the efficacy of drugs with psychogeriatric indications. In Crook T, Ferris S, and Bartus R (eds): Assessment in Geriatric Psychopharmacology. Mark Powley Associates, New Canaan, CT, 1983, pp 1–18.

86. Levin HS and Peters BH: Long-term administration of oral physostigmine and lecithin improve memory in Alzheimer's disease. Letter to the Editor. Ann Neurol 15:210, 1984.

87. Little A, Levy R, Chuaqui-Kidd P, and Hand D: A double-blind, pacebo controlled trial of high-dose lecithin in Alzheimer's disease. J Neurol Neurosurg Psychiatry 48:736–742, 1985.

88. London ED and Coyle JT: Pharmacological augmentation of acetylcholine levels in kainate lesioned rat striatum. Biochem Pharmacol 27:2962–2965, 1978.

89. Maas JW: Biogenic amines and depression — biochemical and pharmacological separation of two types of depression. Arch Gen Psychiatry 32:1357–1361, 1975.

90. Maletta GJ: Medications to modify at-home behavior of Alzheimer's patients. Geriatrics 40:31–42, 1985.

91. Mann DMA, Lincoln J, Yates PO, Stamp JE, and Toper S: Changes in monoamine-containing neurons of the human CNS in senile dementia. Br J Psychiatry 136:533–541, 1980.

92. Masters CL and Beyreuther K: Protein abnormalities in neurofibrillary tangles: Their relationships to the extracellular amyloid deposits of the A4 protein in Alzheimer's disease. In Wurtman RJ, Corkin S, Growdon JH, and Ritter-Walker E (eds): Alzheimer's Disease. Raven Press, New York, 1990, pp 151–161.

93. Mazurek MF, Growdon JH, Beal MF, and Martin JB: CSF vasopressin concentration is reduced in Alzheimer's disease. Neurology 36:1133–1137, 1986.

94. McKhann G, Drachman D, Folstein M, Katzman R, Price D, and Stadlan EM: Clinical diagnosis of Alzheimer's disease: Report of the NINCDS-ADRDA work group under the auspices of HHS Task Force on Alzheimer's Disease. Neurology 34:939–945, 1984.

95. McNair DM, Lorr M, and Droppelman LF: Manual for the Profile of Mood States. Educational and Industrial Testing Service, San Diego, CA, 1971.

96. Mesulam M-M, Mufson EJ, Levey AI, and Wainer BH: Cholinergic innervation of cortex by the basal forebrain: Cytochemistry and cortical connections of the septal area, diagonal band nuclei, nucleus basalis (substantia innominata) and hypothalamus in the rhesus monkey. J Comp Neurol 214: 170–197, 1983.

97. Mesulam M-M, Mufson EJ, and Rogers J: Age-related shrinkage of cortically projecting cholinergic neurons: A selective effect. Ann Neurol 22:31–36, 1987.

98. Meyer JS, Welch KM, Deshmukh VD, et al: Neurotransmitter precursor amino acids in the treatment of multiinfarct dementia and Alzheimer's disease. J Am Geriatr Soc 25:289–298, 1977.

99. Miatto O, Blusztajn JK, Logue M, Gon-

zalez RG, Buonanno F, and Growdon JH: Detection of phospholipids in brain tissue using ^{31}P NMR spectroscopy. In Bazan NG, Horrocks LA, and Toffano G (eds): Phospholipids in the Nervous System: Biochemical and Molecular Pathology. Fidia Research Series, Vol 17. Liviana Press, Padova, 1989.

100. Miatto O, Gonzalez RG, Buonanno F, and Growdon JH: In vitro ^{31}P spectroscopy detects altered phospholipid metabolism in Alzheimer's disease. Can J Neurol Sci 13:535–539, 1986.

101. Mohs RC, Davis BM, Johns CA, et al: Oral physostigmine treatment of patients with Alzheimer's disease. Am J Psychiatry 142:28–33, 1985.

102. Montgomery SA and Asberg M: A new depression scale designed to be sensitive to change. Br J Psychiatry 134:382–389, 1979.

103. Muramoto A, Sugishita M, and Ando K: Cholinergic system and constructional praxis: A further study of physostigmine in Alzheimer's disease. J Neurol Neurosurg Psychiatry 47:485–491, 1984.

104. Nissen MJ, Knopman DS, and Schacter DL: Neurochemical dissociation of memory systems. Neurology 37:789–794, 1987.

105. Palmer AM, Wilcock GK, Esiri MM, Francis PT, and Bowen DM: Monoaminergic innervation of the frontal and temporal lobes in Alzheimer's disease. Brain Res 402:231–238, 1987.

106. Palmert MR, Golde TE, Cohen ML, et al: Amyloid protein precursor messenger RNAs: Differential expression in Alzheimer's disease. Science 241:1080–1082, 1988.

107. Peabody CA, Davies H, Berger PA, and Tinklenberg JR: Desamino-D-arginine-vasopressin (DDAVP) in Alzheimer's disease. Neurobiol Aging 7:301–303, 1986.

108. Peabody CA, Thiemann S, Pigache R, et al: Desglycinamide-9-arginine-8-vasopressin (DGAVP, Organon 5667) in patients with dementia. Neurobiol Aging 6:95–100, 1985.

109. Perry EK, Perry RH, Blessed G, and Tomlinson BE: Necropsy evidence of central cholinergic deficits in senile dementia. Lancet 1:189, 1977.

110. Perry EK, Tomlinson BE, Blessed G, Bergmann K, Gibson PH, and Perry RH: Correlation of cholinergic abnormalities with senile plaques and mental scores in senile dementia. BMJ 2:1457–1459, 1978.

111. Perry RH, Dockray GJ, Dimaline R, Perry EK, Blessed G, and Tomlinson BE: Neuropeptides in Alzheimer's disease, depression and schizophrenia. J Neurol Sci 51:465–472, 1981.

112. Peters BH and Levin HS: Effects of physostigmine and lecithin on memory in Alzheimer's disease. Ann Neurol 6:219–221, 1979.

113. Pettegrew JW, Kopp SH, Minshew NJ, et al: ^{31}P nuclear magnetic resonance studies of phosphoglyceride metabolism in developing and degenerating brain: Preliminary observations. J Neuropathol Exp Neurol 46:419–430, 1987.

114. Phelps CH, Gage FH, Growdon JH, et al: Commentary: Potential use of nerve growth factor to treat Alzheimer's disease. Neurobiol Aging 10:205–207, 1989.

115. Podlisny MB, Lee G, and Selkoe DJ: Gene dosage of the amyloid beta precursor protein in Alzheimer's disease. Science 238:669–671, 1987.

116. Pomara N, Roberts R, Rhiew HB, Stanley M, and Gershon S: Multiple, single-dose naltrexone administrations fail to affect overall cognitive functioning and plasma cortisol in individuals with probable Alzheimer's disease. Neurobiol Aging 6:233–236, 1985.

117. Randels PM, Marco LA, Ford DI, Mitchell R, Scholl M, and Plesnarski J: Lithium and lecithin treatment in Alzheimer's disease. A pilot study. J Clin Psychiatry 6:139–147, 1984.

118. Raskin MA, Peskind ER, Halter JB, and Jimerson DC: Norepinephrine and MHPG levels in CSF and plasma in Alzheimer's disease. Arch Gen Psychiatry 42:343–346, 1984.

119. Reisberg R, Ferris SH, Anand ER, et al: Effects of naloxone in senile dementia: A double-blind trial. [Letter]. N Engl J Med 308:721–722, 1983.

120. Rinne JO, Sako E, Paljarvi L, Molsa PK, and Rinne UK: Brain dopamine D-2 receptors in senile dementia. J Neural Transm 65:51–62, 1986.
121. Risse SC and Barnes R: Pharmacologic treatment of agitation associated with dementia. J Am Geriatr Soc 34:368–376, 1986.
122. Risse SC, Lampe TH, and Cubberley L: Very low-dose neuroleptic treatment in two patients with agitation associated with Alzheimer's disease. J Clin Psychiatry 48:207–208, 1987.
123. Rose RP and Moulthrop MA: Differential responsivity of verbal and visual recognition memory to physostigmine and ACTH. Biol Psychiatry 21:538–542, 1986.
124. Rossor MN, Emson PC, Iversen LL, et al: Neuropeptides and neurotransmitters in cerebral cortex in Alzheimer's disease. In Corkin S, Davis KL, Growdon JH, Usdin E, and Wurtman RJ (eds): Alzheimer's Disease: A Report of Progress in Research. Aging, Vol 19. Raven Press, New York, 1982, pp 15–24.
125. Schildkraut JJ: The catecholamine hypothesis of affective disorders: A review of supporting evidence. Am J Psychiatry 122:509–522, 1965.
126. Schwartz AD and Kohlstaedt EV: Physostigmine effects in Alzheimer's disease: Relationship to dementia severity. Life Sci 38:1021–1028, 1986.
127. Selkoe DJ: Biochemistry of altered brain proteins in Alzheimer's disease. Annu Rev Neurosci 12:463–490, 1989.
128. Serby M, Resnick R, Jordan B, Adler J, Corwin J, and Rotrosen JP: Naltrexone and Alzheimer's disease. Prog Neuropsychopharmacol Biol Psychiatry 10:587–590, 1986.
129. Sims NR, Bowen DM, Allen SH, et al: Presynaptic cholinergic dysfunction in patients with dementia. J Neurochem 40:503–509, 1983.
130. Sitaram N, Weingartner H, Caine ED, and Gillin JC: Choline: Selective enhancement of serial learning and encoding of low imagery words in man. Life Sci 22:1555–1560, 1978.
131. Sitaram N, Weingartner H, and Gillin JC: Human serial learning: Enhancement with arecoline and choline and impairment with scopolamine. Science 201:274–276, 1978.
132. Smith RC, Vroulis G, Johnson R, and Morgan R: Comparison of therapeutic response to long-term treatment with lecithin versus piracetam plus lecithin in patients with Alzheimer's disease. Psychopharmacol Bull 20:542–545, 1984.
133. Soininen H, Koskinen T, Helkala EL, Pigache R, and Riekkinen PH: Treatment of Alzheimer's disease with a synthetic ACTH 4-9 analog. Neurology 35:1348–1351, 1985.
134. Sourander LB, Portin R, Molsa P, Lahdes A, and Rinne UK: Senile dementia of the Alzheimer type with aniracetam: A new nootropic agent. Psychopharmacology (Berl) 91:90–95, 1987.
135. Steele C, Lucas MJ, and Tune L: Haloperidol versus thioridazine in the treatment of behavioral symptoms in senile dementia of the Alzheimer's type: Preliminary findings. J Clin Psychiatry 47:310–312, 1986.
136. Stern Y, Sano M, and Mayeux R: Effects of oral physostigmine in Alzheimer's disease. Ann Neurol 22:306–310, 1987.
137. Sullivan EV, Shedlack KJ, and Corkin S: Physostigmine and lecithin in Alzheimer's disease. In Corkin S, Davis KL, Growdon JH, Usdin E, and Wurtman RJ (eds): Alzheimer's Disease: A Report of Progress in Research. Raven Press, New York, 1982, pp 361–367.
138. Summers WK, Majovski LV, Marsh GM, Tachiki K, and Kling A: Oral tetrahydroaminoacridine in long-term treatment of senile dementia, Alzheimer type. N Engl J Med 315:1241–1245, 1986.
139. Sunderland T, Tariot PN, Mueller EA, Murphy DL, Weingartner H, and Cohen RM: Cognitive and behavioral sensitivity to scopolamine in Alzheimer patients and controls. Psychopharmacol Bull 21:676–682, 1985.
140. Tagliavini F, Giaccone G, Frangione B, and Bugiani O: Preamyloid deposits in the cerebral cortex of patients with

Alzheimer's disease and nondemented individuals. Neurosci Lett 93:191–196, 1988.

141. Tanzi RE, Gusella JF, Watkins PC, et al: Amyloid beta protein gene: cDNA, mRNA distribution, and genetic linkage near the Alzheimer locus. Science 235:880–884, 1987.

142. Tanzi RE, St George-Hyslop PH, Haines JL, et al: The genetic defect in familial Alzheimer's disease is not tightly linked to the amyloid beta protein gene. Nature 329:156–157, 1987.

143. Tariot PN, Sunderland T, Weingartner H, Murphy DL, Cohen MR, and Cohen RM: Naloxone and Alzheimer's disease. Cognitive and behavioral effects of a range of doses. Arch Gen Psychiatry 43:727–732, 1986.

144. Tariot PN, Sunderland T, Weingartner H, et al: Cognitive effects of L-deprenyl in Alzheimer's disease. Psychopharmacology (Berl) 91:489–495, 1987.

145. Thal LK, Fuld PA, Masur DM, and Sharpless NS: Oral physostigmine and lecithin improve memory in Alzheimer disease. Ann Neurol 13:491–496, 1983.

146. U'Prichard D: Biochemical characteristics and regulation of brain alpha-2 adrenoceptors. Ann N Y Acad Sci 430:55–75, 1984.

147. VanWoert MH, Heninger G, Rathey U, and Bowers MB: L-dopa in senile dementia. Lancet 1:573–574, 1970.

148. Weintraub S: The record of independent living: An informant-completed measure of activities of daily living and behavior in elderly patients with cognitive impairment. American Journal of Alzheimer Care 1:35–39, 1986.

149. Wettstein A: No effect from double-blind trial of physostigmine and lecithin in Alzheimer disease. Ann Neurol 13:210–212, 1983.

150. Wettstein A and Spiegel R: Clinical trials with the cholinergic drug RS 86 in Alzheimer's disease (AD) and senile dementia of the Alzheimer type (SDAT). Psychopharmacology (Berl) 84:572–573, 1984.

151. Whitehouse PJ and Kellar KH: Nicotinic and muscarinic cholinergic receptors in Alzheimer's disease and related disorders. J Neural Transm Suppl 24:175–182, 1987.

152. Whitehouse PJ, Martino AM, Antuono PG, et al: Nicotinic acetylcholine binding sites in Alzheimer's disease. Brain Res 371:146–151, 1986.

153. Whitehouse PJ, Price DL, Coyle JT, and DeLong MR: Alzheimer's disease: Evidence for selective loss of cholinergic neurons in the nucleus basalis. Ann Neurol 10:122–126, 1981.

154. Whitson JS, Selkoe DJ, and Cotman CW: Amyloid beta protein enhances the survival of hippocampal neurons in vitro. Science 243:1488–1491, 1989.

155. Wilcock GK, Esiri MM, Bowen DM, and Smith CCT: Alzheimer's disease: Correlation of cortical choline acetyltransferase activity with the severity of dementia and histological abnormalities. J Neurol Sci 57:407–417, 1982.

156. Woods SW, Tesar GE, Murray GB, and Cassem NH: Psychostimulant treatment of depressive disorder secondary to medical treatment. J Clin Psychiatry 47:12–15, 1986.

157. Yarbrough GG and Pomara N: The therapeutic potential of thyrotropin releasing hormone (TRH) in Alzheimer's disease (AD). Prog Neuropsychopharmacol Bio Psychiatry 9:285–289, 1985.

158. Yates CM, Harmar AJ, Rosie R, et al: Thyrotropin-releasing hormone, luteinizing hormone–releasing hormone and substance P immunoreactivity in postmortem brain from cases of Alzheimer-type dementia and Down's syndrome. Brain Res 258:45–52, 1983.

159. Zornetzer SF: Catecholamine system involvement in age-related memory dysfunction. Ann N Y Acad Sci 444:242–254, 1985.

Chapter 14

MANAGEMENT OF PATIENTS WITH DEMENTIA

Nancy L. Mace, M.A.,
Peter J. Whitehouse, M.D.,
  Ph.D., and
Kathleen A. Smyth, Ph.D.

THE PATIENT
THE ENVIRONMENT
THE FAMILY

Because there are few medical interventions that are effective in the treatment of Alzheimer's disease (AD) and related disorders, a sense of therapeutic nihilism shadows the clinical care of these patients.[38] As with other chronic diseases, however, behavioral, psychosocial, and environmental interventions may improve the quality of life for both the patient and the family.[39] Although the role of the physician is key in diagnosis and in the treatment of symptoms and concurrent illness, the acute-care–oriented medical model is not sufficiently broad to address the health needs of patients with dementia: for most patients, an effective response requires assessment and ongoing intervention by physicians, nurses, and social workers, often augmented by input from nutritionists, occupational and physical therapists, and other practitioners, working as consultants or as part of an interdisciplinary team.[11] Further, the spouse, children, and other relatives of the patient with dementia also need care and support throughout the illness.[33,46,63]

This chapter reviews interdisciplinary management strategies for dealing with irreversible dementia, focusing on the patient, the environment, and the family. From the perspective of assisting the patient, issues in both evaluation and ongoing management are addressed, including dealing with problem behaviors and the demands of end-stage care. The interplay of patient and environment is explored and suggestions for assessing and modifying the environment are outlined. Finally, the role and needs of families in dementia care are reviewed.

THE PATIENT

Evaluation

Treatment interventions begin with a comprehensive medical evaluation.[48] (See Chapter 4.) This workup provides the physician with the information needed to help the patient and family understand the nature of the diagnosis and its implications, and any concurrent illness that may affect its progress and management.[59] The nursing diagnostic evaluation focuses on practical issues of care, especially safety and performance of activities of daily living

400

(ADLs) (e.g., feeding, dressing), and on patient and family needs for education. Table 14–1 provides an example of a checklist that could be used to guide the assessment of ADLs in a patient with dementia. Note that it distinguishes problems with initiating activities from problems with carrying them out. An ADL assessment is useful for identifying both problem areas and remaining strengths. The social-work assessment emphasizes family dynamics, previous patterns of coping with stress, access to community services, and financial matters. Other clinicians contribute information on nutritional status, physi-

Table 14–1 ACTIVITIES OF DAILY LIVING CHECKLIST

Bathing
—— Initiates bath/shower with appropriate frequency and at appropriate time
—— Prepares bath/shower
—— Gets in and out of tub or shower
—— Cleans self

Toileting
—— Able to physically control timing of urination
—— Able to physically control timing of bowel movements
—— Recognizes need to eliminate
—— Cleans self after toileting
—— Rearranges clothes after toileting is finished

Personal hygiene/appearance
—— Initiates personal grooming with appropriate frequency and at appropriate time
—— Washes hands and face
—— Brushes teeth
—— Combs hair/shaves (as appropriate)

Dressing
—— Initiates dressing at appropriate time
—— Selects clothes
—— Puts on garments/footwear, etc.
—— Fastens clothing (buttons, shoelaces, zippers, etc.)

Medications
—— Remembers to take medications as scheduled
—— Takes medications in correct dosages

Eating
—— Initiates eating after appropriate length of time since last meal
—— Initiates eating at appropriate times of day
—— Carries out physical acts of eating (including using utensils)
—— Eats with acceptable manners (appropriate speed, not speaking with food in mouth, etc.)

Meal preparation
—— Plans balanced meals
—— Prepares own meals (including cooking on stove)

Mobility
—— Initiates actively moving about environment, as opposed to sitting, not attempting to get about, etc.
—— Actively moves about environment (with or without assisting device)
—— Needs cane, walker, or wheelchair for mobility
—— Gets in and out of bed
—— Gets in and out of chair
—— Gets on and off toilet
   Climbs up and down stairs

continued

Table 14–1 — *Continued*

Shopping
—— Does necessary food shopping, buying appropriate items/quantities
—— Does necessary clothes shopping, buying appropriate items/quantities

Travel
—— Finds way about in familiar surroundings
—— Orients to unfamiliar surroundings without undue difficulty
—— Travels beyond walking distance (driving own vehicle or using public transportation)
—— (If patient drives): Drives alone whenever he/she wishes
—— Drives only under limited circumstances (e.g., certain places, at certain times, or with someone else in car)

Hobbies/personal interests/employment
—— Initiates activities of personal interest
—— Carries out such activities
—— Works for pay

Housework/home maintenance
—— Initiates work around house as needed
—— Carries out work in relatively efficient fashion (e.g., reasonably organized/systematic)
—— Carries out work effectively (e.g., cleanly, neatly, accurately)

Telephone
—— Looks up numbers
—— Dials numbers
—— Answers phone
—— Takes messages

Money management
—— Spends appropriate to means, neither overspending nor being excessively parsimonious
—— Pays for purchases (selecting appropriate amount and determining correct change)
—— Pays monthly bills
—— Manages checking account
—— Handles savings accounts, insurance, will, and so forth

Communication skills
—— Spontaneously expresses thoughts and needs to others
—— Responds accurately to spoken instructions and conversation
—— Reads and understands single words and short phrases (e.g., signs, lists)
—— Reads and understands complex materials (books, newspapers, etc.)
—— Writes short phrases (e.g., lists, brief messages)
—— Writes complex materials (e.g., letters, diary)

Social behavior
—— Shows regard for personal privacy (e.g., dresses and undresses in appropriate seclusion; closes bathroom door; does not intrude on others in such situations)
—— Avoids coarse or vulgar conversation or actions in normal social intercourse
—— When patient has committed any socially inappropriate behavior, he/she is sensitive to effects and attempts to inhibit further such behaviors.

Source: Adapted from the Cleveland Activities of Daily Living Rating Scale. In Martin RJ, Nagley S, and Whitehouse P: ADL Skills in Alzheimer's Disease. Paper presented at the 41st Annual Scientific Meeting of the Gerontological Society of America, San Francisco, November, 1988.

cal functioning, and other effects of the dementia that are crucial to developing a thorough plan of care.

A summary conference attended by the patient, clinicians, and family members involved in the case can be effective in providing families with an integrated diagnostic and prognostic assessment. Because the course of dementing illnesses varies so widely, a realistic but optimistic tone is appropriate. It is important to be aware that families may need considerable time to absorb the information presented in a conference. Patients and families vary both in their awareness of the possibility that the presenting problem is a symptom of irreversible dementia and in their willingness to accept such a diagnosis. Although receiving a diagnosis of Alzheimer's disease or a related dementia can be devastating to patient and family, some clinicians find that patients are relieved to know that they are not "going crazy," and families may experience less guilt concerning their purported role in producing the symptoms.[37]

When the diagnosis is made early, the patient can participate in legal, financial, and care plans. (See Chapter 15.) Before they are faced with a care crisis, families should be encouraged to talk to the patient, with one another, and with their physician about advance directives concerning the patient's wishes for certain types of care (e.g., life-sustaining procedures or autopsy) when he or she is no longer able to make such decisions. Written documentation, such as a living will, can be useful in guiding future care discussion as a reflection of the patient's desires, even though the legal status of these documents varies from state to state.

Ongoing Medical Care

Patients and family caregivers should be reassessed at regular intervals and whenever there is a significant change in the functioning of either. Acute changes in behavior are often the sign of a new illness or psychological stress. Problems can also arise because several health care professionals may share responsibility for ongoing care. This makes coordination of treatment plans critical. For example, changes in medication by one provider may be unknown to another, opening the way for problematic drug interactions. Because they often cannot communicate physical or psychological symptoms, people with dementia are especially vulnerable to conditions that cause excess disability, that is, more cognitive impairment than can be explained by the primary disease itself.[29,43] Monitoring for treatable causes of excess disability (Table 14–2)

Table 14–2 EXCESS DISABILITY IN PATIENTS WITH DEMENTIA: CAUSES, EXAMPLES, AND ASSOCIATED BEHAVIORAL SYMPTOMS

Cause	Examples	Associated Behavioral Symptoms
Illness	Upper respiratory infection	Delirium
	Urinary tract infection	Lethargy
		Increased agitation
Pain	Constipation	Increased agitation
	Arthritis	Stubbornness
	Muscle cramp	Screaming, moaning
	Compression fracture	
Medications	Neuroleptics	Delirium
		Akathisia
		Dystonia
		Tardive dyskinesia
		Parkinsonian symptoms
		Hypotension
	Minor tranquilizers	Depression
		Delirium
	Antidepressants	Tremor
		Dry mouth
		Difficulty with urination
		Delirium
		Hypotension
Poor hearing		Paranoia
Poor vision		Illusions
		Hallucinations

ensures that the patient will function as well as possible throughout the illness.

Managing Problem Behaviors

Problem behaviors result from the combined effects of brain damage and the external environment. They can be exacerbated by excess disability. Once excess disability has been treated, the most successful interventions attempt to circumvent cognitive disabilities and build on remaining skills. The same behavior may have different precipitants in different patients or in the same patient at different times (Table 14–3). Psychiatric symptoms, including depression, hallucinations, delusions, paranoia, or sleeplessness, are common in dementia.[44,47] Many behavior problems, however, such as agitation and wandering, do not fit standard psychiatric categories. These problems are commonly reported by families[50] and by staff of day-care programs[42] and nursing homes,[67] and are major sources of lay and professional caregiver stress.[15,50]

The goal of management of these behaviors is to try nonpharmaceutical approaches first, reserving the use of medications for situations where specific therapeutic goals can be identified.[9,14,23,40] General principles of behavior management include individualized assessment of the patient and the behavior; a focus on here-and-now pleasurable experience for the patient and family; and attention to the safety and security of the patient and those in his or her environment. Depending on the behavior and the circumstances surrounding it, it may be more effective to rechannel or redirect the behavior than to prevent or stop it. In most cases, reassurance will have positive effects. Table 14–4 elaborates on these principles.

In some cases, clinicians may need to help families sort through the behavior management problems they are facing and to target those that are the most upsetting to the caregiver or most detri-mental to the patient. A detailed history, identifying exactly what the patient does when, where, and with whom is essential.[48] This process will usually suggest interventions (such as those listed in Table 14–3). The environment, and the caregivers' capacity for accommodation, described in more detail below, also fluctuate and must be taken into consideration. Family members will need the active support of the clinician as well as concrete suggestions for change if they are to implement interventions successfully.

Interventions such as behavior modification or memory enhancement techniques[20] may be useful in the care of some patients. Behavior-modification approaches attempt to increase desirable behaviors or decrease problem behaviors by appropriately associating the behaviors with reward or punishment. The emphasis is on measuring baseline behaviors, instituting a modification program, and reassessing the behavior to determine the outcome of the intervention. For example, a day-care patient who rummages in other participants' lockers and who likes to draw could be given reinforcement for positive behavior by having access to art material, based on staying away from the locker area. Success is measured by the frequency with which problem behaviors are reduced and desirable behaviors are increased. Memory enhancement techniques range from simple suggestions, such as writing notes, to more sophisticated attempts to improve encoding or retrieval of information, such as visual imagery or verbal mnemonic devices.[58] Interventions that add to the patient's sense of inadequacy or to the caregiver's frustration obviously should be avoided.

The judicious use of medications can improve behavioral problems, although remarkably little scientific literature is available to guide the clinician. Because of the potential for undesirable side effects, particularly the tendency of medication to further cloud cognition, drugs typically should not be used until interpersonal and environmental interven-

Table 14–3 PROBLEM BEHAVIORS: COMMON CAUSES AND INTERVENTIONS

Wandering*

Common Precipitants	Possible Interventions
Feeling lost, searching for something familiar, a desire to return home	Furnish environment with familiar possessions; point out familiar landmarks; provide mementos of family visits
	Acknowledge the feeling; reassure, distract
Need to urinate, pain, discomfort	Recognize signal and assist or treat
Need for exercise	Provide secure area for walking (corridors, yard); Allow behavior to continue if safe
	Make walking area interesting
	Provide escort for a walk
	Offer active tasks: sweeping, dusting, errands
Agitation	Reassure, remove to less stressful setting
	Identify trigger and avoid if possible
	Put away items that may become hazards when the patient is upset
Boredom	Provide active tasks, companionship, group activities
In all cases, regardless of precipitants	Provide supervision or security (keys, locks, latches on doors) to ensure safety
	Close doors or use gates at the top of stairs
	Use an ID bracelet
	Remove throw rugs, other obstacles to reduce risk of falls

Urinary Incontinence

Common Precipitants	Possible Interventions
Infection, other disease process (e.g., congestive heart failure, diabetes mellitus, medications)	Identify, treat if possible
Unable to find toilet, unable to get out of chairs	Avoid restrictive furniture; provide upright chair with arms
	Remove obstacles en route to toilet; make toilet easier to locate
Unable to manage, sequence, or remove clothing	Recognize and assist as needed; use Velcro fasteners, elastic waists; avoid clothing that supports an infantile self-image
Agnosia, failure to recognize that other objects (wastebaskets, chairs) are not toilet	Remove or change target (e.g., lid on wastebasket); improve cues for toilet; use scheduled reminders
Fails to respond to urge; does not respond in time	Use individualized toileting schedule; assist as needed
Depression, hostility	Treat psychiatric symptoms; support social behaviors; allow patient to make appropriate decisions
Underlying neurologic disorder; immobile, bedfast	Use incontinence clothing pads
In all cases, regardless of precipitants	Do complete history and physical
	Do urinalysis
	Consider consult (GYN, urology)
	Ensure appropriate hydration, maintain mobility, use gentle approach, maintain dignity

Note: Only a limited number of potential problem behaviors, precipitants, and interventions are listed here. In all cases, an individualized search for precipitants and a trial-and-error approach to interventions is needed. The reader is referred to *The 36-Hour Day*[37] for additional suggestions on behavior management.

*Apparently aimless walking or pacing (e.g., efforts to leave a home or facility; entering other residents' rooms uninvited).

Table 14-4 THE SIX R'S OF BEHAVIOR MANAGEMENT

Reassess:	When change is observed or when an intervention no longer works.
Restrict:	Prevent a behavior from occurring or stop a behavior from continuing. This is the most common method of intervention and usually the fastest way to ensure safety, but can be unnecessarily restrictive when no one is at risk.
Reconsider:	Ask: From the patient's point of view, is this a reasonable behavior? For example, if the patient does not recognize the context or setting, the patient's actions may seem to us inappropriate.
Rechannel:	Find a way for the patient to continue a behavior in a way that is not disruptive or dangerous.
Redirect:	Divert behavior that is leading toward an outburst. Use distraction, or offer a substitute activity.
Reassure:	Reassure the patient that he/she is safe and that you will see that he/she is not embarrassed or lost. Reassure the patient that you recognize his/her feelings after a catastrophic reaction.

tions have first been tried. (See Chapter 13.)

Stress plays a significant role in behavior problems. Overreactions to minor stresses have been labeled "catastrophic reactions."[21] They are characterized by angry outbursts, agitation, stubbornness, or crying. Fortunately, caregivers can be helped to anticipate and avoid many of the situations that trigger them[41] (Table 14-5).

Late-Stage Care

Much of the current interest in dementia care focuses on patients in the early and middle stages of their illness. Late in the illness, patients may be too impaired to exhibit many problem behaviors or to participate in group activities. These patients may respond to music or other sensory stimulation, however, or to social activities such as visits from family, pets, and children.

Maintenance of general health through passive exercises, nutrition, and body and skin care is important. Those patients who appear to be frightened, anxious, panicky, or in pain should be examined for illness and the environment evaluated for possible causes of distress.

Explicit discussions with family and clinicians about end-of-life care issues (e.g., antibiotics, hospitalization, autopsy) are essential. If there are previously prepared advance directives, these can be used to guide therapeutic decisions. Families who continue to provide care at home will need practical information about the nursing care of the terminal patient.

THE ENVIRONMENT

Whether the patient is living alone, with family or another live-in caregiver, or in a residential facility, a supportive environment is essential for the maintenance of maximum function.[5,32,64] The physical and psychosocial environments can be modified to substitute partially for lost functions and to support remaining abilities. These adaptations can range from simple interventions, such as removing clutter and teaching the caregiver to avoid stressing the confused patient, to a comprehensive "life-prosthetic" environment that provides role-appropriate activities and facilitates the formation of friendships and opportunities for pleasure. The characteristics of the therapeutic environment have not been well researched; nevertheless, we can describe their general outlines.[13,23,27,64,66] Table 14-6 lists steps that may be taken to enhance the fit between patients with dementia and their environment. Studies are under way to document more precisely the effects of specific environmental modifications on patient behaviors. Recent work by Calkins and associates[6] has described the inventive

Table 14-5 CATASTROPHIC REACTIONS: PRECIPITANTS AND INTERVENTIONS

Definition:	Overreaction to minor stress
Early warning:	Flushing
	Restlessness
	Refusal
Precipitants:	Misinterpretation of request
	Misinterpretation of sensory information
	Cognitive overload
	Inability to perform a task
	Fatigue
	Inability to communicate needs, being misunderstood
	Frustration
	Response to demoralizing or infantilizing treatment
Interventions:	Recognize that the behavior is not willful
	Remove precipitant
	Avoid arguing or restraining; be calm and reassuring
Preventive strategies:	Maximize physical health and functioning
	Know patient's limits:
	• Simplify tasks
	• Make environment easier to comprehend
	• Compensate for patient's limitations
	• Fill in when the patient seems to be groping for a word or a skill
	• Take things one step at a time
	• Plan difficult tasks for the patient's best time of day
	Give positive reinforcement only
	Avoid rushing the patient
	Consider that you may be misunderstanding the patient; do not ignore protests
	Maintain familiar routines
	Learn to identify warning signs:
	• Keep a log to help identify what occurred just before an outburst
	• Be alert to the patient's warnings that stress is building and avoid pushing him/her to this point
	• Avoid being too interpretive; the cause of behavior is most likely to be immediate and obvious, rather than psychodynamic or hidden
	Individualize — some interventions will be successful with some patients, but not others
	Be flexible: try things a different way; accept some odd behavior

strategies used by families to adapt home environments to the needs of demented members.

The interpersonal environment can have a profound effect on performance and behavior.[15,41] Even individuals who are severely impaired in verbal skills often remain sensitive to nonverbal messages. Table 14-7 lists some suggestions for improving the patient's psychosocial milieu. Caregiver education courses can help teach necessary skills.[15]

The best environment, whether in the home or in day-care or institutional care programs, also offers sensory and social stimulation.[32] The optimal level and type of stimulation must be deter-mined through an understanding of premorbid life-style and trial and error. The Office of Technology Assessment (OTA)[55] lists 15 areas in which patient improvement has been observed through changes in environment, including beneficial effects on social function, psychiatric symptoms, and disturbed behaviors. No improvements in language skills, motor skills, or memory have been reported. These interventions have proved challenging to implement. They require that the caregiver, whether family member or professional, be well supported, not too stressed, and able to use individualized problem-solving skills creatively and to tolerate difficult behavior.

**Table 14–6 CREATING A THERAPEUTIC
PHYSICAL ENVIRONMENT**

Ensure that glasses and hearing aides are maintained and worn. (Recognize that the patient may not be aware of or be able to compensate for sensory loss.)

Illuminate living areas well. Eliminate bright spots and glare from windows, waxed floors, etc. Use high-contrast colors such as white and bright blue. (The aging eye loses the ability to discriminate between similar tones.)

Reduce clutter.

Avoid or remove things that distract the patient, such as large groups of people or human traffic. The size of group a patient can tolerate is highly idiosyncratic.

Eliminate unnecessary noises such as background music, television, kitchen noise, and machinery.

Use objects that trigger long-term memory or recognition (e.g., mugs or cups instead of styrofoam.)

Make needed items visible (e.g., leave bathroom door open).

Put away toxic or dangerous items (e.g., cleaning products, throw rugs).

Labeling the environment (e.g., signs on bathroom or bedroom doors) will help some patients, but others will not be able to act on what they read.

THE FAMILY

The Caregiving Role

The burden on family caregivers associated with providing ongoing care to a demented family member is enormous and well documented.[25,30,55] Although some aspects of the care required are not different from those associated with other serious illnesses,[34] the loss of person and requirements for constant supervision encountered in dementia care can be uniquely stressful. This so-called "informal" care system provides 80% to 90% of all care.[55] The capacity of families to provide care varies widely. Families dealing with similarly impaired patients may exhibit divergent levels of stress.[64] Variations in measurement and populations studied have made it difficult to generalize about the effects of caregiving.[49] Important ethnic and cultural factors also influence patterns of care and the effects of caregiving.[35] Studies have shown that family care typically is taken on in a hierarchical fashion.[28,61] In most cases, spouses are assumed to be responsible for providing care unless they themselves

**Table 14–7 CREATING A SUPPORTIVE
INTERPERSONAL ENVIRONMENT**

Provide activities that allow the patient to succeed.

Break tasks down into small steps. Take one step at a time.

Use an approach that communicates dignity, respect, and genuine affection.

Use touch. Learn to read and use body language.

Identify and support spared abilities; avoid situations that require lost skills.

Create a relaxed, calm atmosphere.

Use appropriate but not demeaning humor.

are extremely incapacitated. When spouses are unable to provide care, adult daughters and daughters-in-law are generally next in line.[3] Nieces and nephews, siblings, and grandchildren may also take on primary care responsibilities. Although the term "primary caregiver" is commonly used to identify the family member who provides most of the direct care, there are many cases in which family care is a distributed responsibility, with no one person identifiable as primarily responsible for the demented family member. Frequently no family member will or can provide daily care.

Female family members are more likely than male family members to give up or reduce paid employment to provide care.[4] Although there are exceptions, nonspousal male family members typically do not take on the primary caregiving role. Often they handle tasks that do not involve direct care, such as financial and legal matters. Although male caregivers may face particular problems with developing new care and domestic skills, some studies report that male spouses are less stressed by caregiving.[18] Male caregivers have been found to use action-oriented, problem-solving coping styles, which may represent transfer of learning from the workplace.[65]

Spouse caregivers frequently devote all or most of their time to the caregiving role. Numerous studies have documented that spouses will continue to provide care at home, even in the face of their own seriously deteriorating health, and are less likely to use formal services, including nursing homes.[7]

Adult children and other relatives frequently experience role conflict stemming from competing demands of an ill parent, their own children, their spouses, and their job.[45] One consequence is that they tend to place family members in nursing homes sooner than do spouse caregivers.[36] Those who give up jobs to provide care may experience more stress than those who purchase care.[17]

Family caregivers are vulnerable to depression, stress-related illness, and drug and alcohol abuse. Further, they themselves may be suffering from serious chronic illnesses.[19] Recent psychoneuroimmunologic studies suggest that alterations in immune function may mediate the effects of stress on caregiver health.[31] Although the extent of the problem is not known, some caregivers abuse the patient psychologically or physically, often because they do not understand the disease or are under severe stress.[1]

The mental and physical health of the caregiver is an important influence on the likelihood that a demented patient will remain in the home. Unfortunately, support services to aid family caregivers are rarely covered by private or public insurance. Although services for the patient with dementia (e.g., day care, limited overnight care in a residential facility) may often benefit the caregiver, it can be difficult to convince caregivers that sharing the care in these ways is appropriate.

Family Treatment

Care of the family begins with the patient assessment. Families need information about the disease, its symptoms, management, and prognosis. The evaluation provides an opportunity to help the family understand the patient's spared and impaired functions. Families are often confused by the fact that some functions are severely impaired whereas others appear intact. They may therefore place unrealistic demands on the patient. Neuropsychological tests can be helpful in defining the pattern of cognitive impairment so that the clinician can teach the family what to expect of the patient and how to support remaining functions. (See Chapter 5.) An occupational therapist's assessment similarly can offer insights as to how remaining abilities can be channeled into activities that improve self-esteem; maintain adequate nutrition, contact with the community, or involvement in household activities; or promote other appropriate objectives.[66] As noted above, at the time the diagnosis is made many families cannot absorb all the information they need. Written information enables some families to learn at their own pace, but written material is not a substitute for follow-up dialogue with the clinician. Early referral also should be made for legal and financial advice. (See Chapter 15.)

The family needs the physician's support throughout the course of the illness. As the disease progresses, the family will need help to understand the changes likely to take place in patient functioning.[10] Although some caregivers develop behavior management skills on their own or with the help of support groups, others will have difficulty changing their own long-standing behavior patterns with the patient. Many families do not intuitively understand the management of behavioral symptoms; they will need to be shown what prompts the patient to act as he or she does and how to produce desirable changes in behavior.

Perceived social support has been shown to be an important influence on caregiver well-being. Families need to know that they have support from others.[64] Unfortunately, the demands of caregiving can result in reduced contacts with other family members and friends. Further, misunderstandings about the illness and disagreements over care are common and can inhibit the effectiveness of the natural support system. A recent study found that the most burdened caregivers are more likely than other caregivers to perceive their levels of support as inadequate.[8]

Effective interventions may include meetings between clinicians and multiple family members to discuss the demands of caregiving and approaches to supporting the primary caregiver, as well as work with the primary caregiver to enhance abilities to identify sources of support and obtain it effectively.[53] In many cases, the task of caring for a demented family member causes long-term family communication problems to surface. These problems can significantly reduce the capacity of families to tolerate caregiving demands. Social workers have formal training in working with families on such issues,[16] and some families may need referral for short-term therapy.[54]

Support groups can provide families with information and an opportunity to share the positive and negative experiences associated with caregiving. Through its network of chapters, the National Alzheimer's Association (919 N. Michigan Ave., Chicago, IL 60611, 1-800-272-3900) has established support groups throughout the United States. It is important to make family caregivers aware of the availability of support groups and the help they can provide, but it must be recognized that many people will not be inclined to participate in support groups or may find attendance impossible given the press of care and other demands. Nationally, attendance of support groups by caregivers of patients with dementia is under 20%.[55] Few studies have formally evaluated the effects of support groups on participants.[60] One study found no difference in burden level between those in a support group and those on a waiting list.[62] Support group members have been found to evaluate their group experience positively, however, even when no objective effects could be documented.[24] At least one study has found that participation in an education and support group reduced the likelihood that family caregivers would opt for institutional care.[22]

Most Alzheimer's Association chapters also provide newsletters, telephone reassurance, and other forms of caregiver support. The Alzheimer's Association also supports research, advocates public policy change, and provides families with accurate, up-to-date information about new developments. Involvement with the association can provide assurance that all that can be done is being done and an opportunity to fight back against the disease.

Use of Formal Services

Table 14−8 lists health and social services that may be of help to patients with dementia and their families. Little is known about how to effectively link families in need with appropriate services. In a recent survey,[55] caregivers expressed an urgent need for assistance in finding resources, information, respite, and help. Families face formidable barriers to service use, however. Most needed services are not covered by public or private insurance; some services are in short supply or nonexistent in certain geographic areas, with rural areas being particularly problematic; many services are not available when

Table 14−8 CARE SERVICES FOR PERSONS WITH DEMENTIA

Physician services: Diagnosis and ongoing medical care, including prescribing medications and treating intercurrent illness.

Patient assessment: Evaluation of the individual's physical, mental, and emotional status; behavior; and social supports.

Skilled nursing: Medically oriented care provided by a licensed nurse, including monitoring acute and unstable medical conditions; assessing care needs; supervising medications, tube and intravenous feeding, and personal care services; and treating bedsores and other conditions.

Physical therapy: Rehabilitative treatment provided by a physical therapist.

Occupational therapy: Treatment to improve functional abilities; provided by an occupational therapist.

Speech therapy: Treatment to improve or restore speech; provided by a speech therapist.

Personal care: Assistance with basic self-care activities such as bathing, dressing, getting out of bed, eating, and using the bathroom.

Home health aide services: Assistance with health-related tasks, such as medications, exercises, and personal care.

Homemaker services: Household services, such as cooking, cleaning, laundry, and shopping, and escort service to accompany patients to medical appointments and elsewhere.

Chore services: Household repairs, yard work, and errands.

Supervision: Monitoring an individual's whereabouts to ensure his or her safety.

Paid companion/sitter: An individual who comes to the home to provide supervision, personal care, and socialization during the absence of the primary caregiver.

Congregate meals: Meals provided in a group setting for people who may benefit both from the nutritionally sound meal and from social, educational, and recreational services provided at the setting.

Home-delivered meals: Meals delivered to the home for individuals who are unable to shop or cook for themselves.

Telephone reassurance: Regular telephone calls to individuals who are isolated and often homebound.

Personal emergency response systems: Telephone-based systems to alert others that an individual who is alone is experiencing an emergency and needs assistance.

Transportation: Transporting people to medical appointments, community facilities, and elsewhere.

Recreational services: Physical exercise, art and music therapy, parties, celebrations, and other social and recreational activities.

Mental health services: Psychosocial assessment and individual and group counseling to address psychological and emotional problems of patients and families.

Adult day care: A program of medical and social services including socialization, activities, and supervision, provided in an outpatient setting.

Respite care: Short-term, inpatient or outpatient services intended to provide temporary relief for the primary caregiver.

Dental services: Care of the teeth, and diagnosis and treatment of dental problems.

Legal services: Assistance with legal matters, such as advance directives, guardianship, power of attorney, and transfer of assets.

Protective services: Social and law enforcement services to prevent, eliminate, or remedy the effects of physical and emotional abuse or neglect.

Case management: Client assessment, identification and coordination of community resources, and follow-up monitoring of client adjustment and service provision.

Information and referral: Provision of written or verbal information about community agencies, services, and funding sources.

Hospice services: Medical, nursing, and social services to provide support and alleviate suffering for dying persons and their families.

Source: From US Congress, Office of Technology Assessment,[55] p. 202.

they are needed (e.g., nights, week-ends); caregivers may be so burdened and demoralized by the demands of care that they are unable to search for resources; and, in most cases, no effective information and referral mechanism is available to help caregivers find appropriate services. Because few agencies provide coordinated packages of services, establishing an effective plan of service use can be daunting.

An additional problem, particularly vexing to clinicians, is that many families refuse to use formal services, even when they are available at modest cost. Caregivers will frequently assert that recommended services are not needed, even when clinicians observe great need and are convinced that the service would be of great help to the family.[52] A simple referral to use services, without assistance in contacting service providers and follow-up to ensure that the services have been used, is likely to be effective only with highly motivated, compliant, or "system-wise" caregivers.[52] The clinician may need to enlist a second family member or refer the family to someone who can help with this process. Family members can be taught to perform a variety of case management functions,[51] but professional care coordinators or case managers can assume this role of providing access and coordinating service. Caregivers are often reluctant to use respite and may need direct encouragement from the physician.

Some physicians work closely with a social worker who is familiar with the local resource network. Hospitals are developing assessment and care centers for patients with dementia. Many local Alzheimer Association chapters maintain lists of what resources are available and appropriate, and provide this information to families by telephone or mail. Larger cities frequently also have offices on aging, information and referral services, and case managers in private practice, all of possible assistance in connecting families to services.

Most families try for as long as possible to avoid placing their family member in a nursing home or other residential setting, often at great personal cost. One study[17] found that 42% of patients were living at home at the time of death. Often the decision to institutionalize is related as much to the strain experienced by the caregiver as to the objective status of the care recipient.[2,12] According to United States Government Accounting Office estimates,[56] the average cost of a year in a nursing home in 1989 was $25,000. In addition to the cost, the threat to the spouse of impoverishment (now diminished somewhat by new legislation discussed in Chapter 15), the loss of control over the patient's care, problems in access to good facilities, and family values all discourage placement. Access to nursing homes is limited in many states, particularly for minority families and patients who will be dependent on medical assistance.

The stress of caregiving does not end at placement.[26] George[19] found that caregivers continued to report stress in the year following placement. Families who provide care give up friends and hobbies and may find themselves isolated. Some spend most of their time with the patient in the nursing home. Although some caregivers separate emotionally from the patient during the long illness, many will need support during bereavement.

If possible, families should make decisions in advance regarding life-sustaining interventions and autopsy.[57] Because there is no diagnostic test for AD in life and some AD is inherited, many families will wish to have an autopsy to confirm the diagnosis. Contributing brain tissue also offers an opportunity for the family to participate in the research effort. Discussion about long-term legal and financial planning, potential placement, death, and autopsy should be initiated early in the family/clinician relationship and reopened when further declines in the patient's condition make it appropriate. (See Chapter 15.) Preplanning removes the decision-making process from the pressures of hospital discharge or the deathbed and helps the family to prepare for the patient's continued decline.

New respite and residential-care programs for patients with dementia are being developed. Anecdotal evidence suggests that patients in exceptional programs do appear to do better than those in programs that use standard approaches, but research has not identified the most effective interventions or the patients with the greatest potential to benefit from them. Although supportive services aimed at both caregivers and care recipients are intuitively valuable, more information is needed about what forms of help families and patients need and how to deliver this help efficiently and at reasonable cost.

SUMMARY

Therapeutic nihilism is dissipating with regard to Alzheimer's disease and related disorders as clinicians develop skills to maximize patient and family function. Yet there has been little clinical research to identify the interventions that are most effective with specific subgroups of patients. Research is needed in every aspect of care: the prevalence and treatment of psychiatric symptoms; the management of agitation, wandering, and other distressing or dangerous behaviors; the effect of environment on behavior; and the provision of compassionate care of the late-stage patient.

The clinician can do much to improve the quality of life for people with dementia and their families. With good medical care and a supportive environment, these patients can live with less anxiety and can enjoy life from moment to moment. The patient's caregiver often becomes a second victim of the dementia, giving up his or her own freedom, interests, friends, and sometimes health to provide care. The caregiver loses the valued relationship, not to death but to a stranger whose behavior is sometimes familiar and sometimes bizarre. Thus the caregiver needs information, support, respite, and assistance throughout the course of the illness. The patient's well-being and the caregiver's continued ability to cope are critically dependent on good medical care for both individuals.

REFERENCES

1. Ambrogi D and London C: Elder abuse laws: Their implications for caregivers. Generations 10:37–39, Fall 1985.
2. Aronson MK and Lipkowitz R: Senile dementia, Alzheimer's type: The family and the health care delivery system. J Am Geriatr Soc 29(12):568–571, 1981.
3. Brody EM: Parent care as a normative family stress. Gerontologist 25(1):19–29, 1985.
4. Bunting SM: Stress on caregivers of the elderly. Advances in Nursing Science 11(2):63–73, 1989.
5. Calkins MP: Designing special care units: A systematic approach. Journal of Alzheimer's Care and Research, 3(2):16–22, 1987.
6. Calkins MP, Namazi K, Rosner T, Olsen A, and Brodender B: Home Modifications: Responding to Dementia. Research Center, Corinne Dolan Alzheimer Center at Heather Hill, Chardon, OH, 1990.
7. Chenoweth B and Spencer B: Dementia: The experience of family caregivers. Gerontologist 26(3):267–272, 1986.
8. Clipp EC and George LK: Caregiver needs and patterns of social support. J Gerontol: Social Sciences 45(3):S102–S111, 1990.
9. Cohen D and Eisdorfer C: The Loss of Self: A Family Resource for the Care of Alzheimer's Disease and Related Disorders. WW Norton, New York, 1986.
10. Cohen D, Kennedy G, and Eisdorfer C: Phases of change in the patient with Alzheimer's dementia: A conceptual dimension for defining health care management. J Am Geriatr Soc 32(1):11–15, 1984.

11. Colenda CC, Schoedel K, and Hamer R: The delivery of health services to demented patients at a university hospital: A pilot study. Gerontologist 28 (5):659–662, 1988.

12. Colerick EJ and George LK: Predictors of institutionalization among caregivers of patients with Alzheimer's disease. J Am Geriatr Soc 34(7):493–498, 1986.

13. Coons DH: A residential care unit for persons with dementia. Contract report prepared for the Office of Technology Assessment, US Congress, Washington, DC, 1986.

14. Coons DH: The therapeutic milieu: Social and psychological aspects of treatment. In Reichel W (ed): Clinical Aspects of Aging, ed 2. Williams & Wilkins, Baltimore, 1983.

15. Coons DH: Residential care for persons with dementia. In Mace N (ed): Dementia Care: Patient, Family, and Community. Johns Hopkins University Press, Baltimore, in press.

16. Cutler L: Counseling caregivers. Generations 10:53–56, Fall 1985.

17. Enright RB and Friss L: Employed caregivers of brain impaired adults: An assessment of the dual role. Final Report to Gerontological Society of America, Family Survival Project, 1987.

18. Fitting M and Rabins P: Men and women: Do they give care differently? Generations 10:23–26, Fall 1985.

19. George LK: The dynamics of caregiver burden. Submitted to the American Association of Retired Persons, Andrus Foundation, 1984.

20. Gilmore GC, Whitehouse PJ, and Wykle ML (eds): Memory and Aging. Springer Publishing, New York, 1989.

21. Goldstein K: The effect of brain damage on personality. Psychiatry 15:245–260, 1952.

22. Greene VL and Monahan DJ: The effect of a professionally guided caregiver support and education group on institutionalization of care receivers. Gerontologist 27(6):716–721, 1987.

23. Gwyther LP: Care of Alzheimer's Patients: A Manual for Nursing Home Staff. Alzheimer's Disease and Related Disorders Association and American Health Care Association, Washington DC, 1985.

24. Haley WE, Brown SL, and Levine EG: Experimental evaluation of the effectiveness of group intervention for dementia caregivers. Gerontologist 27 (3):376–382, 1987.

25. Haley WE, Levine EG, Brown SL, Berry JW, and Hughes GH: Psychological, social, and health consequences of caring for a relative with senile dementia. J Am Geriatr Soc 35(5):405–411, 1987.

26. Hatch RC and Franken ML: Concerns of children with parents in nursing homes. Journal of Gerontological Social Work 7(3):19–30, 1984.

27. Hiatt LG: Environmental design and mentally impaired older people. In Altman HJ (ed): Alzheimer's Disease and Dementia: Problems, Prospects and Perspectives. Plenum Publishing, New York, 1988.

28. Johnson CL: Dyadic family relations and social support. Gerontologist 23 (4):377–383, 1983.

29. Kahn RL: The mental health system and the future aged. Gerontologist 15:24–31, 1975.

30. Kapust LR: Living with dementia: The ongoing funeral. Soc Work Health Care 7(4):79–91, 1982.

31. Kiecolt-Glaser JK, Glaser R, Dyer C, Shuttleworth E, O'Grocki P, and Speicher CE: Chronic stress and immunity in family caregivers for Alzheimer disease victims. Psychosom Med 49: 523–535, 1987.

32. Lawton MP: Sensory deprivation and the effect of the environment on management of the patient with senile dementia. In Miller N and Cohen GD (eds): Aspects of Alzheimer's Disease and Senile Dementia, Raven Press, New York, 1981.

33. Light E and Lebowitz BD: Alzheimer's Disease Treatment and Family Stress: Directions for Research. US Department of Health and Human Services, National Institute of Mental Health, Rockville, MD, 1989.

34. Liptzin B, Grob MC, and Eisen SV: Family burden of demented and depressed elderly psychiatric inpatients. Gerontologist 28(3):397–401, 1988.

35. Lockery SA: Care in the minority family. Generations 10:27–29, Fall 1985.

36. Lund DA, Pett MA, and Caserta MS: Institutionalizing dementia victims: Some caregiver considerations. Journal of Gerontological Social Work 11 (1–2):119–135, 1987.

37. Mace NL: Self help for the family. In Kelly W (ed): Alzheimer's Disease and Related Disorders: Research and Management. Charles C Thomas, Springfield, IL, 1984.

38. Mace NL: Home and Community Services for Alzheimer's Disease: A National Conference for Families. US Department of Health and Human Services and ADRDA, Washington, DC, May 2, 1985.

39. Mace NL: Dementia Care: Patient, Family, and Community. Johns Hopkins University Press, Baltimore, 1990.

40. Mace NL: Management of problem behaviors. In Mace NL (ed): Dementia Care: Patient, Family and Community. John Hopkins University Press, Baltimore, 1990, pp 74–112.

41. Mace NL and Rabins PV: The Thirty-Six Hour Day: A Family Guide to Caring for Persons with Alzheimer's Disease, Related Dementing Illnesses and Memory Loss in Later Life. Johns Hopkins University Press, Baltimore, 1981.

42. Mace NL and Rabins PV: A Survey of Day Care for the Demented Adult in the United States. National Council on Aging, Washington, DC, 1984.

43. Martin RM and Whitehouse PJ: The clinical care of patients with dementia. In Mace NL (ed): Dementia Care: Patient, Family, and Community. Johns Hopkins University Press, Baltimore, 1990, pp 22–31.

44. Mendez MF, Martin RJ, Smyth KS, and Whitehouse PJ: Psychiatric symptoms associated with Alzheimer's disease. Journal of Neuropsychiatry and Clinical Neurosciences 2:28–33, 1990.

45. Miller DA: The 'sandwich' generation: Adult children of the aging. Soc Work 26(5):419–423, 1981.

46. Morycz RK: An exploration of senile dementia and family burden. Clinical Social Work Journal 8(1):16–27, 1980.

47. Patterson MB, Schnell A, Martin RJ, Mendez MF, Smyth K, and Whitehouse PJ: Assessment of behavioral and affective symptoms in Alzheimer's disease. J Geriatr Psychiatry Neurol 3:21–30, 1990.

48. Patterson MB and Whitehouse PJ: The diagnostic assessment of patients with dementia. In Mace NL (ed): Dementia Care: Patient, Family, and Community. Johns Hopkins University Press, Baltimore, 1990, pp 3–21.

49. Poulshock SW and Deimling GT. Families caring for elders in residence: Issues in the measurement of burden. J Gerontol 39(2):230–239, 1984.

50. Rabins PV, Mace NL, and Lucas MJ: The impact of dementia on the family. JAMA 48:333–335, 1982.

51. Seltzer MM, Ivry J, and Litchfield LC: Family members as case managers: Partnership between the formal and informal support networks. Gerontologist 27(6):722–728, 1987.

52. Smyth KA, Stuckey JC, and Brach LM: Family responses to recommendations for use of formal dementia care. Paper presented at the Annual Scientific Meeting of the Gerontological Society of America, Minneapolis, MN, November, 1989.

53. Springer D and Brubaker TH: Family Caregivers and Dependent Elderly. Sage Publications, Beverly Hills, CA, 1984.

54. Teusink JP and Mahler S: Helping families cope with Alzheimer's disease. Hosp Community Psychiatry 35(2): 152–156, 1984.

55. US Congress, Office of Technology Assessment: Losing a Million Minds: Confronting the Tragedy of Alzheimer's Disease and Other Dementias. Publication No. OTA-BA-323. US Government Printing Office Washington, DC, 1987.

56. US Government Accounting Office: Long-term Care for the Elderly: Issue of Need, Access and Cost. Publication No. GAO/HRD-89-4. US Government Printing Office, Washington, DC, 1989.

57. Volicer L: Need for hospice approach to treatment of patients with advanced progressive dementia. J Am Geriatr Soc 34:655–658, 1986.

58. West RL and Tomer A: Everyday mem-

ory problems of healthy older adults: Characteristics of a successful intervention. In Gilmore GC, Whitehouse PJ, and Wykle ML (eds): Memory, Aging, and Dementia. Springer Publishing, New York, 1989, pp 74–98.

59. Winograd CH and Jarvik LF: Physician management of the demented patient. J Am Geriatr Soc 34:295–308, 1986.

60. Wright SD, Lund DA, Pett MA, and Caserta MS: The assessment of support group experiences by caregivers of dementia patients. Clinical Gerontologist 6(4):35–59, 1987.

61. Zarit SH: New directions. Generations 10:6–8, Fall, 1985.

62. Zarit SH, Anthony CR, and Boutselis M: Interventions with care givers of dementia patients: Comparison of two approaches. Psychol Aging 2(3):225–232, 1987.

63. Zarit SH, Orr NK, and Zarit JM: Working with Families of Dementia Victims: A Treatment Manual. US Department of Health and Human Services, Office of Human Development Services, Administration on Aging, Washington, DC, 1983.

64. Zarit SH, Reever K, and Bach-Peterson J: Relatives of the impaired elderly: Correlates of feelings of burden. Gerontologist 20:649–654, 1980.

65. Zarit SH, Todd PA, and Zarit JM: Subjective burden of husbands and wives as caregivers: A longitudinal study. Gerontologist 26(3):260–266, 1986.

66. Zgola JM: Doing things: A guide to programming activities for persons with Alzheimer's disease and related disorders. Johns Hopkins University Press, Baltimore, 1987.

67. Zimmer JG, Watson N, and Treat A: Behavioral problems among patients in skilled nursing facilities. Am J Public Health 74:1118–1121, 1984.

Chapter 15

LEGAL AND FINANCIAL DECISION MAKING IN DEMENTIA CARE

Roland Hornbostel, M.Div., J.D.

LEGAL INTERVENTIONS
FINANCIAL ISSUES
ADVANCE DIRECTIVES

Because of the chronic and progressive nature of dementing illnesses, early planning for future incapacity on the part of the patient and family will avoid much of the trauma and impoverishment experienced by those who fail to plan. Thoughtful and early planning has the following benefits: (1) Steps can be taken to ensure that spouses and other family members are not impoverished by the costs of medical care incurred by the patient, (2) the patient can retain control over his or her life to the fullest extent possible, (3) decision makers have much greater flexibility in that the need for costly and protracted court intervention is greatly reduced, and (4) the planning process itself assists the family in accepting and understanding the patient's illness. Many agencies can provide information or di-

rect assistance with this planning process (Table 15–1).

LEGAL INTERVENTIONS

In the earlier stages of dementia, assistance with legal decision making may be required. In later stages of the illness, there may be a need for a legal surrogate. Legal interventions are necessary to enable the patient to have access to needed funds, to make treatment decisions, and to carry out estate planning properly. One goal of legal intervention is to use the least intrusive legal mechanism that will provide the necessary level of protection for the patient now and in the future. This is not a platitude to please civil libertarians; rather, it is a matter of practical sense, for as the invasiveness of the legal intervention increases, the cost and difficulty of obtaining it also increase. Therefore the description of various interventions and their relative usefulness in a given situation will start with

Table 15-1 SOURCES OF ASSISTANCE

Alzheimer's Association
National Headquarters
919 North Michigan Avenue, Suite 1000
Chicago, Illinois 60611-1676
1-800-272-3900

American Association of Retired Persons
1909 K Street, N.W.
Washington, DC 20049

American Bar Association
Commission on Legal Problems of the Elderly
1800 M Street, N.W.
Washington, DC 20036

Area Agency on Aging
(coordinates aging activities in local communities)

Legal Aid Society (local)

Local public library

Long-Term Care Ombudsman Program (each state has one; most states have regional programs as well). Check with your State Office on Aging.

National Senior Citizens Law Center
2025 M Street, N.W., Suite 400
Washington, DC 20036

Social Security Office (local, especially for Medicare, SSI, and Representative Payee information)

Society for the Right to Die
250 West 57th Street
New York, 10107

devices one might not regard as legal interventions at all.

Joint Tenancies

The most common form of joint tenancy is the jointly held bank account. Other property, both real and personal, can also be held by joint tenants. A joint tenancy can be created either with or without survivorship rights. A "joint tenant with rights of survivorship" means that upon the death of one tenant, the other tenant becomes the sole owner of the property. Joint tenancies can be beneficial to dementia patients and their families in two basic ways. First of all, if the patient adds a joint tenant to a bank account, then the joint tenant has automatic access to the

funds should the patient become unable to access the funds personally. Second, as an estate planning tool, joint tenancies can be used to pass funds automatically to the joint tenant upon the death of the other tenant, thus avoiding the probate process.

The first advantage of a joint tenancy (Table 15-2) is that little effort is required to establish the tenancy. For example, a bank account will require only a new signature card. For real property, a simple conveyance and new deed are required. A second advantage is that the patient relinquishes little control. The patient can continue to manage the asset while competent, with the joint tenant assuming control when the patient is no longer competent.

The disadvantages of joint tenancies are threefold. First, if the patient holds numerous assets, it will be a cumber-

Table 15–2 WEIGHING THE PROS AND CONS OF LEGAL INTERVENTIONS

Type of Intervention	Positive	Negative
Joint tenancies	Ease of establishment; patient remains in control	Limited amount of protection; hard to identify all assets; high potential for exploitation
Representative payee	Few legal formalities	Protects Social Security or VA income only, not assets; no real monitoring by SSA
Power of Attorney (traditional)	Can be individualized; no court intervention required; low cost	No monitoring; potential for abuse exists; expires when patient becomes mentally incapacitated
Power of Attorney (durable)	Potential for use as an advance directive; same as for Power of Attorney	No monitoring; even higher potential for abuse, as patient may be incapacitated at time of use
Guardianship	Provides total control; oversight	Requires court proceeding; requires cost to establish and maintain; most restrictive to rights of ward; time delay required to establish; monitoring is limited by court resources

some process to identify all these assets and establish separate joint tenancies for each. Second, joint tenancies are less useful as the dementia progresses. Many joint tenancies will require the signature of both joint tenants to liquidate the asset—a problem if the patient is no longer competent to give a valid signature. Thus it may be unwise to set up a joint tenancy that requires more than one signature. A third disadvantage is that joint tenancies are not monitored. Once the patient is no longer competent, there is no check on the activity of the joint tenant. If only one signature is required to withdraw funds from a checking account, for example, the joint tenant may simply remove all the patient's funds.

Even if the joint tenant is scrupulous, joint tenancies may not provide enough protection for the patient. For instance, if the joint tenant is sued, the judgment creditor of the joint tenant may seek to attach the patient's assets. It is important to consider thoroughly the personal, professional, and financial interests of the joint tenant before the tenancy is established. As a practical matter, then, joint tenancies are most useful when used with bank accounts, where speed of access to funds is of paramount importance to pay medical and other living expenses.

Representative Payeeship

Representative payeeship[3] can be used to manage funds received from Social Security or the Veterans Administration (VA). The practical effect of this device is that the patient's monthly checks are sent to and managed by another party, the representative payee, who is responsible for ensuring that the money is used for the patient. A physician or court certification of the need for a payee due to mental or physical incapacity is required. Unlike the case of the joint bank account, the Social Security Administration may intervene in cases in which the representative payee is suspected of misappropriating funds. The Social Security Administration does no ongoing monitoring of the use of funds, however, which limits the usefulness of such protection. In addition, the usefulness of representative payeeship is limited to Social Security and/or

VA income. Other forms of income cannot be controlled through Social Security or VA representative payeeship.

Money Management Programs

Money management programs have been established in some areas. These programs can manage both the income and assets of an individual. They are used primarily for low-income persons who have no family to assist them. The sponsors may be organizations such as social service agencies, churches, or consumer protection agencies.

Powers of Attorney

Conceptually, representative payeeship is a form of surrogate decision making, albeit a very limited one. Power of Attorney, on the other hand, often constitutes a very broad form of surrogate decision making. A Power of Attorney is a type of agency relationship; that is, the one to whom power has been granted acts on behalf and in the stead of the one granting the power. The parties to this arrangement are the Principal, or maker of the Power, and the agent, or Attorney in Fact. Powers of Attorney can be very limited in scope. They are often used for the purpose of making a single transaction. For example, if you wished to sell a certain piece of real estate while at the same time vacationing in Europe, you might give a power of attorney to a trusted friend or agent to make the transaction for you if an offer for the property is made. In another example, if you hate standing in long lines at the license bureau, you could give a friend a limited power of attorney that only allows him to pick up your license plates for you.

Powers of Attorney can also be very broad in scope, conveying wide authority over all of the Principal's assets and even conferring powers to make personal decisions for the Principal. It is in this very broad form that the Power of Attorney becomes an extremely useful device for patients with dementia and their families.

The legal formalities or requirements for establishing a Power of Attorney vary depending on the power to be granted and the state in which the Power is to be used. A Power of Attorney must be in writing and describe the powers granted to the Attorney in Fact. Although a standard-form Power of Attorney may be purchased from any bookstore or stationery shop, it is suggested that a Power of Attorney for a dementia patient be drawn up by an attorney with expertise in this area, to ensure that the Power of Attorney is customized to the individual circumstances of patient and family. Several states, such as New York and California, provide a special statutory form.[1] In such states it is necessary to follow this form carefully to ensure that the Power is honored.

Other requirements for the creation of a valid Power of Attorney vary from state to state. Many states require that a Power be witnessed and that the signature of the Principal be notarized. Some states require that a Power be recorded at a government office in certain circumstances, such as when the Power is to be used to transfer real estate. Prudence, dictated by the mobility pattern of modern society, suggests that the Power be witnessed and notarized even if the patient's current state of residence does not require such formality, as it is possible that the Power may need to be exercised in another state should the patient relocate.

The traditional Power of Attorney is not appropriate for patients with dementia and their families, however, because a Power of Attorney is valid only as long as the Principal or maker is mentally competent. This results from the longstanding legal premise that the Principal should always be able to revoke the Power. When the Principal becomes mentally incapable of revoking the Power, the Power is no longer valid. This obstacle has led every state to recognize the creation of a legal device

Table 15-3 SAMPLE DURABLE POWER OF ATTORNEY

I, [principal], hereby appoint [agent(s) or attorney(s) in fact] to act [jointly/solely] in my name, place and stead in any way which I myself could act with respect to the following financial transactions: Banking transactions, insurance transactions, bond and shareholder transactions, claims and litigation, business operating transactions, and all other similar transactions. I further empower my attorney in fact to make transactions in regard to the following real property: [specify]. My attorney in fact may make such other transactions and enter into such contracts as my attorney in fact deems appropriate. My attorney in fact [may/may not] transfer my property real or personal to himself or herself.

In the event that my attorney in fact is no longer able to exercise this Power, I designate [successor attorneys in fact] to serve in the order listed below.

By this document I intend that my attorney in fact shall be able to make health care decisions for me if and when I am no longer able to make these decisions for myself. My attorney in fact has the power to consent or withhold consent for medical treatment. My attorney in fact is authorized to examine my medical records and speak with medical personnel as necessary to effectuate health care decisionmaking. My attorney in fact shall make health care decisions as I direct, including: [specify desires in regard to treatment and life-prolonging care]. I make the following special provisions and limitations on this power: [specify].

This Power of Attorney shall survive even in the event that I subsequently become incapacitated or disabled. Such incapacity or disability shall not render this Power of Attorney void.

My signature below indicates that I understand the nature of the Powers I have granted to my Attorney in fact.

Signed: _____
Date: _____

First Witness: _____
Date: _____

Second Witness: _____
Date: _____

[It is suggested that witnesses be disinterested nonrelatives who are not beneficiaries of the principal's estate.]

Notary:

---

called a Durable Power of Attorney. Typically, the distinguishing feature of a Durable Power is merely the addition of language to the effect that the Power survives the incapacity or disability of the Principal (Table 15-3). However, several states have established special requirements for the creation of a Durable Power. For that reason, it is recommended that an attorney be consulted to aid in drafting the Durable Power.

A new trend among states is to allow the establishment of a Durable Power for health care decisions.[12] Traditionally, the Power of Attorney was used primarily for conducting financial or business transactions. States have more recently come to see the appointment of a surrogate decision maker, outside the court process, as a desirable end. This has led to the creation of these special Durable Powers. Some states provide that the Durable Power can be a "springing" Power of Attorney. That is, the Power becomes valid only upon the disability or incapacity of the Principal.[12] It is important to note that even in states that have not created a Durable Power of Attorney for health care decisions, there are no reported decisions in which courts refused to honor the surrogate authority granted in the Power.

The major advantages of a Durable Power of Attorney are that, unlike devices previously discussed, they create broad decision-making authority for the patient with dementia. Further, this broad authority is achieved without the expense and delays entailed by court involvement. A final major advantage is that the dementia patient is allowed to choose the surrogate, as opposed to having the court appoint a surrogate who may be a disinterested third party.

Nonetheless, such Powers also involve substantial risk for the dementia patient. The greatest strength of the Durable Power is also its greatest weakness. There is no oversight of the actions or inactions of the Attorney in Fact. Even though in theory the creation of the Power creates a fiduciary relationship between the parties that requires the Attorney in Fact to act with the utmost fidelity to the Principal and the Principal's assets, the real possibility of exploitation of the Principal exists. There may be literally no one to ensure that the Attorney in Fact performs faithfully, especially in situations where the Principal has become incapacitated. One potential way to deal with this problem is to designate more than one Attorney in Fact. The Power of Attorney then provides that the Attorneys in Fact must act jointly. A problem with this technique arises when the Attorneys in Fact are unable to agree, but at least the fear of exploitation of the Principal is greatly diminished. This caution aside, the Durable Power is the simplest and most effective form of surrogate decision making for a majority of dementia patients and their families.

Guardianship

Guardianship is frequently the form of surrogate decision making that first comes to mind when dealing with mentally incapacitated individuals. In some state laws, Guardianship is also called Conservatorship. There are really two types of guardianship: (1) guardianship of the person and (2) guardianship of the estate (frequently called Conservatorship). The Guardian of Person may make personal decisions for the ward, the individual for whom a guardian is appointed. The Guardian of the Estate is restricted to making decisions that only involve the assets of the ward. There is a presumption, often created by state law, that the Guardian has both authorities unless other provisions have been explicitly stipulated by the court. In general, the criteria for the appointment of a Guardian are that the prospective ward must be mentally incapacitated according to state law and that incapacity has rendered the prospective ward incapable of making decisions on his or her own behalf. Some states, however, allow for the appointment of a guardian even when the disability of the ward is only physical incapacity.

Guardianship proceedings are initiated with the filing of a petition with the designated court (ordinarily called probate court). Each state has different formalities that must be observed when filing the petition. A simple guardianship (i.e., uncontested and for a person with low income and no property or significant assets) can usually be managed without an attorney. The guardian can be a family member, a friend, or an attorney. For the more complex guardianships, an attorney is recommended. The amount of compensation for the attorney is regulated by the court and is related to the size of the estate that is being managed. Once a guardianship has been established, the guardian is seen as an officer of the court. Accountings of the ward's assets must be made to the court at periodic intervals. In addition, court permission must be sought before making major decisions such as selling real estate owned by the ward.

The advantages of guardianship as a surrogate decision-making device are that there is no question as to who has decision-making authority and that there is court oversight over the activities of the guardian. The guardian must, in most states, post a bond to ensure that he or she will carry out guardianship activities in the best interests of the ward and with utmost fidelity to the ward.

Guardianship also has disadvantages. In many states, there are time delays as the various statutory requirements for the establishment of guardianships are observed, such as filing the petition, getting the required documentation of incapacity, notice to the ward and other affected parties of the guardianship proceeding, and holding a hearing on the petition. Second, guardianship can be expensive both to initiate and to maintain[12] if it is contested or involves property or significant assets, thereby requiring legal assistance. Third, full guardianship is a restrictive device, stripping the ward of most civil rights. For example, the ward loses the right to marry, to own property, and in some cases, the right to vote. Fourth, guardianships must be revoked through the court process, thus incurring further expense and time delays. Fifth, monitoring of the guardianship by the court is only as effective as court procedures and resources make it. For the most part, overworked courts with crowded dockets do not look behind the papers that are filed in the proceeding. Therefore, despite the requirement for monitoring, there are numerous cases of abuse of the guardianship process by the guardians.

A final concern about guardianships is that the original focus of guardianship law was to protect the *estate* of the ward, not his or her person. This presents two conceptual problems. First, if a guardianship is to be used primarily so that a court-appointed guardian can make a medical decision for a ward, the physician is often frustrated by the time delays incurred as the guardianship process unfolds. Some states have addressed this problem by establishing special expedited procedures to be followed in an emergency. Second, it may be difficult or impossible to find a guardian if the prospective ward has no financial assets. For example, many guardianships by attorneys are terminated when the assets of the ward are exhausted. In the case of persons with dementia, this may occur after the person's mental capacity has deteriorated to the point where a surrogate decision maker is essential, yet all of the patient's assets have now been exhausted.

Extensive difficulties with guardian-ship laws have led many states to attempt reforms of the system to address some of these problems. Some states now allow for the appointment of limited guardians whose powers are specified by the court, while the ward retains those powers not specifically limited by the court. Other states have created public guardians to serve where no other guardian is willing or capable of serving. In some areas, social service agencies are able to provide guardians for persons with no family or assets.

FINANCIAL ISSUES

One of the devastating by-products of a dementing illness is the impoverishment of the patient and often of the patient's family. The reasons for this impoverishment will be explained in this section. In addition, basic information on new Medicaid provisions designed to prevent spousal impoverishment will be presented.

Medicare

Medicare is a government program of health insurance designed to benefit persons over the age of 65, blind persons, and persons who have been totally disabled for 2 years. There are two parts to Medicare. Part A pays for hospitalization and for a limited amount of skilled care in posthospital settings. Part B is designed to pay major medical expenses such as doctor's fees. Every Medicare beneficiary has Part A coverage funded by a payroll tax. Part B is optional and is paid in part by an additional monthly premium borne by the beneficiary. Most individuals are covered by both parts.

Medicare was originally designed to meet acute health care needs. It was not designed to meet the long-term health care needs of beneficiaries who have dementing illnesses — that is, care delivered in settings other than hospitals, such as nursing homes or the patient's own home. The Skilled Care extended benefit under Part A, for care delivered either in a nursing home certified as a Skilled Nursing Facility (SNF) or in the patient's own home by certified home health care agencies, is an extremely limited one. Medicare Part A pays only for a maximum of 100 days of care in an SNF per spell of illness, and it pays the total cost of care for only the first 20 days of SNF care. For day 21 through day 100, there is a coinsurance charge estimated to be over $70 per day in 1990 and $81.50 per day in 1992. Even with this limited benefit, there are some other restrictive requirements. The beneficiary must be hospitalized for at least 3 days prior to receiving care in the SNF. Also, the beneficiary must enter the SNF within 30 days of this hospitalization and be treated for the same condition for which he or she was hospitalized. Finally, the beneficiary must need continuous skilled-care services as defined by the government. By this definition, patients with dementia do not need skilled nursing care (unless the patient also has a hip fracture or some other procedure traditionally covered under Part A). Even though in recent years this stringent definition has been somewhat relaxed, few nursing home residents meet the skilled-care defini-

tion, as evidenced by the fact that less than 2% of nursing home costs in the United States are paid by Medicare.[8]

The situation is similar in the case of home health care, as only skilled services are reimbursable under the terms of the Medicare program. As previously mentioned, the need for skilled services excludes patients with dementing illness as their only diagnosis.

Medicare Supplemental Insurance (Medigap)

This type of insurance usually provides minimal benefits for dementia care. A Medicare supplemental insurance policy is designed to pay the deductibles and coinsurance charges not paid by Medicare for Medicare-covered services. If a medical service such as nursing home care is not covered under the Medicare program, then the supplemental policy will not provide coverage either. It is important for most persons eligible for Medicare to have one (and only one) Medicare supplemental policy (Table 15–4). Very recently, Medicare supplemental insurance has been standardized into 10 policies to ease the task of comparing different policies. For

Table 15–4 WHAT TO LOOK FOR IN MEDICARE SUPPLEMENTAL INSURANCE

Does the policy pay all the deductible and coinsurance amounts you are responsible for under both Medicare Parts A and B?

Do premiuim rates increase with age? (If so, look elsewhere for coverage.)

Is there a limitation on the coverage of preexisting medical conditions? (The shorter this period, the better.)

Is this policy guaranteed renewable? (If not, look elsewhere for coverage.)

Does this policy give you a 10-day period for a "free look" so that you can review the actual policy language and not just a public-relations brochure?

Notes:
- Never buy more than one Medicare supplemental insurance policy.
- Check to see if your employer or pension plan provides Medicare supplemental insurance as a benefit, before you buy an individual policy.
- If your income is less than 80% of the federally established poverty level, you may be eligible to have Medicaid pay your coinsurance and deductibles under Medicare. Thus you may not need to purchase a Medicare supplement.

Medicare beneficiaries with little income and limited assets, the states pay for supplemental charges through their Medicaid programs. A major problem is that many older persons who are eligible for this special coverage, called the Qualified Medicare Beneficiary (QMB) program, do not know that they are eligible and therefore do not apply for the coverage. It is also important to note that indemnity insurance policies sold over the radio or TV by celebrities often are not Medicare supplements.

Long-Term Care Insurance

In the past, "nursing home" insurance, like "cancer" or "dread disease" insurance, was a product to be avoided, as these types of policies rarely pay any benefits. New insurance products, however, are designed to pay for levels of care in nursing homes and in the patient's own home that Medicare does not cover (commonly called intermediate, or custodial, care). Although at present such insurance is not a total answer to the dilemma of the impoverishment of dementia patients and their families, developments in this area are largely positive. Because this type of insurance is so new, however, the old maxim of "let the buyer beware" should be heeded.[16]

At the outset it should be noted that this insurance is expensive and therefore not every older person should consider its purchase. Also, both its strength and its weakness is that it is not tied to Medicare coverage. Therefore, this type of policy should never substitute for a good Medicare supplemental insurance policy.

Premiums are age-based. That is, the premium escalates depending on the age of the insured at the time the coverage is purchased. A policy that would provide coverage to someone age 55 might typically be available for $400 a year. If that person waits until age 74 to purchase the same coverage, the premium might be $3000 per year. Good policies are "guaranteed renewable"; that is, the company may not cancel the individual's coverage. Also, any increase in premium for an existing policy should be based on factors such as inflation, not merely on the increasing age of the insured (Table 15–5).

Table 15–5 WHAT TO LOOK FOR IN LONG-TERM CARE INSURANCE

Is the daily benefit indexed to keep up with inflation?

How long must one wait before preexisting conditions are covered?

Are Alzheimer's disease and other organic and nervous disorders specifically covered?

What is the maximum benefit (or benefit period) payable under the policy? (The longer the better.)

Does it cover all levels of nursing-home care and not just skilled-nursing-facility care? (If no, the policy should not be purchased.)

Does the policy pay for custodial care?

Does the policy pay for in-home care and adult day care? If yes, is a prior nursing-home or hospital stay needed before home care benefits commence?

Does the policy require prior hospitalization?

Is the policy guaranteed renewable?

Is there a waiver-of-premium provision, and how long must benefits be paid before premiums are waived?

Does the premium increase with age? (If yes, look elsewhere for coverage.)

Currently available policies worthy of consideration have strict underwriting requirements. Health screening is done by the insurance companies to exclude applicants with certain disabilities. Thus no company will insure an applicant who has been diagnosed as having a dementing illness. Related to the underwriting requirements are clauses governing "preexisting illnesses." These clauses typically provide that coverage for a disorder of the insured that existed previous to the issuance of the policy will not begin for a period of from 6 months to a year. Obviously, the shorter the duration of this clause's effect, the better for the applicant.

Certain disorders are excluded from coverage entirely. A typical exclusion is for claims arising from "mental illness." Better policies are now available that specify that dementing illness such as Alzheimer's disease is covered under the terms of the policy.

The better policies offer coverage both for nursing-home care and for home health care. Benefits are purchased in increments of $10 per day of coverage. The typical home health benefit is half the benefit payable for confinement in a nursing home. There is a policy limit on maximum total benefits payable over a lifetime, which ranges from 1 to 5 years of coverage.

In summary, long-term care insurance may be an important tool for older persons planning for the future. As the policies become more refined, and as the cost for such insurance drops as more group policies become available, these policies will serve as a partial answer to impoverishment caused by dementing illnesses. These policies are only a partial solution to the massive problem of long-term care financing, however, as experts estimate that less than 20% of long-term care costs will ever be covered by long-term care insurance.[15]

Medicaid

Medicaid is a program jointly funded and administered by the federal and state governments, designed to pay for health care for low-income individuals. Unlike Medicare, which is essentially a health insurance program, Medicaid is a means-tested or "welfare" program. To be covered for medical expenses under the Medicaid program, an individual must fall into one of several groups of "categorically eligible" persons, or in some states, must have medical expenses that make the person eligible under the state's income guidelines. Only 13 states currently lack such a "medically needy" category.[14] Individuals covered are those persons who receive either Aid to Dependent Children or Supplemental Security Income (SSI). Thirty-four states use eligibility criteria for older persons that are derived from the criteria for receipt of SSI. Seventeen states, called "209b states," are allowed to use the more restrictive eligibility criteria in place prior to the passage of Title XVI of the Social Security Act in 1972, which provided for the SSI program.

Also, unlike Medicare, Medicaid pays for significant amounts of long-term care for older persons.[9] Although the federal government sets broad guidelines for the program, each state is responsible for the actual administration of Medicaid. Medicaid covers both skilled and custodial care in nursing homes. Two thirds of the nation's nursing-home residents receive care paid for by Medicaid.[4] In addition, some states, at their option, provide for significant amounts of home health care as well.

Three criteria must be met for a person to receive Medicaid: (1) the individual must medically need the service provided, (2) the individual must meet the maximum income level set by the state, and (3) the individual must have fewer assets than the amount set by each state. The medical necessity requirement is usually not a problem for persons with dementia. Insofar as Medicaid pays for custodial care, the problems discussed earlier in relation to Medicare do not apply.

Maximum income criteria are set by each state. As mentioned earlier, two thirds of the states set the income limit with reference to the limit set by SSI.

These states are permitted to set special income levels for eligibility up to 300% of the current SSI level (currently this would be a total of $1266 per month as the income ceiling). In addition, many of these states allow income levels that are even higher if the patient has higher medical expenses. In the seventeen 209b states, the situation is more complex, as they often use more restrictive criteria than the SSI criteria. However, these states are also required to set up a special eligibility category for those whose income is "spent down" due to a medical expense such as nursing home care.

Medicaid is a supplemental program in that the nursing-home resident's income, after certain permissible deductions, is turned over to the nursing home. The Medicaid program then supplements this payment to the nursing home to make up the difference in the resident's cost of care. Permissible deductions from income allowed by the states include an allowance of at least $30 per month to meet the resident's personal needs, an amount set aside for premium payments on a Medicare supplemental insurance policy, an allowance for a spouse remaining in the community, an allowance for any other dependent family members, and amounts paid for medical services not covered under the terms of a state's Medicaid program (e.g., prescription drugs, eyeglasses, and hearing aids).

The allowable assets vary from state to state; some assets are not countable at all and are, therefore, excluded from the resource calculation. The personal residence of the applicant is exempt from the calculation. Even when the applicant is residing in a nursing home, the home remains exempt as long as there is a chance that the applicant will return from the nursing home (usually for at least 6 months), or as long as the applicant's spouse or dependent child resides there. Personal goods are exempted up to a maximum dollar limit. The value of one automobile is exempted. Life insurance, burial contracts, and burial plots are at least partially exempt from total countable resources. States may provide various other special exemptions as well. A current legal controversy has arisen with regard to whether states must take into account the liabilities of the applicant in determining the total value of countable resources. Thus far, courts have required some SSI states to use such a "resource spend-down" standard.[5]

Assets and resources not exempt from the resource calculation may not be transferred by the applicant for less than fair market value within 30 months of the application without creating a presumption that the transfer was made for the purpose of obtaining assistance from Medicaid. The effect of the presumption, if not rebutted, is to render the applicant ineligible for Medicaid payments for nursing-home care for the number of months the transferred resource would have provided medical care for the applicant, up to a maximum of 30 months. The applicant is still eligible to receive a Medicaid card to pay other health care expenses. This presumption may be rebutted if the applicant is able to prove that the transfer of the resource was for another purpose, such as paying for needed health care or for home improvements. The penalty for improper transfer may also be avoided if its imposition would create an "undue hardship," or when the applicant gives the Medicaid agency the legal right to bring a support action against the party to whom the improper transfer was made.

Numerous critics have charged that the current system is inequitable in that it requires individuals to impoverish themselves and their spouses before the government provides assistance of any kind. In no case is this as true as it is in the case of dementia patients because, as we have seen, traditional insurance pays virtually none of the costs incurred by dementia patients and their families for long-term care. The Medicare Catastrophic Coverage Act (MCCA) of 1988 contained provisions to address this problem, commonly referred to as special impoverishment. These new rules became effective on September 30, 1989 and were not repealed when other aspects of the MCCA were repealed that year. One feature of these new provisions was to standardize to a greater extent the varying eligibility criteria in each state. The basic goal of this new legislation was to provide for a separation of income and assets between spouses at the time one spouse enters a nursing home.

Under the new coverage requirements, the community spouse is entitled to a minimum monthly maintenance-needs allowance equal to 150% of the federal poverty level for a two-person household.[11] This is a significant improvement over the previous situation for community spouses, when virtually all entitlement to the institutionalized spouse's income was surrendered to the nursing home. In certain cases, the community spouse may also be entitled to an excess shelter allowance if shelter costs exceed 30% of his or her allowance. The maximum amount of the total monthly allowance is $1662 unless a greater amount is ordered by a court. This important new income protection applies to all residents in a nursing home with a spouse residing in the community, regardless of when the resident was admitted to the home.

Resource protections, on the other hand, apply only to the community spouses of residents who entered the nursing home on or after September 30, 1989. Some states received approval to enact these resource protections at a later date. It is possible, therefore, that the old resource rules would apply in many situations. For persons admitted to nursing homes on or after September 30, 1989, the assets held by either spouse or both spouses together are aggregated. The community spouse is allowed to protect the first $13,296 of this aggregated amount. If the couple has more than $24,000 in assets, the community spouse is allowed to protect half the assets up to a total of $66,480.[11] These figures will likely increase in future years as they are indexed for inflation.

An example may be useful to illustrate how the new law works. Mary Smith places her husband, John, who has AD, in a nursing home on October 1, 1989. Mary has the right to request that the state Medicaid agency make a determination as to how the couple's assets are to be attributed. The Medicaid agency determines that the couple has $100,000 in total assets. Mary is entitled to keep $50,000; the remainder must be spent down to the resource limit (in most states, $2,000) for John's care before he will be eligible for Medicaid.

The MCCA also permits the transfer of the patient's home without incurring a penalty in cases where the transfer is to the community spouse or a dependent child, to a sibling of the patient who has both an equity interest in the home and was residing in the home for at least a year prior to the patient's admission to a nursing facility, or to a child who both provided care to the patient and was residing in the home for at least 2 years prior to the patient's admission to a nursing facility.[11]

Guidelines for the Medicaid program may be expected to change rapidly during the next several years. Therefore, well-informed advice from attorneys and advocacy organizations such as those listed on Table 15-1 will be important for patients with dementia and their families.

ADVANCE DIRECTIVES

This section will highlight a few of the major ethical dilemmas faced by those who treat patients with dementia and will offer some practical examples of health care decision making. (See also Epilogue).

Consent to Treatment

It is well established that a physician may not treat a patient, except in an emergency, unless that patient consents to such treatment. In fact, the physician who treats a patient without such informed consent may be subject to an action in battery.[10]

The obvious challenge to those who treat dementia patients is that as the dementia progresses, the patient's ability to consent to further treatment is inexorably diminished. Eventually, he or she will no longer be able to understand the course of treatment to weigh its benefits against possible risks. This is the primary reason why advance planning may be more critical for persons with dementing illnesses than for persons with other types of illness.

Types of Advance Directives

In light of the progressive nature of dementia, advance directives are an option that should be considered while the patient is still competent. Advance directives are useful in cases where the patient has decided the extent to which medical procedures should be used to prolong life and where a surrogate decision maker acceptable to the patient is both able and willing to assume the responsibility of acting on the patient's behalf. The use of advance directives is less advisable when the patient is unsure of the course of treatment that should be followed, when the patient has no one with whom he or she is sufficiently close to designate as a surrogate decision maker, or when the motives of the surrogate are questionable. It is important that the physician have enough conversations with the patient to provide a general understanding of the patient's moral and philosophical bases for making decisions.

DURABLE POWER OF ATTORNEY

One major form of advance directive that is often the instrument of choice has been discussed earlier in this chapter the Durable Power of Attorney. As mentioned previously, several states have created specific Durable Powers of Attorney for health care decision making. In these states it is impor-

tant that the instrument creating the Power be executed according to the statutory form provided under that particular state's law.

LIVING WILL

A second type of advance directive is the living will, sometimes called a health care declaration. "Living will" is a term used to describe instruments that provide written instructions concerning the duration, scope, and type of health care that may be provided to the patient in the event of a terminal illness (often defined as illness expected to result in death within a year) or persistent vegetative condition. Although all but six states have enacted that legislation,[12] each has different requirements for the creation of a valid living will. For that reason, a person who moves to another state may need to execute another living will. Some states, including Ohio, allow for "grandfathering" out-of-state living wills. In addition, it is wise to observe the typical format required for the composition of a valid living will, even if the current state of residence of the patient does not specifically require such formalities. Thus living wills should be witnessed by two individuals who are disinterested parties and notarized.

One major advantage of the living will is that, unlike a Durable Power of Attorney, a surrogate decision maker is not required. The patient simply expresses his or her wishes in the document itself. There are some serious limitations to the use of living wills by patients with dementia, however. First, the patient with dementia may not be considered to have a terminal illness at all, in that the patient is typically not expected to die within 1 year. This is a classic Catch-22 situation. By the time the dementia has progressed to the point that the patient is expected to die within 1 year, the patient is no longer competent to make a valid living will. Second, many states provide that the living will is valid only in cases where the care provided is "extraordinary." Thus many states categorically prohibit the use of a living will to withhold food and fluids from terminally ill patients.[12] Finally, a living will may not be valid when executed in a different state. As a result of these difficulties, it would be advisable for most patients to execute both types of advance directives. It should be emphasized, though, that there are no reported cases holding a physician or other medical practitioner liable for following the wishes of a patient as set forth in a living will. There are cases, however, holding doctors liable for failing to follow patients' wishes, even without a living will.[10]

The Patient Self Determination Act

The American Association of Retired Persons has estimated that only 15% of adult Americans have a valid advance directive. Even when there is an advance directive, it is only effective if the treating physician and the health care facility know that it exists and have a copy of it. These two problems led to the passage of the Patient Self Determination Act as part of Omnibus Budget Reconciliation Act (OBRA) 1990.

This new law requires Medicare and Medicaid certified providers (hospitals, nursing homes, home health agencies, hospices, and health maintenance organizations) to provide information to all adult patients on the laws governing their rights to accept or refuse care and execute an advance directive. In addition, these health care providers are required to (1) develop policies and procedures for implementing such rights and notify patients of these policies and procedures, (2) ask whether the patient has an advance directive and incorporate the advance directive into the patient's record, and (3) ensure that patients will not be discriminated against on the basis of having or not having an advance directive.

Each state, and each health care provider, is to develop a written pamphlet for patients so as to properly implement the terms of the Patient Self Determination Act.

Cessation of Treatment

One of the areas of greatest controversy in medicine today is the debate over when it is proper to withhold or withdraw treatment from a patient.[6,13] In particular, in regard to patients with dementia, the debate has centered on the issues of nutrition and hydration.

The complex set of issues in regard to the withdrawal of food and fluid are best illustrated by the leading court case on the subject concerning an elderly demented person, *In re Conroy*.[7]

Claire Conroy was an 84-year-old nursing home resident suffering from dementia. At the time her case came to the attention of a New Jersey court in 1983, Ms. Conroy was unable to respond to almost all external stimuli. She was sustained by nasogastric feeding. Her nephew sought a court order to withdraw the feeding tube so that she might be allowed to die. Though Ms. Conroy did, in fact, die before the New Jersey Supreme Court rendered its opinion in the case (the same court that years earlier heard the famous case of Karen Ann Quinlan[8]), the *Conroy* case broke important new legal ground in the analysis of when it might be permissible to withhold nutrition and hydration from a patient.

Although the complexities of the process detailed by the court in *Conroy* cannot be fully treated in this chapter, it is important to note the decision-making criteria spelled out. First, the court discusses a subjective test directed at ascertaining the wishes of the incompetent patient. These wishes may be ascertained by examining the prior declarations of the nursing-home resident (e.g., a living will). This type of decision making is frequently referred to as "substituted judgment."

If the incompetent patient's prior wishes cannot be ascertained, the *Conroy* court discusses the application of a more objective test based on the "best interests" of the patient. The inquiry here is directed at determining whether the benefits of the patient's continued existence are outweighed by the burdens imposed by continued treatment.[7] The *Conroy* court further discusses a "limited objective" test to be employed when there is some trustworthy prior expression of the patient's aversion to continued medical treatment, but not enough of an expression to allow application of the doctrine of "substituted judgment."

The problem that is not satisfactorily answered by *Conroy*, as evidenced by the continued involvement of New Jersey courts in similar cases, is determining who is to apply the criteria. That is, Do the courts always have to be involved? As previously discussed in the section on guardianship, resort to the processes of any court results in time-consuming delays and potentially expensive legal proceedings. This is especially true in cases that are appealed to one or more higher courts. The answer to this dilemma will evolve as the use of advance directives and alternative decision-making processes, such as ethical review teams, expands.

A final problem with the rationale of the court in *Conroy* is that the court limited its application to cases in which two doctors concurred that death was likely to occur within 1 year. The difficulties in predicting when the life of a patient with dementia will end are such that the answer provided by *Conroy* will be inapplicable to many situations involving such patients.

The recent decision of the United States Supreme Court in *Cruzan v. Director, Missouri Dept of Health*[2] is further illustration of the practical need for patients to make a written record of their wishes in regard to life-sustaining treatment and to provide copies to any medical professional or institution that is providing ongoing treatment. Like Ms. Conroy, Nancy Cruzan was in a persistent vegetative state, in this case resulting from an automobile accident. Her parents went to court to have the artificial provision of food and fluids halted. The Supreme Court ruled that the state could protect its legitimate interest in human life by requiring that a patient's wishes in regard to life-sus-

taining treatment be proved by clear and convincing evidence. The Supreme Court remanded the case to the Missouri State Court to determine whether Ms. Cruzan's oral expressions in regard to not wishing to be kept alive unless she could lead a[11] halfway-normal existence[11] did constitute clear and convincing evidence of her intent.

As a practical matter, patients should record in writing their wishes in regard to life-sustaining treatment and should share these written wishes with all medical practitioners who are providing treatment to ensure that the patient's wishes are honored. *Cruzan* provides one more reason for the necessity of early advance planning by those with dementing illnesses and their families.

SUMMARY

Early legal and financial planning is essential to minimize the devastating impact of dementia on patient and family. Each family with a member affected by dementia needs to have access to the latest information concerning laws affecting health care and the availability of community resources. A variety of legal mechanisms may be used to assist the caregiver in managing the financial and medical affairs of the patient. These devices include joint tenancy, power of attorney, guardianship, and living wills. Federal and state regulations concerning Medicare and Medicaid change fairly frequently, and early planning is particularly important to avoid impoverishment. New forms of long-term care insurance are being developed by private companies and need to be carefully evaluated.

In the future, the issues highlighted in this chapter are likely to create further change in the courts, the insurance industry, state and federal bureaucracies, the long-term–care delivery system, and, of course, the health professions themselves. We will all be challenged by the issue of how to finance long-term care for an ever-increasing aging population. Closely coupled with this issue is an ethical one: How much health care is an individual entitled to, and does this entitlement change with age or physical condition? The network of services available to the aged will have to respond to the needs of those who not only need the delivery of services, but also need someone to manage how and when these services are delivered. Such case management for persons with dementia will need to expand to create viable alternatives to the costly and time-consuming court process. Finally, both the medical and the social-service communities will need to be more responsive to the planning needs of dementia patients and their families. Building awareness on the part of the general public of the need for careful and thoughtful planning for the later years will have to become the responsibility of all of us.

REFERENCES

1. California Civil Code §§ 2410–2443.
2. Cruzan v Director, Missouri Dept of Health, 1990 US Lexis 3301 (US June 25, 1990).
3. 20 CFR § 404.2001 ff.
4. General Accounting Office: Medicaid and nursing home care: cost increases and the need for services are creating problems for states and the elderly. Publication GAO/IPE 84–1. U.S. Government Printing Office, Washington, DC, 1983.
5. Haley v Commissioner of Public Welfare 394 Mass 466, 476 NE2d 572 (1985).
6. Hastings Center Report, various issues, see esp. 13(5) (Oct. 1983) and 16(1) (Feb 1986).
7. In re Conroy, 486 A2d 1209, NJ Supreme Ct, 1985.
8. In re Quinlan, 355 A2d 647, NJ Supreme Ct, 1976.
9. Kane R and Kane R: Long Term Care: Principles, Programs, and Policies. Springer Publishing, New York, 1987, p 76.
10. Leach v Shapiro, 469 NE2d 1047, Summit Co, Ohio, 1984.
11. Medicare Catastrophic Coverage Act of 1988, §§ 1924 ff.
12. Mishkin B: A Matter of Choice: Planning Ahead for Health Care Decisions. American Association of Retired Persons, Washington, DC, 1987.
13. Post S, Binstock R, and Whitehouse PJ (eds): Dementia: Moral Values and Policy Choices in an Aging Society. Johns Hopkins University Press, Baltimore (in press).
14. Public Citizen Health Research Group: Poor Health Care for Poor Americans: A Ranking of State Medicaid Programs. Author, Washington, DC, 1987.
15. Weiner JM: We can run but we can't hide: Financing options for long term care. Testimony before the Budget Committee, US House of Representatives, October 1, 1987.
16. Who can afford a nursing home? Consumer Reports, May 1988, pp 300–308.

Part IV
CONCLUSION

EPILOGUE

Peter J. Whitehouse, M.D.,
Ph.D., and
Robert M. Cook-Deegan, M.D.

BIOLOGIC PERSPECTIVES
PSYCHOLOGICAL PERSPECTIVES
SOCIOLOGIC PERSPECTIVES

The concept of dementia has a short history and a long future. In the preface to this book we outlined the challenges that dementia creates for scientists, clinicians, families, and all other members of society. The intervening pages have presented the state of knowledge; the remaining pages examine, primarily from an ethical framework, the issues we will face in the future. Addressing the biologic, psychological, and social challenges from the perspective of either the individual or society as a whole will demand an exploration of the values underlying the creation and use of new knowledge. Setting goals to improve the plight of victims of dementia will require making tough decisions based on finding a balance among the moral values of autonomy, beneficence, and justice. Scientific progress and health care reform promise change and, with it, a better future, but we must be sure our efforts are well informed and targeted on finding long-term solutions to the critical problems of dementia.

Grasping the magnitude of the dementia problem is difficult. Even words such as "epidemic of the century" cannot fully capture the extent of the challenge.[8] How can one comprehend a disease that destroys mind but not body and creates a funeral that never ends? And what of the cost of this funeral in societies around the world, which have fewer and fewer young people to support growing populations of elderly, particularly the very old, who are most at risk for dementia?

For the scientist no disease more ably permits the demonstration of new, powerful tools yet taunts the mind with our inability to construct a unified model of pathogenesis. Bridges need to be built between molecular, cellular, and systems neuroscience to span the chasms of ignorance about how the brain actually works. Dementia offers the opportunity to try to cross the grand canyon of neuroscience — how brain function relates to human behavior. Dementia promises, too, the chance to span astronomical gaps of knowledge concerning human mortality — why we age in the first place and what the genetic essence of *Homo sapiens* is.

The division of our challenges into biologic, psychological, and sociologic creates a framework that allows the intellectual dissection of dementia into fragments manageable by different professionals. Such categorization, however, can distort the phenomenon whose essence we want to understand and whose challenges we wish to meet. The frequently issued clarion call for interdisciplinary research into dementia is echoed in the demand for more coordination in our health care system. Such holistic viewpoints are appealing for their attempts to unify fragmented knowledge bases and care systems, but they are not yet clear enough to support their claims of superiority over more traditional compartmentalization of re-

435

search and clinical work. Nevertheless, it is likely that in the future the organization of scientific and clinical endeavors to meet the challenges of dementia will be profoundly different from our current system, reflecting the need to create new knowledge at the interface of classically defined academic and clinical disciplines. Moreover, coordinated strategic planning and information exchange among government, business, and academia will be critical in determining the success of efforts to develop better biologic or sociologic interventions to cure or care for demented patients.

Despite the limitations of the divided approach, we will use biology, psychology, and sociology as categories to examine the issues we face in the future.

BIOLOGIC PERSPECTIVES

Molecular genetics offers our best hope to trace the causal chain that leads to the most common form of dementia, Alzheimer's disease (AD), as well as rarer conditions such as Huntington's disease (HD). A piece of DNA on chromosome 21 — in some cases maybe a specific point mutation on that chromosome — clearly causes AD.[6,9] Identifying the specific events linking the genetic change to the subsequent death of cells will undoubtedly help us to understand all AD, as well as likely help us to understand normal age-related changes in the central nervous system. Yet this challenging job depends on serendipity to an extent not often appreciated, as illustrated by the initial rapid progress in locating the HD gene and the subsequent, frustratingly slow search. The quest for human disease genes such as those that cause dementia should be a major motivation for undertaking a carefully planned analysis of the human genome. Yet the goal of the Human Genome Project should not be the mapping itself, but rather the information it will bring to solve real human problems. Perhaps more critical study of the development of modern science will teach us to build better

bridges between basic science and medical problems such as dementia.

Although molecular genetics is on the threshold of defining the inherited dementias in precise biologic terms, its full impact is on the disease as a human experience. Consider the ethical implications of the presymptomatic testing now available to patients at risk for HD; combined with the use of selective abortion (already a controversial aspect of human life), such testing could theoretically eliminate the HD gene from the human gene pool. The patient and then the professional will determine how near we can come to that goal and even whether we choose it as a goal. Our understanding of the genetics of the more common forms of AD is more limited, as the analysis is complicated by the strong likelihood of genetic heterogeneity. Yet in the rare families with point mutations on the amyloid precursor protein (APP) gene, we can now theoretically offer genetic counseling on an individual basis without performing family linkage studies.[6] Thus, today a member of these pedigrees can know whether he or she will suffer from an early progressive loss of cognitive abilities, by examination of DNA from lymphocytes from that individual alone.

The application of such genetic technologies raises other questions: What will be the financial and emotional costs? Who will have a right to know an individual's genetic makeup, when such knowledge allows reasonable prediction of the individual's health and potential burden on society — the present or future spouse, children, insurers, physician, or society? Will understanding the genetics of central nervous system disease allow us a glimpse of the controls over normal brain aging? How might such clues lead us to think about research into extending human lifespan?

Short of revolutions in therapy based on an understanding of the cause of dementia, we are likely to be able to develop biologic treatments to relieve symptoms or perhaps even to slow progression. Drugs to treat the symptoms of dementia are now available in some countries, although most, if not all, are little more than placebos. Yet for the first time in modern neuropsychopharmacology, a New Drug Application for a proposed treatment of cognitive impairment in AD, tacrine, has been submitted to the Food and Drug Administration in the United States, thus facing one of the highest national standards for demonstrating drug efficacy.

How good must such a drug be in order for it to be approved? Most informed individuals believe that the drug must do more than just improve performance on a paper-and-pencil test of memory, but how much more? Should we let the physician decide whether the drug is beneficial at a clinically meaningful level, or should the family decide based on the effect of the drug on an Activities of Daily Living Scale or another assessment instrument? Should policymakers and bill payers decide how much drug effect is enough to warrant approval and reimbursement, based on comparisons with other drugs or with behavioral interventions?

Also likely is the development of better drugs to treat the noncognitive symptoms in dementia such as agitation and psychosis. Efforts are under way in nursing homes to eliminate or at least diminish the use of these drugs, particularly tranquilizers, labeled by some as "chemical strait jackets." But these same drugs can be used to keep patients in day care, so they can live with their families rather than be admitted to a nursing home, or can permit a patient to stay in a special unit for dementia rather than be transferred to a state institution. The science to guide such policy-making is not adequate, unfortunately, as few studies of the effects of drugs on behavior in dementia have been reported.

PSYCHOLOGICAL PERSPECTIVES

The individual with AD is labeled by many and understood by few. "Patient," "client," "subject," and "vic-

tim" are terms used to describe such an individual, who is first and foremost a *person* experiencing a tragic disease.[5] The variability of personal experience with dementia is now becoming apparent to clinicians. Such heterogeneity undoubtedly reflects both the individual's biology and life history. Preliminary studies suggest that premorbid personality affects the psychopathology after onset of the disease.[2] Yet it also seems likely that the full nosologic richness of the dementias has not been recognized. Attempts to define subtypes of the degenerative dementias abound, but they have not yet been convincing enough to replace traditional eponyms. Improved disease classification tests our conceptual abilities and will likely be more successful when biologic and clinical variability can be correlated.

Dementia challenges an individual's (and a family's) autonomy like no other life condition. The defense of autonomy needs to be balanced with other, often competing, ethical principles. Beneficence (acting in an individual's best interest) must contend with patient autonomy and with justice (for example, distributing health care fairly). Our culture in the United States seems to overvalue autonomy while ignoring broader concepts such as dignity. One example of the power of the autonomy issue is the current focus on advance directives such as the living will and power of attorney. Certainly there is a need for us all to think about our future as individuals and to consider the possibility of diseases that rob us of the ability to plan for ourselves. Advance directives are not the panacea they seem to be, however. Who can foresee all the possible events to account for in such a document, let alone all the new medical procedures that will undoubtedly appear in the future? And can we really speak best for our future demented self at an earlier point in life, without the experience and wisdom that may be gained later?[3] Certainly such directives are important to consider both for ourself and with our patients, at very least —and perhaps mostly—to facilitate discussion about the value we find in life and the attitudes we have toward death.

At the center of discussions of care for the demented person is the concept of quality of life. Our goal as clinicians and researchers is to improve the quality of life of our patients. Yet such a concept, although the subject of much current attention, remains elusive. Our society's concern for the quality of *goods* in the current economic climate perhaps represents a recognition that resources are finite; goods must be made to fit consumer needs and to function well and long. So too, we as a society and as individuals are coming to realize that *quantity* of life is no longer the primary goal, but rather *quality* of life. Yet our acute health care system remains devoted to the preservation of life with little regard for quality. Consider its epitome, the intensive care unit, where the consequence and cost of actions are often little considered in the fray of the battle to save lives. This care system has little relevance for the demented patient. The National Chronic Care Consortium is an example of a group of providers attempting to build health care systems with an appropriate balance between acute and chronic care.

The many dimensions of quality of life include health, intellectual abilities, social relations, and financial means, as well as another key component — subjective well-being.[7] Biologic and behavioral interventions will be assessed by their impact on all these dimensions. Thus the newly proposed guidelines for antidementia drugs stress the importance of the effect of a drug on patients' lives rather than solely on their performance on clinical laboratory tests. The Institute of Medicine's report on improving the quality of care in nursing homes[7] is driving a revolution concerned with measuring and improving the impact of care on the patient's functional abilities and life activities.

How can we assess the quality of life of a person with dementia? In the early stages we can measure such quality in the same way as in cognitively intact persons, but later we must rely on other guidelines. For example, should caregivers be considered in determining goals for therapy? Such a question illustrates that in many respects the family is as much a victim of dementia as the patient, an idea to be regarded in a sociologic framework.

Before considering a sociologic perspective on the future of dementia, however, we must face fully the issue of euthanasia. When does the quality of life become so poor that death is preferable? Physicians have been assisting death for centuries by, for example, withdrawing life-support technologies in terminal patients. But what of active euthanasia? Ironically, a so-called suicide machine developed by a pathologist in Michigan was first used to assist the death of a patient said to have very early AD.[10] Normally, AD patients lose the ability to perceive their plight and cannot take an active role in planning suicide. If nursing care is extraordinarily good, patients with AD may survive the ravages of being bedridden and enter the persistent vegetative state. As Nancy Cruzan's plight illustrates, members of society differ in their criteria for what constitutes a medical treatment (for example, are food and fluid given through a tube placed in the stomach medical therapy or not?) and for when therapy should be stopped when judged futile.[1,10] (See Chapter 15.) More assisted suicide is occurring in the Netherlands, especially in terminal illness such as cancer. But is dementia a terminal illness, and how can suicide be assisted in an individual who cannot communicate his or her own wishes? Should an advance directive be written that specifies a fatal injection to be administered if the patient can no longer recognize a spouse? It is important to consider our views about passive and not-so-passive euthanasia before health care costs put pressure on us to further limit care to patients in the advanced stages of dementia, or perhaps even to patients with mild dementia who require costly operations.

SOCIOLOGIC PERSPECTIVES

Families provide an estimated 80% of all care to demented patients, an enormous burden considering that over $50 billion is spent in the formal or professional health care system.[11] Yet is this not the role of families? Should we professionalize the care of demented patients to remove this responsibility from the family? Some caregivers wish to provide care without using formal support services or, on the other hand, may not know about available services. As a result, community services to caregivers may be undersubscribed. Whether this lack of utilization will change in the future will depend on the marketing of such services as well as on changes in attitudes of the next generations of caregivers.

Some individuals resent the term "caregiver" as a label provided by professionals to describe a job that these lay persons see as part of being a wife, husband, or child. Professionals have even invented a new disease, caregiver burden or stress, in their efforts to be helpful to their clients, but whatever the outcome of attempts to label the state of the caregiver, it is obvious that the formal health care system cannot and should not replace the family as the basic organizational unit for caring. No army of well-meaning case managers or care coordinators can replace family commitment to provide mutual help or alter the fact that we as families (or at least our spouses) are, as a rule, our own best case managers. Nevertheless, recognition that a dementing illness is a family problem and not just an individual matter should be recognized in health care planning by such means as reimbursement for services used by the caregiver.

The prospect of dementia is genuinely frightening not only to individuals in their later years and to younger family members (who may be prospective caregivers) but also to health service providers and planners. One third of families in the United States are already affected by dementia in a family member or close friend.[11] A study in East Boston was recently used to increase the estimate of currently affected individuals with AD to 4 million, although not everyone would agree that the Boston rates can be generalized to the entire country.[4] Nevertheless, with the rapid increase of those over age 85, who are most at risk for dementia, the problem of AD and related disorders will grow enormously. By the middle of the next century, 10 to 15 million people may well be affected.[11]

The challenge of dementia is global, and our likelihood of success will be greater if we learn from international experience. Some countries, notably Japan and other nations in Asia, are aging even more rapidly than the United States. Worldwide, there may be hundreds of millions of demented patients in the years to come.

Such numbers clearly dictate the need to invest now in basic research to develop interventions that will modify the impact of the disease on the individual and society. Yet the promise of basic research breakthroughs is not guaranteed, and we must not ignore the need for health care reform while awaiting fundamental biologic remedies.

The discussion of health care reform must begin not with resources but with goals. What would ideal care be for the demented individual? Clearly the goals will change as the disease evolves. For the mildly affected patient, the goals are perhaps the same as for the rest of us, but for the patient who can no longer recognize a spouse of 50 years or who has gone further and developed a persistent vegetative state, the goals must be quite different—for example, the relief of immediate pain and suffering. Such goals compete for finite resources, however, not only with other kinds of health care such as childhood vaccinations, but also with broader societal goals like environmental quality and educational opportunities.

Currently, goals for the health care of patients with dementia are based on several general principles. Efforts are being made to enhance services that permit the patient to stay at home in the community rather than be placed in an institution. New organizational forms and physical environments are being created that are more congruent with the needs of patients with cognitive impairment, such as special care units in nursing homes. As innovative care programs emerge, we must use objective outcome studies to assess their impact on patient and caregiver. Educational programs are being developed to inform lay individuals about dementing diseases and the services available to affected persons. The role of family members and other volunteers is being considered in relation to the formal health care system. Lay organizations, particularly the Alzheimer's Association, are defining positions in the health care system beyond advocacy and education, as they make forays into providing or supporting actual service delivery.

Access to services and their coordination lie at the center of efforts to improve the quality of care for individuals with dementia. Even in wealthy communities, knowledge of the many services available, and thus access to them, is often limited. Overlapping services have proliferated, with varied eligibility and sources of payment. Administrative waste of resources is already occurring and may increase if we are not careful in planning new systems of health care. Acute care hospitals, community services, and long-term care facilities must be integrated into a coherent system to improve the quality and cost of care through better coordination. The information management system will be the glue that binds the components together and promotes organizational effectiveness.

SUMMARY

Dementia is both a lonely personal experience and a shared, worldwide crisis. We must work now by investing in basic research to find the roots of biologic solutions as well as by examining carefully what the goals of our care system should be. The biologic, psychological, and social challenges of dementia are enormous. Addressing them will require not only intelligence but also integrity; answering them offers not only a better life for victims of dementia but also a more human life for all.

REFERENCES

1. Battin MP: Euthanasia in Alzheimer's? Philosophy, fiction, and the development of social policy. In Binstock R, Post SG, and Whitehouse PJ (eds): Dementia and Aging: Ethics, Values, and Policy Choices. Johns Hopkins University Press, Baltimore (in press).
2. Chatterjee A, Strauss M, Smyth K, and Whitehouse PJ: Personality changes in Alzheimer's disease. Arch Neurol (submitted).
3. Dresser RC: Autonomy revisited: The limits of anticipatory choices. In Binstock R, Post SG, and Whitehouse PJ (eds): Dementia and Aging: Ethics, Values, and Policy Choices. Johns Hopkins University Press, Baltimore (in press).
4. Evans DA, Funkenstein HH, Albert MS, et al: Prevalence of Alzheimer's disease in a community population of older persons: Higher than previously reported. JAMA 262:2551–2556, 1989.
5. Foley JM: The experience of being demented. In Binstock R, Post SG, and Whitehouse PJ (eds): Dementia and Aging: Ethics, Values, and Policy Choices. Johns Hopkins University Press, Baltimore (in press).
6. Goate AM, Haynes AR, Owen MJ, et al: Predisposing locus for Alzheimer's disease on chromosome 21. Lancet 1:352–355, 1989.
7. Institute of Medicine: Improving the Quality of Care in Nursing Homes. Report of the Committee on Nursing Home Regulation. National Academy Press, Washington, DC, 1986.
8. Plum F: Dementia as an approaching epidemic. Nature 279:269, 1979.

9. St George-Hyslop PH, Tanzi RE, Polinsky RJ, et al: The genetic defect causing familial Alzheimer's disease maps
on chromosome 21. Science 235:885–
890, 1987.

10. Thomasma DC: Mercy killing of elderly
people with dementia: A counterpropo-
sal. In Binstock R, Post SG, and Whitehouse PJ (eds): Dementia and Aging:

Ethics, Values, and Policy Choices.
Johns Hopkins University Press, Baltimore (in press).

11. US Congress, Office of Technology Assessment: Losing a Million Minds: Confronting the Tragedy of Alzheimer's
Disease and other Dementias. Publication OTA-BA-0323. US Government
Printing Office, Washington, DC, 1987.

INDEX

A "T" following a page number indicates a table; an "F" indicates a figure.

443

Venezuelan equine encephalitis, 239, 239T
Ventricle-to-brain ratio (VBR), schizophrenia
    and, 365
Ventricular system, compliance of,
    hydrocephalus and, 341
Ventriculoperitoneal shunting, hydrocephalus
    and, tuberculous meningitis and, 285
Verbal fluency, 142–143, 145T, 146
    Alzheimer's disease and, 173
Vidarabine, in management of herpetic
    encephalitis, 240
Viral dementias, 237–238. See also specific type
Viral-mediated gene transfer, 46
Vision, assessment of, 100–101, 132–133
    multi-infarct dementia and, 221
Visual Reproduction, 138T
Visually guided stylus mazes, 149T
Visuospatial function
    assessment of, 105, 148–151, 149T, 150F,
        151F
    HIV-1 encephalopathy and, 244
    Parkinson's disease and, 185
Vitamin B_{12} deficiency, metabolic dementia due
    to, 329–330

WAIS. See Wechsler Adult Intelligence Scale
Waldenstrom's macroglobulinemia, 325
Wandering, 405T
Washington University Clinical Dementia
    Rating (CDR) scale, 6–7
WCST. See Wisconsin Card Sorting Test
Wechsler Adult Intelligence Scale (WAIS,
    WAIS-R), 104, 106T

Block Design in, 149T
Picture Arrangement in, 145T
Similarities in, 145T
Vocabulary subtest of, 142T
Wechsler Memory Scale (WMS), 105–106
    Visual Reproduction, 149T
Wernicke-Korsakoff syndrome, 95–96, 315,
    328–329
Western equine encephalitis, 238, 239, 239T
White matter
    CT of, 110
        Binswanger's disease and, 226F, 226–227
        HIV-1 encephalopathy and, 246, 246F
        multi-infarct dementia and, 222, 222F
    MRI of, 114
        Binswanger's disease and, 227, 227F
        HIV-1 encephalopathy and, 246–247, 247F
        multi-infarct dementia and, 222, 223F
    multiple sclerosis and, 348, 349, 350F
Wilson disease, 195T, 197T
Wisconsin Card Sorting Test (WCST), 145T,
    146–147
    schizophrenia and, 365–366
WMS. See Wechsler Memory Scale
Word association, 107
Word-List Learning, 137T
Word problems, 145T, 147
Word-Stem Completion, 138T
World Health Organization, ICD of. See
    International Classification of Diseases

Xanthomatosis, cerebrotendinous, 194T, 197T